ENT SECRETS

2nd edition

Editors

BRUCE W. JAFEK, MD, FACS, FRSM
Professor and Former Chair (1976–1998)
Department of Otolaryngology–Head and Neck Surgery
University of Colorado School of Medicine
Denver, Colorado

BRUCE WILLIAM MURROW, MD, PHD
Faculty
Department of Otolaryngology
University of Colorado School of Medicine
Denver, Colorado

HANLEY & BELFUS, INC. / Philadelphia

Publisher: HANLEY & BELFUS, INC.
            Medical Publishers
            210 South 13th Street
            Philadelphia, PA 19107
            (215) 546-7293; 800-962-1892
            FAX (215) 790-9330
            Web site: http://www.hanleyandbelfus.com

Note to the reader: Although the information in this book has been carefully reviewed for correctness of dosage and indications, neither the authors nor the editors nor the publisher can accept any legal responsibility for any errors or omissions that may be made. Neither the publisher nor the editor makes any warranty, expressed or implied, with respect to the material contained herein. Before prescribing any drug, the reader must review the manufacturer's current product information (package inserts) for accepted indications, absolute dosage recommendations, and other information pertinent to the safe and effective use of the product described. This is especially important when drugs are given in combination or as an adjunct to other forms of therapy.

Library of Congress Cataloging-in-Publication Data

ENT secrets / edited by Bruce W. Jafek, Bruce W. Murrow.—2nd ed.
    p. ; cm. — (The Secrets Series®)
  Includes bibliographical references and index.
  ISBN 1-56053-473-7 (alk. paper)
  1. Otolaryngology—Examinations, questions, etc. I. Jafek, Bruce W. II. Murrow,
Bruce W. III. Series.
  [DNLM: 1. Otorhinolaryngologic Diseases—Examination Questions. WV 18.2
E61 2001]
RF57.J34 2001
617.5'1'0076—dc21

2001024737

ENT SECRETS, 2nd edition   ISBN 1-56053-473-7

Last digit is the print number: 9 8 7 6 5 4 3 2 1

CONTENTS

XII. CONCLUSION

CONTRIBUTORS

Mona Abaza, MD
Laryngologist and Assistant Professor, Department of Otolaryngology, University of Colorado School of Medicine, Denver, Colorado

Wendy Marie Ahlbrandt, MS IV
Medical Student, University of Colorado School of Medicine, Denver, Colorado

Steven B. Aragon, MD, DDS
Clinical Professor, Department of Otolaryngology, University of Colorado School of Medicine, Denver, Colorado

Stephen G. Batuello, MD
Private Practice, Aurora, Colorado

Jon M. Braverman, MD
Associate Clinical Professor, Department of Ophthalmology, University of Colorado School of Medicine, Denver, Colorado

John P. Campana, MD
Assistant Professor, Department of Otolaryngology, University of Colorado Health Sciences Center, Denver, Colorado

Stephen P. Cass, MD, MPH
Associate Professor, Department of Otolaryngology, University of Colorado School of Medicine, Denver, Colorado

Kenny H. Chan, MD
Chief of Pediatric Otolaryngology, The Children's Hospital of Denver; Professor, Department of Otolaryngology, University of Colorado School of Medicine, Denver, Colorado

James I. Cohen, MD, PhD
Director, Head and Neck Oncology, and Associate Professor, Department of Otolaryngology, Oregon Health Sciences University, Portland, Oregon

Anne K. Cosgriff, MD (formerly Stark)
Manager of Regulatory Affairs, Cochlear Corporation, Englewood, Colorado

Brennan Thomas Dodson, MS IV
Medical Student, University of Oklahoma College of Medicine, Tulsa, Oklahoma

Timothy J. Downey, MD
Madigan Army Medical Center, Tacoma, Washington

Vincent D. Eusterman, MD, DDS
Madigan Army Medical Center, Tacoma, Washington

Brenda Fishman, MS III
Medical Student, University of Colorado School of Medicine, Denver, Colorado

Matthew Flaherty, MD
Department of Anesthesiology, North Colorado Medical Center, Greeley, Colorado

Carol Ann Foster, MD
Assistant Professor, Departments of Otolaryngology, and Audiology and Rehabilitation Medicine, University of Colorado Health Sciences Center, Denver, Colorado

Vincent D. Franco, Jr, MS III
Medical Student, Department of Otolaryngology, University of Colorado School of Medicine, Denver, Colorado

Sandra A. Gabbard, PhD
Audiologist and Assistant Professor, Department of Otolaryngology, University of Colorado Health Sciences Center, Denver, Colorado

Jeffrey R. Gagliano, MS III
Medical Student, University of Colorado School of Medicine, Denver, Colorado

Kent E. Gardner, MD
Otolaryngologist–Head and Neck Surgery, Private Practice (Dixie Regional Medical Center), St. George, Utah

Mari Gardner, MS IV
Medical Student, University of Colorado School of Medicine, Denver, Colorado

Joseph A. Govert, MD
Director, Medical Intensive Care Unit, Duke University Hospital, and Assistant Professor, Department of Pulmonary and Critical Care Medicine, Duke University, Durham, North Carolina

James A. Harris, MD, FACS
Assistant Clinical Professor–Hair Transplantation, Department of Otolaryngology, University of Colorado School of Medicine, Denver, Colorado

David A. Hendrick, MD
Otolaryngology, Private Practice, Salina, Kansas

Caroline L. Hollingsworth, MD
Department of Radiology, Duke University Medical Center, Durham, North Carolina

John W. Hollingsworth II, MD
Fellow, Department of Pulmonary and Critical Care Medicine, Duke University Medical Center, Durham, North Carolina

Bruce W. Jafek, MD, FACS, FRSM
Professor and Former Chair (1976–1998), Department of Otolaryngology, University of Colorado School of Medicine, Denver, Colorado

Herman Arthur Jenkins, MD
Professor and Chair, Department of Otolaryngology, University of Colorado School of Medicine, Denver, Colorado

David W. Johnson, MD
Assistant Clinical Professor, Department of Ophthalmology, University of Colorado School of Medicine, Denver, Colorado

Madeleine Ann Kane, MD, PhD
Professor, Departments of Medicine and Medical Oncology, University of Colorado Health Sciences Center, Denver; Chief, Department of Medical Oncology, Denver VA Medical Center, Denver, Colorado

Kayla E. J. Kirkpatrick, BA
Graduate Student, American Sign Language, Boston University, Boston, Massachusetts

David M. Kleinman, MD
Chief, Division of Ophthalmology, Department of Surgery, Denver Health Medical Center, Denver; Assistant Professor, Department of Ophthalmology, University of Colorado Health Sciences Center, Denver, Colorado

Ben Lee, MD
Assistant Clinical Professor, Department of Otolaryngology, University of Colorado School of Medicine, Denver, Colorado

Jay H. Lee, MD
Chief Resident, Department of Family Practice, Denver Health Track at the University of Colorado, Denver, Colorado

Michael Leo Lepore, MD, FACS
Medical/Surgical Director, Division of Otolaryngology, Denver Health Medical Center, Denver; Professor, Department of Otolaryngology, University of Colorado School of Medicine, Denver, Colorado

Tyler M. Lewark, MD
Chief Resident, Department of Otolaryngology, University of Colorado School of Medicine, Denver, Colorado

Kjell N. Lindgren, MS, MS IV
Medical Student, University of Colorado School of Medicine, Denver, Colorado

Miriam Roswitha Linschoten, PhD
Instructor, Department of Otolaryngology, University of Colorado Health Sciences Center, Denver, Colorado

Betty Luce, RN, MA
Clinical Nurse, University ENT Specialists, Denver, Colorado

Gregory J. Martin, MD

Phillip L. Massengill, MD
Chief Resident, Department of Otolaryngology–Head and Neck Surgery, Madigan Army Medical Center, Tacoma, Washington

Anne L. Matthews, RN, PhD
Associate Professor, Department of Genetics, and Director, Genetic Counseling Program, Case Western Reserve University, Cleveland, Ohio

Arlen D. Meyers, MD, MBA
Professor, Department of Otolaryngology, University of Colorado Health Sciences Center, Denver, Colorado

Mark Edward Miller, MS III
Medical Student, University of Colorado School of Medicine, Denver, Colorado

Mark R. Mount, MD
Otolaryngologist, Centennial Lakes Medical Center, Edina; and Fairview Southdale Hospital, Minneapolis, Minnesota

Bruce William Murrow, MD, PhD
Faculty, Department of Otolaryngology, University of Colorado Health Sciences Center, Denver, Colorado

Jerry L. Northern, PhD
Editor, American Academy of Audiology, McLean, Virginia

J. Honey Onstad, MS IV
Medical Student, University of Colorado School of Medicine, Denver, Colorado

Marvin Pomerantz, MD
Professor of Surgery; Chief, Section of General Thoracic Surgery, Department of Cardiothoracic Surgery, University of Colorado Health Sciences Center, Denver, Colorado

Sheri Ann Poznanovic, MD
Resident, Department of Otolaryngology, University of Colorado Health Sciences Center, Denver, Colorado

B. Burton Putegnat, MD
Department of Radiology, University of Texas Medical Branch, Galveston, Texas

Rachel Rabinovitch, MD
Associate Professor, Department of Radiation Oncology, University of Colorado Cancer Center, Denver, Colorado

Amir A. Rafii, MS IV
Medical Student, University of California School of Medicine, Davis, California

Chitra Rajagopalan, MD
Associate Professor, Department of Pathology, University of Colorado Health Sciences Center, Denver; Chief, Pathology and Laboratory Medicine Service, Veterans Affairs Medical Center, Denver, Colorado

Arvin K. Rao, MS IV
Medical Student, Department of Otolaryngology, University of Colorado Health Sciences Center, Denver, Colorado

Kay Rhew, MD
Assistant Professor, Department of Otolaryngology, University of Colorado School of Medicine, Denver, Colorado

Gresham Richter, MD
Resident, University of Arkansas School of Medicine, Little Rock, Arkansas

Matthew L. Robertson, MD
Resident, Department of Otolaryngology—Head and Neck Surgery, University of Cincinnati College of Medicine, Cincinnati, Ohio

Nathaniel H. Robin, MD
Associate Professor, Department of Genetics, Case Western Reserve University, Cleveland, Ohio

Scottie B. Roofe, MD
Chief, Department of Otolaryngology—Head and Neck Surgery, Bayne-Jones Army Community Hospital, Fort Polk, Louisiana

David C. Roska, DO
Flight Surgeon, Unites States Navy, Departments of Aviation and Primary Care Medicine, Kaneohe Marine Corps Base, Kaneohe Bay, Hawaii

David Rubinstein, MD
Associate Professor, Department of Radiology, University of Colorado School of Medicine, Denver, Colorado

Richard E. Schaler, MD, FACS
Assistant Clinical Professor, Department of Otolaryngology, University of Colorado School of Medicine, Denver; Attending Physician, Swedish HealthOne Medical Center, Porter Memorial Hospital, and University of Colorado Hospital, Denver, Colorado

Nicolas G. Slenkovich, MD
Chief Resident, Department of Otolaryngology, University of Colorado School of Medicine, Denver, Colorado

Douglas M. Sorensen, MD, FACS
Staff, Department of Otolaryngology–Head and Neck Surgery/Oncology, Madigan Army Medical Center, Tacoma, Washington

Michael F. Spafford, MD
Assistant Professor, Department of Surgery/ENT, University of New Mexico Health Sciences Center, Albuquerque, New Mexico

Margaret K. T. Squier, MD
Research, University of Colorado School of Medicine, Denver, Colorado

Michelle Stanford, MD
Chief Resident, Department of Pediatrics, University of Colorado School of Medicine, Denver, Colorado

Sylvan E. Stool, MD
Pediatric Otolaryngologist, and Professor, Department of Otolaryngology, University of Colorado School of Medicine, Denver, Colorado

Lynnette C. Telck, MS III
Medical Student, University of Colorado School of Medicine, Denver, Colorado

Richard D. Thrasher, MD
Resident, Department of Otolaryngology, University of Colorado School of Medicine, Denver, Colorado

Douglas H. Todd, MD, FACS
Assistant Clinical Professor, Departments of Otolaryngology–Head and Neck Surgery, and Family Practice, University of Oregon Health Sciences Center, Klamath Falls, Oregon

Ryan L. Van De Graff, MD
Resident, Department of Otolaryngology, University of Colorado School of Medicine, Denver, Colorado

Mark A. Voss, MD
Otolaryngologist, Wausau Hospital, Wausau, Wisconsin

Daniel W. Watson, MD
Staff Otolaryngologist, Department of Otolaryngology, Brooke Army Medical Center, Houston; Clinical Instructor, Department of Otolaryngology, University of Texas, San Antonio, Texas

Mark K. Wax, MD
Director, Microvascular Reconstruction, and Associate Professor, Department of Otolaryngology, Oregon Health Sciences University, Portland, Oregon

Leah Suzanne Widger, MS IV
Medical Student, University of Colorado School of Medicine, Denver, Colorado

William H. Wilson, MD
Senior Instructor, Department of Otolaryngology, University of Colorado School of Medicine, Denver, Colorado

Catherine P. Winslow, MD
Chief, Facial Plastic Reconstructive Surgery, Section of Otolaryngology, Walter Reed Army Medical Center, Washington DC

Joel H. Witter, MD
Department of Internal Medicine, University of Colorado School of Medicine, Denver, Colorado

Bozena Wrobel, MD
Resident, Department of Otolaryngology, University of Colorado School of Medicine, Denver, Colorado

PREFACE TO THE SECOND EDITION

It's hard to believe that it's been 5 years since the first edition of *ENT Secrets*. There have been a number of advances in the field of otolaryngology, all of which we've attempted to include while maintaining a readable, affordable text. Otolaryngology is still an exciting, viable, challenging specialty.

ENT Secrets, 2nd edition remains committed to the Socratic approach, posing those questions that really do face clinicians and really do demand an answer. The text is focused upon the needs of the both the neophyte (medical student or person wishing an overview of the field) and the primary care clinician or resident preparing for his or her initial Board examination. Additionally, the material now becomes of value for the practicing otolaryngologist preparing for the recertification examination or simply wishing to update his or her practice. Pertinent references have been completely updated, retaining a few "classic" sources.

Any errors are unintended and have survived a meticulous review process. We hope that you will find our efforts useful!

Bruce W. Jafek and Bruce W. Murrow
Editors
Denver, Colorado

ACKNOWLEDGEMENTS

The editors wish to thank Mr. Jim Gough for his outstanding cartoons, which we feel add important respite from the science in this second edition of *ENT Secrets*. We also wish to thank the many otolaryngology residents and medical students at the University of Colorado School of Medicine (and rotators from other institutions) whose inquisitiveness through the years raised many of the included questions. Our gratitude to Ms. Joyce Vernon, our departmental secretary, without whose encouragement and editorial assistance this project would have been greatly delayed. Ditto for our editor, Ms. Jacqueline Mahon, who patiently oversaw the entire project. Finally, the senior editor (BWJ) wishes to thank his ever-supportive wife, Mary, for her encouragement as he pursued his academic career, and his equally supportive children, Lynette, Rob, Tim, Britta, Kayla, and Kristen.

PREFACE TO THE FIRST EDITION

Daily, the physician is asked to make decisions in the face of inadequate data. Asking questions and investigating possibilities are intuitive processes for the accomplished physician. In addition to explicating details and specifics, training should refine the student's ability to formulate the appropriate questions. *ENT Secrets,* in the Socratic spirit, should guide the reader toward questions that stimulate discussion and sharpen the focus of inquiry.

Because otolaryngology involves perhaps the most challenging surgical anatomy, *ENT Secrets* addresses this complexity, as well as its broad scope of practice, in an approachable manner suitable for the medical student. *ENT Secrets* is also appropriate of otolaryngology residents, presenting broad practical concepts and "bullets" of information that may be used in the operating room, in the clinics, and on the wards. *ENT Secrets* should also be useful for primary care practitioners, as the evolution of medicine dictates that these providers become increasingly proficient in all specialties.

We hope this book will stimulate the reader to investigate more comprehensive textbooks and current literature pertaining to the immense field of otolaryngology.

Bruce W. Jafek, M.D.
Anne K. Stark, M.D.

I. Introduction

I. INTRODUCTION TO OTOLARYNGOLOGY

Bruce W. Jafek, M.D., FASC, FRSM

---

1. What is otolaryngology?

Otolaryngology, pronounced with an initial long "o" (ōtōlaryngology, *not* "auto-" laryngology) is the specialty that deals with diseases of the head and neck region, or, in simplified terms, the region from the eyebrows to the collarbones. The American Academy of Ophthalmology and Otolaryngology was established in 1896, one of the earliest specialties to organize on a national basis. American board certification examination and recognition followed approximately 25 years later. The specialty originally included the treatment of eye conditions and was commonly identified as EENT (eyes, ears, nose, and throat). However, as a result of the explosion of medical knowledge, ophthalmology split from otolaryngology many years ago. The American Academy of Otolaryngology recognized this expanded breadth and adopted a more anglicized qualification when it changed the name to "otolaryngology–head and neck surgery." Of course, not even this qualification solves the problem of the specialty's definition, but it is a significant improvement. Calling an otolaryngologist an "ENT" is no more appropriate than calling a cardiologist a "heart" or an oncologist a "cancer." (We'll leave the description of a colon and rectal surgeon to *your* imagination!)

2. What subdivisions exist within the specialty?

Initially, otology, laryngology, rhinology, and bronchoesophagology were recognized. With increased medical knowledge, however, pediatric otolaryngology, otolaryngologic allergy, facial plastic and reconstructive surgery, and "head and neck" (primarily cancer) surgery have been identified. "Otology" has been expanded to include otology, neurotology, and skull-base surgery. Even this is not all encompassing, as otolaryngologists are interested in neurolaryngology, microvascular surgery, chemosensation (taste and smell disorders), audiology, and speech disorders. Truly, the specialty deals with the comprehensive management of *all* diseases of the head and neck region, including the manifestations of systemic processes affecting this area.

3. Is otolaryngology a medical or a surgical specialty?

Actually, it is both. Many conditions are managed medically and require no surgery, whereas others require surgery. In common practice, for every 13 patients needing medical care, only one will require surgery. It is important to note that this ratio has been altered somewhat by the advent of managed care, in which much medical management of otolaryngologic conditions has been assumed by the primary care physician. The otolaryngologist is therefore now more of a "tertiary care specialist." He or she cares for adults and children, males and females, young and old. The breadth of the field and the complexity of the patients' conditions make it both challenging and stimulating, as well as extremely satisfying for the practitioner.

4. Why is the otolaryngology match an "early match"?

Resident positions are offered through the Otolaryngology Matching Program, a program separate from the "general match." The San Francisco Matching Programs administer this match. Medical students who are interested in otolaryngology should complete their applications no later than September of their senior year. Interviews are usually conducted in November and December. Rank lists are due the first week in January, and the match is completed in mid-January. However, postgraduate year 1 positions are determined through the general match. Because the otolaryngology match is so competitive, it is an "early match." Those who do not find a position in otolaryngology have time to find another position in another discipline through the "general match."

5. How many students and graduates are interested in otolaryngology?

In 2000, 520 medical students and graduates applied to the otolaryngology match. Each applicant subsequently applied to an average of 37 otolaryngology programs and received an average of 8.9 interviews.

6. How many resident positions exist in the United States?

There are about 1000 otolaryngology residents in the United States. In 2000, 244 resident positions were available at a postgraduate year 2 level. All positions consistently and competitively fill with the match.

7. Overall, what is the likelihood of a match?

Of those who submitted a rank list in 2000, 83% of U.S. seniors matched. Fifty percent of U.S. graduates matched (i.e., those students who graduated and started a preliminary surgical internship, etc.) and 6% of foreign medical graduates matched.

8. How do I request an application for the otolaryngology match?

Write to:
Central Application Service of the Otolaryngology Matching Program
P.O. Box 7999
San Francisco, CA 94120-7999
Better yet, contact the office through its website at http://www.sfmatch.org. This website also contains the history of the match and up-to-date information on the comparative statistics of the match. The San Francisco Match also offers a computerized match for plastic surgery, neurosurgery, ophthalmology, and neurology, in addition to otolaryngology.

9. Have the Match statistics remained stable with the ongoing changes in the health care system?

Although many students are considering primary care today, otolaryngology remains a highly desirable and competitive field. In general, these statistics have fluctuated very little over the last 10 years.

10. What kind of training does an otolaryngologist–head and neck surgeon receive?

To qualify for board examination, following graduation from medical school, the resident first completes 1 year of preliminary training in general surgery followed by 4 years of training in otolaryngology–head and neck surgery, for a total of 5 years of training. Some programs are longer, but this defines the minimum training necessary to sit for the certification examination.

11. Is recertification required?

Not at this time. Ten-year, time-limited certificates will be first issued in 2002. A recertification examination is currently under development, and a pilot examination has been conducted. A voluntary recertification examination is expected to be available by 2001.

12. What about subspecialization?

Fellowships are offered in pediatric otolaryngology, facial plastic surgery, Mohs surgery, otolaryngologic allergy, and otology/neurotology and craniofacial surgery through the San Francisco match (see Question 9). In addition, fellowship training in rhinology and sinus surgery, head and neck surgery, and otolaryngologic allergy is also available.

13. How long are subspecialization training programs?
One or 2 years of additional training are offered, depending on the program. Many programs are currently moving toward 2-year training periods.

14. Do these programs lead to subcertification?
The American Board of Otolaryngology is authorized to issue subspecialty certificates in pediatric otolaryngology, otology/neurotology, and plastic surgery within the head and neck. Examinations are currently being developed in all areas. No certificates have been issued and specific dates for administration of these examinations are not available at this time. (American Board of Otolaryngology, December 2000)

HISTORY OF OTOLARYNGOLOGY

References to diseases of the ear, nose, and throat can be traced back to Egyptian (frankincense in goose grease into the ear for a draining ear), Hindu (acrid vapors or oil instillation into the nose for atrophic rhinitis), Chinese (discovery of a narcotic nectar as one of the earliest forms of anesthesia), and Greek civilizations. Important early observations and contributions were also made by the Romans, Alexandrians, Arabians, and Indians.

~Weir N, Otolaryngology: An Illustrated History, 1990

BIBLIOGRAPHY

1. American Academy of Otolaryngology-Head and Neck Surgery, Inc. http://www.entnet.org/
2. American Board of Otolaryngology http://www.aboto.org/
3. Frequently Asked Questions, American Board of Otolaryngology, December 2000 http://www.aboto.org
4. San Francisco Matching Programs http://www.sfmatch.org/

2. THE HEAD AND NECK EXAMINATION

Leah S. Widger, M.S. IV, Anne K. Stark, M.D., and Bruce W. Jafek, M.D.

1. What are the 10 components included in a comprehensive examination of the head and neck region?

Ears	Larynx
Nose	Nasopharynx
Oral cavity	Face and scalp
Oropharynx	Neck
Hypopharynx	General and neurologic examination, as indicated

2. Should the head and neck examination be performed in a specific order?

Yes, a general order should be followed, to insure completeness of the examination. The complete examination almost always starts with ears, then nose, then oral cavity and throat; interestingly, the order matches the acronym ENT. Finally, the neck and neurologic examination are completed. In examining a given area, proceed from outside in so as not to miss something. For example, proceed from the pinna to the external canal and then the tympanic membrane (TM), instead of going right to the TM and possibly missing lesions in the external canal.

Unlike many examinations, a complete head and neck examination requires several instruments, including an otoscope, a head mirror, a light source, and various specula. Much of the examination requires practice and patience. To ensure that you do not miss any portion of the examination on any patient, become familiar with the otolaryngologic instruments, organize them before you begin the examination, and establish a comfortable, orderly routine for yourself.

3. What should be evaluated when examining the external ear?

The outer ear inspection begins with evaluation of the auricle and external meatus. The external ear, pinna, or auricle, is assessed for lesions, masses, infection, or deformities. Compare the ears bilaterally for symmetry. The **auricle** and **tragus** of each ear are moved gently to assess for pain, which may be a sign of otitis externa or inflammation within the external auditory canal. The area overlying the **mastoid** should also be palpated. Tenderness with palpation may indicate otitis externa, with lymphatic nodal involvement, or mastoiditis.

4. What size speculum is used in the otologic examination?

Select the largest speculum that will fit comfortably into the patient's ear; a variety of sizes should be available for the examination. This insures optimal visualization and a tight seal for pneumatic otoscopy. (See Question 7.)

5. Describe the proper technique for otoscopic examination.

The patient's head should be tilted toward his or her opposite shoulder, away from the examiner. With a firm but gentle grasp on the auricle, retract the auricle upward and backward while inserting the speculum. This maneuver straightens the auditory canal and provides the best visualization of the TM. Inspect the auditory canal from the meatus to the TM by checking for discharge, scaling, erythema, lesions, foreign bodies, and cerumen. The speculum is inserted approximately 1.0 to 1.5 cm, to a point just beyond the last canal hair, which marks the junction between the *lateral* cartilaginous canal and the *medial* bony canal. If the inner or medial two thirds of the auditory canal, the bony portion, is touched with the speculum during the examination, it will be painful to the patient. Once the speculum is positioned properly, the otoscope can be gently tilted in various directions so that the entire TM can be inspected.

6. Describe the appearance of a normal tympanic membrane.

The normal TM (eardrum) is oval, pearly gray, and translucent; it is approximately 1 cm in diameter. The periphery is thickened for the inferior 90% of the circumference, constituting the **annulus.** Superiorly, the annulus is deficient, overlying the area of the **Notch of Rivinius.** This part of the TM without the annulus is called the **pars flacida,** whereas the remaining TM with annular support is the **pars tensa,** which is the vibratory part. The most prominent landmark of the TM is the **manubrium** of the malleus. It appears as a white streak running down the middle of the superior half of the eardrum. The contour of the TM membrane is conical, with the center attached to the end of the malleus at the **umbo.** Another useful landmark is the **short process** of the malleus, which appears as a small superior-anterior projection in the inferior aspect of the Notch of Rivinius. The manubrium of the malleus is oriented in an *anterosuperior* direction from the umbo to the short process.

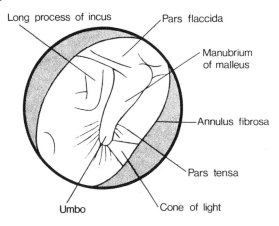

Structural landmarks of the normal tympanic membrane. (From Marshall KG, Attia EL: Disorders of the Ear: Diagnosis and Management. Boston, John Wright, PSG Inc., 1983, p 4, with permission.)

7. What is pneumatic otoscopy?

The pneumatic attachment to the otoscope may be used to evaluate the mobility of the TM. The speculum must form a gentle, tight seal between the canal and instrument. Gentle puffs of alternating positive and negative pressure applied to the normal TM cause it to shift slightly. Positive pressure causes the TM to retract inward, toward the patient, and negative pressure causes the TM to bulge outward, toward the examiner. If a middle ear is under negative pressure, applied positive pressure will not further shift the TM inward, but applied negative pressure will cause it to bulge outward. On the other hand, if a middle ear, is under positive pressure from a Valsalva maneuver or acute otitis media, the TM will move outward with applied positive pressure but not inward with applied negative pressure.

8. How do you properly use a head mirror?

The otolaryngologic head mirror is a valuable tool in the examination of the nasal cavity, oral cavity, larynx, and nasopharynx. If you are a right-handed examiner, sit in front of the patient or to the patient's right side. You must be able to see the same area through the hole in the mirror with your left eye as you see with your right eye to maintain depth perception to properly place mirrors for the examination. Therefore, secure the head mirror around your head so that the back of the mirror is as close to your left eye as possible. You should be able to see clearly through the hole in the mirror with your left eye, even if your right eye is closed (but keep your right eye open, as just described). A light source (e.g., light bulb) placed over the patient's right shoulder is directed into your mirror. The examining chair should be raised so that the light source, head mirror, and patient are all at the same horizontal level.

Position the patient so that he or she is leaning forward with the chin extended. Most mirrors have a focal length of approximately 20 cm. The light is reflected from your mirror onto the patient's face. Often, moving the patient toward you will help to focus the beam. Adjust the patient, light source, and your mirror so that the point of maximally focused light is on the area to be examined. Always examine with both eyes open. The best head mirror has a larger (~1.5 cm diameter) observer hole in the center.

9. What should the clinician look for when examining the external nose?

The external nose should be inspected for evidence of previous trauma, such as scars or deformities, as well as external symmetry. The skin should be examined for lesions. The nares and columella are examined for symmetry. External deviation may be associated with an underlying septal deviation.

10. How do you properly use a nasal speculum?

Position the patient and focus the light from the mirror; the light source is behind the patient's right ear and shining toward the examiner's mirror (for the right-handed examiner). With the nasal speculum in your right hand (hand away from the side of the light source, to avoid blocking the light beam), put your left hand on the patient's shoulder with the thumb on his or her mandible and index finger on the occiput (to give "three-point fixation" and to move the head; the right hand on the nose provides the third point). With the speculum closed, insert it into the nasal cavity, lift the ala and gently open the nare vertically, to facilitate examination of the upper and lower nasal cavity. Avoid touching the septum with the speculum, as this will cause the patient discomfort. Rotate the patient's head on the reflected light beam to view inside the nasal cavity. Remove the speculum while it is open (otherwise you may pull out nasal hairs). Without changing hands, inspect the other side, using the same procedure. Rotating the patient's head slightly on the light beam achieves this.

11. Describe the examination of the internal nose.

With the speculum in place, the examiner should first focus on the **nasal septum** and **nasal cavities.** The cavities should be fairly symmetrical, and the inferior septum should be without spurs. A deviated septum may produce asymmetry of the posterior nasal cavities. Evaluate the septum for any perforations. When examining a patient with a history of epistaxis, special attention should be given to enlarged anterior blood vessels or crusting.

Next, the examiner focuses on the **turbinates,** inspecting the mucosa for color, discharge, masses, lesions, and swelling. The turbinates are rarely the same size because of the normal nasal cycle; however, significant differences between the sides should be noted. Only the inferior and middle turbinates are easily visualized. With the patient's head in the erect position, examine the vestibule and inferior nasal turbinate. Then tilt the patient's head back to more clearly visualize the middle meatus and middle turbinate. Turbinates should be firm and the same color as the surrounding mucosa. Swollen, boggy turbinates, which are bluish gray or pale pink, are often associated with allergies. Polyps may appear as round or elongated masses protruding from the middle meatus.

12. What is included in the oral cavity examination?

First the **lips** are assessed for color, symmetry, texture, and lesions including plaques, vesicles, nodules, and ulcerations. Ask the patient to clench the teeth and smile. This maneuver allows the examiner to simultaneously evaluate for **facial nerve (VII) function** and occlusion of the teeth. Ask the patient to remove all dental appliances so that you can inspect the buccal mucosa, gums, and teeth. You can use one or two tongue blades to move tissues gently aside to evaluate **all mucosal surfaces.** The mucosal surface should be pink, smooth, moist, and free of lesions or masses. Patchy, dark pigmentation may be a normal variation in dark-skinned patients. Examine the floor and **roof of the mouth,** as well as the **tongue** (see below). With a gloved hand, palpate the mucosal surfaces for induration, tenderness, or masses. Note loose, missing, or carious teeth. Finally, do not forget to inspect and palpate the soft and hard palate, the floor of the mouth, and the tongue.

13. Describe the physical examination of the tongue.

First inspect the dorsum of the tongue for smoothness, color, and health of the papillae. Ask the patient to stick out the tongue, and inspect it for **symmetry,** as 12th nerve lesions and cancer may cause an asymmetric protrusion. **Fasciculation** of the tongue, in which the surface appears as "moving worms," is often seen with amyotrophic lateral sclerosis and may be, along with **dysartria,** the first sign of the disease. **Cancer** most commonly occurs on the sides of the tongue and at the base, where lesions may not be easily identified. With a gloved hand and gauze, gently pull the tongue to either side and inspect it for lesions. Gently palpate the entire tongue, including its base, evaluating for any suspicious induration.

14. How is a tongue blade used to examine the oral cavity?

Position the patient so that the headlight is focused on the oral cavity. Stand on the patient's right side (again, for the right-handed examiner), and put your right hand on the top of the patient's head. Do not ask the patient to stick out the tongue. This maneuver can raise the base of the tongue and exposes more of the gag area. With the tongue blade in your left hand, place the tip of the blade in the center of the tongue, depressing it and gently pulling forward. Focus the light on the oropharynx. To view the entire oral cavity, move the patient's head into the path of the light. Do not move your head or the light will be defocused.

15. Describe the oropharyngeal examination.

With the tongue blade in place, observe the **tonsillar pillars** and note the size of the **tonsils.** The tonsillar mucosa should be the same pink color as the surrounding pharyngeal mucosa. The tonsils normally do not project beyond the tonsillar pillars. An arbitrary grading system, 1+ to 4+ describes how far the tonsil projects from the fossa. With the anterior pillar as a starting point, the tonsil is described by the number of "fourths" it projects toward the midline. For example, a tonsil that projects halfway (two-fourths) toward the midline is 2+, and tonsils that meet in the midline (termed "kissing tonsils") are 4+. Crypts may be present on the tonsils where debris may collect **("tonsiloliths").** Infected tonsils may appear erythematous, hypertrophied, or covered with exudate. The posterior wall should be smooth and without lesions. Postnasal drip may be associated with a yellowish mucoid film running down the back of the pharynx. By touching the posterior wall of the pharynx, you can elicit the gag reflex (cranial nerves IX and X).

16. How do you use a laryngeal mirror?

Warm a #4 laryngeal mirror. This is done to prevent fogging of a cold mirror by the patient's breath, not to sterilize it. Position the patient so that he or she is leaning slightly forward with the head slightly extended. Ask the patient to stick out the tongue. With gauze in your left hand, grasp the tongue. With the laryngeal mirror in your right hand and your hand stabilized against the patient's chin, place the mirror against the soft palate. Focus the light of your head mirror onto the laryngeal mirror. Firmly slide the mirror back along the soft palate, rotating the mirror until the larynx is visualized. If the patient gags, spray the pharynx with 10% lidocaine and try again after a few minutes.

17. How do you perform a nasopharyngeal examination?

The nasopharyngeal examination is one of the most technically difficult examinations. This examination is done to assess the nasopharynx for adenoid hypertrophy, nasopharyngeal tumors, or posterior nasal polyps. Again, optimally position the patient. Depress the tongue with a tongue blade held in your left hand and expose the oropharynx. Grasp a warmed #0 nasopharyngeal mirror with the thumb and index finger of your right hand. Stabilize this hand against the patient's chin. With the patient breathing through the nose, slip the mirror behind the soft palate, focus your head mirror, and look up to view the nasopharynx and up and anteriorly to see the posterior choanae. This examination is largely being replaced by the use of rigid and flexible fiberoptic scopes.

18. What is the correct procedure to prepare the patient for fiberoptic laryngoscopy?

A fiberoptic endoscope allows the examiner to visualize the laryngeal structures in greater detail with minimal discomfort to the patient. Inform the patient that the flexible scope will be gently passed through the nose and into the throat. To begin with, tell the patient that you will be spraying two solutions into the nose, a topical decongestant and a topical anesthetic. These solutions may "taste bitter and may produce a numb tongue." Following the spraying, the patient may feel as if he or she cannot swallow or talk, but both functions are unaffected; reassure the patient as the examination proceeds. Repeating the technique used for the nasal examination, determine which nasal cavity is the most patent and use this for the insertion. Hold the nasal speculum in place and tilt the patient's head back. Use atomizers to first spray the nose with 0.5% phenylephrine followed by 4% lidocaine. Alternatively, a 4% cocaine spray may be used as a single spray to both anesthetize and vasoconstrict the nose. Allow several minutes for these solutions to take effect.

19. Describe the structures seen during the fiberoptic laryngoscopy.

As you insert the scope, you will be able to visualize the **entire nasal cavity.** This includes the turbinates, superior nasal cavity and olfactory area, eustachian tube orifice, and adenoids. As the scope is focused downward, through the posterior choanae, the **oropharynx** is visible, including the soft palate, uvula, posterior pharyngeal wall, and base of the tongue. As the scope reaches the **hypopharynx,** the valleculae and epiglottis appear. The epiglottic folds, arytenoids, and pyriform fossae are visualized. Finally, as the scope is advanced deep into the pharynx, the **false vocal cords, ventricles,** and **true vocal cords** are seen. At this point, the patient is asked to phonate, and the examiner can evaluate vocal cord motion.

20. Describe the examination of the face.

The face should be assessed for symmetry, motion, and any masses or edema. The scalp should be examined (including areas covered with hair) for masses or ulceration.

21. How are the sinuses evaluated on physical examination?

When the nasal examination reveals polyps or drainage suggestive of sinus disease, the sinuses should be thoroughly evaluated. The evaluation includes direct examination, palpation, percussion, and transillumination of sinus walls. Walls that are directly available for examination include the maxillary floor (from the palate), anterior maxillary wall (from the cheek), lateral ethmoid wall (from the medial canthus), frontal floor (from the roof of the orbit), and anterior frontal wall (from the supraorbital skull). Palpation and percussion of these areas may demonstrate tenderness in the presence of acute inflammation. In contrast, discomfort is rarely elicited in the presence of chronic sinusitis.

22. How is transillumination of the nasal sinuses performed?

Transillumination is used to assess the health of the maxillary and frontal sinuses. In a darkened examination room, you evaluate the maxillary sinus by illuminating it with a light placed medial to the nose and then inspecting the palate. Placing the light at the upper and inner angle of the orbit illuminates the frontal sinus. Comparing the sinuses bilaterally, decreased brightness on one side suggests sinus disease, but this is only valid if the premorbid status of the transillumination is known. Lack of transmission may mean that the patient has an aplastic sinus.

23. Describe the neck examination.

The neck should be visually inspected for symmetry, masses, or scars. Palpate the neck, taking care to cover all areas. Finally, the thyroid and trachea should be assessed.

24. What are the 10 classic lymph node groups?

Your examination should note the size, consistency, shape, and tenderness of palpable lymph nodes. It is important to determine whether the nodes are discrete, fixed, or matted. The 10 groups of lymph nodes are:

Preauricular	Submental
Posterior auricular (postauricular)	Superficial cervical
Occipital	Posterior cervical chain
Tonsillar	Deep cervical chain
Submaxillary	Supraclavicular

25. Explain the physical examination of the trachea and thyroid.

The **Adam's apple,** or thyroid notch, is often the most prominent landmark in males. Inferior to this landmark lies the **cricoid,** which can be felt as a firm ring and is often the more prominent landmark in females. Inferior to the cricoid, the **tracheal rings** are palpable. Deviation of these rings is suggestive of a mass. The **thyroid isthmus** lies between the cricoid cartilage and the sternal notch. Asking the patient to swallow may allow the identification of the isthmus as it moves up and down with the trachea. The **thyroid** can be palpated on either side of the trachea just superior to the sternal notch. It may be difficult to feel the thyroid distinctly; asymmetric masses or nodules suggest a pathologic condition.

26. What should be assessed in the general and neurologic examination?

If not done previously, cranial nerves II through XII should be evaluated. An extended neurologic examination may be indicated, depending on findings of the history and initial otolaryngologic examination. The patient's cognitive status and overall health, including nutrition and self-care, can be assessed during the history taking process and throughout the head and neck examination.

27. How does the head and neck examination differ in children from that in adults?

In newborns, the ears, nose, mouth, and throat are common areas of congenital malformations and therefore require thorough evaluation for deformities, skin tags, and clefts. In older children, the key to a successful examination is trust. To achieve this, the examination may be more effective if the clinician dispenses with the use of many of the otolaryngologic instruments. Often a child's ears and nose can be successfully examined without speculums. You can examine the ear by gently retracting the pinna backward while drawing the tragus forward, and the nose by slightly lifting the nasal tip. Review also Chapter 10, Otitis Media and Associated Complications, for more specific information on the examination of the child's ear. Children's differing anatomy, along with the lesser amount of historical information, requires closer attention by the examiner. For example, children's ear canals are more horizontal, as compared with the more vertical ear canal of the adult.

CONTROVERSIES

28. What is the diagnostic significance of an otologic "light reflex"?

A light reflex is often described in the normal ear as a cone of light that reflects from the umbo of the malleus on otoscopic examination. Although some practitioners believe that an aberrance of this finding signifies disease, the light reflex generally has no diagnostic importance. This finding may be present in a severely diseased ear, and it may be absent or abnormal in a normal ear.

29. Who should perform fiberoptic laryngoscopy?

Traditionally, otolaryngologists remain experts at the evaluation of the larynx and may be the most experienced with fiberoptic laryngoscopy. However, primary care physicians and emergency medicine physicians can be trained to perform this examination safely and effectively. Most emergency departments possess a fiberoptic laryngoscope, and clinicians may find them useful in their office practice. Complex problems, however, may necessitate an otolaryngologist.

―――>●<―――

THE NASAL SPECULUM

One of the earliest references to a nasal speculum was made by **As Sayzari** (?–1193) in a demonstration of an Arabian collection of instruments of the 12th century. Subsequent modifications were made by **Guy de Chauliac** (1300–1368), **Giovanni Savonarola** (1384–1482), and even **Gabriel Fallopius** (1523–1562). The nasal speculae most commonly used today were designed by **Sir St Clair Thomson** (1859–1943) and **Gustav Killian** (1860–1921).

~Weir N, Otolaryngology: An Illustrated History, 1990

―――>●<―――

BIBLIOGRAPHY

1. Ballenger JJ, Snow JB Jr (eds): Diseases of The Nose, Throat, Ear, Head, and Neck, 15th ed. Philadelphia, Lea & Febiger, 1996.
2. Bickley LS: The head and neck. In Bickley LS (ed): Bates Guide to Physical Examination and History Taking, 7th ed. Philadelphia, Lippincott, 1999, p 163–244.
3. Cummings CW, Frederickson JM, Harker LA (eds): Otolaryngology: Head & Neck Surgery, 3rd ed. St. Louis, Mosby-Year Book, 1998.
4. Duncavage JA: Outpatient evaluation and diagnosis. In Bailey BJ, Calhoun KH (ed): Head & Neck Surgery-Otolaryngology, 2nd ed. Philadelphia, Lippincott-Williams & Wilkins, 1998, p 235–242.
5. Hawthorne MR (ed): Synopsis of Otolaryngology, 6th ed. London, Butterworth-Heinemann, 1999.
6. Lee KJ: Essential Otolaryngology: Head and Neck Surgery, 7th ed. New York, McGraw-Hill, 1999.
7. Lucente FE, Har-El G (eds): Essentials of Otolaryngology, 4th ed. Philadelphia, Lippincott Williams & Wilkins, 1999.
8. Maran AGD: Logan Turner's Diseases of the Ear, Nose and Throat. London, Butterworth-Heinemann, 2001.
9. Scott-Brown WG, Kerr AG (eds): Scott-Brown's Otolaryngology, 6th ed. London, Butterworth-Heinemann Medical, 1997.

II. Otology

3. ANATOMY AND PHYSIOLOGY OF THE EAR

Bruce W. Murrow, M.D., Ph.D.

1. What structures compose the external ear?

The external ear consists of the pinna and external auditory canal and is bounded medially by the tympanic membrane. The lateral one third of the canal is cartilaginous and has hair follicles, along with ceruminous and sebaceous glands. The medial two-thirds of the canal is bony and free of hairs and adenexal structures. The external ear serves to collect and direct the sound toward the tympanic membrane (TM). The length of the external canal, about 2.5 cm in adults, gives it a resonance frequency of 3–4 kHz.

2. What is the middle ear?

The middle ear is a 1 to 2-cm³ air-filled cavity that houses the **ossicles,** the **stapedius** and **tensor tympani muscles,** and the **chorda tympani nerve** (containing taste fibers from the anterior two-thirds of the tongue and parasympathetic fibers to the submandibular and sublingual glands). The middle ear is bounded laterally by the tympanic membrane and medially by the lateral wall of the inner ear (labyrinth capsule). It is continuous with the mastoid air cells via the antrum and the nasopharynx via the eustachian tube. The facial nerve runs very close to the middle ear in a bony canal, which can be dehiscent and increase the risk that a middle ear pathologic lesion could affect the facial nerve. The tympanic membrane and ossicular chain most efficiently transmit frequencies between 500 and 3000 Hz with a resonance around 1 kHz.

3. Name the three ossicles in the middle ear.

The **malleus, incus,** and **stapes** form the ossicular chain. The malleus is positioned between the TM and the incus. The incus is connected to the stapes. The stapes subsequently connects to the oval window of the inner ear.

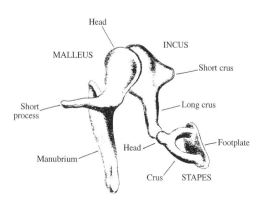

Ossicles. (From Seidel HM: Mosby's Guide to Physical Examination. St. Louis, Mosby, 1991, p 224, with permission.)

4. What role do the tensor tympani and stapedius muscles play?

The tensor tympani and stapedius muscles dampen middle ear mechanics. Loud sounds (about 80 dB) cause the stapedius muscle to contract, which limits the movement of the stapes. Although the acoustic reflex may provide a protective role, it also may serve as a gain-control mechanism to keep cochlear input more constant and expand the dynamic range of the system. Alternatively, contraction of the stapedius muscle has been noted with chewing and vocalization, and thus, it may reduce self-generated noise.

5. Which structure provides aeration of the middle ear?

The eustachian tube, by its connection to the nasopharynx, aerates and drains the middle ear. Its dysfunction can cause a plugged feeling in the ear and/or otitis media. The immature function of the eustachian tube in children predisposes them to ear infections.

6. How does the middle ear maximize the transfer of sound stimuli to the cochlea?

As sound travels from air to a fluid medium, the final stimuli is greatly diminished because of impedance mismatching. The middle ear minimizes this problem amplifying the sound energy by the **area effect** of the tympanic membrane and the **lever action** of the ossicular chain. The effective vibrating area of the tympanic membrane is about 17 times the area of the stapes footplate, resulting in a 17-fold increase in sound energy. The handle of the malleus is about 1.3 times the length of the short process of the incus, so the force at the stapes is increased by 1.3-fold. The combination of these two effects creates a 22:1 mechanical advantage, which provides a 25-dB increase in sound energy arriving to the cochlea.

7. What is the inner ear?

The inner ear is a membranous labyrinth system that is embedded in bone. This system consists of the auditory end organ (**cochlea**), which is responsible for detection of sound, and the vestibular end organs (**utricle, saccule,** and **semicircular canals**), which sense acceleration and gravitional forces.

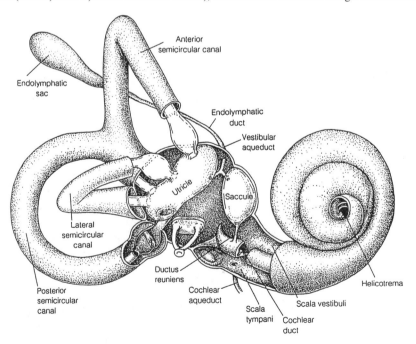

The membranous labyrinth. (From Pender DJ: Practical Otology. Philadelphia, J.B. Lippincott Company, 1992, p 7, with permission.)

8. Describe the tonotopic organization of the cochlea.

A **tonotopic gradient** exists in the cochlea. Higher frequency sounds are detected at the base of the cochlea, whereas lower frequency sounds are detected at the apex. The mechanical properties of the basilar membrane shape this tonotopic gradient.

9. What is the "traveling wave"?

G. von Bekesy is credited with describing the pattern of movement of the basilar membrane, or traveling wave, in response to sinusoidal sound. Each point on the basilar membrane moves at the same frequency as the stimulus. However, the amplitude and phase differ considerably along the length of the cochlea. As a result, the movement of the basilar membrane appears as a traveling wave moving from the base to the apex. The tonotopic map of the basilar membrane determines where the largest peak of the wave occurs.

10. Describe the anatomy of the cochlea.

The cochlea is a snail-like tube that is divided along its length into three compartments: the **scala vestibuli** (top), the **scala media** (middle), and the **scala tympani** (bottom). **Reissner's membrane** separates the scala vestibuli from the scala media. The **basilar membrane** separates the scala media from the scala tympani. **Perilymph,** a fluid similar to extracellular fluid, fills the scala vestibuli and tympani, and **endolymph,** a fluid similar to intracellular fluid, fills the scala media. The scala media houses the **organ of Corti**.

11. What is the organ of Corti?

The organ of Corti contains the auditory receptor cells, called hair cells, and a host of other structural and supporting cells. The hair cells sit on the basilar membrane and are overlaid by the tectorial membrane. There are two types of hair cells in the cochlea, **inner hair cells** and **outer hair cells.** The inner hair cells form one row of cells that spirals up the cochlea near the central axis. Three to four rows of adjacent outer hair cells spiral up the cochlea further from the central axis.

12. Why are auditory receptor cells called hair cells?

Receptor cells have evaginations of the membrane on their apical surfaces called **stereocilia.** At low magnification, stereocilia appear as hairs. The stereocillia contain the mechanically activated ion channels opened by the sound stimuli.

13. How are the cochlear hair cells stimulated?

The tectorial and basilar membranes are connected centrally. Sound moves these two structures differentially, causing a **shear force** that bends the stereocilia. Movement of the stereocilia opens and closes ion channels, producing a receptor potential in the inner hair cell. The receptor potential in turn releases neurotransmitters onto afferent nerve fibers, essentially signaling the brain to the presence of a specific sound frequency. The specific hair cells stimulated by a given sound depend on the tonotopic map of the basilar membrane.

14. What is the function of the inner hair cells?

The inner hair cells are thought to be the classic auditory receptor cells that are responsible for signaling the brain as to the presence of specific sound frequencies.

15. What is the function of the outer hair cells?

The outer hair cells are located further from the central axis than the inner hair cells. These outer hair cells are thought to provide an amplifying effect of the sound stimuli to their adjacent inner hair cells, as well as sharpening the frequency response of the adjacent inner hair cells. Outer hair cells have been shown to shorten and lengthen when stimulated by sound. This pumping motion may affect the inner hair cells by altering the basilar membrane motion and increasing the sensitivity and frequency selectivity of the cochlear output. Recently, a protein called prestin was isolated that gives outer hair cells their ability to contract. However, some feel that the amplifying effect in the cochlea may originate in the stereocilia of the hair cells.

16. What recordable features are associated with outer hair cell function?

The outer hair cells produce the **cochlear microphonic effect** of electrochleography. They also are thought to be responsible for producing **otoacoustic emissions,** which is energy that can be recorded with a microphone in the external auditory canal. These emissions can be used clinically to screen newborns for hearing loss or to test the hearing of patients who are uncooperative or difficult to test by standard audiometry.

17. How does the innervation of inner and outer hair cells differ?

Inner hair cells are predominantly *afferently* innervated. Afferent nerve fibers carry information from the hair cells to the brain. In contrast, outer hair cells are predominantly *efferently* innervated. Efferent fibers carry information from the brain to the hair cells. Efferent stimulation of the outer hair cells may be responsible for decreasing the responsiveness of the cochlea.

18. What are the major neurotransmittors released at the hair cell–neural synapses?

Glutamate is thought to be responsible for carrying the signal from the inner hair cells to the afferent neural fibers. **Acetylcholine** is the neurotransmittor found at the efferent synapses onto the outer hair cells.

19. Trace the neural sound pathway from the cochlea to the brain.

Stimulation begins at the hair cells and travels through the afferent nerves, cochlear nuclei, superior olive complexes, lateral lemnisci, inferior colliculi, and medial geniculate bodies to arrive in the auditory cortex. At the level of the superior olivary complex and above, there is significant crossover between the left and right sides.

20. Name the five vestibular end organs and their stimuli.

One utricle, one saccule, and three semicircular canals (lateral or horizontal, superior, and posterior). The **semicircular canals,** lying at right angles to each other, detect angular acceleration such as head rotation. The **utricle** and **saccule** detect linear acceleration, such as gravity and straight line motion. The utricle has receptor cells oritented in a horizontal plane, and the saccule has receptor cells oriented in the vertical plane.

21. How are the receptor cells in the semicircular canals, utricle, and saccule stimulated?

Each semicircular canal contains hair cells with stereocilia embedded in the jelly-like substance of the cupola. This substance has the same density as endolymph. Angular motion moves the endolymph, as well as the cupola, bending the stereocilia and stimulating the hair cell. The saccule and the macule of the utricle contain hair cells that are overlaid by an otolithic membrane made of calcium carbonate crystals. This otolithic membrane is denser than the endolymph. Thus, gravity and linear acceleration move the membrane relative to the hair cells, bending the cells' stereocilia and causing stimulation.

22. Describe the firing patterns of the semicircular canals upon stimulation.

The neural fibers from each canal fire at a basal rate. In the horizontal canal, displacement of the hair cell's steriocillia *toward* the vestibule (ampullopetal) increases the firing rate, whereas displacement *away* from the vestibule (ampullofugal) decreases the rate. The opposite situation exists in the posterior and superior canals.

23. Why are vestibular reflexes important?

The vestibulo-ocular, vestibulospinal, and cerebellovestibular reflexes link the vestibular system with a number of other systems. Vestibular reflexes contribute to maintaining posture and muscle tone. In addition, they generate transient muscle contractions that contribute to equilibrium and eye stability while a person is moving.

CONTROVERSIES

25. Can auditory receptor cells regenerate?

Classic teaching has held that once auditory receptor cells are destroyed, they cannot be regenerated. This notion has begun to be challenged with the recent findings that hair cells in the avian system are in fact capable of regeneration. Likewise, similar results have recently been reported to occur to a limited degree in some mammalian auditory systems. The significance of these findings for humans has yet to be elucidated.

26. What important players may mediate hair cell destruction in ototoxicity or sound induced trauma?

A review of the recent literature supports the notion that reactive oxygen species (i.e., free radicals) may play a common role in the destruction of hair cells from both ototoxicity and loud sound exposure.

THE EAR

Medieval superstition held that the conception of the Virgin Mary occurred through the breath of the Holy Ghost into her ear and that the ear was the female organ of conception. This was depicted by medieval artists and in icons of the period. Belief in this unusual method of conception is also found in Indian, Mongolian, and Persian legends. Early Greeks, on the other hand, attributed a more masculine role to the ear, as they felt that the veins of the ear conveyed the semen from the head, where it was generated, to the male genitalia. With this belief, the ears of thieves were amputated to interrupt the veins and render them sterile.

~Weir N, Otolaryngology: An Illustrated History, 1990

BIBLIOGRAPHY

 1. Bailey BJ, Calhoun KH (ed): Head & Neck Surgery-Otolaryngology, 2nd ed. Philadelphia, Lippincott Williams & Wilkins, 1998.
 2. Bekesy GV: Experiments in Hearing. New York, McGraw-Hill, 1960. *(An earlier classic)*
 3. Contache DA: Structural recovery from sound and aminoglycoside damage in the avian cochlea. Audiol Neurootol 4(6):271–285, 1999.
 4. Cummings CW, Frederickson JM, Harker LA (eds.): Otolaryngology: Head & Neck Surgery, 3rd ed. St. Louis, Mosby-Year Book, 1998.
 5. Feghali JG, et al: Mamalian auditory hair cell regeneration/repair and protection: A review and future directions. Ear Nose Throat J 77(4):276, 280, 282–285. 1998.
 6. Hackney CM: Active forces in hearing. Trends Neurosci 23(6):233–234, 2000.
 7. Kopke R, et al: A radical demise: Toxins and trauma share common pathways in hair cell death. Ann NY Acad Sci 884:171–191, 1999.
 8. Lee KJ: Essential Otolaryngology: Head and Neck Surgery, 7th ed. New York, McGraw-Hill, 1999.
 9. Lucente FE, Har-El G (eds): Essentials of Otolaryngology, 4th ed. Philadelphia, Lippincott Williams & Wilkins, 1999.
10. Nobili R, Mammano F, Ashmore: How well do we understand the cochlea? J Trends Neurosci 21:159–167, 1998.
11. Pasha R: Otolaryngology Head and Neck Surgery, Clinical Reference Guide. Canada, Singular, 2000.

4. THE HEARING EVALUATION

Catherine Winslow, M.D., and Jerry L. Northern, Ph.D.

1. What questions do you ask of a patient presenting with a hearing loss?

As with any evaluation, first obtain a detailed history of the problem. Details such as onset, course since onset, ear involved, exacerbating and relieving factors, and related symptoms are important. Also note the presence of tinnitus, vertigo, and aural fullness. Ask for a detailed family, medical, and social history, including noise exposure, to search for risk factors. Patients should also be asked about temporary or permanent functional changes involving other cranial nerves, in addition to a thorough cranial nerve examination. Recent trauma, either blunt or penetrating, may also produce hearing loss.

2. What are the two general types of hearing loss and how are they different?

Conductive hearing loss (CHL) results from any disruption in the passage of sound from the external ear to the oval window. Anatomically, this pathway includes the ear canal, tympanic membrane, and ossicles. Such a loss may be due to cerumen impaction, tympanic membrane perforation, otitis media, or otosclerosis. Conductive losses are often correctable with medical or surgical treatment.

Sensorineural hearing loss (SNHL) results from otologic abnormalities beyond the oval window. Such abnormalities may affect the sensory cells of the cochlea or the neural fibers of the 8th nerve. Presbycusis is an example of an SNHL. Tumors of the 8th nerve may also lead to such a loss. Sensorineural losses are generally permanent and more difficult to manage medically. Patients may also have a mixed hearing loss, for example resulting from chronic otitis media coexistent with cochlear damage.

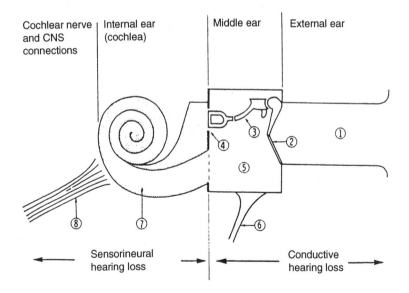

Conductive and sensorineural hearing loss. Examples: (1) wax, inflammatory swelling; (2) perforated eardrum; (3) necrosed or immobile ossicles; (4) stapes fixation by otosclerosis; (5) otitis media; (6) eustachian tube block; (7) sensory presbycusis, mumps, noise injury; (8) neural presbycusis, acoustic tumors. (From Coleman BH: Diseases of the Nose, Throat and Ear, and Head and Neck. Edinburgh, Churchill Livingstone, 1992, p 196; with permission.)

3. What is the Weber tuning fork test? How is it performed and interpreted?

The Weber test is a basic test of hearing. In the Weber test, a 512-hertz (Hz; a unit of measure formerly defined as cycles/second) tuning fork is struck, and its base is placed midline on the patient's skull. The patient is first asked where the tone is perceived and next whether the tone is louder in one ear or the other. In a conductive loss, the tone is louder and localizes to the poorer hearing, affected ear. In an SNHL, the patient perceives the tone to be louder in the better hearing or unaffected ear. Patients with equal hearing or bilaterally symmetrical hearing problems will localize the sound to the skull midline.

4. What is the Rinne tuning fork test? How is it done?

The Rinne test is also used to differentiate between CHL and SNHL. This test is performed by alternately placing the prongs of a vibrating tuning fork at the patient's ear canal and the base of the tuning fork on the patient's mastoid bone. The patient is asked whether the tone is heard louder at the ear canal or on the mastoid. In a patient with normal hearing and normal middle ear status, the tuning fork is heard louder at the ear canal or equally loud in both positions. Similar findings are expected from a patient with an SNHL. Patients with conductive loss, however, hear the tuning fork sound louder at the mastoid position, a *negative* Rinne test result. A negative test result is obtained when the hearing loss is at least 25 decibels hearing level (dB HL).

5. Describe the Schwabach tuning fork test.

The Schwabach test is a crude estimation of sensorineural hearing deficit. The base of a vibrating tuning fork is placed on the patient's mastoid bone. When the tone decays to the point that the patient is unable to perceive it, the examiner quickly transfers the tuning fork to his or her own mastoid. If the examiner is able to hear the tone, the test indicates that the patient has an SNHL. The test result is then reported as "diminished," reflecting the patient's hearing status. Note that this test, of course, requires that the examiner has normal hearing.

6. How wide is the frequency range for normal hearing?

The human ear reportedly can detect sound in the frequency range of 20–20,000 Hz. However, the typical adult can only detect frequencies between 200 and 10,000 Hz. The speech frequency spectrum ranges from 400–3000 Hz.

7. What is a decibel?

A decibel is an arbitrary unit of measurement that is logarithmic in nature. Several decibel scales are used to measure sounds and hearing, and it is necessary to identify each reference scale when presenting a value in decibels. For example, hearing is measured on a biologic scale in decibels hearing level (dB HL), whereas environmental sounds are measured on a physical scale in decibels sound pressure level (dB SPL). The normal human ear is not equally sensitive to all frequencies, and it is able to hear high frequencies better than low frequencies. Normal hearing, for example, at 125 Hz is about 45 dB SPL, but normal hearing at 1000 Hz is about 7 dB SPL. A reference level of 0 dB HL represents normal hearing across the entire frequency spectrum.

8. What is an audiogram?

An audiogram is a *relative* measure of the patient's hearing as compared to an established "normal" value. An audiogram is a graphic representation of auditory threshold responses that are obtained from testing a patient's hearing with pure-tone stimuli. The parameters of the audiogram are frequency, as measured in cycles per second (Hz), and intensity, as measured in decibels (dB). The typical audiogram is determined by establishing hearing thresholds for single-frequency sounds at 250, 500, 1000, 2000, 4000, and 8000 Hz; the primary speech thresholds are 500, 1000, and 2000 Hz. (See figure and table next page.)

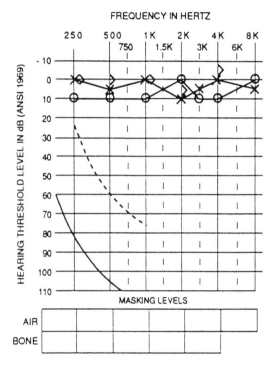

A normal audiogram. (From Lee KJ: Essential Otolaryngology–Head and Heck Surgery. Norwalk, CT, Appleton & Lange, 1995, p 37; with permission.)

Commonly Used Audiogram Symbols

LEFT EAR (BLUE)	INTERPRETATION	RIGHT EAR (RED)
×	Unmasked air conduction	○
□	Masked air conduction	△
>	Unmasked bone conduction	<
]	Masked bone conduction	[
\	No response	/

9. What is normal hearing?

Practically speaking, normal adult hearing is represented as a biologic range between −10 and 20 dB HL. The measurement of hearing is based on threshold responses, with a threshold defined as that point at which a patient perceives a sound stimulus 50% of the time. Patients with hearing loss have audiograms with poorer thresholds (larger numbers in decibels) at the involved frequencies. This is generally considered to be >20 dB.

Hearing Threshold Levels

< 20 dB HTL	Normal hearing
20–40 dB HTL	Mild hearing loss
40–60 dB HTL	Moderate hearing loss
60–80 dB HTL	Severe hearing loss
> 80 dB HTL	Profound hearing loss

10. What is the pure-tone average?
The pure-tone average is an estimate of the patient's ability to hear within the speech frequencies. The value is calculated by averaging the air conduction hearing thresholds at 500, 1000, and 2000 Hz.

11. When an audiologist says that a hearing loss in one ear is elimated with masking, what does this mean?
Sound that is presented to the test ear can travel via bone conduction through the head and be perceived in the opposite, nontest ear. This phenomenon, called **crossover,** can obscure measurement results in the test ear. Therefore, the nontested ear must be eliminated from the test. Air conduction sounds cross over when a 50-dB difference exists between the air conduction threshold of the test ear and the bone conduction threshold of the nontest ear. In contrast, however, bone conduction sounds may cross over when as little as 0-dB difference exists between the bone conduction thresholds of the two ears. **Masking** is the presentation of sound to the nontest ear and serves to prevent the nontest ear from interfering with true sound perception in the test ear.

12. How does the audiologist distinguish between air and bone conduction deficits?
In measurements of air conduction hearing thresholds, headphones deliver sound to the patient. If a hearing loss is noted on testing air conduction, bone conduction hearing thresholds are subsequently measured. You test bone conduction by placing a vibrating device behind the ear on the mastoid. This vibrating device presents the sound to the inner ear, thus bypassing the middle ear system. Patients with SNHL have equal hearing thresholds by air and bone conduction measurements. Patients with CHL have normal cochlear function; therefore, these patients show normal hearing thresholds by bone conduction but poor hearing thresholds by air conduction.

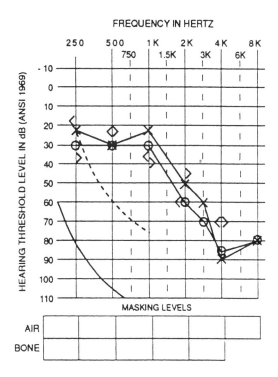

Audiogram showing sensorineural hearing loss. (From Lee KJ: Essential Otolaryngology–Head and Neck Surgery. Norwalk, CT, Appleton & Lange, 1995, p 38; with permission.)

13. What do you look for on an audiogram to tell whether a hearing loss is sensorineural or conductive?

Look for an air-bone gap. An air-bone gap is the difference in decibels between the hearing threshold levels for air and bone conduction. Significant air-bone gaps represent conductive hearing loss. Because the patient hears better through bone conduction than with headphones, a gap exists between the two measurements. With normal hearing, the air and bone conduction thresholds are approximately equal (< 15 dB HTL). With SNHL, the air and bone conduction thresholds are approximately equal but, overall, show a deficit.

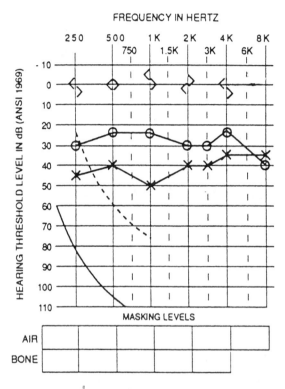

Air-bone gap typical of a conductive hearing loss. (From Lee KJ: Essential Otolaryngology–Head and Neck Surgery. Norwalk, CT, Appleton & Lange, 1995, p 37; with permission.)

14. What is the speech reception threshold (SRT) test?

This test is performed to confirm the pure-tone threshold findings. A specific set of bisyllabic words, known as **spondees,** are presented to the patient at decreasing intensities. Spondees are two-syllable compound words that are pronounced with equal emphasis on each syllable — e.g., oatmeal, popcorn, shipwreck. The SRT is the lowest intensity at which the patient correctly identifies the word in 50% of the presentations. The SRT should be within ± 6 dB of the three-frequency pure-tone average.

15. Describe the speech discrimination test.

The speech discrimination test utilizes word recognition to assess the patient's understanding of speech. A standardized list of single-syllable words are presented 30–40 dB above the SRT. The patient repeats each word, and the score is determined according to the percentage of words that are correctly identified. For example, a patient may understand the test word *knee* as *me*. A score > 90% is considered to represent normal word recognition and speech understanding.

16. What do you do when your patient's tuning fork test results did not agree with the audiogram?

Consider a number of factors. Has the audiometry equipment recently been producing questionable results? Do both headphones work? Is the examiner properly using the tuning forks? Is the examiner comfortable with the anatomy? Does the patient understand the instructions? Does the patient have a secondary gain? If available, old audiograms should be obtained for comparison. Re-testing the patient in the presence of both the otolaryngologist and audiologist may help to identify the cause of the discrepancy. Most importantly, the inconsistency needs to be resolved.

17. What is the immittance test battery?

The **immittance test battery** is not a hearing test, per se, but rather an electroacoustic testing procedure that is used to evaluate the status of the auditory system. The test battery typically includes tympanometry, the physical volume measurement of the ear canal, and ipsilateral and contralateral acoustic reflex measurements.

18. How is the examiner's *subjective* evaluation of tympanic membrane mobility quantified *objectively*?

Tympanometry can be thought of as electronic pneumatic otoscopy. Tympanometry is an objective test that measures the mobility, or **compliance,** of the tympanic membrane and the middle ear system. A seal is formed between the instrument probe and the external canal. Air pressure is manipulated into the space bound by the probe, the external ear canal, and the tympanic membrane. Tympanometry results are represented by air pressure/compliance graphs known as tympanograms. The compliance of the tympanic membrane is at its maximum when air pressure on both sides of the eardrum is equal. The peak air pressure of the tympanogram is equal to the patient's middle ear pressure. The range of normal middle ear pressures is between 0 and -150 mm H_2O and represents normal eustachian tube function. Middle ear pressures that are more negative than -150 mm H_2O are indicative of poor eustachian tube function. Home tympanometers are now available for parents to follow their childrens' effusions.

19. The chart of a patient says she had a type B tympanogram on her last visit. What does this mean?

Tympanograms are classified into five general configurations:
- Type A — Normal middle ear function
- Type A_s — Tympanic membrane is stiffer than normal (lower compliance) in the presence of normal middle ear pressures (e.g., otosclerosis)
- Type A_d — Tympanic membrane is more flaccid than normal (higher compliance) in the presence of normal middle ear pressure (e.g., ossicular discontinuity)
- Type B ("flat" tympanogram) — Shows no pressure peak and indicates nonmobility of the tympanic membrane (e.g., middle ear effusion or perforated tympanic membrane)
- Type C — Shows a peak in the negative pressure range (< -150 mm H_2O); indicates poor eustacian tube function

20. How can I tell if a patient's type B tympanogram results from fluid or from a perforation?

Look at the middle ear volume, normally recorded next to the tympanogram. This test is conducted with an immittance meter and measures the volume that is medial to a hermetically sealed probe. The result, typically reported in cm^3, is the absolute volume of the ear canal when the tympanic membrane is normal. However, in situations where the tympanic membrane is perforated or not intact, the measurement is quite large, because the volume of the middle ear space is also included. Pressure equalization tubes will therefore result in a large volume measurement.

21. What is the function of the stapedius muscle?

The stapedius muscle, attached to the posterior crus of the stapes, contracts reflexively at the onset of a loud sound. The muscle contracts bilaterally, even when only one ear is stimulated. The stapedius muscle can provide some protection to the inner ear in the presence of potentially damaging intense sound. The acoustic reflex causes immediate stiffening of the ossicles and increased compliance of the middle ear system and tympanic membrane. Testing the contraction of the stapedius muscle and the acoustic reflex is an important part of the immittance test battery.

22. Describe the acoustic reflex neural pathways.

The acoustic reflex has both an ipsilateral and a contralateral pathway. The majority of neurons run through the ipsilateral pathway. The **ipsilateral** pathway begins at the cochlea and proceeds through the 8th nerve, cochlear nucleus, trapezoid body, superior olivary complex, and facial motor nucleus to the ipsilateral stapedial muscle. The **contralateral** pathway crosses the brainstem to continue to the opposite cochlear nucleus, trapezoid body, contralateral olivary complex, motor nucleus of the facial nerve, and opposite stapedius muscle.

23. How is the acoustic reflex measured?

The acoustic reflex is measured with the immittance meter. The change in compliance of the middle ear is caused by contraction of the stapedial reflex and is time-locked to the presence of a loud acoustic stimulus. When the ipsilateral reflex is measured, the stimulus is presented through a sealed probe. When the contralateral reflex is measured, the stimulus is presented through an earphone on the opposite ear. Measurement of the acoustic reflex is a valuable screening technique that is used to determine the integrity of the neural pathways. This measurement is also used to detect 8th nerve tumors, sensory cell impairment of the cochlea, and loudness tolerance for patients with SNHL.

24. What is auditory brainstem response audiometry?

Auditory brainstem response (ABR) is an objective, physiologic measurement of hearing. This computerized audiometric test is also useful in the identification of retrocochlear pathologic lesions and can detect lesions that interfere with the main neural hearing pathways—tumors of the 8th nerve, internal auditory meatus, and cerebellopontine angle.

You conduct an ABR by using scalp electrodes to pick up the minute electroencephalographic activity created when sound is perceived. A series of clicks are delivered to the patient through earphones. When an acoustic signal stimulates the ear, it elicits, or "evokes," a series of small electrical events, or "potentials," along the entire peripheral and central auditory pathway. This minute electrical activity is picked up by the electrodes, amplified, and averaged with a computer.

The electrical activity is displayed as a waveform with five latency-specific wave peaks. The latency of each wave peak corresponds to sites in the neural auditory pathway. In basic terms, each peak represents one anatomic structure in the auditory pathway. A tumor will slow the neural circuit and delay the waveform at the site of the lesion.

The ABR can also be used to determine hearing thresholds. As the amplitude of the stimulus click is decreased, the peaks of the waveform will eventually disappear. The ABR test is especially useful in testing hearing in infants and young children who cannot be tested by conventional methods.

25. How do you interpret an auditory brainstem response?

The mnemonic **E COLI** will help you to remember the ascending order of structures that corresponds to each wave form.

Wave I	Eighth nerve action potential
Wave II	Cochlear nucleus
Wave III	Olivary complex (superior)
Wave IV	Lateral lemniscus
Wave V	Inferior colliculus

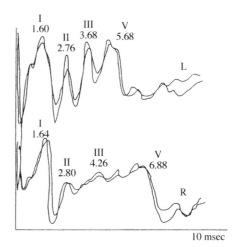

I
1.60
II
2.76
III
3.68
V
5.68
L

I
1.64
II
2.80
III
4.26
V
6.88
R

10 msec

Normal and abnormal ABRs. ABR tracing from left ear *(top)* is normal. Right ear *(bottom)* is abnormal. (From Glasscock ME, Cueva RA, Thedinger BA: Handbook of Vertigo. New York, Raven Press, 1990, p 24, with permission.)

26. How do you evaluate hearing in a pediatric patient?

The hearing evaluation of infants and children poses a challenge. Audiologists use special techniques, adapted to the age level of the child, to obtain valid and reliable test results.

In **behavioral observation audiometry,** sounds are presented to the child at various intensity levels, and an audiologist watches for a movement or reaction. Positive reinforcement is typically incorporated into the test procedure. For example, when the child reacts appropriately to the presence of the auditory stimulus, a visual reinforcement is utilized, such as a lighted toy. An older infant or young child may be conditioned to look toward the source of sound where they expect to see the illuminated toy.

During **play audiometry,** used for children over 3 years of age, a game is incorporated into the test. Each time the child hears the stimulus tone, the child responds by picking a marble out of a bucket, putting a peg into a board, or performing another simple but fun task.

In **speech audiometry,** the audiologist presents spondee words along with pictures, and the child points to the appropriate picture. The intensity level of the spondee word is adjusted to determine the speech reception threshold.

Objective tests, such as immittance measurements and ABRs, are of particular value in determining the hearing status of young children who are difficult to test with conventional methods.

27. What are the pediatric high-risk factors commonly associated with hearing loss?
- Family history of childhood hearing impairment
- Congenital perinatal infection, such as cytomegalovirus, rubella, herpes, toxoplasmosis, syphilis
- Anatomic malformation of head or neck
- Birth <1500 g
- Hyperbilirubinemia at level exceeding indications for exchange transfusion
- Bacterial meningitis, especially *Haemophilus influenzae* infection
- Severe asphyxia, including infants with Apgar scores of 0–3 who fail to institute spontaneous respiration by 10 minutes and those with hypotonia persisting to 2 hours of age

High-risk newborns should be screened for hearing with ABR prior to hospital discharge.

CONTROVERSIES

28. When should a primary care physician be concerned about a patient's hearing complaint?

Always. All patients with hearing loss need further evaluation. Often patients with conductive hearing problems can be successfully treated by medical or surgical means. Patients with SNHL need to be medically evaluated prior to audiologic fitting with hearing aids. Patients with a history of sudden-onset hearing loss, trauma, infection associated with the loss, or asymmetrical hearing loss should be given thorough hearing tests and concurrent otolaryngologic evaluation. Symptoms of tinnitus, aural fullness, vertigo, or ear drainage also require a complete otolaryngologic evaluation.

THE HEARING TEST

The "norms" for the most widely used hearing test or evaluation were established by testing normal subjects during 1935–1936, including, legend has it, a number of randomly selected Iowa State Fair-goers. The results of testing this subject group, assumed to be normal, were used to establish the bell-shaped curve that represents "normal" hearing.

~*ANSI Standards, 1938*

BIBLIOGRAPHY

1. Chodzko-Zajko WJ: Normal aging and human physiology. Sem Speech Lang 18:95–104; quiz 104–105, 1997.
2. Evans P, Halliwell B: Free radicals and hearing: Cause, consequence, and criteria. Ann NY Acad Sci 884:19–40, 1999.
3. Hudspeth AJ: How hearing happens. Neuron 19:947–1950, 1997.
4. Lee KJ: Essential Otolaryngology: Head and Neck Surgery, 7th ed. New York, McGraw-Hill, 1999, p 57.
5. Lefebvre PP, Van De Water TR: Connexins, hearing and deafness: Clinical aspects of mutations in the connexin 26 gene. Brain Res Brain Res Rev 32:159–162, 2000.
6/ Lim DJ, Kalinec F: Cell and molecular basis of hearing. Kidney International (suppl) 65:S104–113, 1998.
7. Martini A, Mazzoli M, Kimberling W: An introduction to the genetics of normal and defective hearing. Ann N Y Acad Sci 830:361–374, 1997.
8. Meurer J, Malloy M, Kolb M, et al: Newborn hearing testing at Wisconsin hospitals: A review of the need for universal screening. WMJ 99:43–46, 2000.
9. Northern J (ed): Hearing Disorders, 3rd ed. Needham Heights, MA, Allyn & Bacon, 1995.
10. Robertson NG, Morton CC: Beginning of a molecular era in hearing and deafness. Clin Genet 55:149–159, 1999.
11. Sataloff RT, Sataloff J: Audiologic testing: An overview for occupational physicians. Occup Med 12:433–447, 1997.
12. Silverman CA: Audiologic assessment and amplification. Prim Care 25:545–581, 1998.
13. Stein LK: Factors influencing the efficacy of universal newborn hearing screening. Pediatr Clin North Am 46:95–105, 1999.

5. CONDUCTIVE HEARING LOSS

Bruce W. Murrow, M.D., Ph.D.

1. What is conductive hearing loss?

A conductive hearing loss (CHL) involves a pathologic lesion located between the opening of the external auditory canal and the cochlea—i.e., the ear canal, tympanic membrane (TM), and/or middle ear. Essentially, the conduction of the auditory stimulus is hindered from reaching the cochlear receptor cells.

2. In the evaluation of a conductive hearing loss, what should the history and physical examination address?

History: age of onset; progression of hearing loss; unilateral versus bilateral effect; ear fullness; ear pain; ear discharge; tinnitus; vertigo/dizziness; trauma; visual, speech, or other neurologic problems; medication used and family otologic history.

Physical examination: complete head and neck examination with focus on the external ear, TM, and middle ear; pneumatic otoscopy; tuning fork tests.

3. Describe the results of tuning fork tests in a purely conductive hearing loss.

With the **Weber test,** the sound "lateralizes" toward the ear with the CHL. If the CHL is > 20 dB, the **Rinne test** will demonstrate bone conduction louder than air conduction.

4. How is the Weber test useful after otologic surgery to verify that the operated ear has not become a dead ear?

During otologic surgery, extreme care is taken as not to cause hearing loss from injury to neurosensory structures. Often after surgery, a CHL is expected in the operated ear due to packing placed in the middle ear or external canal or the removal of structures such as the ossicles. Consequently, the Weber test often is expected to lateralize to the operated ear, and, if such is the case, this indicates that at least some neurosensory hearing is present and the ear is not a dead ear.

5. What is an "air-bone gap" on an audiogram? What does it indicate diagnostically?

The air-bone gap represents a response discrepancy between air- and bone-conducted stimuli and is indicative of a CHL. The bone-conducted stimuli, placed directly on the mastoid, bypasses the conductive mechanisms of the external and middle ear, whereas the air-conducted stimuli must pass through these structures and will be diminished by the conductive related pathologic lesion.

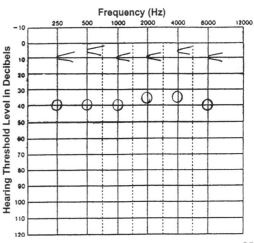

Audiogram of a right ear with pure conductive hearing loss. The difference between the air conductive response *(circles)* and the bone conductive response *(arrows)* is referred to as the air-bone gap. (From Lee KJ: Essential Otolaryngology–Head and Neck Surgery, 6th ed. Norwalk, CT, Appleton & Lange, 1995, with permission.)

6. What is the greatest loss that a conductive hearing loss can produce?

Apure and complete CHL can result in a 60 dB deficit. Ossicular discontinuity should be considered with losses > 50 dB.

7. How does tympanometry help with the diagnosis of conductive hearing loss?

Tympanometry measures the compliance of the TM to different pressure changes. In the absence of a TM pathologic condition, low compliance (type A_s) occurs with fixation of the ossicles, as in otosclerosis, whereas high compliance (type A_d) is found with ossicular discontinuity. The tympanogram in cases of otitis media also has decreased compliance (type B or C) because of the fluid in the middle ear. Pneumatic otoscopy in association with tympanometry as needed is thought by many practitioners to be the gold standard for the clinical diagnosis of otitis media with effusion.

8. What audiometric tests can be confounded by conductive hearing loss?

Measurement of the **stapedial reflex** can be useful in evaluation for retrocochlear pathologic lesion (e.g., acoustic neuroma). CHL greater than 40 dB can eliminate the stapedial reflex, which makes interpretation of this test difficult. Also, CHL can block the recording of **otoacoustic emissions,** which is useful in newborn audio screening and to evaluate difficult-to-test patients. Finally, unilateral CHL, if large enough, can interfere with accurate measurements of air and bone lines in the opposite ear, consequently requiring masking techniques to accomodate these problems.

9. Which imaging modality is most useful for evaluating conductive hearing loss?

Computed tomographic (CT) scan of the temporal bone in general is the imaging choice for CHL, specifically for examination of middle ear disease and temporal bone fractures.

10. List the pathologic conditions of the external ear that produce conductive hearing loss.
- Impacted cerumen
- Foreign bodies
- External otitis
- Exostosis (bony projections into the canal)
- Osteomas
- Tumors
- Congenital aplasia or stenosis
- Cysts

11. List the pathologic conditions of the middle ear that produce conductive hearing loss.
- Otitis media
- TM perforations
- Cholesteatoma
- Otosclerosis
- Ossicular malformations
- Ossicular discontinuity
- Previous ear surgery
- Hemotympanum
- Eustachian tube dysfunction
- Retracted TM
- Tumors
- Tympanosclerosis

12. What is the most common cause of conductive hearing loss?

Cerumen impaction is probably the most prevalent cause of CHL. Excluding cerumen, the most common cause between the ages 15 and 50 is otosclerosis. Approximately 1% of the population is affected by otosclerosis.

13. What amount of hearing loss can be attributed to cerumen impaction?
Impacted cerumen that completely occludes the canal may lead to a 30–40 dB hearing loss.

14. Which is the most common cause of conductive hearing loss in children?
Otitis media with effusion.

15. What procedure is commonly undertaken to offset conductive hearing loss due to otitis media?
Myringotomy and placement of tympanostomy tubes are often employed in patients with a CHL due to otitis media. A tympanostomy tube is also known as a pressure equalization tube. A small incision (myringotomy) is made in the TM, and a tube is placed into the incision. This tube allows drainage and aeration of the middle ear space.

16. What is the significance of addressing conductive hearing loss in children at an early time point?
CHL in early childhood development can result in inconsistent and distorted speech audiotory signals. Subsequently, language development is compromised, combined with academic, psychosocial, and emotional problems. Some practitioners also stress the effect of even "minimal" or "mild" hearing losses in young children on developmental issues.

17. What is otosclerosis? How does it cause conductive hearing loss?
Otosclerosis is an abnormality of bone metabolism and turnover affecting the ossicles. Stiffening and fixation of the stapes footplate occurs secondary to the dense sclerosis and cause a CHL. **Stapedectomy** has a 90–95% success rate for improving hearing.

18. How do tympanic membrane perforations cause conductive hearing loss?
The efficiency of transferring sound from the external auditory canal to the cochlea relies heavily on the larger surface area of the TM in relation to the area of the stapes footplate. This physical advantage is reduced by a perforation, which decreases the sound-receiving area of the TM. However, to obtain a maximal hearing loss with ossicular discontinuity, the TM must be intact, because otherwise sound is able to get through the perforation and present at the oval window directly to cause cochlear stimulation.

19. What is tympanosclerosis? What contribution can it make toward conductive hearing loss?
Tympanosclerosis involves collagen changes and calcerous deposition in the TM, tympanic cavity, and/or ossicular chain. This condition is called myringosclerosis if it is restricted to the TM and appears as chalky white patches. Myringosclerosis, unless involving an extensive amount of the membrane or adherence to the handle of the malleus, is relatively asymptomatic. The intratympanic type often produces a CHL secondary to ossicular chain restrictive movement. Tympanosclerosis is thought to be a reactive change to inflammation and changes related to bouts of otitis media.

20. How do temporal bone fractures result in conductive hearing loss?
Longitudinal fractures through the temporal bone tend to produce bloody otorrhea, fractures of the external auditory canal, perforation of the TM, and disruption of the ossicular chain. Transverse fractures are likely to produce a hemotympanum.

21. How does a cholesteatoma produce conductive hearing loss?
A cholesteatoma is a nest of epithelial cell growth that can occur in the middle ear. It causes CHL by a mass effect that impairs movement of the ossicles. If untreated, cholesteatoma can erode the ossicles, leading to ossicular dysfunction or discontinuity.

22. What other surgical treatments are used for conductive hearing loss?
Myringoplasty involves the closure of the TM perforation with a tissue graft, most often temporalis fascia. Small perforations can be closed with a paper patch, allowing re-epithelialization over the perforation.

If repair of the ossicles is needed, as in ossicular discontinuity, an **ossiculoplasty** is performed.

Stiffening and fixation of the stapes footplate in otosclerosis are surgically treated with a **stapedectomy,** which involves replacement of the stapes with a prosthesis. Alternatively, a **stapedotomy** involves drilling a hole through the stapes footplate and placing a movable prosthesis through the hole.

Treatment of cholesteatoma requires removal of the involved bone and cholesteatoma and reconstruction of the damaged middle ear structures via a **mastoidectomy** and **tympanoplasty.**

CONTROVERSIES

23. In middle ear exploration, if both a fixed stapes (otosclerosis) and tympanosclerosis are found, should a stapedectomy be performed?
Tough call (which is why this is included in the Controversies section)! In this situation, judgment is required to differentiate "burned out," mature tympanosclerosis (see also Question 19), which presumably is no longer contaminated or infected, from "active" tympanosclerosis, which presumably still harbors infective organisms. Stapedectomy, or even stapedotomy with piston placement, in an actively infected ear has a much higher incidence of a "dead ear" postoperatively. Therefore, stapedectomy should probably not be performed. On the other hand, the ear might subsequently be re-explored after 6–12 months, assuming that there was no sign of active infection during the intervening months, and stapedectomy/stapedotomy might then be considered, assuming that the tympanosclerosis continued to appear inactive (uninfected and uncontaminated).

JOSEPH TOYNBEE (1815–1866)

Toynbee developed an artificial tympanic membrane, which consisted of a disc of gutta-percha attached to a fine silver wire (quite similar to a modern total ossicular reconstruction prosthesis). In describing his results, he noted that one patient "was obliged to move to a quieter street, as the noise of the traffic was so well heard on using the artificial membrane"—an early "optimal result" that might better be characterized as a "sequella." His experimental treatment for tinnitus was not quite as successful. Believing that it might be relieved by the inhalation of the vapors of hydrocyanic acid and chloroform, with a subsequent Valsalva insufflation, he fatally subjected himself to the test, and died at the age of 51.

~ *Weir N, Otolaryngology: An Illustrated History, 1990*

BIBLIOGRAPHY

1. Allexander AE Jr, et al: Clinical and surgical application of reformatted high-resolution CT of the temporal bone. Neuroimag Clin NA 8:631–650, 1998.
2. Asiri S, et al: Tympanosclerosis. JLO 113:1076–1080, 1999.
3. Austin DF: Acoustic mechanisms in middle ear sound transfer. Otol Clin North Am 27:641–654, 1994.

4. Bailey BJ (eds): Head and Neck Surgery—Otolaryngology. Philadelphia, Lippincott, 1998.
5. Coker NJ, Jenkins HA: Atlas of Otologic Surgery. Philadelphia, WB Saunders, 2001.
6. Cummings CW, Frederickson JM, Harker LA (eds): Otolaryngology: Head & Neck Surgery, 3rd ed. St. Louis, Mosby-Year Book, 1998.
7. Briggs RJ, Luxford WM: Correction of conductive hearing loss in children. Otolaryngol Clin North Am 27:607–620, 1994..
8. Hannley MT: Audiologic characteristics of the patient with otosclerosis. Otolaryngol Clin North Am 26:373–387, 1993.
9. Katz J: Handbook of Clinical Audiology, 4th ed. Baltimore, Williams & Wilkins, 1994.
10. Lee KJ: Essential Otolaryngology: Head and Neck Surgery, 7th ed. New York, McGraw-Hill, 1999.
11. Nadol JB Jr: Hearing loss. N Engl J Med 329:1092–1102, 1993.
12. Pasha R: Otolaryngology Head and Neck Surgery; Clinical Reference Guide. Canada, Singular, 2000.
13. Tharpe AM, Bess FH: Minimal, progressive, and fluctuating hearing losses in children. Ped Clin North Am 46:65–78, 1999.

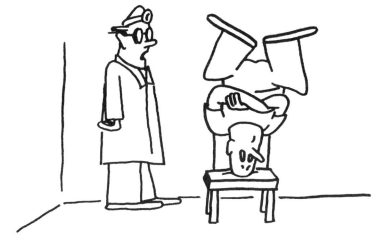

"It looks like an inner ear problem."

Jim Gough

6. SENSORINEURAL HEARING LOSS

Mari Gardner, M.S. IV and Nicolas G. Slenkovich, M.D.

1. What is sensorineural hearing loss?

Sensorineural hearing loss (SNHL) is due to defects either in the *sensory* end-organ of the cochlea or in *neural* transmission to the central nervous system (CNS). A defect exists either in the conversion of acoustic energy by the sense organ of the inner ear or in the transmission of neural impulses centrally.

2. Describe the audiogram in sensorineural hearing loss.

An audiogram in SNHL shows similar air and bone conduction lines, which are both below normal hearing thresholds. Pure SNHL shows no air-bone gap. (See also Chapter 4.)

3. What are the major etiologies of sensorineural hearing loss?

Ototoxicity	Syphilis
Hereditary	Sudden idiopathic hearing loss
Meniere's disease	Multiple sclerosis
Noise-induced	Trauma
Presbycusis	Diabetes mellitus

4. What pathophysiologic mechanisms are responsible for sensorineural hearing loss?

Sensory loss can be due to degenerative, toxic, immune-mediated, infectious, or traumatic damage to the cochlea, as well as genetic or vasculopathic etiologies. **Neural transmission impairment** is most commonly due to either traumatic nerve damage or nerve impingement from a neoplastic lesion. Central neural transmission includes bilateral pathways from each ear. Central defects, therefore, are difficult to detect and generally cause subtle findings, such as impaired sound localization.

5. List the essential elements of the history and physical examination for patients presenting with hearing loss.

- Elicit a history that includes events surrounding the hearing loss, such as infection, trauma, strain, and medication usage.
- Assess the nature of the onset of symptoms, including the timing, side involved, and fluctuation, as well as associated otologic symptoms of pain, discharge, tinnitus, vertigo, and cranial nerve or other neurologic disturbance.
- Obtain a history regarding prior hearing loss, otologic surgery, noise exposure, and family history of hearing loss.
- Physical examination includes a complete head and neck evaluation, including cranial nerves, pneumatic otoscopy, and tuning fork tests.
- A neurologic examination is performed when indicated.

6. What treatments are available for sensorineural hearing loss?

SNHL is most commonly treated with hearing aids. Directed treatment is for treatable cases, such as patching of a perilymphatic fistula, surgical excision of an acoustic neuroma, or antibiotic and corticosteroid therapy for a syphilitic infection. Steroid therapy is advocated for cases of suspected immune-mediated hearing loss and for idiopathic sudden SNHL. Cochlear implantation is an option in cases of profound SNHL.

7. How can the Weber and Rinne tests determine whether hearing loss is conductive or sensorineural?

In the **Weber test** (tuning fork placed on top of head), sound will lateralize to the side toward a conductive deficit. This occurs because on the side with a conductive loss, the background noise is blocked out, and only the sound from the tuning fork can be heard. This makes the side with the conductive loss seem louder to the patient. In unilateral sensorineural hearing loss, sound is heard in the good ear more than the bad ear because the impaired inner ear or cochlear nerve is less able to transmit impulses regardless of how the sound reaches the cochlea.

When a patient with normal hearing takes the **Rinne test** (tuning fork placed on mastoid process and then in air next to ear), he or she should hear the sound from the fork louder when it is removed from the mastoid and put in the air. Normally, air conduction is greater than bone conduction. A person with conductive hearing loss will hear the sound louder when it is on the process rather than in the air. This is because, like the background noise in the Weber test, the sound from the fork is now blocked out. With SNHL, the Rinne test shows the normal pattern of air conduction lasting longer than bone conduction, because the inner ear or cochlear nerve is less able to transmit the impulses regardless of how the vibrations reach the cochlea.

8. Name the major cause of preventable hearing loss in the United States.

Noise-induced hearing loss. Ten million Americans have hearing loss caused in part by excessive noise exposure in the workplace or during recreational activities. Noise-induced hearing loss is the second most common cause of SNHL after presbycusis. Both the intensity and duration of noise exposure determine the possibility for damage to the hair cells of the inner ear. Often, sounds perceived as "comfortable" to the listener can be harmful. Hearing loss is usually gradual in onset with an audiogram pattern of bilateral or unilateral high-frequency loss, showing a notch at 3000 to 4000 Hz. There are no medical or surgical treatments that can reverse noise-induced hearing loss. Accordingly, the patient should be carefully counseled regarding hearing protection (use of "personal protective devices," such as ear plugs) to avoid further hearing loss from noise exposure.

9. What symptoms suggest that a person is receiving potentially hazardous noise levels?

People exposed to potentially damaging amounts of noise may complain that they need to shout to converse in their workplace. They may have symptoms of aural fullness, tinnitus, or muffled hearing after work. Depression is often a concurrent symptom with hearing loss because it can interfere with speech discrimination and social functioning. Patients report that words run together and high-pitched sounds may not be perceived at all. They hear words but cannot recognize the correct word. They often guess what is said or pretend to understand.

10. How does acoustic trauma cause sensorineural hearing loss?

Sound exerts a shearing force on the stereocilia of the hair cells lining the basilar membrane of the cochlea. When sound is excessive, this force leads to cellular metabolic overload, cell damage, and cell death. Thus, excessive "wear and tear" on the delicate inner ear structures is indicated. Outer hair cells are damaged first, followed by inner hair cells and neural degeneration.

11. What is the cause of the ringing and muffled feeling after excessive noise exposure?

A temporary threshold shift is the transient hair cell dysfunction that occurs in patients who have been exposed to excessive noise. Repeated temporary threshold shift may result in a permanent hearing loss.

12. What is the most common nonoccupational cause of noise-induced hearing loss?

Gunfire produces 140 to 170 dB of noise. An audiogram typically documents a hearing loss in the 4000 Hz range. A right-handed rifle or shotgun shooter tends to sustain a left-sided hearing loss, since the right ear is semiprotected by being tucked to the shoulder while the rifle is aimed and fired.

13. List other levels of noise.
Jet takeoff (140 dB)
Rock concert, chain saw (110–120 dB)
Diesel locomotive, stereo headphones (100 dB)
Motorcycle, lawnmower (90 dB)
Some isolated intensive care unit (ICU) alarms (92 dB)
Average ICU noise levels (71–77 dB)
Conversation (60 dB)
A quiet room (50 dB)
A whisper (30–40 dB)

14. Discuss some preventative strategies for noise-induced hearing loss.
• Educate the patient about the hazards of excess noise and the cumulative effect of noise exposure over time.
• Hearing protection should be used correctly and consistently during exposure to excessive noise, even if it is not causing "pain" in the person.
• Patients should be told where they can get hearing protection and instructed about the proper way to wear it.
• Assist the patient and family in coping with the hearing loss.

15. What is the dB A scale?
The dB A scale is a noise-level scale weighted toward high-frequency noises (1000–5000 Hz), as high-frequency noises tend to cause more hearing damage than equivalent levels of low-frequency noise. Workplace exposures > 85 dB A are concerning if these levels are sustained for long periods. Federal occupational regulations require hearing protection for workers who are exposed to 90 dB A for 8-hour periods each day.

16. Define presbycusis.
Presbycusis is a slowly progressive, symmetric SNHL presenting in people over age 60. More than one-third of persons over age 75 are affected by presbycusis. Although studies have attempted to link noise, ototoxicity, diet, metabolism, arteriosclerosis, and hereditary factors to this disorder, the cause remains unclear. Hearing loss is usually greatest at frequencies > 2000 Hz and tends to be accompanied by a significant decrease in speech discrimination. Often patients can hear conversation but are unable to interpret the words, regardless of how loud the speech is presented. Hearing aids may be helpful.

17. Which drugs may produce ototoxic hearing loss?
Salicylates, aminoglycosides (gentamicin, tobramycin, amikacin), erythromycin, and loop diuretics (furosemide, ethacrynic acid, bumetanide) are commonly used drugs associated with hearing loss. Hearing loss is typically bilateral and can be permanent.

18. Who is at special risk for ototoxicity?
Patients receiving more than one ototoxic drug or patients with compromised renal function are at increased risk of hearing loss. Prevention of hearing loss in these patients requires special care in administering known ototoxic drugs. Such a patient should undergo serum drug level monitoring in addition to serial audiometric evaluations. Any patient with elevated peak and trough ototoxic drug levels, for either nonintentional or therapeutic reasons, must be strictly monitored for hearing loss.

19. Describe the mechanism of ototoxic drugs.
Aminoglycosides damage cochlear hair cells, whereas loop diuretics damage the stria vascularis. The stria vascularis is a region of specialized epithelium in the organ of Corti that is responsible for maintaining ionic balance.

Careful examination of the eyes may show congenital fissures or defects of the iris, termed coloboma, in infants with sensorineural hearing loss. Hazy discoloration of the cornea or opacification of the lens in infants with congenital sensorineural hearing loss would be pathognomonic for congenital syphilis and congenital rubella, respectively.

Infants with midline neck masses suggestive of a goiter may have sensorineural hearing loss, which would indicate Pendred's syndrome.

28. What is the most common cause of pediatric sensorineural hearing loss?

Otitis media with persistent effusion.

29. What is the role of neuroradiographic imaging in pediatric hearing loss?

Radiographic evaluation to identify inner ear malformations in infants with sensorineural hearing loss should be considered, although retrospective studies have shown that computed tomographic scans reveal temporal bone malformations in only 7% of infants with sensorineural hearing loss. Enlarged vestibular aqueduct syndrome is the most common imaging abnormality detected in children with sensorineural hearing loss. Temporal bone imaging can detect bony defects that may allow aberrant communication between the subarachnoid space, the inner ear, and the middle ear. The presence of such defects in images of the temporal bone may help to identify patients at risk for perilymphatic fistula or stapes gusher and may explain recurrent bouts of meningitis, or hearing loss caused by minor head trauma.

Imaging of the central nervous system rarely is necessary to evaluate infants with sensorineural hearing loss because central nervous system tumors, including acoustic neuromas, are extremely rare in infants and congenital anomalies or infections involving the brain are diagnosed on the basis of other neurologic sequelae. Indications for neuroradiographic imaging include the following: infants undergoing evaluation for cochlear implantation, infants with a history of recurrent meningitis, infants with a history of progressive or sudden sensorineural hearing loss, especially when it is related to head trauma, and infants with hearing loss in whom imaging results may have some impact on genetic counseling or family planning.

30. Which immune-mediated disorders can cause sensorineural hearing loss?

Immune-mediated hearing loss is poorly understood. Systemic and locally mediated immune disorders have been implicated in SNHL, including Cogan's syndrome, Wegener's granulomatosis, Behçet's disease, and systemic lupus erythematosus. Additionally, multiple sclerosis causes SNHL resulting from demyelination in central auditory pathways.

31. What signs and symptoms suggest immune-mediated sensorineural hearing loss?

Immune-mediated SNHL most often presents as an unexplained, bilateral, rapidly progressive hearing loss in the 20- to 50-year-old age group. Patients may exhibit coexistent systemic immune disease. Results of the otoscopic examination is typically normal. The audiogram is variable, often showing poor speech discrimination relative to the hearing loss.

32. How is immune-mediated sensorineural hearing loss diagnosed?

Although histopathologic temporal bone study has demonstrated inflammatory vasculitis and infiltration in patients with these disorders, it is difficult to make a definitive diagnosis in clinical cases. Serologic tests to rule out syphilis are obtained. Cellular and humoral antigen-specific immune laboratory tests, such as lymphocyte transformation testing and Western blot, may be more helpful than nonspecific immune testing. Antibodies to type II collagen are often identified in the serum of patients with Meniere's disease and in patients affected by idiopathic bilateral sensorineural hearing loss.

33. How is immune-mediated hearing loss treated?

Steroid therapy is indicated in most cases. Cytotoxic drugs and plasmapheresis may be indicated when hearing loss progresses despite steroids.

34. What are the causes of sudden sensorineural hearing (SSNHL) loss?

Only 10–15% of sudden hearing loss cases are found to have a specific etiology. Most cases are attributed to **infectious** causes, **vascular** causes, or **otologic membrane rupture.** Patients have a high rate of seroconversion to viruses such as mumps, rubeola, varicella zoster, cytomegalovirus, and influenza B. One-third of patients report symptoms of upper respiratory infection within 1 month of the hearing loss. Rare infectious causes of SSNHL include otosyphilis and Lyme disease.

Because the cochlea receives its entire blood supply from the cerebellar artery, vascular compromise may lead to SSNHL. Vascular associations include embolic events during cardiopulmonary surgery and hypercoagulable states. However, it is notable that the population of SSNHL patients is not skewed toward persons with vascular risk factors.

Cochlear membrane rupture can be caused by external barotrauma from diving or ascending to altitude rapidly or from a rapid increase in cerebrospinal fluid (CSF) pressure from straining. Fistulas of the oval or round window cause a leak of perilymphatic fluid. Rupture of Reissner's membrane or the basilar membrane causes ionic fluid imbalance from mixing of perilymphatic and endolymphatic fluids. Acoustic neuromas, causing impingement of cranial nerve VIII within the internal auditory canal, are rare causes of SSNHL but should be kept in the differential diagnosis.

35. Do any factors influence the prognosis in sudden sensorineural hearing loss?

It is reported that 40–70% of patients with SSNHL experience recovery of hearing without treatment.

36. Should sudden sensorineural hearing loss be evaluated differently from hearing loss of gradual onset?

The initial work-up for sudden SNHL should include studies to rule out the possibility of an acoustic neuroma in the internal auditory canal. Either an auditory evoked brainstem response test or, in cases of high suspicion, a gadolinium-enhanced magnetic resonance imaging scan of the internal auditory canal is performed. About 1–3% of sudden hearing loss is due to acoustic neuroma. Roughly 10% of patients with acoustic neuromas present with sudden hearing loss. In "suspicious cases," radiographic evaluation should be performed whether or not recovery occurs. Additionally, electronystagmometry with a fistula test to document vestibular findings and a screen for a perilymphatic fistula is performed. Depending on the cause, treatment for sudden SNHL includes steroids, rest, antiviral drugs, or avoidance of noise exposure.

37. Describe traumatic causes of sensorineural hearing loss.

Barotrauma, blunt trauma, and penetrating trauma can all cause hearing loss. Barotrauma can cause sufficient pressure transmission to cause rupture of the oval or round windows and a leak of perilymphatic fluid from the inner ear. Additionally, an acute increase in CSF pressure from physical strain is thought to be capable of causing inner-cochlear membrane rupture via pressure transmission through the cochlear aqueduct. Trauma to the temporal bone can cause a conductive hearing loss by disrupting the external canal, tympanic membrane, or ossicular chain or by creating a hemotympanum. Sensorineural loss occurs from damage to the cochlea or auditory nerve.

38. Describe the infectious causes of sensorineural hearing loss.

Infections may impair the cochlear labyrinth or eighth nerve. Bacterial meningitis, spread of otitis media, congenital and acquired syphilis, and viral infections have all been implicated in infectious labyrinthitis or neuritis leading to hearing loss. Additionally, opportunistic infections of the temporal bone or cerebellopontine angle in immunocompromised patients may cause SNHL.

39. Discuss sensorineural hearing loss as it is related to human immunodeficiency virus (HIV).

The prevalence of SNHL in HIV-infected patients ranges from 21–49%. This condition is usually characterized by a high-frequency hearing loss with speech discrimination scores greater than 90%. Auditory brainstem response testing implicates a central auditory abnormality in many cases. The cause may be iatrogenic, an opportunistic infection, malignancy, or primary infection of the CNS by HIV. Ototoxic medications, such as amphotericin B, vincristine, inosine pranobex (Isoprinosine), aminoglycosides, erythromycin, and azidothymidine, can also be a contributing factor. Hearing loss is associated with cryptococcal infection in 27% of patients.

Otosyphilis develops more rapidly in HIV-infected patients (2–5 years versus 15–30 years for non-HIV-infected patients). The diagnosis is suggested by history, demonstration of a unilateral or bilateral low-frequency sensorineural hearing loss, and hydropic labyrinthine symptoms and is confirmed by blood or cerebrospinal fluid testing.

Other possible causes for a SNHL in HIV-infected patients include progressive multifocal leukoencephalopathy, cytomegalovirus infection, herpes simplex virus, herpes zoster virus, primary or metastatic central nervous system neoplasms (e.g., lymphoma), and direct infection by HIV.

CONTROVERSIES

40. Are any additional diagnostic tests merited in patients with sudden sensorineural hearing loss?

Hematologic studies, viral studies, syphilis serologies, and metabolic and autoimmune work-up are controversial in terms of cost-effectiveness and usefulness in changing outcomes.

41. How should sudden hearing loss be treated?

To date, only corticosteroid therapy has been proved efficacious for idiopathic SSNHL. A number of other treatments have been advocated, including antivirals, carbogen (5% carbon dioxide in oxygen), vasodilators, diuretics, anticoagulants, thrombolytics, plasma expanders, and intravenous contrast therapy. When specific lesions are suspected or diagnosed, such as when history suggests oval or round window rupture, then directed surgical or other treatments may be indicated.

SPIRITUS AURIS

Middle Ages physicians such as the Italian **Hieronymus Mercalis** (1530–1606) differentiated conductive hearing loss (*solutio continui* —"in the bone or tympanic membrane") from sensorineural hearing loss (*mala intemperies* —"in the brain") according to the presence or absence of *spiritus animales,* necessary for normal ear function. Loud noises drove off the spiritus and were incurable. The loss of hearing in older patients was attributed to infrequent and weak passage of the spiritus from the brain to the ear.

~Politzer, History of Otology, 1981

BIBLIOGRAPHY

1. Berrocal JRG: Immune response and immunopathology of the inner ear: an update. J Laryngol Otol 114:101–107, 2000.
2. Brookhouser PE, Beauchaine KL, Osberger MJ: Management of the child with sensorineural hearing loss. Medical, surgical, hearing aids, cochlear implants. Pediatr Clin North Am 46:121–141, 1999.
3. Feghali JG, Lefebvre PP, Staecker H, et al: Mammalian auditory hair cell regeneration/repair and protection: A review and future directions. Ear Nose Throat J 77:276, 280, 282–285, 1998.

4. Halpern NA: Hearing loss in critical care: An unappreciated phenomenon. Crit Care Med 27:211–219, 1999.
5. Mills JH, Adkins WY: Anatomy and physiology of hearing. In Bailey BJ, Calhoun KH (ed): Head & Neck Surgery—Otolaryngology, 2nd ed. Philadelphia, Lippincott Williams & Wilkins, 1998.
6. Pickett BP: Early identification and intervention of hearing-impaired infants. Otol Clin North Am 32:1019–1035, 1999.
7. Rabinowitx PM: Noise-induced hearing loss. Am Fam Phys 61:2749–2756, 2000.
8. Seidman M: Biologic activity of mitochondrial metabolites on aging and age-related hearing loss. Am J Otol 21:161–167, 2000.
9. Thurmond M, Amedee RG: Sudden sensorineural hearing loss: Etiologies and treatments. J Louisiana State Med Soc 150:200–203, 1998.
10. Tomaski SM: Hearing loss in children. Pediatr Clin North Am 46:35–53, 1999.
11. Truitt TO: Otolaryngologic manifestations of human immunodeficiency virus infection. Med Clin North Am 83:303–315, 1999.
12. Veldman J: Immune-mediated sensorineural hearing loss. Auris Nasus Larynx 25:309–317, 1998.

7. DEAFNESS

Kayla E. J. Kirkpatrick, B.A.

Regardless of the etiology or severity, there are a number of considerations in the management of deafness, especially in the face of now not-so-recent legislation. Some of these are obvious and some are not so obvious to the clinician. Kayla Kirkpatrick is an interpreter and deaf educator who presents important insights into this condition. ~*Editors*

1. Is "deaf" a proper term?

The term "Deaf," with a capital "D," refers to a group of people who identify themselves as a cultural and linguistic minority. They are members of the Deaf community, sharing a culture and a manual language. The term "deaf," with a small "d," refers to a pathologic condition or audiologic loss, and deaf people are not categorically members of the Deaf community. Don't use "the D/deaf" to describe deaf people. The term "Deaf people" is more positive.

"Hearing impaired" is a new term and was thought to be more politically correct and sophisticated. Hearing people, who thought this term sounded less obtrusive and threatening, made it up. It doesn't provide necessary cultural information. The word "Deaf" has symbolic connotations and carries with it cultural information.

2. How do you characterize a Deaf person?

It is impossible to characterize a Deaf person because of the large number of background factors that affect deafness. These include the **age of onset** (for example, post-lingual deaf persons have heard language, and this exposure makes it easier for them to acquire a new language); **accumulated educational background** (mainstream, residential school, etc.); **family climate** (Deaf, hearing, how they deal with it, socioeconomic status, etc.); **degree of hearing loss** (dB loss) (the greater the loss, the more subnormal the experience); and **etiology** (especially as associated with other handicaps). Four of five leading causes of deafness cause other handicaps, and one-third of Deaf people have some other handicap (e.g., rubella, Rh factor incompatibility, premature birth, meningitis). This will also effect the family climate.

3. What is "Deaf culture"?

Quite simply, Deaf culture is the culture of Deaf people who use American Sign Language (ASL). The avenues of access to the Deaf community are as follows:
- Audiologic (some type of hearing loss—the specific dB loss is not important to Deaf culture members)
- Social (participating in Deaf social activities, having Deaf friends, etc.)
- Linguistic (expressive and receptive knowledge of and use of ASL)
- Political (supporting the goals of the Deaf community and working for their success)

Some items of interest and explanation as to why Deaf culture is so valued:
- In the Deaf culture, there is potential for 100% understanding and language comprehension.
- ASL is the shared language (speaking for the Deaf culture of the United States).
- There is a sense of fairness, due to similar experiences and frustrations.
- Values are shared.

Cultural considerations conclude that Deaf people are a minority group with shared lifestyle, beliefs, and technology. Deaf people have a rich culture complete with folklore, jokes, poetry, customs, rules for turn taking, and so on. Most Deaf people want children like them, just as you want children like you. Family similarities facilitate bonding through shared experiences. Mutual values maintain the Deaf culture.

Most congenitally Deaf people feel that, given the option, they would rather stay deaf than become hearing. Deaf people often have a pride that is created out of bonding and coming together and overcoming adversity; some hearing people lack this, as they don't share the same experiences.

Deaf people marry other Deaf people at a high rate. This provides a refuge from the hearing world. There are social clubs to join, and Deaf clubs are a place where the Deaf experience is passed to future generations. There is ease of communication, a common language.

4. In what sense is Deaf culture a reaction to the perception of hearing people?

It isn't. However, negation by hearing people causes Deaf people to turn to each other to survive in a hearing world. Deaf people are normal, but striving to adapt to a hearing society. Deaf people have a disability—*not a handicap*—that causes them to deal with the world differently than hearing people.

5. What categories of hearing people are most accepted by the Deaf culture? What group is closest and what group is most distant? Why?

The people who know the most about Deaf culture, children of Deaf adults (called CODAs), are the most accepted. They are bicultural and emotionally involved, and ASL generally is their first language. ASL interpreters are the second closest. The people who believe deafness is something that needs to be "fixed" are furthest away; this, of course, defines most medical professionals. Ironically, these professionals often think they are closest because of client/patient relationships and their understanding of the need to fix the handicap and help the Deaf person, but there is often misunderstanding and lack of trust or friendship.

6. Why is the Deaf community unlike other ethnic groups in terms of location and recruitment?

There is no legal definition for deafness or geographic separation. Anyone can become deaf. Deaf people are an invisible minority: You can't tell a person is deaf until there is interaction.

7. What is the role of "the School For the Deaf"?

Schools for the Deaf are a source of pride among members of the Deaf community and have a huge role in the preservation of Deaf culture. Preserving the language means preserving the culture. It is in these schools that a true Deaf culture exists. The residential school teaches language and culture and gives the opportunity to participate in sports. It is a home, and students learn to have fun and how to relate to others. It creates a sense of unity. However, not all residential school experiences are good. In the past, some Deaf schools did not allow signing, and slapping of hands was common. Also, it is sometimes difficult to deal with hearing parents in this situation because they usually can't communicate well enough to tell the child where he or she is going. The parents may also have feelings of abandoning their child.

In summary, a School For the Deaf is important because:
• Deaf people often feel it is home.
• It provides a strong sense of identity and relation.
• It provides for social interaction among Deaf people.
• It facilitates full communication immersed in language and culture.
• It allows involvement in sports and other extracurricular activities.
• It provides the opportunity for learning experiences outside of the classroom and incidental learning.
• It allows free and open communication among Deaf people.

8. What is American Sign Language?

The language of the Deaf community in the United States is American Sign Language, or ASL. ASL is a natural language created by Deaf people, for Deaf people, and is passed down from generation to generation in the same way any other language is—by native users. Linguists recognize ASL as a true language. Like English and other spoken languages, ASL possesses rules regarding syntax, semantics, pragmatics, morphology, and phonology. It is not just gestures or pictures in the air, but a system of arbitrary symbols with grammar and syntax, agreed on by the culture. ASL does not use English word order, just as Spanish does not use English word order. Other sign languages are used in other nations. For example, France has its own sign language.

ASL has evolved over time, similarly to how "English" has evolved in different areas of the United States. ASL is roughly 200 years old, and some research suggests that signed languages were in existence before spoken languages, since, in human development, the gross motor functions came before fine motor functions necessary for speech.

ASL is not superior to English, nor is English superior to ASL. Spoken language is *not* the "hallmark of being human." True deprivation does not lie in loss of sound, but in loss and lack of language. Linguists, including Noam Chomsky, recognize ASL as a true language.

9. Parents of deaf children are sometimes told to avoid signing. What are some of the reasons given?
- "If you want your child to learn to speak, don't learn to sign. It's a crutch. Signing detracts from the ability to speak."
- "Signing will give your child the ability to be *in* the society, but not *of* the society." (assimilation and bilingual issue)
- "If your child learns to sign, he or she will refuse to speak."

Research has proved these statements to be false.

10. Should Deaf children be mainstreamed?
Mainstreaming limits exposure of Deaf children to ASL and does not allow the child to get his or her education directly, because it comes via an *interpretation* of what the teacher is saying. The child's education is only as good as the interpretation, and schools often do not pay interpreters well, so mainstream schools are often where new interpreters find jobs. Mainstreaming creates an identity crisis for Deaf children by isolating them, forcing friendships, and creating a confused feeling about which world the child belongs in. In addition, in a mainstream classroom, there is a lot of incidental information that the Deaf child misses because the interpreter cannot hear it or is interpreting something else. Most mainstream classrooms lack the highly visual stimulation a Deaf learner requires. Further, the child cannot have direct communication with his or her peers. Thus, a mainstream education does not provide a full experience.

11. How have psychological tests frequently overlooked the intellectual capacity of Deaf persons?
Standard tests are given based on hearing cues and culture. When given a perceptual test (visual), Deaf people do just as well as their hearing counterparts. The results of standard tests are therefore skewed, because the test is culturally biased and tends to underrepresent the intellectual ability of the Deaf testee.

12. What are some issues in medical interpreting?
The interpreter in a medical setting, along with the clinician and patient, can be faced with life and death situations. In this setting, medical service and medical care are the first priority, not communication. The illness can affect language, so a Deaf/hearing team is a good idea, especially with trauma patients. For example, the patient may be under physical or emotional stress, the injury hinders communication, medication hinders communication, and the patient can't interpret if his or her eyes aren't open!

Medical interpretation may lead to misunderstandings, so it is important to define roles to medical personnel clearly.

13. What misconceptions might medical personnel have about Deaf patients?
- All Deaf people can lip-read.
- Interpreters know all medical terminology, and it is their responsibility to explain it to the patient. Actually, the interpreter should know meanings for words like "chronic" and "acute," but the clinician, just to be safe, should explain all specifics related to medicine.
- Written communication is good enough.

- Interpreters know the patient's medical history — mental, physical, emotional status.
- Interpreters will be involved in patients' treatment in ways other than to facilitate communication.
- The interpreter is an expert on deafness and hearing loss.
- The interpreter will try to take over.
- The interpreter will be in the way of medical procedures and limit access to the patient.

14. What misconceptions might members of the Deaf community have regarding interpreters in a medical setting?

- Interpreters are cold and unfeeling. Deaf patients want comfort; the interpreter is a provider in this situation.
- Taking notes home from the appointment will be enough. Patients don't realize that the interpreter can help get more in-depth information.
- Privacy (physical or emotional) will be lost.

15. What misconceptions might a medical interpreter have?

- Feeling that they have to fight medical personnel for communication.
- Thinking simultaneous communication is best. Actually consecutive is better sometimes.
- Believing that they are 100% responsible for medical terminology. Actually, the medical professional carries this responsibility.
- Picking and choosing jobs in an attempt to stay out of the emergency room (ER). Life-threatening things happen in the entire medical field, even outside the ER, so this experience expands the interpreter's capabilities.

16. What physical factors should an interpreter consider when taking a job in a medical setting?

Medical sights, sounds and smells aren't for everyone. The interpreter may become ill.

Medical interpreting can get very hot.

Medical equipment presents a lot of obstacles, and interpreters may have difficulty positioning themselves so that they remain in the patient's line of sight. If the patient can't see the interpreter, the patient can't receive the interpreter's message.

Privacy must be maintained, as far as possible.

Strategies and codes must be developed for communicating during radiography, since the patient will be alone.

In the isolation setting with masks, gowns, and gloves, signing is difficult. In such a setting, it may be better to write, but only if the patient clearly comprehends English.

17. What can an interpreter do to maintain a patient's privacy?

Be the same sex as the patient whenever possible.

Position yourself for utmost privacy (the patient's), usually at the level of the patient's shoulders.

Maintain eye contact. This lets the patient know that you are with them for communication only.

Break eye contact for the patient's emotional privacy, but stay there in case the patient starts talking again.

Dynamics. Eye contact can determine whether the patient needs support. The desire for contact can be voiced so that the doctor can initiate it.

Leave the room, but be sure to explain that you are right outside and can come back at any-time.

18. How can an interpreter prepare for a medical appointment?

Get information on the background of the patient's condition(s) and what the appointment is about.

19. What is the interpreter's role in pre and post sessions (usually on phone)?

Be sure the patient knows about his or her medications.

Be sure clear communication has occurred.

20. What roles does the interpreter *not* serve in a medical setting?

The interpreter is not a patient advocate. The hospital can provide these.

The interpreter is not available to pass information on to Deaf family members.

The interpreter does not speak for the patient. The Deaf consumer needs to be fully involved.

CONTROVERSIES

21. What facilities are available to assist deaf people?

This is a difficult question, as different areas offer different services. Developmentally, deaf people get much less environmental input and have different pressures and demands placed on them. The absence of sound creates differences in the sociocultural environment (doorbells, spoken language, sirens, telephones); the human environment (simply the act of sharing between two people); interpersonal environment (the interaction with others); the education environment (the presence of interpreters, assignment to special education); labels (stereotypes, stigma, the negative connotation of "deaf"); and intrapersonal environment (how a person *responds internally* to other environments).

There is also the implication that this question is asking what services are available to help deaf people get their hearing. Many culturally Deaf people don't miss what they never had and are not interested in those kinds of services. As far as learning life skills, getting employment training, interpreters, and so on, an individual would have to check services in his or her area. It should be noted that just because someone can sign, it does not mean that he or she is an interpreter or can function as one.

Finally, Deaf people are a protected class under the Americans with Disabilities Act.

22. Should a child receive a cochlear implant?

Prior to making this decision, the parents must carefully consider unbiased information related to all of the available education and communication options. These include:

- Auditory-Verbal
- Cued Speech
- American Sign Language (ASL)
- Signed English
- Magnet/Charter School
- State School for the Deaf
- Mainstream School

Often, hearing parents are so distraught over the diagnosis of deafness that they have a difficult time considering any option that will not restore their child to "perfection." Deafness is harder to deal with than other disabilities because it can't be seen—the child still looks perfect—and hearing people value speech so much. Because the child appears normal and hearing is difficult to determine in the infant, a delay in the diagnosis often occurs, compounding the problem of acceptance by the parents. But "hearing" does not necessarily equate with perfection, and there are many Deaf people who lead happy, satisfying lives, never missing what they never had.

Cochlear implantation of children is a controversial issue, and both sides make partially valid claims. The dissenters say that to implant a child who is less than 2 years old, subjecting them to invasive surgery, is no less than abuse. However, otolaryngologists will tell you that this surgery is only invasive to the extent that the child is put under general anesthesia and bone is shaved to make space for the implant pedestal, but it is not a "life-threatening" surgery. The dissenters also say that the training is too intense for children and a high percentage of children fail anyway. Also, the surgery is expensive and the dissenters will say that a person with a cochlear implant is not accepted by the Deaf community or the hearing community and therefore fits in nowhere. The supporters of early implantation counter that this is the closest to hearing that a child without hearing can get and that the child's central processing is more "plastic" and they can therefore adapt to using the implant better than if it is delayed until the child is older.

Currently, many parents who ultimately make the decision to implant their children are first exposing them to ASL via Magnet/Charter Schools and State Schools for the Deaf, in addition to their English training that goes along with the cochlear implant. This way, the child will have exposure to both languages during the critical early language period. The important thing is to get the child exposed to "language" as much and as often as possible during the early language period.

A good, complete cochlear implant team should contain (at the very minimum) the doctors, an audiologist, and a Deaf person; I would not trust a team that did not include a culturally Deaf member.

A postlingually deafened person, on the other hand, is usually a perfect candidate for a cochlear implant.

DEMOGRAPHIC CHARACTERISTICS OF DEAFNESS

Ninety percent of parents of deaf children are hearing. Twenty million American people have a hearing impairment. As a gender, males are more likely to become deaf (postlingually) because of a number of risk factors such as military service or occupational exposure. Deafness is correlated with age, because the older you are, the greater your chance of becoming deaf.

BIBLIOGRAPHY

1. Barnett S: Clinical and cultural issues in caring for deaf people. Fam Med 31:17–22, 1999.
2. Grundfast KM, Atwood JL, Chuong D: Genetics and molecular biology of deafness. Otolaryngol Clin North Am 32:1067–1088, 1999.
3. Jacobson JT: Nosology of deafness. J Am Acad Aud 6:15–27, 1995.
4. Lenarz T: Cochlear implants: Selection criteria and shifting borders. Acta Otorhinolaryngol Belg 52:183–199, 1998.
5. Marschark M, Mayer TS: Interactions of language and memory in deaf children and adults. Scand J Psych 39:145–148, 1998.
6. McLeod RP, Bently PC: Understanding deafness as a culture with a unique language and not a disability. Adv Pract Nurs Q 2:50–58, 1996.
7. Padden C: Deaf in America: Voices from a Culture—Tom Humphries and Carol Padden. Cambridge, Mass: Harvard University Press, 1988.
8. Parasnis I: Cognitive diversity in deaf people: Implications for communication and education. Scand Aud Suppl 49:109–115, 1998.
9. Reamy CE, Brackett D: Communication methodologies: Options for families. Otolaryngol Clin North Am 32:1103–1116, 1999.
10. Robinson K: Implications of developmental plasticity for the language acquisition of deaf children with cochlear implants. Int J Pediatr Otorhinolaryngol 46:71–80, 1998.
11. Rotenberg J: Adapting the clinical encounter for the deaf patient. RI Med 77:81–83, 1994.
12. Stebnicki JA, Coeling HV: The culture of the deaf. J Transcult Nurs 10:350–357, 1999.
13. Steel KP: Science, medicine, and the future: New interventions in hearing impairment. Br Med J 320:622–625, 2000.
14. Wilcox S (ed): American Deaf Culture: An Anthology. Boston, Linstok Press, 1989.

8. HEARING AIDS AND COCHLEAR IMPLANTS

Bozena Wrobel, M.D., and Sandra A. Gabbard, Ph.D.

1. Name the major components of a hearing aid. How do these components work?

A traditional hearing aid consists of five main components: microphone, amplifier, receiver, volume control, and battery power source. The function of a hearing aid is to amplify acoustic signals, which it accomplishes in three basic stages that correspond to the major hearing aid components. In the first stage, the diaphragm of the microphone converts acoustic energy, or sound, into mechanical energy. The microphone then converts this energy into electrical energy. The second stage involves the amplifier, which boosts the electrical signal. In the final stage, the receiver transforms the boosted electrical signal back into an acoustic signal, which is then broadcast into the ear.

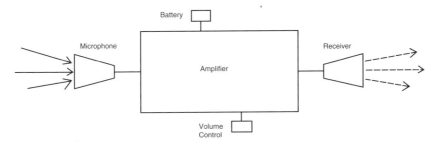

Block diagram of a simple hearing aid. (From Pollack MC (ed): Amplification for the hearing impaired, 3rd ed. Orlando, Grune and Stratton, Inc., 1988, p 25, with permission.)

2. When does a patient with a hearing loss need a hearing aid?

Patients with hearing loss who manifest communication difficulties, either objectively or subjectively, may benefit from hearing amplification. Because of current technology, audiologists are able to fit almost all patients with variable types and degrees of hearing loss.

3. Define saturation sound pressure level, acoustic gain, output limiting, frequency gain response, and distortion.

These terms describe the different electroacoustic properties of a hearing aid. **Saturation sound pressure level** is the maximum amount of sound pressure output, or power, that a hearing aid can produce. **Acoustic gain (input-output)** refers to the difference in the output of a hearing aid relative to its input. For example, if a tone at 1000 Hz is presented to the microphone at 60 dB, and if the measured output is 100 dB, then the gain of the hearing aid at this frequency is 40 dB. Input-output function can be linear or nonlinear. **Output limiting** refers to the maximum intensity of the amplified signal. **Frequency gain response** is the amount of gain as a function of frequency. **Distortion** refers to the clarity of signal produced by a hearing aid.

4. What are the input-output characteristics?

Input-output function can be linear or nonlinear. Linear amplification means that the relationship between input and output is proportional: for every dB increase in the input, there is corresponding dB increase in the output. Both soft and loud sounds are amplified indentically. Problem with this type of amplification is that it does not address the nonlinearity of loudness growth that occurs with sensorineural hearing impairment. Nonlinear amplification means that the relationship between input and output is not proportional, so that, for example, low-intensity sounds are amplified to a greater extent than high-intensity sounds.

5. How can hearing aids be prevented from amplifying sound past a comfort level?

Hearing aids are not tolerated if they amplify sound beyond a level that is comfortable to the patient. There are two strategies for output limiting: peak clipping and compression. Compression means that as the hearing input increases, the amount of gain is automatically reduced to avoid reaching an uncomfortable output level. This concept can be applied across the entire frequency range (single-band compression) or can be applied to specific frequencies at which the patient experiences recruitment or loudness discomfort (multiple-channel compression).

- **Peak clipping:** a traditional strategy for output limitation; creates distortion when the hearing aid is in saturation (reached maximum output)
- **Compression:** can be used in limiting of input, output, or both; does not create distortion when the hearing aid is in saturation (reached maximum output)

6. What are the circuit options in hearing aids?

Currently available circuit option in hearing aids are analog, digitally controlled analog, digital (all are programmable), programmable (meaning hearing aid can be plugged to the computer and adjusted), and multimemory. The digital strategy in hearing aids provides better sound quality and improved understanding in noisy situations thanks to more precise and flexible frequency shaping, better acoustic feedback reduction, and more sophisticated compression algorithms.

7. Name the seven common types of hearing aids.

Behind-the-ear (BTE) aids   In-the-ear (ITE) aids
In-the-canal (ITC) aids   Completely-in-the-canal (CIC) aids
Body aids   Eyeglass aids
CROS and BICROS aids

8. What are the advantages and disadvantages of behind-the-ear (BTE) hearing aids?
Advantages
- They generate enough power to adequately accommodate a patient with severe to profound hearing loss.
- They are more cosmetically appealing than body aids.
- They are large enough to accommodate multiple controls for electroacoustic properties, allowing for adjustment flexibility.
- The microphone and receiver are more easily separated in BTE aids than in ITE and ITC models, which allows for less feedback.

Disadvantages
- In patients with severe to profound hearing loss, the earpiece must fit tightly in the canal to eliminate feedback problems.
- More manual dexterity is required than with body aids.
- They require a relatively normal pinna, are easily affected by perspiration, and may be less cosmetically appealing than ITE and ITC aids.

9. What are the advantages and disadvantages of in-the-ear (ITE) hearing aids?
Advantages
- They are more cosmetically appealing than BTE aids.
- Increased amplification provided by the pinna boosts gain in high frequencies.
- They improve localization of sound sources.
- They are made of only one component.

Disadvantages
- The amount of gain is limited because of problems with acoustic feedback.
- They are appropriate only for patients with mild, moderate, and moderately severe hearing loss.
- The small size limits the number of adjustment controls.
- They are more fragile than BTE aids.

10. **What are the advantages and disadvantages of in-the-canal (ITC) hearing aids?**

Advantages
- They are more cosmetically appealing than most hearing aids.
- Increased amplification provided by the pinna boosts gain in high frequencies.
- Placement of the microphone improves sound localization.

Disadvantages
- They are appropriate only for patients with mild to moderate hearing loss.
- Models are fragile and difficult to use for patients with manual dexterity problems.
- The small size limits the number of controls for adjustments.
- They have limited venting options.

11. **What are the advantages and disadvantages of completely-in-the-canal (CIC) hearing aids?**

Advantages
- They are barely noticeable because they are placed deep in the canal.
- They provide full or partial resolution of the occlusion effect.
- Use with telephones is improved because they do not need a vent.
- The wind-noise problem is resolved.
- Gain in high frequencies is improved due to pinna effect.
- They have Secure fit, reduced acoustic feedback due to minimal venting, and good sound localization.

Disadvantages
- They provide adequate amplification only for patients with mild to moderate hearing loss.
- Fragile aids need frequent repairs, and shell modifications are expensive.
- More extensive counseling is required to teach use.
- Some dispensers are reluctant to perform deep canal impressions.
- Small batteries are difficult for patients with inadequate dexterity.
- They can develop feedback with jaw movement.
- They cannot be used in patients with unfavorable external auditory canals.

12. **What are CROS-type and BiCROS hearing aids?**

CROS stands for **contralateral routing of sound.** These hearing aids are used in individuals with usable hearing in one ear but no hearing, very poor hearing, or unaidable hearing in the other ear. A microphone is placed on the side of the patient's poorer ear. The signal received through this microphone is routed to the opposite ear and amplified. The signal is routed by either an electrical cord worn behind the head and neck or by wireless FM radio signals. These aids improve the patient's ability to hear sounds that originate on the side of the poorer-hearing ear.

BiCROS, or **bilateral CROS**, is used for bilateral hearing loss when only one ear is aidable. A CROS system is combined with conventional hearing aid; the better ear receives inputs from microphones on both the better side (conventional fitting) and the poorer side (CROS).

13. **Explain the occlusion effect.**

The occlusion effect occurs when the body of the hearing aid blocks the external auditory canal. To the patient, this occlusion causes a muffled sensation due to a shift in the peak of the natural resonance of the ear canal. The result of this shift is an increase in low-frequency amplification. In individuals with normal low-frequency hearing, this amplification is not desired. The occlusion is lessened by the use of aids that do not occlude the canal, contain a vent, or have electronic filtering of low frequencies. The larger the vent, the less low frequencies will be heard by the patient. Not all hearing aids can be vented: digital hearing aids cannot be vented as well as small hearing aids.

14. **How does acoustic feedback occur?**

Acoustic feedback results when amplified sound leaks from the receiver back into the microphone. The result is an unpleasant high-pitched squeal. Short microphone-to-receiver distance, wax in the canal, vents, and poor hearing aid fit are all associated with increased feedback problems. ITE or ITC hearing aids are more likely to have these problems than BTE aids.

15. Are patients with sensorineural hearing loss candidates for hearing aids?

Yes. Until the last few decades, it was believed that only patients with conductive hearing losses were candidates for hearing amplification. It was thought that boosting the volume would not improve clarity or speech discrimination. It is now well accepted that patients with sensorineural hearing loss benefit from hearing aids. Although the processing component of a sensorineural hearing loss cannot be overcome, the heightened volume increases audibility and reduces the strain of understanding sound in daily listening situations.

16. Do patients with bilateral hearing loss need monaural or binaural amplification?

In most cases, patients with bilateral hearing losses do better with binaural amplification. Binaural amplification is advantageous because it eliminates the "head shadow" effect—i.e., the 6-dB loss in sound intensity that occurs when sound has to cross the head to the contralateral ear. This effect is amplified in a noisy environment. Additional benefits include better speech discrimination, improved ease of listening, heightened speech localization, and avoidance of sensory deprivation. Retrospective studies have shown that when only one ear is aided, the unaided ear suffers a reduction in word-recognition score.

17. What are assistive listening devices (ALDs)? Why are they needed?

ALDs assist the hearing impaired in specific "difficult listening situations" (e.g., lecture halls, theaters, television). Most of these difficult listening situations involve a sound source that is located far from the listener. The intensity of a sound signal decreases by 6 dB each time the distance between the listener and the sound source doubles. This leads to a decreased signal-to-noise ratio. Some ALDs maintain a normal signal-to-noise ratio by transferring the sound signal, at the original intensity level, directly to the listener or hearing aid microphone via FM, infrared, or inductance loop transmission devices. Other available ALDs include telephone amplifiers, vibrating alarm clocks, TV closed-caption decoders, and visual alarm systems.

18. What is the earliest age at which a child can benefit from hearing amplification?

When needed, children should be fitted for hearing aids at the earliest possible age. Although determining the exact nature of an infant's hearing loss is challenging, an infant can be fitted initially with a nonspecific hearing aid based on available audiometric data. Hearing amplification can be adjusted as the child grows and more reliable testing can be performed. Caution should be exercised in infants to prevent further hearing damage with overamplification. Infants with congenital atresia or microtia of the pinna may be fit as young as 2 months of age.

19. How do prelingual and postlingual hearing loss differ?

Prelingual deafness refers to hearing loss prior to the development of basic spoken language skills. *Postlingual* deafness refers to the loss of hearing after the development of basic language skills. The development of basic spoken language skills usually occurs at 2 to 3 years of age. The classification of patients into prelingual and postlingual categories has prognostic significance when predicting how a patient will respond to cochlear implantation.

20. What is a cochlear implant (CI)?

A cochlear implant is a highly sophisticated listening device that can restore auditory abilities to deafened individuals who do not benefit from hearing aids. The first device was developed for clinical use in Australia in the 1970s. Early cochlear implants were single electrode devices. Current implants tend to have multiple electrodes, which transmit more sound information. These devices require surgical implantation and extensive postoperative therapy.

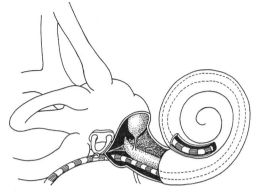

Internal view of cochlear implant. (From Pender DJ: Practical Otology. Philadelphia, J.B. Lippincott Co., 1992, p 65, with permission.)

21. Name the components of a cochlear implant.

Cochlear implants have internal and external components. The internal components consist of one or more electrodes, placed in or onto the cochlea, as well as a receiver, usually a coil, that transmits the electrical signal to the electrode. The external components consist of a speech processor, a behind-the-ear microphone, a decoding unit, and the coil (transmitter or a percutaneous plug). The transmitter is magnetically secured over the mastoid to the magnet in the implanted portion of the device. External components continue to undergo size reduction.

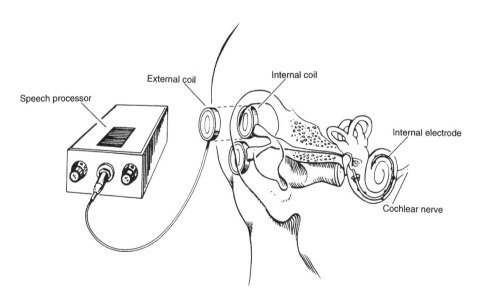

The cochlear implant system. (From Cummings CW, et al: Otolaryngology–Head and Neck Surgery, 3rd ed. St. Louis, Mosby, 1998, with permission.)

22. Who is a candidate for auditory brainstem implant?

Patients with the diagnosis of NF-2, patients whose auditory nerve has been damaged during acoustic tumor removal are candidates for auditory brainstem implant. These patients require placement of the electrode over the cochlear nuclei.

23. What are the different sites of cochlear implant electrodes placement?

Several locations are used for the placement of the CI electrodes

Intracochlear: electrodes placed in the scala tympani of the cochlea

Extracochlear: electrodes placed outside the cochlea in the promontory, round window

Intraneural: electrodes placed directly in the modiolus

24. Who can benefit from cochlear implantation?

Cochlear implants are currently indicated for patients at least 18 months of age (with a trend to implant children as young as 12 months of age) who have binaural severe to profound sensorineural hearing loss, have intact 8th cranial nerve function, and show little or no benefit from hearing aids (should have at least 6 months experience with high-powered binaural amplification). Audiologic criteria: pure tone average at 0.5, 1, and 2 kHz higher than 90 dB or word understanding of up to 30% on open-set testing. Postlingual patients tend to do better than prelingual ones. Other important prognostic variables include general health, level of motivation, expectations, and quality of the patient's support group.

25. Is the cochlear malformation a contraindication to cochlear implant?

Cochlear malformations are not a contraindication for CI, but modification of conventional implantation is necessary. Bony malformations of the cochlea (cochlear hypoplasia, common cavity deformity-combined cochlea and vestibule with no internal structure, incomplete partition such as in Mondini malformation) are associated with the absence of the round and oval windows and with aberrant course of the facial nerve. Risk of cerebrospinal fluid leak and electrode migration is higher. Facial nerve monitoring should be used.

26. How do cochlear implants work?

The behind-the-ear microphone receives sound and converts it into electrical signals. These signals are delivered to the external signal processor worn on the belt. The signal processor modifies the signal and delivers it to the transmitter over the mastoid. The transmitter then delivers the signal to the implanted receiver/stimulator either directly or indirectly. Directly, the signal may be carried via a hard-wired percutaneous connector. Indirectly, the signal may be carried by an FM radio frequency or magnetic induction. The receiver/stimulator, implanted under the skin in the mastoid, further modifies the signal and delivers it to electrodes implanted in the scala tympani. These electrodes stimulate the remaining neural tissue, usually spiral ganglion cells, in the cochlea.

27. How is sound perceived by a patient with a cochlear implant?

Sounds produced by CIs are not like normal hearing. The electrical stimulation provided by the implant is perceived as auditory sensations that vary in pitch and loudness. The speech processor of the implant selects out specific characteristics of sound that are important for speech understanding. The quality of these sounds is such that most patients are able to develop improved communication skills. A few patients are even able to understand speech without visual cues.

28. What are the surgical risks and complications of cochlear implant?

- *Intraoperative:* partial insertion of the electrode (ossified cochlea), insertion trauma (penetration of the electrode through basilar membrane, fracture of the osseous spiral lamina), perilymphatic gusher (in presence of Mondini malformation)
- *Postoperative:* postauricular flap edema, necrosis (the most common complication), transient vertigo, facial nerve stimulation or paralysis, meningitis, extrusion of the implant

29. What are the future challenges in improving the cochlear implants?

The range of performance across the CI users is large even with the indentical type of speech processor and electrode array. The mechanism of this variability is unknown. Research is in progress to indentify this mechanism. Another challenge is to provide more help for CI users in listening to speech in background noise.

30. What are the results in cochlear implant users?
More than 75% of adults and children are able to understand a significant amount of open-set speech. Sentence recognition is 80% to 90%.

31. Is magnetic resonance imaging (MRI) contraindicated in patients with cochlear implant?
Yes, MRI is contraindicated in patients with conventional cochlear implants because of the risk of implant movement. However, a nonmagnetic version of multichannel cochlear implant is available for use in patients who are candidate for CI and require repeat MRI for monitoring of central nervous system disease.

CONTROVERSIES

32. Should a child receive a cochlear implant?
Optimal comprehensive management of a child with SNHL involves constructive dialogue and coordination with the child's family and teachers. Not all children with SNHL benefit from conventional amplification, even after parents have invested significant amounts of money in hearing aids. Parents may encounter frustration and disappointment if their children fail to achieve communicative and academic goals they have established in their own mind. If the child is a potential candidate for cochlear implantation, this decision not only involves the risks (albeit modest) of surgery but also often a substantial financial commitment to help defray the cost of this sophisticated electronic device. The parents may encounter conflicting advice from friends and members of the adult deaf community about the benefit of cochlear implantation. Throughout the course of all of these difficult considerations, the health professionals caring for a child with hearing loss should be a source for information, guidance, and support to the family. (See also Chapter 7.)

ALESSANDRO VOLTA (1745–1827)

Volta might be considered the father of electrical stimulation of the ear. Along with his seminal electrical experiments, he reportedly placed metal rods into both of his ears and heard "bubbling water"—*just before he lost consciousness*!

~*Weir N, Otolaryngology: An Illustrated History, 1990*

BIBLIOGRAPHY

1. Clark GM: Cochlear implants in the Third Millennium. Am J Otol 20:4–8, 1999.
2. Cohen NL: An overview of cochlear implants for the general otolaryngologist. PROHNS 8–2, August 2000.
3. Gantz BJ, Tyler RS, Rubenstein JT: Seventh symposium on cochlear implants in children. Ann Otol Rhinol Laryngol Suppl 185. 109 (Pt 2):1–125, 2000.
4. Graham JM, Phelps PD, Michaels L: Congenital malformations of the ear and cochlear implantation in children: Review and temporal bone report of common cavity. JLO Suppl 25:1–14, 2000.
5. Hodges AV, Butts S, Dolan-Ash S, et al: Using electrically evoked auditory reflex thresholds to fit the CLARION cochlear implant. Ann ORL Supp 177:64–68, 1999.
6. Johnson I, O'Donoghue G: Who benefits from cochlear implantation? Practitioner 242:434, 437–438, 444, 1998.

7. Laszig R, Aschendorff A: Cochlear implants and electrical brainstem stimulation in sensorineural hearing loss. Curr Opin Neurol 12:41–44, 1999.
8. Lenarz T: Cochlear implants: Selection criteria and shifting borders. Acta Otorhinolaryngol Belg 52:183–199, 1998.
9. Linstrom CJ: Cochlear implantation. Practical information for the generalist. Prim Care Clin Off Pract 25:583–617, 1998.
10. Marzella PL, Clark GM: Growth factors, auditory neurones and cochlear implants: A review. Acta Oto Laryngol 119:407–412, 1999.
11. Mukherjee N, Roseman RD, Willging JP: The piezoelectric cochlear implant: Concept, feasibility, challenges, and issues. J Biomed Mat Res 53:181–187, 2000.
12. Niparko J: Cochlear Implants. Philadelphia, Lippincott Williams &Wilkins, 2000.
13. Rizer FM, Burkey JM: Cochlear implantation in the very young child. Otol Clin North Am 32:1117–1125, 1999.
14. Rubinstein JT, Miller CA: How do cochlear prostheses work? Curr Opin Neurobiol 9:399–404, 1999.
15. Slattery WH 3rd, Fayad JN: Cochlear implants in children with sensorineural inner ear hearing loss. Pediatr Ann 28:359–363, 1999.
16. Truy E: Neuro-functional imaging and profound deafness. Int J Pediatr Otorhinolaryngol 47:131–136, 1999.

9. DISEASES OF THE EXTERNAL EAR AND TYMPANIC MEMBRANE

Bruce W. Jafek, M.D., Douglas M. Sorensen, M.D., and Catherine Winslow, M.D.

1. Identify the parts of the auricle.

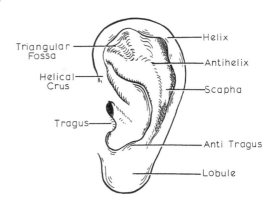

Anatomy of the auricle. (From Lee KJ: Essential Otolaryngology–Head and Neck Surgery. Norwalk, CT, Appleton & Lange, 1995, p 2, with permission.)

2. Name the six hillocks of His. What is their clinical significance?

In the embryo, the first and second branchial arches each give rise to three hillocks. The **first arch** gives rise to the first three hillocks that form the tragus, the helical crus, and the helix. The **second arch** gives rise to the second three hillocks that form the antihelix, the scapha, and the lobule. If these primitive ear hillocks fail to fuse, preauricular pits result. Preauricular pits may become recurrently infected, requiring excision.

3. What are the complications of an auricular hematoma if left untreated?

This blunt injury commonly occurs in wrestlers and boxers. Characteristically, as the ear swells, it becomes large and blue and loses the outline of its conchal folds. Because a hematoma accumulates between the cartilage and perichondrium, the proper name for this injury is **sub-perichondrial hematoma**. This hematoma deprives the cartilage of nutrients and predisposes the ear to necrosis and infection. The principal complication is the "**cauliflower ear**" deformity, which results from cartilage loss. Subtler ear deformities may result from an infection or fibrosis.

4. How should an auricular hematoma be managed?

The goal of management is to prevent deformity. First, the skin overlying the hematoma should be anesthetized with 1% lidocaine. The clinician should then evacuate the hematoma by making an incision with a no. 15 scalpel (use of a large bore needle is an alternative, but is often unsuccessful, as the hematoma is organized). Next, the cavity should be irrigated with saline. Finally, this evacuated space should be bolstered with 4–0 nylon suture and dental rolls. The dental rolls compress the wound and prevent reaccumulation of blood. An anti-staphylococcal antibiotic should be prescribed, and the rolls should be left in place for 1 week.

5. What is perichondritis of the auricle? How is it treated?

Perichondritis and **chondritis** are infections that involve the perichondrium and cartilage of the auricle, respectively. Usually, these infections result from an auricle laceration, although non-infectious causes, such as **relapsing polychondritis,** may also lead to this disorder. They are more commonly seen in the diabetic condition or other conditions with compromised microvasculature.

These infections present with diffuse painful erythematous swelling of the auricle. The treatment begins with surgical debridement of the devitalized cartilage, and intravenous antibiotics that cover aerobic and anaerobic bacteria should be administered. Oral antibiotics are less efficacious. *Pseudomonas* and *Staphylococcus* are the most common causative organisms, with *Pseudomonas* being more common in the diabetic patient.

6. What is keratitis obturans?

Keratitis obturans, also known as cholesteatoma of the external auditory canal, is an uncommon condition. A conductive hearing loss results from the thickened skin, which "peels off" as a sheet or cast of the external auditory canal (including the tympanic membrane) under the operating microscope. Pain is due to bony erosion of the external auditory canal from a cholesteatoma. Steroidal otic drops may be helpful in slowing the process, and methotraxate has also been advocated. Usually, however, periodic débridement is required to prevent retention of fluids (e.g., from sweat or showering) with subsequent recurrent otitis externa. This condition is frequently associated with disorders such as chronic obstructive pulmonary disease, bronchiectasis, and sinusitis.

7. Describe the clinical signs and symptoms of frostbite to the external auricle.

Frostbite may progress clinically from cyanosis to ischemia with pallor, edema with vesicle formation, and finally, tissue necrosis. Temperatures $< 10°C$ block sensory nerve conduction and therefore pain. Treatment involves rapid rewarming.

8. What is otitis externa?

Otitis externa is a common inflammatory condition involving the skin of the external auditory canal. It can be localized or diffuse and acute or chronic. A history of antecedent ear canal trauma or water exposure is common, hence the term "swimmer's ear." Other predisposing conditions include loss of the canal's protective coating, maceration of the skin from water or humidity, and glandular obstruction. Symptoms include otalgia, pruritus, and foul-smelling otorrhea. The ear canal may appear mildly erythematous. If the infection is severe, edema may completely obstruct the canal. The ear and its canal may be exquisitely tender. *Pseudomonas aeruginosa* and *Staphylococcus aureus* are the primary pathogenic organisms. Treatment begins with local débridement and the administration of antibiotic steroid drops. In cases of severe canal swelling, a wick impregnated with an anti-inflammatory agent should be placed carefully in the canal and left there for 2–7 days.

9. What is the general approach to otitis externa?

The management of patients with otitis externa includes debridement, topical therapy with acidifying and antimicrobial agents, and systemic antimicrobial therapy when indicated (uncommon).

Patients with **chronic otitis externa** require cleansing and debridement, accompanied by topical acidifying and drying agents. This is followed by topical antibiotics and corticosteroid preparations. Surgery (again, uncommon) is mainly used to allow cleansing and aeration and/or removal of the scarred tissue. Patients with **acute localized otitis externa** (furunculosis) are treated with local heat and systemic antibiotics in the inflammatory stage, and drainage in the abscess state. **Mycotic external otitis** is managed with topical acidifying and antifungal agents (e.g. Gentian violet), whereas viral (herpes) infection is treated with topical and systemic aciclovir (acyclovir). Patients with **necrotizing (malignant) external otitis,** which is mainly caused by *P. aeruginosa and S. aureus,* are treated with systemic antibiotics and, rarely, by surgical débridement. Therapy for **eczematous otitis externa** is first directed at the secondary infection and thereafter at the primary dermatologic condition.

Prevention of recurrent external otitis is aimed at minimizing ear canal trauma and avoiding exposure to water. Preventative use of topical acidifying agents or 70% alcohol is also advocated. A 50:50 mixture of white (distilled) vinegar and isopropyl alcohol (drying) can be made by the patient and carried in a dropper bottle.

10. Are systemic antibiotics useful in the treatment of otitis externa?

Prompted by rising rates of antibiotic resistance, lack of standardized treatment regimens, and new treatment alternatives, the American Academy of Otolaryngology–Head and Neck Surgery convened an expert consensus panel to consider recommendations for the responsible use of antibiotics in chronic suppurative otitis media, tympanostomy tube otorrhea, and otitis externa. The Panel concluded that in the absence of systemic infection or serious underlying disease, topical antibiotics alone constitute first-line treatment for most patients with these conditions. The Panel found no evidence that systemic antibiotics alone or in combination with topical preparations improve treatment outcomes compared with topical antibiotics alone. Topical preparations should be selected on the basis of expected bacteriology and informed knowledge of the risks and benefits of each available preparation. The use of nonototoxic preparations in treating acute otitis externa (when the tympanic membrane is perforated or its status is unknown), chronic suppurative otitis media, and tympanostomy tube otorrhea should be considered.

11. Does allergy cause otitis externa?

Allergy may affect the outer, the middle, or the inner ear. Although the otologic manifestations of allergy are not by themselves diagnostic, the history, including family history and associated symptoms in other target organs, will often help lead to the correct diagnosis and institution of therapy. Patients with significant and chronic symptoms, including those with labyrinthine symptoms of allergy, will respond well to specific immunotherapy and/or dietary elimination.

12. An elderly, insulin-dependent diabetic woman with a history of chronic otitis externa presents to your clinic with severe otalgia and auricle edema. Examination shows granulation tissue in the external auditory meatus, at the junction between the cartilaginous and bony canal. What is your working diagnosis? What treatment do you prescribe?

Malignant otitis externa refers to a progressive and necrosing *Pseudomonas* infection of the ear (although *Staphylococcus* is also uncommonly the offending organism). This infection does not remain localized to the skin of the ear canal but instead extends to the deeper tissues and invades medially along the floor of the ear canal to produce an osteomyelitis. This medial and posterior extension leads to invasion of the mastoid, facial nerve, and base of the skull. The typical patient is elderly, diabetic, and has severe otalgia. Management begins with gaining control of the patient's diabetes. Local ear canal débridement or mastoidectomy may be necessary. Intravenous antipseudomonal antibiotics should be given early. Response to therapy can be determined by decreasing pain, but the mortality of this seemingly "slight" condition may approach 50%. Serial sedimentation rates are also helpful in following the course of the condition.

13. How is otomycosis recognized and managed?

Otomycosis, or externa mycotica, refers to a fungal or candidal infection of the external auditory canal. Symptoms are similar to those of otitis externa; however, pruritus is a more common symptom than otalgia. Upon examination of the ear canal, the disease may be recognized easily by visualization of the fungal mycelia. Moisture, high temperature, poor hygiene, and immunosuppression appear to contribute to the development of this condition. The offending organisms usually are *Aspergillus albicans, Aspergillus niger,* and *Candida albicans.* Treatment begins with débridement of the ear canal. A topical fungicide, such as nystatin powder, cresylate, 4% boric acid powder, or 1% gentian violet, should be applied. Applying Cortisporin drops or other antimicrobials may exacerbate otomycosis.

14. How are exostoses differentiated from an auditory canal osteoma?

Exostoses are benign periosteal outgrowths that occur in the bony canal. They are often associated with multiple exposures to swimming in cold water. Clinically, they appear as hard nodules next to the annulus and frequently are multiple and bilateral. Exostoses are usually small enough that they do not obstruct the canal, although a patient may suffer from secondary otitis externa. An **osteoma** is usually single and unilateral, often occurring at the bony cartilaginous junction of the tympanomastoid suture line. Surgical removal of either may be required if they interfere with insertion of a hearing aid or produce recurrent otitis externa secondary to fluid retention or lead to a conductive hearing loss, but these are all very uncommon.

15. What is Ramsay Hunt syndrome?

Ramsay Hunt syndrome, also known as **herpes zoster otiticus,** is due to infection of the geniculate ganglion and other cranial nerve ganglia, probably by the chickenpox virus. The chief symptom stems from painful herpetic lesions in the external auditory meatus and auricle. If the virus affects the seventh nerve, cutaneous herpes and ipsilateral facial paralysis (Bell's palsy) may result. If the virus affects the 8th nerve, vomiting, vertigo, nystagmus, and hearing loss may result.

16. What is microtia?

Microtia is a term used to describe hypoplasia of the external ear, often associated with atresia of the external auditory canal. Microtia typically presents as a rudimentary auricle with maldeveloped cartilage. In the place of a normal ear, an S-shaped skin fold is often positioned vertically. This external ear anomaly presents a challenge to the reconstructive surgeon as it is often displaced anteriorly and inferiorly. Four degrees, ranging from "mild" (I) to complete absence (IV, or "anotia") are described.

17. What is aural atresia?

Aural atresia is a congenital deformity of the auricle and middle ear and is accompanied by inner ear deformity in up to 30% of cases. Atresia is more commonly unilateral, occurs more often in males, and is more common on the right. The degree of abnormality may be minor, moderate, or severe. Treatment involves fitting the patient with bone-conduction hearing aids until the patient is old enough for surgery.

18. What are the predisposing factors to aural atresia?

The incidence of congenital aural atresia is increased if there is a positive family history, prenatal teratogenic drug ingestion, or a viral illness during pregnancy.

19. Does the degree of external deformity correlate with the degree of middle ear derangement?

Yes, it appears that the degree of internal functional derangement is proportional to the degree of external deformity, but additional specific anatomical correlations are not apparent.

20. Are additional congenital malformations more common with microtia and atresia?

Yes, additional congenital malformations will be found in over 50% of patients, ranging from simple preauricular tags to the complex syndromes of achondroplasia or rubella embryopathy. The most common systemic abnormalities were skeletal and cardiac, with epithelial and structural abnormalities more common in the head and neck region. Multiple malformations are common.

21. Where do keloids develop?

A keloid is a common benign tumor often affecting the auricle that commonly forms after ear piercing, trauma, or surgical ear procedures. Often, these tumors do not develop until long after the initial insult to the ear. Keloids present a difficult problem because their surgical excision usually results in a larger, more-deforming tumor recurrence. Keloids are often treated with intralesional steroids.

22. How do you clean a cerumen impaction?

Because cerumen has an acidic pH, it is bacteriostatic and fungistatic. If the tympanic membrane is obscured by cerumen, the canal must be cleaned for proper evaluation. Cleaning with warm water irrigation is often the preferable approach, especially in children. However, if you suspect a tympanic membrane perforation, the ear should never be irrigated. You should consider a perforation based on a suspicious history, odor, blood, or discharge within the auditory canal.

A cerumen spoon may also be used; however, the skin of the auditory canal is fragile and bleeds easily. Small abrasions may cause the patient significant pain. If you are unable to remove tightly impacted cerumen, you may advise the patient to use mineral oil or Cortisporin drops daily for 1 week to soften the impaction. You may need to remove such impactions with the aid of an otolaryngologist's working microscope.

23. A 3-year-old child presents with a small calculator battery in his right ear. The child is crying and upset. What is the proper management?

Foreign bodies in the ear are usually confined to children. Management can be divided into two categories: those cases that should be irrigated and those that should not. Most foreign bodies can be removed easily with gentle syringe irrigation. In certain cases, however, irrigation is contraindicated. Small batteries, such as calculator and watch batteries, are dangerous because they may leak acid into the ear. Irrigation of this acid only aggravates the problem. Batteries should be removed with the aid of a microscope and a small hook. Often children insert peas or other vegetable material into their ears. Irrigation in these cases is also inappropriate, as water will cause the vegetables to swell, leading to excruciating pain. Again, this material should be removed with a small hook. Occasionally, removal is inhibited when the child is extremely upset. General anesthetic is reserved for very small or uncooperative children with deeply embedded foreign bodies.

24. Describe abnormal signs that may be found on examination of the tympanic membrane and their associated conditions.

Tympanic Membrane Signs and Associated Conditions

SIGNS	ASSOCIATED CONDITIONS
Mobility	
Bulging, no mobility	Fluid or pus in middle ear
Retracted, no mobility	Obstruction of eustachian tube
Mobility on negative pressure only	Obstruction of eustachian tube
Excessive mobility in one small area	Healed perforation
Color	
Amber	Serous fluid in middle ear
Blue or deep red	Blood in middle ear
White	Infection in middle ear
Red (with crying)	Infection in middle ear
Dullness	Fibrosis
White plaques	Healed inflammation
Contents	
Air bubbles	Serous fluid in middle ear

25. What are the most common causes of traumatic tympanic membrane perforations?

Perforations may be caused by foreign bodies, such as hairpins or Q-tips. Trauma to the ear may cause sufficient air compression in the external meatus to rupture the drum. Gunfire may also cause sufficient air displacement, leading to tympanic membrane rupture. The drum generally heals spontaneously, but residual perforations can be repaired with surgery.

26. Where is Prussak's space?

Prussak's space, or the superior recess of the tympanic membrane, is an area behind the tympanic membrane. It is bound laterally by the flaccid portion of the tympanic membrane, or the pars flaccida, and medially by the neck of the malleus. The lateral malleolar fold in the middle ear encloses Prussak's space.

27. Why is Prussak's space significant?

A retraction or perforation in the pars flaccida may allow keratinous debris to enter the middle ear space, resulting in infection, osteitis, and erosion. This leads to the progression of a cholesteatoma.

28. In patients with chronic otitis media, how are tympanic membrane perforations classified?

Perforations resulting from chronic otitis media are classified as central or marginal. In central perforations, the fibrous annulus remains unaffected, and the tympanic membrane circumscribes the entire intact ring. In *marginal* perforations, the fibrous annulus is involved. In these cases, the defect is usually seen posteriorly on the drum. Occasionally, destruction of the drum's margin leads to abnormal epithelial growth. If squamous epithelium grows into the middle ear cavity, a subsequent cholesteatoma may form. Marginal perforations are generally more difficult to repair than central perforations.

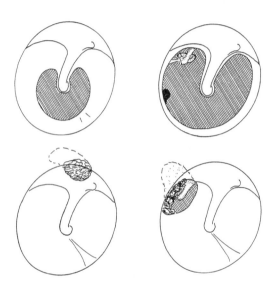

Tympanic membrane perforations. *Top,* Central perforations. There is a margin of eardrum around the periphery. The perforation may be small or subtotal. It may be posterior, inferior, or anterior. *Bottom,* Marginal perforations. An attic perforation *(left)* may harbor a small or large cholesteatoma. In the posteromarginal defect *(right)* granulations are present, and the incus will soon necrose. Again, there may be a small or large cholesteatoma. (From Coleman BH: Diseases of the Nose, Throat and Ear, and Head and Neck. Edinburgh, Churchill Livingstone, 1992, p 220, with permission.)

29. Name the three layers of the tympanic membrane.

The outermost layer, or the *lateral squamous layer,* is continuous with the skin of the external auditory meatus. Directly under it lies the *middle fibrous layer,* also known as the lamina propria. Finally, the *medial mucosal layer* is continuous with the mucosa of the tympanic cavity.

30. Which tympanic membrane layers will regenerate after a perforation?

The epithelial and endothelial layers will regenerate to seal the perforation. However, the fibrous mesothelial layer does not regenerate. Although the new membrane has two layers, the newly formed membrane is called a **monomeric membrane.** Actually, this is probably more properly characterized as a "dimeric" membrane, reflecting the lateral and medial epithelial regeneration, but this term is not used. Occasionally, the new membrane will be very translucent and resemble a perforation to the untrained eye. On pneumoscopic examination the monomeric membrane appears hypermobile with positive and negative pressure.

31. How do you "paper patch" a tympanic membrane?

For small to moderate-sized perforations that will not heal spontaneously, a paper patch can be applied to the tympanic membrane. This patch acts as a scaffold for the re-epithelialization process. Prior to the procedure, the ear must be dry with no infection or exudate. The edges of the perforation can be abraded with an instrument or with chemical cautery (e.g., trichloroacetic acid) to stimulate migration. A circular patch of cigarette or rice paper is made with a paper punch and is placed over the opening. Because the patch is frequently displaced with the resultant epithelial migration, the patient should be followed monthly, and the procedure may be repeated as necessary. The patient should be cautioned not to blow his or her nose.

32. A whitish plaque is seen on the tympanic membrane of an otherwise normal ear. Is further evaluation needed?

In **myringosclerosis,** also known as **tympanosclerosis,** whitish plaques form in the fibrous layer of the tympanic membrane in response to infection or inflammation. Alone, this process generally does not lead to a hearing loss. However, a concurrent otitis may certainly lead to a conductive deficit.

33. What is bullous myringitis?

Bullous myringitis is a viral infection that involves the tympanic membrane and its adjacent deep canal. This condition is associated with viral and bacterial upper respiratory tract infections. Previously it was thought to be indicative of mycoplasma infection associated with atypical pneumonia, but it is now known to be a nonspecific indication of middle ear infection. Severe otalgia is usually present. Examination of the tympanic membrane reveals reddish vesicles on the surface that enlarge to form bullae. Treatment includes antibiotic steroid drops, oral antibiotics, and analgesics.

CONTROVERSIES

34. Can the tympanic membrane heal after perforations?

Tympanic membrane perforations usually heal well, although not all perforations heal. Marginal perforations, involving the annulus, are less likely to heal than central ones. Epithelial migration proceeds from the umbo outward at a rate of 0.05 mm/day.

JOHN HARRISON CURTIS (1778–1860)

Curtis was one of the more notorious practitioners of quackery in hearing restoration with the artificial ear in the 1800s. Practicing in an exclusive area of London, his patrons included George VI. Distinguishing between "Spanish and French ears," Curtis recommended "the silver German ear" as the finest.

~Weir N, Otolaryngology: An Illustrated History, 1990

BIBLIOGRAPHY

1. Boustred N: Practical guide to otitis externa. Austral Fam Phys 28:217–221, 1999.
2. Brook I: Treatment of otitis externa in children. Paed Drugs 1:283–289, 1999.
3. Chandler JR: Malignant external otitis and osteomyelitis of the base of the skull. Am J Otol 10:108–110, 1989. *(Still a classic)*
4. Derebery MJ, Berliner KI: Allergy for the otologist. External canal to inner ear. Otol Clin North Am 31:157–173, 1998.
5. Hannley MT, Denneny JC III, Holzer SS: Use of ototopical antibiotics in treating 3 common ear diseases. Otol Head Neck Surg 122:934–940, 2000.
6. Hern JD, Almeyda J, Thomas DM, et al: Malignant otitis externa in HIV and AIDS. J Laryngol Otol 110:770–775, 1996.
7. La Rosa S: Primary care management of otitis externa. Nurse Pract 23:125–128, 131–133, 1998.
8. Ostrowski VB, Wiet RJ: Pathologic conditions of the external ear and auditory canal. Postgrad Med 100:223–228, 233–237, 1996.
9. Rea P, Joseph T: A GP strategy for otitis externa. Pract 242:466–468, 470–471, 1998.
10. Shohet JA, Scherger JE: Which culprit is causing your patient's otorrhea? Postgrad Med 104:50–55, 59–60, 1998.
11. Vogelin E, Grobbelaar AO, Chana JS, et al: Surgical correction of the cauliflower ear. Br J Plast Surg 51:359–362, 1998.

10. OTITIS MEDIA AND ASSOCIATED COMPLICATIONS

Douglas H. Todd, M.D., Sylvan E. Stool, M.D. and Bruce W. Jafek, M.D.

1. Explain the terminology used to describe ear infections.

Historically, the terminology used to describe ear infections has been confusing and has resulted in miscommunication among patients and physicians. When describing infections of the ear, the terminology should define the anatomic location of the process and its chronicity.

Otitis externa—inflammatory process of the external auditory canal or auricle

Myringitis—inflammatory process of the tympanic membrane

Otitis media (OM)—inflammatory process of the middle ear space. The presence or absence of a middle ear effusion (OME) should be noted.

Otitis media with effusion (OME)—OM accompanied by fluid in the middle ear (often can be visualized through the intact TM). This fluid may be purulent or "sterile." Sterile fluid may remain after the causative organism has been killed or may merely reflect our inability to culture organisms that may still be present (e.g., viruses).

Mastoiditis—inflammatory process of the mastoid cavity

Labyrinthitis—inflammatory process of the inner ear

Note that acute (AOM) processes last < 3 weeks. Subacute processes last between 3 weeks and 3 months. Chronic processes persist > 3 months.

2. What are the functions of the eustachian tube?

The eustachian tube can be considered as a valve that connects the middle ear cleft to the nasopharynx. This structure ventilates the middle ear and protects the middle ear from nasopharyngeal secretions. Fluid found in the middle ear or mastoid usually drains via the eustachian tube. Conditions that alter eustachian tube function may lead to the accumulation of fluid in the middle ear and mastoid. This accumulation may subsequently lead to infection, secondary to ascending infection via the eustachian tube, resulting in otitis media and possibly mastoiditis.

3. How is otitis media diagnosed?

Common signs and symptoms of acute otitis media may include **otalgia,** often associated with ear tugging or irritability in young children, **otorrhea,** indicating perforation or patent tympanostomy tubes, and **fever,** indicating an acute infection. Less commonly seen are postauricular swelling, facial paralysis, vertigo, and tinnitus. The tympanic membrane should be evaluated for position, mobility, and color. Decreased mobility indicates an effusion or perforation, and erythema indicates infection. Perforation of the tympanic membrane, retraction pockets, or other pathologic lesion should be noted and documented.

4. Why are younger children predisposed to otitis media?

At birth, the eustachian tube is in a horizontal plane and has a relatively small lumen. In adults, this structure is at a 45-degree angle with the ear. The adult eustachian tube is higher than the nose and has a relatively large lumen. Children are predisposed to otitis media because secretions from the nasopharynx can readily pass through a horizontal patent eustachian tube, introducing pathogens into the middle ear. Additionally, a small amount of inflammation can obstruct a child's already small lumen, aggravating the infectious process.

5. What environmental risk factors are associated with otitis media with effusion?

- Bottle-feeding of infants instead of breast-feeding
- Propping a bottle in a supine infant's mouth (resulting in milk reflux into the middle ear through the eustachian tube)

- Passive smoking
- Attendance in a child care facility

Risk factors for resistant pathogens include recent antibiotic treatment of acute otitis media, children in daycare facilities, wintertime infections, and acute otitis media in children less than 2 years of age.

6. Which organisms are most commonly found in otitis media?

The most common organisms found in **acute** otitis media are *Streptococcus pneumoniae, Haemophilus influenzae,* and *Moraxella (Branhamella) catarrhalis.* Although rare in older patients, gram-negative enteric bacilli are isolated in 20% of infants with middle ear effusions. Viruses can be isolated in approximately 4% of middle ear effusions, with respiratory syncytial virus and influenza virus being the most common.

Organisms isolated in **chronic** otitis media vary considerably. The predominant organisms are gram-negative bacilli, such as *Pseudomonas aeruginosa, Proteus* sp., and *Escherichia coli,* and anaerobes such as *Bacteroides fragilis.* These organisms, along with *Staphylococcus,* are also more common in nosocomial (hospital-acquired) infections.

7. What is the role of viruses in the pathogenesis of acute otitis media?

Acute otitis media (AOM) is often considered a simple bacterial infection that can be effectively treated with antibiotics. However, despite the extensive use of broad-spectrum antibiotics, poor clinical response to treatment of acute otitis media is common in children. Numerous studies ranging from animal experiments to extensive clinical studies have clearly demonstrated that respiratory viruses play a critical role in the etiology and pathogenesis of acute otitis media. Viral infection of the upper respiratory tract initiates the whole cascade of events that finally leads to the development of acute otitis media as a complication. Respiratory viruses induce a release of inflammatory mediators in the nasopharynx, increase bacterial colonization and adherence, and have a suppressive effect on the host's immune defense.

Recent data indicate that at least some types of viruses actively invade the middle ear. Viruses also seem to enhance the inflammatory process in the middle ear and impair the outcome of the disease. Vaccines against the major viruses predisposing to acute otitis media hold a great promise for the prevention of this disease.

8. How common is otitis media?

Acute otitis media affects at least 80% of children younger than 2 years of age and is responsible for one-third of physician visits of children younger than 5 years of age.

9. What is the role of pneumatic otoscopy?

To enhance the likelihood of accurate diagnosis of AOM, pneumatic otoscopy is the preferred method of examination generally available to clinicians. It is the "gold standard" for the diagnosis of otitis media. The findings on pneumatic otoscopy should be correlated, of course, with the presence or absence of symptoms and signs to confirm (or rule out) the diagnosis of AOM or OME.

10. What type of hearing loss is expected in otitis media with effusion?

In OME, the middle ear cleft contains fluid that decreases tympanic membrane mobility. This results in a conductive hearing loss with a type B tympanogram and normal external auditory canal volume.

11. How is the development of acute otitis media or otitis media with effusion related to tonsil or adenoid infection?

- Adenoid inflammation leads to inflammatory obstruction of the eustachian tube.
- Early colonization of the adenoid with the three major bacterial pathogens of otitis media is the most important factor in the early pathogenesis of otitis media.

- The local immune system in the adenoid, particularly specific secretory IgA, directed against both viruses and bacterial pathogens, is probably genetically controlled and represents the primary immunologic factor in protecting the host against invasion of these agents in the eustachian tube and middle ear. Failure of this protection contributes to AOM.
- Two triggers are viral infections and upper respiratory tract allergy, both of which affect the tonsils and adenoids locally.

12. At what age is adenoidectomy useful in the treatment of otitis media with effusion?

Adenoidectomy decreases the morbidity of otitis media in children 4 years of age or older. Adenoidectomies in younger children have not been demonstrated to control otitis media and are generally not recommended.

13. Why is otitis media more difficult to manage now than it was in the past?

AOM has become increasingly difficult to treat in the 1990s, the decade of drug-resistant *Pneumococcus*. Throughout the world, drug-resistant strains of this pathogen are being recovered from 20 to 50% of cases of untreated AOM, and from 45 to 90% of refractory AOM. Almost as alarming is that beta-lactamase-producing strains of *Haemophilus influenzae* are currently being isolated in 40 to 50% of cases of AOM. It is now imperative that clinicians become aware of the regional prevalence of drug-resistant bacteria and, just as importantly, their patterns of antibacterial resistance.

Although some authors would hold that any antibacterial agent, or even placebo, should be adequate for most cases of AOM, clinical practice appears to suggest otherwise. Amoxicillin, still the first-line therapeutic choice for the initial treatment of AOM, will often fail. The real dilemma begins when clinicians begin to search for clinical data to select an antibacterial for therapeutic failures. To give optimal treatment to a patient who has failed antibacterial therapy—the true actual indication for all second-line antibacterials—the clinician must instead become familiar with the following in vivo and in vitro data:

- In vivo sensitivity data: otherwise known as bacteriologic efficacy, in which repeat tympanocentesis is performed in mid-therapy. This should reveal the sensitivity.
- Clinical efficacy data: analysis of rates of clinical resolution after therapy in comparative trials that use a single tympanocentesis initially and a gold standard antibacterial.
- "Bug to drug" data: comparison of reported middle ear concentrations for each individual antibacterial agent relative to the respective minimum inhibitory concentrations of isolates, particularly drug-resistant *Pneumococcus* and *H. influenzae* (if possible, obtained from the pediatric respiratory tract).

The selection of an antibacterial agent for AOM in any particular case can no longer be merely a random process.

14. What is the appropriate medical management for *acute* otitis media?

Treatment options for otitis media are controversial and include antimicrobials, decongestants, antihistamines, corticosteroids, immunizations, and allergy hyposensitization. Standard medical therapy for acute otitis media includes antimicrobial agents given for 10–14 days, although recent studies suggest that a shorter course (5 days) may be curative. Amoxicillin has been considered the drug of choice, although many effective agents are readily available. The selected agent should be active against *S. pneumoniae, H. influenzae,* and *M. catarrhalis.* It should also have a convenient dosing schedule, produce minimal side effects, be cost-effective, and taste good.

15. How should the proper antibiotic be selected?

Overall, the choice of antibiotics for treatment of otitis media should take into consideration their in vitro activity against the **locally prevalent organisms,** especially **resistant organisms,** and results obtained from studies in which **bacteriologic outcome** was used as the endpoint.

Amoxicillin remains the antibiotic of first choice, although a higher dosage (80 mg per kg per day) may be indicated to ensure eradication of drug-resistant *S. pneumoniae* (DRSP). Oral cefuroxime or amoxicillin-clavulanate and intramuscular ceftriaxone are suggested second-line choices for treatment failure. For patients with clinically defined treatment failure after 3 days of therapy, useful alternative agents include oral amoxicillin-clavulanate, cefuroxime axetil, and cefpodoxime proxetil. Intramuscular ceftriaxone should be reserved for severe cases or patients in whom noncompliance is expected. Many of the 13 other Food and Drug Administration—approved otitis media drugs lack good evidence for efficacy against DRSP. Currently, local surveillance data for pneumococcal resistance that are relevant for the clinical management of AOM are not available from most areas in the United States. The management of otitis media has entered a new era with the development of DRSP. Tympanocentesis for identification of pathogens and susceptibility to antimicrobial agents is recommended for selection of third-line agents.

16. How long can middle ear effusions persist after an episode of otitis media?

Research has shown that in 80% of children aged 2–6 years, OME clears within 2 months. Without medical intervention, approximately 60% of children recover within 3 months.

17. Describe the medical management for *chronic* otitis media with effusion.

Medical management of otitis media with effusion initially includes watchful waiting, control of environmental risk factors, and antimicrobial therapy. Research indicates that middle ear effusions following acute otitis media usually resolve within 3–6 months. Therefore, watchful waiting may be appropriate therapy. Other studies indicate that antibiotics help about 15% of children to hasten clearance of effusion within a 1-month period. Corticosteroid therapy remains controversial. Antihistamines and decongestants are not recommended for isolated OME.

18. What are the surgical options for treatment of otitis media?

Surgical options include tympanocentesis, myringotomy, and tympanostomy tube insertion (pressure equalization tube). Complications from otitis media may necessitate tympanoplasty, ossiculoplasty, and mastoidectomy.

19. What are tympanocentesis and myringotomy?

Tympanocentesis is needle aspiration of fluid from the middle ear space. It is used to identify organisms in middle ear effusions of children who appear toxic or unresponsive to antimicrobial therapy. Myringotomy is an incision into the tympanic membrane that allows drainage of middle ear secretions. It is usually preceded by tympanocentesis. Indications for myringotomy include complications of purulent otitis media, such as severe otalgia, meningitis, or facial paralysis.

20. List the indications for myringotomy and tympanostomy tube insertion.

- History of severe otitis media
- Chronic otitis media with effusion (present for > 3 months with associated hearing loss of > 30 dB in the better ear)
- Poor response to antibiotic therapy
- Impending complication of otitis media
- Recurrent acute otitis media (three episodes in 6 months or four episodes in 12 months)
- Chronic retraction pockets of the tympanic membrane or tympanic membrane atelectasis
- Barotitis media
- Autophony secondary to eustachian tube dysfunction

21. Are there any potential complications of tympanostomy tube insertion?

Complications from tympanostomy tube insertion are uncommon with experienced surgeons. Potential morbidity can include external auditory canal laceration, persistent otorrhea, granuloma formation, cholesteatoma, and chronic tympanic membrane perforation. Structural changes, such as tympanic membrane retraction, flaccidity, and myringosclerosis, may also occur. Myringosclerosis is felt to be of little clinical or functional importance. Tympanostomy tube insertion into the posterior superior quadrant should be avoided, as this is the most compliant part of the pars tensa and may result in chronic perforation, atrophic scarring, or retraction. Likewise, injury to the ossicles may occur. Insertion of a tube under the tympanic annulus may result in cholesteatoma. The sequel of insertion is the need to limit water exposure in the intubated ear (See also Question 30, Controversies.)

22. What are the intratemporal complications of untreated otitis media?

Conductive hearing loss	Mastoiditis
Sensorineural hearing loss	Petrositis
Tympanic membrane perforation	Labyrinthitis
Retraction pocket	Perilymphatic fistula
Cholesteatoma	Facial paralysis
Tympanosclerosis	Cholesterol granuloma
Ossicular chain fixation or discontinuity	

23. What organisms are found in mastoiditis?

Mastoiditis is the inflammation of the mastoid cavity. **Acute** mastoiditis is most likely caused by the same organisms that cause acute otitis media, including *S. pneumoniae, Staphylococcus pyrogenes,* and *Staphyloccus aureus*. *H. influenzae* is less common. **Chronic** mastoiditis is most likely to be caused by the organisms that cause chronic otitis media.

24. List intracranial complications of untreated otitis media.

Meningitis	Brain abscess
Extradural abscess	Lateral sinus thrombosis
Subdural empyema	Otitic hydrocephalus
Focal otitic encephalitis	

25. When are ototopical drops used to treat ear infections?

The American Academy of Otolaryngology–Head and Neck Surgery convened an expert consensus panel to address this question. The panel concluded that in the absence of systemic infection or serious underlying disease, ototopical antibiotics alone constitute first-line treatment for most patients diagnosed with chronic suppurative otitis media, tympanostomy tube otorrhea, and otitis externa.

26. What is the significance of unilateral otitis media in an adult?

Unilateral otitis media in the adult may indicate the presence of a nasopharyngeal mass obstructing the eustachian tube orifice. Unilateral otitis media in the adult should be considered neoplastic until proved otherwise by examination of the nasopharynx.

CONTROVERSIES

27. Is steroid therapy useful in the treatment of otitis media with effusion?

Although this is a controversial treatment, the literature regarding the use of corticosteroid agents is growing rapidly. Currently, steroids are not recommended for the treatment of otitis media in children of any age.

28. Does otitis media with effusion affect subsequent speech development?

It would appear so. In one study, recently available speech analysis programs, lifespan reference data, and statistical techniques were implemented with three cohorts of children with OME and their controls originally assessed in the 1980s. Early recurrent OME was not associated with an increased risk for a speech disorder in this sample but was associated with approximately 4.6 times increased risk for subclinical or clinical speech disorder in children.

29. Is there an association between second-hand smoke and otitis media?

Overall, there is a very consistent picture with odds ratios for respiratory illnesses and symptoms and middle ear disease of between 1.2 and 1.6 for either parent smoking, the odds usually being higher in preschool- than in school-aged children. For sudden infant death syndrome, the odds ratio for maternal smoking is about 2. In addition, studies of the effects of environmental tobacco smoke on children with cystic fibrosis and asthma conclude from the limited evidence that there is a strong case for a relationship between parental smoking and admissions to hospital. Policies need to be developed that reduce smoking among parents and protect infants and young children from exposure to environmental tobacco smoke.

30. Can a child with tympanostomy tubes swim?

Yes, although different clinicians advise different precautions. At one end of the spectrum, swimming is forbidden or occlusive ear plugs are used under a bathing cap. On the other hand, some clinicians allow swimming but no diving, without any protective device, believing that water cannot come through the small tubes because of the cohesive nature of the molecules. These clinicians, however, usually advise the avoidance of soapy water.

MASTOIDITIS

Called to the bedside of the young King Charles II of France, the great French medieval surgeon, Ambrose Paré, recommended an operation on the skull to drain away the pus. The boy-king's bride, Mary, Queen of Scots and France, consented, but the king's mother, Catherine de' Medici, forbade an operation, so Mary lost her first husband and her first throne while she was still only 18 years old.

~Shambaugh GE, Surgery of the Ear, 1974

BIBLIOGRAPHY

1. Block SL: Strategies for dealing with amoxicillin failure in acute otitis media. Arch Fam Med 8:68–78, 1999.
2. Bluestone CD: Clinical course, complications and sequelae of acute otitis media. Pediatr Infect Dis J 19(5 Suppl):S37–46, 2000.
3. Cook DG, Strachan DP: Health effects of passive smoking—10: Summary of effects of parental smoking on the respiratory health of children and implications for research. Thorax 54:357–366, 1999.
4. Daly KA, Giebink GS: Clinical epidemiology of otitis media. Pediatr Infect Dis J 19(5 Suppl):S31–36, 2000.
5. Dowell SF, Butler JC, Giebink GS, et al: Acute otitis media: Management and surveillance in an era of pneumococcal resistance—a report from the Drug-resistant *Streptococcus pneumoniae* Therapeutic Working Group [published erratum appears in Pediatr Infect Dis J 18:341, 1999] [see comments]. Pediatr Infect Dis J 18:1–9, 1999.
6. Hannley MT, Denneny JC 3rd, Holzer SS: Use of ototopical antibiotics in treating three common ear diseases. American Academy of Otolaryngology–Head and Neck Surgery Foundation. Otol Head Neck Surg 122:934–940, 2000.
7. Heikkinen T, Chonmaitree T: Increasing importance of viruses in acute otitis media. Ann Med 32:157–163, 2000.
8. Jung TT, Hanson JB: Classification of otitis media and surgical principles. Otol Clin North Am 32:369–383, 1999.
9. Klein JO: Review of consensus reports on management of acute otitis media. Pediatr Infect Dis J 18:1152–1155, 1999.

10. Maw AR, Bawden R: Spontaneous resolution of severe chronic glue ear in children and the effect of ade-noidectomy, tonsillectomy and insertion of ventilation tubes. Br Med J 306:756–760, 1993.
11. Pelton SI, Klein JO: The promise of immunoprophylaxis for prevention of acute otitis media. Pediatr Infect Dis J 18:926–935, 1999.
12. Pichichero ME: Acute otitis media: Part II. Treatment in an era of increasing antibiotic resistance. Am Fam Phys 61:2410–2416, 2000.
13. Ramilo O: Role of respiratory viruses in acute otitis media: Implications for management. Pediatr Infect Dis J 18:1125–1129, 1999.
14. Stool SE, Berg AO, Berman S, et al: Otitis Media with Effusion in Young Children. [Clinical Practice Guideline, no. 12.] Rockville, MD, Agency for Health Care Policy and Research, Public Health Service, U.S. Department of Health and Human Services, July 1994, p 41. [AHCPR Publication no. 94–0622.]
15. Teele DW: Acute otitis media: antimicrobial therapy in an era of resistant bacteria and suceptical meta-analysticians. N Z Med J 113:284–286, 2000.
16. Todd DH, Stool SE: Otitis media with effusion: A condensed review. Ambul Child Health 1:44–54, 1995.

11. DISEASES OF THE MIDDLE EAR

Douglas M. Sorensen, M.D. and Bruce W. Jafek, M.D.

1. How does eustachian tube dysfunction affect the middle ear?

The three classic functions of the eustachian tube are aeration, clearance, and protection of the middle ear. The hallmark of eustachian tube dysfunction is a **middle ear effusion.** However, the signs and symptoms vary from patient to patient. Patients may experience intermittent ear popping in the absence of middle ear effusion. Those with middle ear effusions may report otalgia, fullness in the ear, hearing loss, or vertigo. Patients may even be asymptomatic. Signs of middle ear effusion include limited mobility on pneumatic otoscopy and loss of normal landmarks.

2. What is a retraction pocket?

Aretraction pocket is an invagination of the tympanic membrane that usually occurs in the pars flaccida, or posterosuperior quadrant. It may appear to be a perforation to the untrained eye. This disorder results from negative middle-ear pressure that is often secondary to otitis media and its associated inflammation. As a retraction pocket deepens, desquamated keratin cannot be cleared from the recess and a cholesteatoma results. Specifically, this type of cholesteatoma is termed a **primary acquired cholesteatoma.**

3. What is a cholesteatoma? Where do they occur?

Acholesteatoma is an epithelial cyst that contains desquamated keratin. It is located medial to the normal position of the tympanic membrane. The suffix *-oma* may suggest that it is a tumor, but this is not the case. However, as more debris accumulates in the cyst, the cholesteatoma expands, which can erode bony structures.

4. Name the two basic types of cholesteatoma.

Congenital and acquired.

5. Describe a congenital cholesteatoma.

A congenital cholesteatoma is generally discovered in children. Potential sites include the middle ear, petrous apex, and cerebellopontine angle. Most congenital cholesteatomas are visible behind the tympanic membrane.

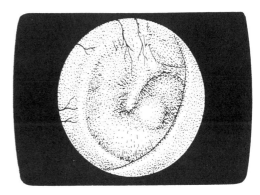

Congenital cholesteatoma pearl. (From Pender DJ: Practical Otology. Philadelphia, J.B. Lippincott Co., 1992, p 168, with permission.)

6. What are the two types of acquired cholesteatoma?

An acquired cholesteatoma generally occurs as a consequence of otitis media and eustachian tube dysfunction. The accumulation of keratin debris within the middle ear may be associated with a conductive hearing loss or chronic otorrhea. The hearing loss may be secondary to erosion of involved ossicles, with resulting discontinuity, a mass effect of the cholesteatoma, due to impingement on the ossicles.

A **primary acquired cholesteatoma** occurs as the consequence of a retraction pocket of the tympanic membrane and negative pressure within the middle ear. Once the retraction pocket invaginates so deeply that keratin fails to clear from the pocket, the debris accumulates.

A **secondary acquired cholesteatoma** occurs with the ingrowth of squamous epithelium from the margin of a perforation. Such a perforation is most commonly caused by an infectious process.

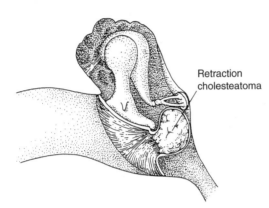

Retraction cholesteatoma

Retraction cholesteatoma. (From Pender DJ: Practical Otology. Philadelphia, J.B. Lippincott Co., 1992, p 156, with permission.)

7. How do patients with cholesteatomas present clinically?

Patients with a cholesteatoma generally present with repeated infections or progressive conductive hearing loss. Infection of the keratin debris is usually due to *Pseudomonas aeruginosa*. When infection is present, a mucopurulent, malodorous discharge can be detected. A primary acquired cholesteatoma usually presents as an invagination in the superior region of the tympanic membrane. Patients with congenital cholesteatomas present with a hearing loss and have an intact tympanic membrane (TM), or the condition may be an incidental finding on an imaging study.

8. What are the complications of cholesteatomas?

Cholesteatomas destroy bone. Therefore, any bony structure in or near the middle ear and mastoid cavity may be eroded and subsequently infected. In addition to hearing loss, complications include
- Semicircular canal erosion/fistula and dizziness
- Extradural or perisinus abscess
- Serous or suppurative labyrinthitis
- Facial nerve paralysis
- Meningitis
- Epidural, subdural, or parenchymal brain abscess
- Sigmoid sinus thrombosis/phlebitis

9. How are cholesteatomas managed?

Treatment is primarily surgical. Surgery is directed at eradication of the entrapped keratinizing epithelium and keratin from the middle ear and mastoid spaces. Medical management is indicated in preparation for a definitive surgical procedure. Infections should be controlled preoperatively with microscopic débridement of the ear canal and topical antibiotic solutions, such as tobramycin and ciprofloxacin. The primary goal of surgery is to create a disease-free, or "safe," ear. Reconstruction of the hearing mechanism is secondary.

10. What is a cholesterol granuloma of the middle ear?

The hallmark of a cholesterol granuloma is **idiopathic hemotympanum,** or a dark bluish discoloration of the tympanic membrane that is not associated with antecedent trauma. Cholesterol crystals cause a foreign-body reaction of the temporal bone. An initial hemorrhage in the middle ear is followed by drainage interference and leads to this foreign-body reaction. Bony erosion is rare in the setting of a cholesterol granuloma.

11. What is the role of imaging in the evaluation of middle ear disease?

The foundation of middle ear surgery has traditionally been a thorough knowledge of the anatomy and familiarity with landmarks, constant alertness to detect unsuspected complications and the experience to tailor the surgery to the pathologic lesion encountered. While not indispensable, computed tomography (CT) scanning may be a useful adjunct in the evaluation of certain types of middle ear disease (e.g., cholesteatoma) and in the evaluation of congenital middle ear pathology.

12. What is tympanosclerosis?

Clinically, tympanosclerosis is apparent as a whitish "plaque" of the TM. Pathologically, it is submucosal hyaline degeneration in the TM and middle ear mucosa. Extensive involvement of the TM and ossicles may result in conductive hearing loss. On rare occasions, middle ear surgery is advised to restore hearing. Medical therapy and pressure equalization tubes (PETs) do not prevent progression of disease. In fact, it is seen in as many as 40% of children with PETs tubes. When the tympanosclerosis affects both the TM and the middle ear, the majority of patients have an air-bone gap > 40 dB. When the whitish tympanosclerotic plaques involve the TM, this is termed **myringosclerosis..**

13. What is glomus tympanicum?

A glomus tympanicum is a tiny tumor that usually presents as pulsatile tinnitus. It is otoscopically visualized as a reddish-blue mass behind the tympanic membrane. It may be difficult to differentiate a glomus tympanicum from a larger **glomus jugulare** that has extended into the middle ear cavity. CT scans can be obtained to distinguish these two tumors. A glomus tympanicum is exclusively contained within the middle ear cavity. This tumor is usually small enough to be excised surgically without embolization. Glomus tumors also occur along the course of the vagus nerve **(glomus vagale).**

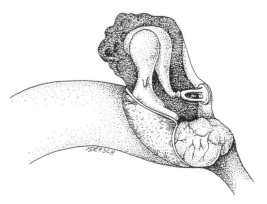

Glomus tympanicum. (From Pender DJ: Practical Otology. Philadelphia, J.B. Lippincott Co., 1992, p 160, with permission.)

14. What are the clinical features of otosclerosis?

Otosclerosis is due to the fixation of the stapes where it articulates with the oval window. Hearing loss is the major symptom, with the initial conductive hearing loss progressing over months to years. Fixation of the stapes may result in a maximum 50–60 dB air-bone gap. Vertigo may occur in up to 50% of patients with otosclerosis. Audiologic features include a conductive hearing loss that is frequently unilateral, normal speech discrimination, and absence of recruitment. Results of a physical examination are usually normal. **Schwartze's sign,** visualized through the TM, is hyperemia of the promontory mucosa that is due to increased vascularity. However, this physical sign is present in only a minority of patients and often disappears as the otosclerosis progresses.

15. How frequently does otosclerosis occur?

In autopsy studies, otosclerotic disease is found in temporal bones of 7.3% of white males and 10.3% of white females. Therefore, for every person with a hearing loss caused by otosclerosis, approximately nine people have asymptomatic histologic disease. In blacks, otosclerosis is found in only 1% of temporal bones. Overall, the female-to-male ratio of patients with symptomatic otosclerosis is about 2:1. The disease usually presents in patients aged 30–49 years. Patients usually delay seeking medical advice for an average of 2–3 years after symptomatic hearing loss begins.

The predominant audiometric finding in a patient with otosclerosis is a conductive hearing loss. Early in the disease process, these conductive losses typically involve the low frequencies, producing a "stiffness tilt" to the hearing loss. As the disease progresses, conductive losses in the higher frequencies become evident, resulting in a "mass tilt." Sensorineural losses may also develop with advanced disease, apparently due to involvement of the otic capsule. The bone conduction curve often demonstrates a distinctive notch of hearing loss at 2000 Hz. This notch is referred to as **Carhart's notch** and is believed to be associated with mechanical impedance changes in the middle ear transformer due to stiffness, friction, and the mass effect of an otosclerotic lesion.

16. What is cochlear reserve?

Otosclerosis falsely decreases sensorineural levels on audiometry. These deceptive levels often show that a patient has greater sensorineural losses than are truly present. We know that this is true because of the surprising audiogram results after otosclerosis surgery. Surgery on the stapes is intended to improve only the conductive defects, but sensorineural levels may also improve or return to normal. Cochlear reserve refers to the true sensorineural thresholds in a patient with otosclerosis prior to surgery. The true sensorineural levels prior to surgery can be estimated by adding 0 dB at 250 Hz, 5 dB at 500 Hz, 10 dB at 1000 Hz, 15 dB at 2000 Hz, and 10 dB at 4000 Hz to the obscured sensorineural levels.

17. If a parent has otosclerosis, what is the chance that his or her child will develop the disease?

The child of a parent with otosclerosis has a 20% chance of developing the disease. Some practitioners believe that otosclerosis is transmitted in an autosomal recessive pattern, whereas others believe that it is transmitted in an autosomal dominant pattern with variable penetrance. A positive family history can be obtained in over 50% of patients with otosclerosis. In women, pregnancy tends to exacerbate the development and progression of otosclerosis and hearing loss.

18. What are the signs and symptoms of ossicular dysfunction?

The hallmark of ossicular dysfunction is **hearing loss.** Physical findings may be normal, except in those cases in which TM perforation has occurred with ossicular damage. The Weber tuning fork test lateralizes to the side of the conductive hearing loss. In the case of ossicular discontinuity, a maximum conductive hearing loss of 55–65 dB may be present.

19. What are the possible etiologies of ossicular dysfunction?

There are many **congenital malformations** involving the ossicles: malleus ankylosis; congenital stapes fixation; malformation of the malleus, incus, and stapes; and incudostapedial joint disruption. Isolated congenital anomalies of the ossicles are rare. The majority of cases of congenital conductive hearing loss secondary to middle ear anomalies have other associated defects, such as atresia, microtia, and craniofacial deformities. **Ossicular fixation** physically restricts normal ossicular motion and is associated with otosclerosis, hyalinized connective tissue in tympanosclerosis, and scar tissue after surgery or infection. **Ossicular discontinuity** occurs when the incudostapedial joint is separated completely. In this condition, maximal conductive hearing loss occurs when the tympanic membrane is intact. In general, ossicular dissociation presents as a flat conductive loss. The incudostapedial joint is at risk of devascularization when trauma or infection occurs.

20. How can you reconstruct the ossicular chain?

The goal of functional ossicular reconstruction is to obtain permanent restoration of hearing. When the stapes is normal, a carefully fitted ossicular prosthesis can be implemented. The **incus** is the most readily available ossicle to use as an autogenous graft to restore the ossicular continuity. The incus (shaped or sculptured) can be placed between the handle of the malleus and the head of the stapes. **Cartilage** can also be used. A total or partial ossicular reconstruction prosthesis can be used if an autograft is neither available nor appropriate.

22. What is a partial ossicular reconstruction prosthesis (PORP)?

Prostheses are composed of porous Plastipore that is bioinert. If a stapes arch exists, the PORP is interposed between the capitulum of the stapes and the posterior tympanic membrane. To decrease the likelihood of extrusion, cartilage is used to cover the platform of the prosthesis.

23. What is a total ossicular reconstruction prosthesis (TORP)?

TORP is used when the stapes superstructure is missing. The TORP can be placed directly from the mobile footplate to the tympanic membrane. A cartilage interface may also prevent extrusion through the tympanic membrane.

24. How do you place a pressure equalization tube in an adult?

In contrast to children, adults rarely require general anesthesia for PET insertion. The adult patient is placed in the supine position under the clinic microscope. Prior to the myringotomy, local anesthesia can be achieved with either 1% lidocaine injections or topical phenol dotted onto the tympanic membrane at the site of incision. A four-quadrant injection with 1% lidocaine is performed at the external auditory meatus. After successful local anesthesia has been obtained, a myringotomy is placed in either the anteroinferior or the posteroinferior quadrant. If middle-ear fluid is present, gentle suctioning is performed. The ventilation tube is inserted, and the procedure is complete.

25. What are perilymph fistulas? How do they occur?

Spontaneous perilymph fistulas are very rare occurrences, and the majority are likely incited by a pressure-altering event (e.g., weightlifting). They result from ruptures of the round window membrane or, less commonly, a leak around the stapes footplate. Current methodologies do not provide sufficient specificity and sensitivity to accurately diagnose these. The results of endoscopic studies of the middle ear in the evaluation of perilymphatic fistula suggest a low incidence compared with the large number of fistulas reported in the literature. A high index of suspicion must be maintained, and appropriate preoperative counseling should reflect the current controversies. Questions must continue to be asked and further research pursued to help distinguish reality from myth.

26. Are implantable hearing aids feasible?

Implantable hearing aids represent a technically attractive and clinically promising challenge. Yet, the mechanical complexity of biotechnical interfaces in the middle ear and technical problems are immense and perhaps not even fully understood. Currently available devices still leave many biomechanical questions unanswered. The three mainly technical issues, in addition to size, are positioning the receiver, connecting the amplifier to the patient, and recharging the unit. Candidates should be carefully selected to avoid unsuccessful implantations, to prevent premature abandonment of this new technique.

CONTROVERSIES

27. Can sodium fluoride therapy help to treat otosclerosis?

Sodium fluoride (with calcium and vitamin D) is used as a controversial treatment for otosclerosis. Although otosclerosis tends to cause a conductive hearing loss, it may also cause a sensorineural hearing loss. Sodium fluoride appears to retard the development of this sensorineural component. Because most patients with otosclerosis do not have a significant sensorineural component, sodium fluoride is usually not indicated. Sensorineural hearing loss or vestibular symptoms are the primary indications for the use of sodium fluoride in otosclerosis.

28. What is the best technique for reconstruction of the middle ear ossicles?

Middle ear reconstructive techniques have increased to such an extent that the otolaryngologist is faced with a large number of surgical options. The literature, however, has yet to demonstrate any technique to be optimal in every surgical scenario. This is because of the lack of direct comparisons between techniques and dissimilar criteria for measuring success.

MAGNIFICATION IN EAR SURGERY

Holmgren was the first to introduce the magnifying loupe and binocular microscope for operations on the labyrinth for otosclerosis. Howard House and Jack Urban, engineers working primarily with Storz Instruments, made major advances in the development of a reliable operating microscope.

~Shambaugh GE, Surgery of the Ear, 1974

BIBLIOGRAPHY

1. Albino AP, Reed JA, Bogdany JK, et al: Increased numbers of mast cells in human middle ear cholesteatomas: Implications for treatment. Am J Otol 19:266–272, 1998.
2. Asiri S, Hasham A, al Anazy F, et al: Tympanosclerosis: Review of literature and incidence among patients with middle-ear infection. J Laryngol Otol 113:1076–1080, 1999.
3. Benton C, Bellet PS: Imaging of congenital anomalies of the temporal bone. Neuroimag Clin North Am 10:35–53, vii–viii, 2000.
4. Chole RA, Skarada DJ: Middle ear reconstructive techniques. Otol Clin North Am 32:489–503, 1999.
5. Coker NJ, Jenkins HA: Atlas of Otologic Surgery. Philadelphia, W. B. Saunders, 2001.
6. Friedland DR, Wackym PA: A critical appraisal of spontaneous perilymphatic fistulas of the inner ear [published erratum appears in Am J Otol 20(4):560, 1999]. Am J Otol 20:261–76; discussion 276–279, 1999.
7. Goycoolea MV: Mastoid and tympanomastoid procedures in otitis media: Classic mastoidectomy (simple, modified, and radical) and current adaptations; open-cavity, closed-cavity, and intact-bridge tympanomastoidectomy. Otol Clin North Am 32(3):513–523, 1999.
8. Huttenbrink KB: Current status and critical reflections on implantable hearing aids. Am J Otol 20:409–415, 1999.
9. Karmody CS, Byahatti SV, Blevins N, et al: The origin of congenital cholesteatoma. Am J Otol 19:292–297, 1998.

10. Mancini F, Taibah AK, Falcioni M: Complications and their management in tympanomastoid surgery. Otol Clin North Am 32:567–583, 1999.

11. Miyanaga S, Morimitsu T: Prussak's space: Chronological development and routes of aeration. Auris Nasus Larynx 24:255–264, 1997.

12. Mutlu C, da Costa SS, Paparella MM, et al: Clinical-histopathological correlations of pitfalls in middle ear surgery. Eur Arch Otol-Rhino-Laryngol 255:189–194, 1998.

13. Pisaneschi MJ, Langer B: Congenital cholesteatoma and cholesterol granuloma of the temporal bone: Role of magnetic resonance imaging. Top Mag Res Imag 11:87–97, 2000.

14. Roger G, Denoyelle F, Chauvin P, et al: Predictive risk factors of residual cholesteatoma in children: A study of 256 cases. Am J Otol 18:550–558, 1997.

15. Tange RA, Grolman W, Woutersen DP, et al: The prevalence of allergy in young children with an acquired cholesteatoma. Auris Nasus Larynx 27:113–116, 2000.

16. Watts S, Flood LM, Clifford K: A systematic approach to interpretation of computed tomography scans prior to surgery of middle ear cholesteatoma. J Laryngol Otol 114:248–253, 2000.

17. Zhao F, Wada H, Koike T, et al: The influence of middle ear disorders on otoacoustic emissions. Clin Otol Allied Sci 25:3–8, 2000.

12. EVALUATION OF THE DIZZY PATIENT

Carol A. Foster, M.D.

1. On the initial approach to the patient, what categories of dizziness should be considered in the differential diagnosis?

You will want to determine whether the dizziness is **vestibular** in origin or **nonvestibular.** Next you will want to define the illness as **emergent, acute,** or **chronic.** For vestibular illnesses, you will need to determine whether the problem is **peripheral** (limited to the ear or 8th nerve), or **central** (in the brainstem or brain). Once a peripheral disorder is diagnosed, you will attempt to determine whether one or both ears (**unilateral** or **bilateral**) are involved. Ideally, you will be able to determine which ear is affected in unilateral disorders.

2. Which lesions necessitate urgent treatment?

Central nervous system (CNS) hemorrhages and infarcts are the most serious causes of acute dizziness and require immediate intervention. Trauma to the inner ear or temporal bone, bacterial labyrinthitis, and acute perilymphatic fistulas also require urgent treatment. Your evaluation should rule out these processes immediately.

3. List the main peripheral vestibular disorders that cause dizziness.

The most common peripheral disorders causing dizziness are benign positional vertigo, viral neurolabyrinthitis, and, in children, acute otitis media. Trauma to the labyrinth can cause an acute syndrome of vertigo, and Meniere's disease is common in otologic practices. Ototoxic drug exposure is less common and usually occurs in hospitalized patients or those on long-term intravenous antibiotic treatment. Autoimmune disorders and vasculitis can damage the inner ear as well.

4. What are the main central vestibular disorders causing dizziness?

Migraines are the most common central disturbances associated with dizziness. Trauma can result in a postconcussive syndrome or direct brain injury. Other central processes include vertebrobasilar transient ischemic attacks (TIAs), cerebrovascular accidents, intracranial vasculitis or vascular lesions, and demyelinating CNS lesions such as multiple sclerosis. Neoplasms in the posterior fossa, such as acoustic neuroma, are an important cause of dizziness or hearing loss.

5. Your patient claims he is "dizzy." How should you explore this during your history taking?

Vertigo is the illusion that the body or environment is spinning or tumbling. Often, patients use the word *dizzy* to describe a general sensation of altered spatial orientation, such as unsteadiness, dysequilibrium, or lightheadedness. As you take a patient's history, it is important to distinguish lightheadedness or presyncopal dizziness from a sensation of motion. For example, upon standing quickly, an elderly patient is probably experiencing dizziness due to an orthostatic problem, not vestibular disease. Vertigo usually indicates a vestibular problem. Any sensation of motion, such as the sensation of tilting or falling, can also be vestibular in origin.

6. Which elements of the patient's history are useful in diagnosing lesions of the peripheral vestibular system?

A history of a chronic draining ear, acute ear pain, previous ear surgeries, hearing loss, or barotrauma suggests a peripheral lesion. Acute systemic infections can cause peripheral vertigo if the inner ear becomes involved. Patients with a history of collagen disease should be evaluated for autoimmune disease affecting the inner ear. Vertigo after head trauma is more likely to be peripheral than central in origin, since benign positional vertigo is often triggered by trauma.

7. Which elements of the history suggest a central vestibular disorder?

When a CNS lesion is suspected, you should inquire about headaches and any new visual, sensory, or motor losses. Diplopia or visual field cuts are often indicative of injury to the central visual system. Facial weakness or paresthesias, incoordination, or unilateral extremity weakness or paresthesias also usually indicate a central process.

8. What elements of the history are important to rule out nonvestibular disease?

You should obtain a detailed drug history. Neuroleptics, antihypertensives, and street drugs commonly cause dizziness. An irregular heartbeat, faintness, fatigue, or irregular thought processes in combination with the dizzy episodes suggest a systemic problem. Extreme hypertension may cause dizziness in association with a severe headache, whereas hypotension can cause presyncopal dizziness. Nonspecific dizziness can occur when a patient is experiencing hypoglycemia.

9. What elements of the history raise the possibility of dizziness related to a psychiatric disorder?

Look for a history of panic attacks or phobias, depression, and pending litigation or disability applications. Panic attacks can cause a floating, detached feeling. If you suspect that the patient's dizziness is associated with anxiety, you should not immediately rule out vestibular disease, since acute vertigo often causes extreme fearfulness. Depression and poor sleep patterns often coexist and can cause mild, chronic lightheadedness. Patients with sources of secondary gain, such as pending litigation, frequently magnify dizziness symptoms.

10. You know very little about the dizzy patient in your examination room, but you have time for only one more question in your history. What should you ask?

Of course, a diagnosis is never based on the reply from one question. However, knowing the *duration of symptoms* often helps the clinician broadly categorize the cause of vertigo. Therefore, it is important to ask, "How long do your dizzy spells last?"

Seconds: benign paroxysmal positional vertigo (BPPV)
Minutes: TIA
Hours: Meniere's disease
Days: viral neurolabyrinthitis
Variable: migraine

11. When evaluating a dizzy patient, what should your neurologic examination include?

A complete neurologic examination should always be performed and includes an evaluation of cranial nerves; examination of cerebellar function by testing of coordination, gait, and balance; observation for nystagmus, and a check of the ears and hearing. The neck should be evaluated for carotid artery bruits. Also, the clinician should always perform a Dix-Hallpike maneuver.

12. How do you properly examine a patient for nystagmus?

Nystagmus has slow and quick components. The slow component is generated by the vestibular system and causes the eye to deviate slowly. The fast phase represents a corrective response, which quickly returns the eyes to their original position. By convention, the direction of the nystagmus is named by its fast component. When testing a patient for gaze-evoked nystagmus, you should not bring the patient's eyes to the extremes of lateral gaze, as this frequently induces normal "end-point nystagmus." Instead, evaluate for spontaneous nystagmus with the eyes centered, then 20–30 degrees to the left and 20–30 degrees to the right. **First-degree nystagmus** is present if the nystagmus beats on lateral gaze in only one direction. **Second-degree nystagmus** is present if the nystagmus is present with the eye centered and increases on gaze laterally in the direction of the fast component. **Third-degree nystagmus** is present if there is a nystagmus beating in only one direction that is evident in all three positions of gaze. If nystagmus reverses direction with gaze to the right and left, it is a central, **gaze-evoked nystagmus.**

13. Name the five general categories of nystagmus.

Gaze-evoked nystagmus is present if the nystagmus occurs when the patient looks to the left and right and/or up and down.

Positional nystagmus occurs in certain head or body positions when the patient is supine.

Positioning nystagmus occurs when the patient is abruptly moved (the Dix-Hallpike maneuver).

Spontaneous nystagmus is present when the patient is upright with the eyes open.

Induced nystagmus is elicited by stimulation with caloric or rotational tests.

14. How is the Dix-Hallpike maneuver performed?

The Dix-Hallpike maneuver is a test for BPPV. The patient is seated lengthwise on the examination table and reassured that he or she will not fall during the dizzy spell. Emphasize to the patient that he or she should keep his or her eyes open throughout the maneuver, so that you can observe the eyes for nystagmus. Hold the patient's head turned 45 degrees to the right and then swiftly move the person into the supine position until the head overhangs the table edge. Continue to support the patient's head throughout the test. After at least 30 seconds, assist the patient in reassuming the sitting position. The test is then repeated on the left.

15. What constitutes an abnormal Dix-Hallpike maneuver?

Although this test has many implications, it is most valuable when used to diagnose BPPV. A rotatory nystagmus and sensation of vertigo that begins several seconds after assuming the head-

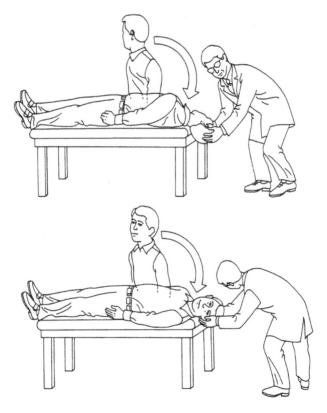

Dix-Hallpike maneuver. (From Cummings CW, et al (eds): Otolaryngology–Head and Neck Surgery, 3rd ed. St. Louis, Mosby, 1998, with permission.)

hanging position is characteristic of benign positional vertigo. The nystagmus fades after < 1 minute, reverses direction upon sitting, and "fatigues" with repeated testing. For example, if the patient has a left pathologic ear, he or she will manifest a mixed vertical and rotatory nystagmus when positioned with the left ear down, and the upper poles of the eyes will appear to you as if they are beating toward the floor. A different type of BPPV, horizontal canal BPPV, causes a violent, purely horizontal paroxysm of nystagmus on Dix-Hallpike that can last for as long as a minute and often causes vomiting.

16. Do other disorders cause nystagmus with the Dix-Hallpike maneuver?

Other disorders of central or peripheral vestibular pathways may cause positional nystagmus. This kind of nystagmus usually does not fade away while the head remains in the hanging position, nor does it fatigue on repeated testing. If nystagmus is vertical, lacking the torsional component that is found in BPPV, it indicates a central disorder.

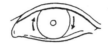
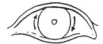

Clockwise rotatory nystagmus

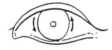

Counterclockwise rotatory nystagmus

Rotatory nystagmus. (From Lee KJ: The vestibular system and its disorders. In Lee KJ (ed): Essential Otolaryngology–Head and Neck Surgery. Norwalk, CT, Appleton & Lange, 1995, p 97, with permission.)

17. Describe the doll's eye test.

This test of the vestibular system uses quick head rotation to demonstrate high-grade vestibular lesions in awake or comatose patients. Awake patients should be asked to stare into your eyes during the test. Face the patient while holding the patient's head and then briskly turn the head to the right and to the left. Normally, the patient's gaze remains "locked" straight ahead on your eyes. The test is abnormal if the patient's gaze can be jerked away from yours by the quick head turn. In patients with lesions, a series of "catch-up" saccades may occur as the eyes attempt to regain focus on you. If the patient has an abnormal response with a right head turn, the patient has right vestibular injury. If the patient has an abnormal response with a left head turn, the patient has a left vestibular impairment.

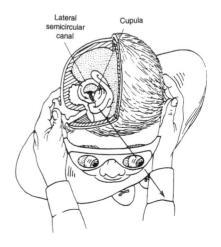

Doll's eye test. (From Pender DJ: Practical Otology. Philadelphia, J.B. Lippincott Co., 1992, p 108, with permission.)

18. On physical examination, what findings suggest a peripheral lesion?

An acute otitis media, an attic perforation with a cholesteatoma, or unilateral hearing loss should lead the clinician to suspect a peripheral lesion. Viral inner ear infections are frequently associated with a concurrent upper respiratory infection, but nystagmus, although present initially, may disappear before the patient is evaluated. A classically positive Dix-Hallpike examination diagnoses the most common peripheral disorder, BPPV.

19. What physical findings suggest a central lesion?

A central vestibular lesion causing dizziness without other neurologic findings is rare. Most central lesions exhibit some type of neurologic deficit, such as cranial nerve abnormalities, smooth pursuit difficulties, ataxia, a positive Romberg sign, dysrhythmia, extremity weakness, or sensory deficits. In contrast to peripheral lesions, central disorders can cause persistent and unusual nystagmus. Central nystagmus may be purely vertical, and eye movements can be dissociated. Patients with central disorders often have more findings than symptoms, whereas peripheral disorders usually cause more symptoms than findings.

20. You suspect your patient is malingering. What findings will increase your suspicion?

A malingerer will usually reveal a source of secondary gain in the history, such as pending disability claims or lawsuits. The examination of the ears, cranial nerves, and results of tests for dysrhythmia and dysdiadochokinesia are normal, but there is a positive Romberg sign and unusual gait instability. On Romberg testing, the malingerer may sway backward and lift the toes off the floor, or lean heavily on the examiner rather than attempting to correct the sway. During ambulation, the patient may cross the feet scissors-fashion, dip down at the knees, flail the arms, or drop to the floor in such a way as to avoid striking the head. This type of exaggerated pattern of imbalance is often called **phobic postural vertigo.**

21. Should other systems be checked in patients with dysequilibrium?

Vision and proprioception assist the vestibular system in maintaining balance. Macular degeneration, glaucoma, cataracts, and abnormalities of ocular tracking can worsen dizziness and imbalance. Peripheral neuropathy with diminished sensation of proprioception in the legs and feet also worsens balance.

22. What studies should be performed on the dizzy patient?

Initially, an audiogram and an electronystagmogram should be obtained. If either of these studies or the neurologic examination shows an asymmetric or localizing finding, further studies are indicated. At this point, you should perform magnetic resonance imaging (MRI) with gadolinium contrast to include the posterior fossa and internal auditory canals. If a congenital disorder of the temporal bone is suspected, an enhanced fine-cut computed tomographic (CT) scan without contrast would be the most useful study. If the patient has long (> 1 hour) spells of vertigo, laboratory studies may be beneficial, including a complete blood count, sedimentation rate, free treponemal antibody test, and human immunodeficiency virus (HIV) testing. Tests to rule out diabetes and lipid abnormalities may also be useful.

23. What is an electronystagmogram (ENG)?

This is a method of evaluating the visual tracking and vestibular systems. In the traditional ENG, electrodes on the patient's face record eye movements by measuring the changing electrical potential between the cornea and retina. Newer test methods may use infrared-sensitive video cameras to record eye movements in darkness. A battery of tests is performed, including tests of saccade function and visual tracking, gaze, positional and positioning tests for nystagmus, and caloric testing.

24. Describe the normal caloric response.

When the left ear is stimulated with water that is cooler than body temperature, a right-beating nystagmus (directed toward the opposite ear) results. When the left ear is stimulated with water that is warmer than body temperature, a left-beating nystagmus (directed toward the irrigated ear) occurs. Similar but oppositely directed responses occur for the right ear. You can remember the expected direction of nystagmus with the helpful mnemonic COWS:

Cold = **O**pposite

Warm = **S**ame

The symmetry of the paired responses is then calculated, giving two results, both expressed as a percentage: (1) canal paresis or unilateral weakness, describing the side and extent of a peripheral vestibular impairment; and (2) directional preponderance, suggesting an underlying tendency to nystagmus.

25. What is the major limitation of caloric testing?

Caloric tests reveal abnormalities by comparing the two ears to each other. If both ears have identical impairments, the test result may appear normal. Thus ENG is unable to detect bilateral but incomplete loss of vestibular function. This type of loss is better evaluated using rotational chair testing.

CONTROVERSIES

26. How significant is an isolated abnormal directional preponderance on ENG testing?

A directional preponderance of greater than 30% is considered abnormal and, in the absence of other ENG findings, is often interpreted as indicating a vestibular abnormality. True directional preponderance indicates an underlying nystagmus and is often accompanied by positional or spontaneous nystagmus or a canal paresis on caloric testing. When the remainder of the ENG findings are perfectly normal, the peak caloric responses for all four caloric tests should be examined. If one test shows an unusually vigorous response compared with the other three, it will often cause a spurious appearance of directional preponderance. In this case, the results of the ENG should be considered normal.

27. When is posturography indicated in the work-up of dizziness?

Posturography is a test of the vestibulospinal system in which standing sway is measured with a force plate. Although it has been advocated as a means of diagnosing vestibular disorders, it is not able to localize disease precisely to the central or peripheral vestibular system. It has proved most useful in following the recovery of balance in vestibular rehabilitation programs, in medicolegal evaluations, and in diagnosing multisensory imbalance.

———————

THE OTOSCOPE

Although earlier "aurists" (the name given to early specialists in diseases of the ear), such as Fabricus Hildanus (1560–1634) of Germany, developed ear "specula," which were hinged, similar to modern nasal specula, Joseph Toynbee (1815–1866) is regarded as the inventor of the modern otoscope.

~Politzer A, History of Otology, 1981

———————

BIBLIOGRAPHY

1. Baloh RW: Differentiating between peripheral and central causes of vertigo. Otolaryngol Head Neck Surg 119:55–59, 1998.
2. Baloh RW, Halmagyi GM (eds): Disorders of the Vestibular System. New York, Oxford University Press, 1996.
3. Baloh RW, Honrubia V: Clinical Neurophysiology of the Vestibular System. Philadelphia, F.A. Davis Co., 1990.
4. Bhansali SA, Honrubia V: Current status of electronystagmography testing. Otolaryngol Head Neck Surg 120:419–426, 1999.
5. Buttner U, Helmchen C, Brandt T: Diagnostic criteria for central versus peripheral positioning nystagmus and vertigo: a review. Acta Oto laryngol 119:1–5, 1999.
6. Dobie RA: Does computerized dynamic platform posturography help us care for our patients? Am J Otol 18:108–124, 1997.
7. El-Kashlan HK, Telian SA: Diagnosis and initiating treatment for peripheral system disorders: imbalance and dizziness with normal hearing. Otolaryngol Clin North Am 33:563–578, 2000.
8. Foster CA, Baloh RW: Episodic vertigo. In Rachel RE (ed): Conn's Current Therapy. Philadelphia, W.B. Saunders, pp 837–841, 1995.
9. Lempert T: Vertigo. Curr Opin Neurol 11:5–9, 1998.
10. McNaboe E, Kerr A: Why history is the key in the diagnosis of vertigo. Practitioner 244:648–653, 2000.
11. Singleton GT: Evaluation of the dizzy patient. In Bailey BJ (ed): Head and Neck Surgery—Otolaryngology. Philadelphia, J.B. Lippincott Co., 1998, pp 1870–1876.
12. Solomon D: Distinguishing and treating causes of central vertigo. Otolaryngol Clin North Am 33:579–601, 2000.
13. Waterston J: Neurology. 3: Dizziness. Med J Aust 172:506–511, 2000.

13. VESTIBULAR DISORDERS

Carol A. Foster, M.D.

1. What is the most common treatable cause of vertigo?

Benign paroxysmal positional vertigo (BPPV). Characteristically, sudden episodes of vertigo are precipitated by specific head movements, usually in bed at night. For example, the patient may complain of vertigo precipitated by rolling over in bed or by sitting up from reclining. These episodes are brief, lasting < 1 minute. Hearing loss or tinnitus is not typical. Although BPPV occurs most commonly in the elderly, it can occur in any age group. This condition is usually self-limited and resolves spontaneously over weeks to months in most cases. Treatment maneuvers can result in immediate resolution of symptoms.

2. Discuss the pathophysiology of benign paroxysmal positional vertigo.

In 1969, Schucknecht described the underlying pathophysiology of BPPV as **cupulolithiasis.** In his classic study of two diseased temporal bones, he found that otoconial material was lodged on the cupula of the posterior/inferior semicircular canal. To further support this theory, patients suffering from BPPV exhibited immediate relief on sectioning of the posterior ampullary nerve. Over time, other researchers have noted that cupular deposits should cause long-lasting nystagmus, rather than paroxysmal spells. A newer theory, **canalithiasis,** posits that debris such as displaced otoliths becomes lodged in the lumen of the posterior semicircular canal and acts as a piston to cause paroxysmal nystagmus. Recent intraoperative findings of chalky material in the posterior canal lumen of affected patients support this theory. Particles can also enter the lateral/horizontal canal, often as a consequence of previous treatment maneuvers.

3. How is benign paroxysmal positional vertigo treated?

This disorder usually disappears without treatment over a few weeks, but the course can often be shortened dramatically by using therapeutic head maneuvers designed to rotate the particles out of the affected canal. The **Epley maneuver,** also called the canalith repositioning procedure, has proved very useful, with a success rate near 90%. A different, log-rolling maneuver is necessary if the particles are in the horizontal canal. Vestibular rehabilitation programs in which patients repeatedly trigger attacks of vertigo have also proved effective. If the condition persists, surgical ablation of the ear or blockage of the affected canal will stop the spells.

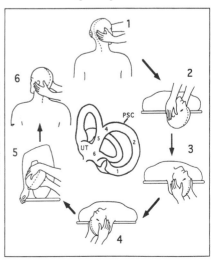

Treatment maneuver for BPPV affecting the right ear. The procedure is reversed to treat the left ear. The numbers in the posterior semicircular canal (PSC) represent the position of the particles in each head position as they are moved toward the utricle (UT). Each position change should be performed as rapidly as possible. Positions 2 and 3 are the same for the patient; the examiner moves from the side of the patient to the end of the table behind the patient's head to continue the maneuver. Repeat the sequence until no nystagmus can be elicited.

4. You suspect that a patient's vestibular symptoms are due to migraine. On what grounds do you base your diagnosis?

Migraine is the most common cause of chronic dizziness in young adults. Although this disorder often has a benign course between attacks, it also causes serious debility. The age of onset is between 5 and 30 years in 85% of cases, and > 50% of patients have a positive family history. Vertigo may occur as part of an aura, as part of the headache phase, or between the headaches. Headaches may be accompanied by an aura, often consisting of visual illusions such as a scintillating scotoma, or may occur without aura. Typically the headaches are moderate to severe, last for hours, and are associated with nausea, photophobia, or phonophobia. There is an association between migraine and certain other vertigo disorders, particularly Meniere's disease.

5. How is migraine-associated dizziness treated?

Migraine with vertigo can be treated with suppressants such as meclizine or promethazine if attacks are infrequent. However, prophylactic treatment is necessary if attacks are occurring more than once every few weeks. Tricyclic antidepressants such as amitryptylline are a good first-line choice; beta-blockers, calcium channel blockers, divalproate, and acetazolamide are also effective in some individuals. Medications should be tried for at least 1 month before another type is tried, since the effect often builds over several weeks. Newer migraine treatments aimed at the headache phase, such as sumatriptan, are generally not effective for migraine-associated vertigo spells.

6. What is the most common cause of dizziness and imbalance in the elderly?

Normal balance depends on a normal vestibular system, normal vision and visual tracking, and normal sensation and proprioception in the lower extremities. People with impairments in each of these areas have **multisensory imbalance.** Typically vision, visual tracking, and sensation in the feet become impaired with age. When coupled with any vestibular disorder, or with a gradual age-related decline in vestibular function, multisensory imbalance occurs. Patients usually feel dizzy only when ambulating, and their symptoms are relieved when using a grocery store cart. Symptoms are reduced by treatment of any correctable deficits in vision or sensation, provision of vestibular rehabilitation, and the use of a four-wheeled rolling walker with hand brakes.

7. What is Ménière's triad?

In its classic form, the triad of Ménière's disease includes (1) a fluctuating, low-tone, **sensorineural hearing loss;** (2) fluctuating **tinnitus;** and (3) **episodic vertigo.** A feeling of aural fullness is also common. The frequency of the attacks is variable, and long remissions from the symptoms can occur. Vertigo is usually the most distressing feature to patients; it can range in severity from episodic impaired balance to the intense illusion of spinning surroundings associated with vomiting. The onset of vertigo is usually sudden, reaching a maximum intensity within minutes and then persisting for 30 minutes to several hours. Also distressing is the character of the tinnitus, which is often described as roaring or buzzing. The symptoms typically subside completely after the episode, but some patients have dysequilibrium for days after the attack. As the disease progresses, the tinnitus may become constant and often is so irritating that this symptom becomes the chief complaint. Permanent hearing loss usually develops in the affected ear, and the vertigo often ceases when hearing loss is complete. About one-third of patients go on to develop bilateral disease, usually within the first few years after diagnosis.

8. Can Ménière's disease be treated medically?

Because it is impossible to predict when Ménière's disease will go into remission, several medical therapies are employed. Medical therapy is directed at slowing the progression of hearing loss and alleviating the uncomfortable symptoms. Traditional treatment has included dietary sodium restriction and the use of a diuretic. Steroids can be given orally or by injection into the middle ear.

Vertigo spells may be treated with vestibular suppressors such as promethazine, diazepam, or meclizine.

9. When is Ménière's disease treated surgically?

About 10% of patients with Ménière's disease become severely disabled because of recurrent vertigo, despite medical management. Although controlling vertigo is the primary goal of treatment, preserving hearing is the secondary goal. Most surgeries destroy vestibular function in the affected ear. When the patient has no residual hearing, a labyrinthectomy is extremely effective in abolishing the debilitating episodes. When the patient has useful hearing, common effective surgeries include vestibular nerve section and transtympanic aminoglycoside treatment to the inner ear. Procedures to decompress the hydropic endolymphatic sac have been used with variable results.

10. What is viral neurolabyrinthitis?

This unilateral vestibular disorder is usually preceded by a nonspecific viral illness. Within hours to days, the patient experiences the sudden onset of vertigo. This vertigo reaches a peak rapidly and then gradually declines over a few days to weeks. Cochlear symptoms are variable, ranging from normal hearing to a mild high-frequency hearing loss to sudden profound deafness in one ear. If there is no hearing loss, the disease is called **vestibular neuritis.** Total destruction of all auditory and vestibular function in one ear can occur after certain viral infections, such as measles, mumps, or herpes zoster. After the severe symptoms have subsided, the patient may experience mild light-headedness with sudden movement. These mild symptoms may persist for months. With time, however, the patient's vestibular system compensates, and the dizziness usually clears.

11. How are viral inner ear infections treated?

If hearing loss does not occur, most patients are managed symptomatically. Vestibular suppressant medication, such as meclizine, diazepam, or promethazine, are used to control vomiting. These medications should be discontinued after a week because they interfere with the normal process of compensation to vestibular injuries. Patients who are still symptomatic at that time are good candidates for vestibular rehabilitation. If hearing loss occurs, steroids are often given in an attempt to prevent deafness in the affected ear.

12. What neuro-otologic complications occur in patients with acquired immunodeficiency syndrome (AIDS)?

Opportunistic infections can give rise to a sudden unilateral vestibular impairment similar to viral neurolabyrinthitis. These infections may result in a progressive syndrome of repeated attacks, similar to Ménière's disease, and hearing loss can occur. Ototoxic drug exposure during treatment for other infections can cause bilateral vestibular loss.

13. What is oscillopsia?

Oscillopsia is the illusion that the environment is moving. Objects may appear to "jump" or "bob" spontaneously or with head movement. Two mechanisms can lead to this symptom. After vestibular injuries, there may be impairment of the vestibulo-ocular reflex, leading to the inability of patients to successfully stabilize an image on the retina during head motion. Vision blurs with rapid head movement, like that of a video camera. This head-movement-dependent oscillopsia is a classic symptom of aminoglycoside toxicity. When patients see the room spinning because of nystagmus, they are also describing oscillopsia. In this case, oscillopsia is due to abnormal spontaneous eye movement.

14. Discuss ototoxicity and its relationship to bilateral vestibular loss.

Loss of vestibular function in both ears is due most frequently to aminoglycoside ototoxicity, usually from gentamicin. Ototoxicity can occur if high blood levels of aminoglycosides occur, so monitoring serum levels is important during treatment. However, toxicity also increases with cumulative exposure to these drugs, even if blood levels are in the acceptable range. Patients should have a hearing test and be questioned regarding symptoms of dizziness or imbalance on a weekly basis if aminoglycosides are continued beyond 2 weeks. If hearing loss, dizziness, or oscillopsia occur, the aminoglycoside should be stopped immediately. There will often be further impairment of hearing or balance over the ensuing days or weeks. Vestibular rehabilitation is an effective treatment for imbalance due to ototoxicity.

15. How are permanent vestibular injuries treated?

A simple list of vestibular exercises, developed by Cawthorne in the 1940s, has been used successfully for years to assist patients recovering from vestibular injuries. However, physical therapy programs for vestibular rehabilitation are generally more effective in shortening the duration and severity of symptoms. These programs provide exercises aimed at improving balance and eye-head coordination. Exercises to habituate the patient to feelings of dizziness are also included. Balance and coordination are gradually retrained, beginning with very simple exercises that can be performed while sitting or supported, and progressing to more complex exercises while standing and walking as the patient improves. For uncomplicated vestibular injury in young adults, a course of 4–8 weeks is usually sufficient.

16. What are the symptoms of vertebrobasilar insufficiency?

Vertebrobasiliar insufficiency can cause transient vertigo that usually lasts for several minutes. The vertigo may be accompanied by other brainstem symptoms, such as headache, diplopia, loss of vision, perioral numbness, or dysarthria. These attacks are referred to as **transient ischemic attacks (TIA).** If the symptoms persist for more than an hour, a stroke is likely.

17. Describe the pathophysiology of transient ischemic attacks.

TIAs are due to a transient decrease in cerebral blood flow, frequently attributed to atherosclerosis. Vestibular symptoms are due to ischemia of the lateral part of the medulla where the vestibular nuclei are situated, or they are due to ischemia involving the labyrinthine artery that supplies blood to the ear. Cerebellar ischemia can also result in vertigo.

18. How can a posterior circulation stroke be differentiated from an acute peripheral vertigo problem?

Patients with acute strokes involving the cerebellum or brainstem are usually competely unable to walk, in contrast to persons with peripheral vertigo who are usually able to ambulate, even though they may drift or stagger. Patients with vertigo who are unable to ambulate should be hospitalized and examined for other signs of stroke, such as other cranial nerve lesions, dysrhythmia, dysdiadochokinesia, and altered sensation to pain or temperature on the face and extremities. It is common for stroke to be associated with total loss of hearing and balance function in the ipsilateral ear, so unilateral deafness does not reliably indicate that the problem is peripheral in origin.

19. What causes motion sickness?

Motion sickness, or kinetosis, is a condition characterized by nausea, vomiting, pallor, and sweating. Motion sickness is not a disease but rather a physiologic response to a mismatch between vestibular and visual information about the moving environment. For short exposures to motion, preventive medication includes diphenhydrinate or diphenhydramine. For exposures longer than 1 day, meclizine or transdermal scopolamine may be used.

20. What is persistent mal de debarquement?

After a boat trip, normal individuals will feel a rocking sensation for several hours after disembarkation, called mal de debarquement. When this symptom persists for weeks, months, or years after the exposure to motion, it is called persistent mal de debarquement. Usually results of the neuro-otologic examination and caloric tests are normal, and no new symptoms develop over time. The condition can resolve spontaneously. There is an association with migraine, and some patients respond to migraine prophylactic medications or to vestibular rehabilitation. A similar rocking vertigo can occur without prior exposure to boat travel; the course and treatment of this syndrome are similar.

21. What is Cogan's syndrome?

Cogan's syndrome is a systemic autoimmune disorder that preferentially affects the inner ear and eye. Vestibuloauditory symptoms are severe and bilateral and include fluctuating hearing loss, episodic vertigo, tinnitus, and aural fullness. Such symptoms closely precede or follow ocular inflammation. On vestibular evaluation, caloric responses are decreased or absent.

22. What is Behçet's disease?

Behçet's disease, also an autoimmune disorder, exhibits a clinical triad of oral and genital ulcers, iritis or uveitis, and progressive sensorineural hearing loss. Vertigo is often associated with this disease. An underlying vasculitis is thought to be responsible for these symptoms.

CONTROVERSIES

23. Do vascular loops cause vertigo?

Controversy surrounds the relationship of vascular loops in the cerebellopontine angle and vestibular symptoms. A vascular loop may be formed by the anterior inferior cerebellar artery or a branch that intrudes into the internal auditory canal. This causes compression of the 8th nerve. However, vascular loops in this area are commonly found in normal individuals. There is also considerable overlap between the reported symptoms of vascular loop and other inner ear diseases, such as Meniere's. If patients who suffer from brief attacks of positional vertigo and tinnitus are responsive to carbamazepine, they are likely candidates for the diagnosis of vascular compression.

24. What is cervical vertigo?

Also known as whiplash vertigo, this condition was previously a common diagnosis given to people with concomitant neck pain and vertigo. This diagnosis has largely gone out of fashion. Injury to the cervical joints and muscle receptors of the neck can cause a persistent floating sensation; however, the truly vertiginous accident victim is likely to have post-traumatic BPPV (the most common cause of post-traumatic vertigo), concussion, or direct trauma to the inner ear. Once a cervical fracture is ruled out, a Dix-Hallpike examination, audiogram, electronystagmogram, and magnetic resonance imaging should be considered in the setting of trauma.

―――⇒●⇐―――

MÉNIÈRE'S DISEASE

Prospere Ménière (1799–1862), in 1861, described a young girl who developed acute vertigo, vomiting, and deafness. This syndrome was named for him. Although later evaluation has shown that this patient definitely did *not* have Ménière's disease, or endolymphatic hydrops, as we currently understand the condition, Ménière's report did establish that vertigo, which had always been considered to be a symptom of an intracranial pathologic lesion, could be caused by an inner ear pathologic lesion. It seems most likely, given her acute death and "bloody exudate" in the inner ear, that this young girl had acute leukemia.

~Shambaugh GE, Surgery of the Ear, 1974

―――⇒●⇐―――

BIBLIOGRAPHY

1. Baloh RW: Differentiating between peripheral and central causes of vertigo. Otolaryngol Head Neck Surg 119:55–59, 1998.
2. Baloh RW: Vertigo [see comments]. Lancet. 352:1841–1846, 1998.
3. Baloh RW: The dizzy patient. Postgrad Med 105:161–164, 167–172, 1999.
4. Baloh RW, Halmagyi GM (eds): Disorders of the Vestibular System. New York, Oxford University Press, 1996.
5. Brandt T: Benign paroxysmal positioning vertigo. In Buttner U (ed): Vestibular Dysfunction and Its Therapy. Adv Otorhinolaryngol 55:169–194, 1999.
6. El-Kashlan HK, Telian SA: Diagnosis and initiating treatment for peripheral system disorders: Imbalance and dizziness with normal hearing. Otolaryngol Clin North Am 33:563–578, 2000.
7. Foster CA, Baloh RW: Episodic vertigo. In Rachel RE (ed): Conn's Current Therapy. Philadelphia, W.B. Saunders, pp 837–841, 1995.
8. Foster CA: Vestibular rehabilitation. Baillieres Clin Neurol 3(3):577–592, 1994.
9. Hornibrook J: Treatment for positional vertigo [see comments]. N Z Med J 111:331–332, 1998.
10. Johnson GD: Medical management of migraine-related dizziness and vertigo. Laryngoscope 108 (Supp 85):1–28, 1998.
11. Lempert T: Vertigo. Curr Opin Neurol 11:5–9, 1998.
12. Rosenberg ML, Gizzi M: Neuro-otologic history. Otolaryngol Clin North Am 33:471–482, 2000.
13. Staab JP: Diagnosis and treatment of psychologic symptoms and psychiatric disorders in patients with dizziness and imbalance. Otolaryngol Clin North Am 33:617–636, 2000.
14. Whitney SL, Rossi MM: Efficacy of vestibular rehabilitation. Otolaryngol Clin North Am 33:659–672, 2000.

14. TINNITUS

Bruce W. Jafek, M.D. and Mark A. Voss, M.D.

1. What is tinnitus?

Tinnitus comes from the latin word *tinnire,* which means "to ring." It is described as a sound sensation that originates in the head and is not attributable to any perceivable external sound. Tinnitus is a condition that impinges on the lives of sufferers to varying degrees. In some people, it is a fairly minor irritation, but for many, the tinnitus intrudes to such a degree that it affects their ability to lead a normal life, and in some very extreme cases has resulted in suicide. Insomnia, inability to concentrate, and depression are commonly reported to accompany the condition.

2. How common is tinnitus?

As many as one-third (32%) of Americans experience tinnitus sometime in their lives. These data are supported by similar studies performed in Europe. It is estimated that approximately 18 million Americans seek medical attention for their tinnitus. Nine million report being seriously affected by their condition, and 2 million are disabled because of the elusive sounds. Patients who suffer from this chronic symptom report a dwindling in their quality of life, primarily because of the annoyance factor associated with tinnitus. Activities of daily living are affected in proportion to the intensity of the tinnitus. Tinnitus is the 10th most common presenting complaint among the elderly in primary care.

3. What is the origin of subjective tinnitus?

One opinion regarding its site of origin is that it is primarily a central nervous system pathologic condition. One theory is that an initial auditory insult is translated into a central neurologic perception of tinnitus. Plastic changes arising from sensory deprivation are thought to trigger a change in synaptology and neurotransmission, with a consequent change in receptor configuration. From neuroanatomical considerations and analogies with other clinical conditions, it is postulated that serotonin (5-HT) is involved in these plastic changes, although the mechanism is unknown.

4. How do you quantify tinnitus?

Actually, we can't. In 1981, four tinnitus measures were recommended: pitch, loudness, maskability, and residual inhibition. Since then, psychoacoustic research into all four topics has proliferated, yielding many valuable insights and controversies concerning the details of measurement techniques. A consensus has emerged that neither the loudness nor other psychoacoustic measures of tinnitus bear a consistent relation to the severity or perceived loudness of tinnitus. Nevertheless, quantification is needed in clinical trials of proposed treatments and in a variety of other types of tinnitus research. Standardization of techniques for specifying the acoustic parameters of tinnitus thus continues to be an important research goal.

5. How do you classify a patient's tinnitus?

A historical classification schema for tinnitus that persists in contemporary literature revolves around objective versus subjective tinnitus. **Objective tinnitus** refers to those uncommon conditions that produce tinnitus that can be heard by an observer. **Subjective tinnitus** encompasses all other patients who experience a sound that defies detection. A more useful classification schema that is finding favor among otolaryngologists focuses on categorizing tinnitus by its etiology. These categories are vascular, external and middle ear, myogenic, peripheral sensorineural, and central sensorineural.

6. When evaluating a patient with tinnitus, what questions are asked to facilitate the patient's description of the ringing?

Most patients are able to localize the tinnitus to one ear. **Quality** (popping, clicking, pulsing, pure or multiple tones) gives insight into possible vascular or myogenic origins. It is important to document **progression** and **frequency** of symptoms as a gauge of disease, as these patients are typically followed for months or years. Daily or monthly **cycling** as well as **associated events** or symptoms can give important clues for determining etiologies.

7. List the key topics in obtaining an otologic history.

Accompanying audiovestibular disease
Trauma
Noise exposure
Family history
Ototoxic chemicals/medications
Systemic diseases
Infection (local, systemic)
Otologic surgery

8. What instruments would you place in your black bag before going to evaluate a patient with tinnitus?

A sharp eye and skillful hands are invaluable when performing a thorough head and neck examination, though you can't put these in your bag. A sphygmomanometer and stethoscope will help to detect a potential vascular cause. Pneumotoscopy is mandatory when observing the external and middle ear. Tuning forks (512 and 1024 Hz) are used in performing the Weber and Rinne tests. An ophthalmoscope will help to rule out a carotid-cavernous fistula. Tongue blades are a must for examining the palate and dental occlusion in suspected myogenic or temporomandibular joint-related causes. A flexible nasopharyngoscope would be helpful (but expensive) when looking for myogenic etiologies. Depending on the size of your black bag, an audiometer, tympanometer, computed tomographic (CT) scanner, and/or a magnetic resonance imaging (MRI) unit would be useful adjunctive equipment to evaluate suspected peripheral or central sensorineural tinnitus. A peek at the contents of your patient's medicine cabinet is often quite revealing.

9. What historical or physical findings would make you suspect a vascular cause for tinnitus?

A pulsatile or throbbing quality that parallels the heartbeat should raise your index of suspicion. A reddish or blue mass behind the tympanic membrane may indicate a glomus tumor arising within the middle ear cleft or a dehiscence of the jugular bulb or carotid artery. A hemotympanum may follow a history of head trauma. Arteriovenous malformations are uncommon but may occur between the occipital artery, arising from the external carotid artery and passing medial to the mastoid process, and the transverse sinus. A venous hum may represent one of the more common causes of vascular tinnitus. It may signify impingement of the jugular vein by the second cervical vertebra or suggest an underlying high output cardiac condition, such as anemia, exercise, pregnancy, or thyrotoxicosis.

10. In attempts to define the extent of a patient's tinnitus, how much sound pressure should mask the symptoms?

Approximately 80% of patients will have their tinnitus masked with 6 dB or less of sound pressure.

11. What is the best imaging study to evaluate tinnitus?

Tinnitus may be pulsatile or continuous (nonpulsatile). This distinction, with the detailed clinical evaluation, determines the most appropriate imaging study. For patients with **nonpulsatile tinnitus,** MR imaging is the study of choice to exclude a vestibular schwannoma or other neoplasm of the cerebellopontine angle cistern.

Pulsatile tinnitus suggests a vascular neoplasm, vascular anomaly, or vascular malformation (although the cause may be as simple as transient otitis media). Glomus tumors are the most common type of neoplasm. Vascular anomalies may also cause pulsatile tinnitus, but the mechanism is unknown, and another cause should be sought. Most neoplasms and anomalies are best seen on bone windows of the CT studies. Dural vascular malformations are often elusive on all cross-sectional imaging studies, and conventional angiography may be necessary to make this diagnosis. Flow-sensitive MR images show vascular loops compressing the eighth cranial nerve. Carotid dissections, aneurysms, atherosclerosis, and fibromuscular dysplasia can all be identified on both MR imaging or MR angiographic studies and CT or CT angiographic studies. Otosclerosis and Paget's disease may be seen on CT scan. Benign intracranial hypertension often has no abnormal imaging findings. Multiple sclerosis is a rare cause of pulsatile tinnitus and is best seen on MR studies. Many patients with tinnitus have no abnormal imaging findings.

12. Can foreign bodies in the external auditory canal cause tinnitus?

Yes. Cerumen, hair, or foreign bodies in contact with the tympanic membrane have been associated with tinnitus. The close proximity of the mandibular condyle with the external auditory canal should also be ruled out with a careful history and focused examination.

13. Palatal myoclonus is known to produce a tinnitus. What is the best way to detect this condition?

Using flexible nasopharyngoscopy in the awake clinical patient allows examination of the palate from a superior perch in the nasopharynx. Examining the palate from an oral cavity approach may lead to temporary extermination of the myoclonus while the mouth is stretched open. From a practical approach, both methods of examination should be employed.

14. What systemic diseases may be associated with myoclonus?

Multiple sclerosis, cerebrovascular accidents, intracranial neoplasms, and various psychogenic causes.

15. What is the association of tinnitus with hearing loss?

Eighty-five percent of tinnitus patients have audiometrically documented hearing loss in the 250–8000 Hz range. However, the presence of tinnitus does not absolutely imply hearing loss.

16. How is the ototoxicity caused by salicylates different from that due to aminoglycosides?

High serum concentrations of salicylates and some nonsteroidal anti-inflammatory drugs (NSAIDs) cause a flat, bilateral hearing loss and tinnitus. The hearing loss is a mild to moderate sensorineural hearing loss of about 20–40 dB. No otologic histopathologic condition has been consistently demonstrated. Both the hearing loss and the tinnitus are reversible within 24–72 hours of discontinuation of the offending medication. Aminoglycoside ototoxicity occurs in up to 15% of patients and can occur at therapeutic serum concentrations. Effects can include cochlear toxicity, yielding hearing loss and tinnitus, or vestibulotoxicity, yielding vertigo. Hearing loss is also heralded by tinnitus. Ototoxic effects that are still present 2–3 weeks after therapy termination are likely to be permanent.

17. Name some common medications that can cause tinnitus.

Angiotensin-converting enzyme (ACE) inhibitors: enalapril, fosinopril (Monopril)

Anesthetics: dyclonine, bupivacaine (Marcaine, Sensorcaine), lidocaine

Antibiotics: aztreonam, ciprofloxacin, erythromycin estolate, erythromycin ethylsuccinate/ sulfisoxazole (Pediazole), gentamicin (Garamycin), imipenem-cilastatin (Primaxin), sulfisoxazole, trimethoprim-sulfamethoxazole, vancomycin

Antidepressants: alprazolam (Xanax), amitriptyline (Elavil), desipramine, doxepin, fluoxetine (Prozac), imipramine, maprotiline (Ludiomil), nortriptyline (Pamelor)

Antihistamines: aspirin-promethazine-pseudoephedrine (Phenergan), chlorpheniramine-

phenylpropanolamine (Triaminic), clemastine (Tavist), pseudoephedrine-chlorpheni-
ramine (Deconamine), pseudoephedrine-triprolidine (Actifed)

Antimalarials: chloroquine, pyrimethamine-sulfadoxine (Fansidar)

Beta-blockers: betaxolol (Kerlone), carteolol (Cartrol), metoprolol (Lopressor), nadolol
(Corgard), timolol (Timoptic)

Calcium channel blockers: diltiazem (Cardizem), nicardipine (Cardene), nifedipine (Procardia)

Diuretics: acetazolamide (Diamox), amiloride, ethacrynic acid

Narcotics: dezocine (Dalgan), pentazocine (Talwin)

NSAIDs: diclofenac (Voltaren), diflunisal (Dolobid), flurbiprofen (Ansaid), ibuprofen, in-
domethacin, meclofenamate (Meclomen), naproxen (Naprosyn), sulindac (Clinoril), tol-
metin (Tolectin)

Sedatives/hypnotics/anxiolytics: azatadine (Optimine), buspirone (BuSpar), chlorpheni-
ramine-phenylpropanolaomine (Ornade)

Miscellaneous: albuterol (Proventil), allopurinol, bismuth subsalicylate (Pepto-Bismol), carbamazepine (Tegretol), cyclobenzaprine (Flexeril), cyclosporine, diphenhydramine (Be-
nadryl), flecainide, hydroxychloroquine (Plaquenil), iohexol (Omnipaque), isotretinoin
(Accutane), lithium, methylergonovine (Methergine), nicotine polacrilex (Nicorette),
prazosin, omeprazole (Prilosec), quinidine, recombinant hepatitis B vaccine (Recom-
bivax), salicylates, sodium nitroprusside (Nipride), sulfasalazine (Azulfidine), tocainide

18. Will acupuncture cure tinnitus?

Two unblinded studies showed a positive result, whereas four blinded studies showed no significant effect of acupuncture. Thus, acupuncture has not been demonstrated to be efficacious as
a treatment for tinnitus on the basis of rigorous randomized controlled trials.

19. What percentage of patients with acoustic neuromas have tinnitus as the presenting symptom?

Ten percent of these patients present with tinnitus. In patients with an acoustic neuroma, over
80% will have tinnitus during the course of their disease.

20. How is tinnitus treated?

Sixty-nine research clinical trials (RCTs) evaluated tocainide and related drugs, carbamazepine, benzodiazepines, tricyclic antidepressants, 16 miscellaneous drugs, psychotherapy,
electrical/magnetic stimulation, acupuncture, masking, biofeedback, hypnosis, and miscellaneous
other nondrug treatments. Despite the many drugs now available, none has been approved by the
United States Food and Drug Administration for the treatment of tinnitus. Many surgical therapies have been advocated but are directed toward the treatment of concurrent vertigo or for tumors of the cerebellopontine angle, with tinnitus sometimes being relieved by the operation. Specific surgical procedures such as cochlear resection and microvascular decompressions lack
clear-cut efficacy. Despite author bias and a myriad of treatment modalities at present, there is
still no specific therapy that definitively relieves tinnitus clinically.

Nonspecific support (see also Question 23) and counseling are probably helpful, as are tricyclic antidepressants in severe cases. Benzodiazepines, newer antidepressants, and electrical
stimulation deserve further study. Examples of nonpharmacologic management include hearing
aids for those with hearing loss, hypnotherapy, counseling, and masking. Future tinnitus therapeutic research should emphasize adequate sample size, open trials before RCTs, careful choice
of outcome measures, and long-term follow-up. Clinical research remains hampered by the absence of a reliable objective assessment of the tinnitus and by the variable nature of the complaint.

21. How do anesthetics such as lidocaine act to decrease tinnitus?

Lidocaine and several related anesthetics act as central nervous system depressants by inhibiting the influx of sodium and therefore reducing the number of action potentials. One theory
to explain tinnitus pertains to the high baseline spontaneous firing rate of the normal auditory sys-

tem and the loss of its natural inhibitors. Anesthetics are thought to augment or replace this natural inhibition process, holding tinnitus in check. At present, intravenous lidocaine is the only medication that can reliably stop tinnitus in many patients. However, it is impractical because of the short duration of action and its method of administration.

22. What role does surgery play in tinnitus?
Only a few of the many causes of tinnitus lend themselves to surgical intervention: persistent middle ear effusion, foreign body of the external auditory canal, otosclerosis, Ménière's disease, and tumors of the cerebellopontine angle.

CONTROVERSIES

23. List some alternative nonsurgical treatments for tinnitus.
Several controversial treatments exist for the control of tinnitus. Hypnotherapy has been shown to improve coping skills in approximately one-third of patients. Control of inhalants and food allergies has alleviated tinnitus in approximately 30% of patients with these conditions. Biofeedback has a high success rate (70–90%) for improving patients' ability to cope with their disease. Acupuncture has not been shown to be beneficial. Tinnitus correlates with levels of stress, and therefore support groups and stress-reduction tactics play important therapeutic roles. The American Tinnitus Association produces a quarterly newsletter. Their address is P.O. Box 5, Portland, OR 97207; tel. 800-634-8978.

24. Does tinnitus occur in children?
Tinnitus in childhood is appears quite common when children are directly asked about the symptom. However, children rarely spontaneously complain of tinnitus. Little is known about effective management strategies for pediatric tinnitus.

25. What laboratory tests should you consider in the evaluation of the patient with tinnitus?
One or more of the following tests may be indicated if the history of tinnitus or a review of systems suggests a possible cause. Except in highly suspicious cases, their limited cost-effectiveness makes their use controversial.
Complete blood count
Fluorescent treponemal antibody absorption test
Screening for ototoxic drugs and environmental pollutants (including heavy metals and carbon monoxide)
Thyroid stimulating hormone
Blood glucose
Cholesterol, lipid profile
Autoimmune screening (rheumatoid factor, antinuclear antibody, total complement)

TINNITUS

Instillation of a variety of potions into the external auditory canal has been recommended for the treatment of tinnitus. The many folklore remedies included ant eggs, bull urine (how this was to be collected is not indicated), crab juice, moles' blood, and snail "juice." Wines, salt, and mercury were also recommended.

~*Politzer A, History of Otology, 1981*

BIBLIOGRAPHY

1. Baguley DM, McFerran DJ: Tinnitus in childhood. Int J Pediatr Otorhinolaryngol 49:99–105, 1999.
2. Billue JS: Subjective idiopathic tinnitus. Clin Excel Nurse Pract 2:73–82, 1998.
3. Dobie RA: A review of randomized clinical trials in tinnitus. Laryngoscope 109:1202–1211, 1999.
4. Ernst E, Stevinson C: Ginkgo biloba for tinnitus: a review: Clin Otolaryngol & Allied Sci 24:164–167, 1999.
5. Hart CW: Medicolegal aspects of tinnitus. Int Tinnitus J 5:63–66, 1999.
6. Henry JA, Meikle MB: Psychoacoustic measures of tinnitus. J Am Acad Audiol 11:138–155, 2000.
7. Park J, White AR, Ernst E: Efficacy of acupuncture as a treatment for tinnitus: A systematic review. Arch Otolaryngol Head Neck Surg 126:489–492, 2000.
8. Parnes SM: Current concepts in the clinical management of patients with tinnitus. Eur Arch Otorhinolaryngol 254:406–409, 1997.
9. Peifer KJ, Rosen GP, Rubin AM: Tinnitus: Etiology and management. Clin Geriatr Med 15:193–204, viii, 1999.
10. Simpson JJ, Davies WE: A review of evidence in support of a role for 5-HT in the perception of tinnitus. Hear Res 145:1–7, 2000.
11. Teixido MT, Connolly K: Explosive tinnitus: An underrecognized disorder. Otolaryngol Head Neck Surg 118:108–109, 1998.
12. Tyler RS: Perspectives on tinnitus. Br J Audiol 31:381–386, 1997.
13. Weissman JL, Hirsch BE: Imaging of tinnitus: A review. Radiol 216:342–349, 2000.

15. EAR INJURIES AFTER FLYING AND DIVING

Mark R. Mount, M.D.

1. What is Boyle's law and why is it important in otolaryngology?

Most otolaryngologic problems that are caused by scuba diving or air travel can be understood by applying Boyle's law. The air-occupied spaces in the middle ear and sinuses are susceptible to changes in pressure. Unlike air, water is incompressible. Boyle's law states that at a constant temperature, the volume of a gas is inversely proportional to pressure. In other words, volume decreases as pressure increases. So while increases in pressure do not affect blood, bone, or cellular fluid, they do affect air-containing spaces. These spaces must add or remove air during pressure changes to maintain equilibrium.

2. Discuss the other air pressure principle that is important in understanding ear problems.

Henry's law states that "at a given temperature, the mass of a gas dissolved in a given volume of solvent is proportional to the pressure of the gas with which it is in equilibrium." This application becomes important when considering the increased amount of nitrogen that dissolves in the body fluids and tissues during descent and is released during ascent. Too much nitrogen released from blood will form bubbles in the bloodstream and cause decompression sickness, otherwise known as "the bends." These bubbles may ultimately reach the inner ear microvasculature, producing deafness, vertigo, or both.

3. Is the eustachian tube normally open or closed? Why is this important in diving?

Normally, the eustachian tube is closed, opening only when there is positive pressure in the nasopharynx or by muscular action of the tensor veli palatini, levator palatini, or salpingopharyngeus. It has been shown, however, that as a diver descends, the eustachian tube acts as a flutter valve, which remains closed under pressure unless it is reflexively or voluntarily opened by the diver. If the tube fails to open, this may result in middle ear barotrauma, or a "squeeze effect."

4. Which nerves supply sensation to the ear?

Innervation of the external canal is through three cranial nerves: the auriculotemporal (V3), the facial nerve (VII) through the tympanic plexus, and Arnold's nerve (auricular branch of X). The auriculotemporal nerve (V3) innervates the tympanic membrane. The middle ear is supplied by Jacobson's nerve (IX), the auriculotemporal nerve (V3), and Arnold's nerve (X).

5. Why does ear pain occur during changes in ambient pressure, such as during diving or flying?

Air spaces in the head, such as the middle ear and paranasal sinuses, must maintain pressure equilibrium with ambient air. According to Boyle's law, as pressure increases, gas volume decreases. The pressure increases linearly, and so every 10 m of descent in water causes a pressure increase of 14.7 psi, or 100 kpa, or 1 atm. Air pressure at 18,000 ft is one-half of that at sea level. Pressure changes much more slowly in the air compared with underwater. However, a pressurized aircraft that suddenly loses pressurization may have an extremely rapid pressure change and cause problems similar to those associated with ascending too quickly from a dive. Sea-level pressure is doubled at 33 ft (10 m) below the surface. Therefore, as the middle ear descends in air or water, the existing air shrinks. This shrinkage creates a negative pressure inside the cavity, causing pain. During ascent, the gas in the cavity expands and must ventilate, or it will cause pressure on the middle ear mucosa and tympanic membrane.

6. Other than middle ear barotrauma, what can cause ear pain during flying or diving?

External ear barotrauma or "canal squeeze" often occurs in divers with impacted cerumen. The air deep to the occlusion remains the same as the surface pressure, while the surrounding pressure and middle ear pressure increase as the diver descends. A relative vacuum develops, resulting in the development of ear pain and congestion of the canal skin and tympanic membrane.

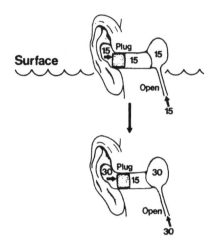

Canal squeeze, resulting from an ear plug in the external auditory canal. During descent, the pressure in the canal remains at seal-level pressure, whereas the middle ear and external to the ear are at ambient pressure. The resultant negative pressure in the canal pulls the plug inward and bulges the eardrum outward. A tympanic membrane perforation can occur if there is a great enough pressure differential. (From Reuter SH: Underwater medicine: Otolaryngologic considerations of the skin and scuba diver. In Paparella MM, Shumrick DA, Gluckman JL, Meyerhoff WL (eds): Otolaryngology, 3rd ed. Philadelphia, W.B. Saunders, 1991, pp 3231–3257, with permission.)

7. What is meant by "reversed squeeze"?

On ascent, if the eustachian tube remains blocked, the pressure within the middle ear will increase as its volume of air expands. This results in severe ear pain, sometimes associated with dizziness. This reversed squeeze can be severe enough to result in rupture of the tympanic membrane, middle ear hemorrhage, and even permanent hearing loss.

8. At what depth do most divers terminate a dive because of pain?

More than 75% of divers terminate their dive within 33 ft of the surface. During the first 33 ft, the pressure doubles, demonstrating the greatest change in both density and pressure that the diver experiences.

9. Is it more common to have ear pain during ascent or during descent while flying?

During ascent, the relative pressure in the middle ear increases, causing the tympanic membrane to bulge out. Air escapes passively through the eustachian tube if the pressure differential is 15 mm Hg or more. During descent, the relative pressure in the middle ear decreases, causing the tympanic membrane to bulge inward. Passive venting through the eustachian tube is more difficult, and passengers usually must take active measures to equalize pressure, such as the Valsalva maneuver. More people develop pain in the plane's descent than in the ascent.

10. Is it okay to fly with myringotomy tubes in place?

Yes. The presence of myringotomy tubes or a tympanic membrane perforation creates an artificial pressure-equalization system that bypasses the eustachian tube. Therefore, no pressure buildup should occur. Anxious parents often need reassurance that tubes are ideal for flying. It is important, however, to ensure that the tubes are patent.

11. At what pressure differential does the tympanic membrane rupture during flying?

At an approximately 60 mm Hg pressure differential, passengers begin to feel fullness within the middle ear. As the pressure differential increases to 90 mm Hg, the eustachian tube becomes locked. Any attempts to equalize become futile. Finally, as the pressure differential increases between 100 and 500 mm Hg, the tympanic membrane ruptures.

12. In a diver who develops ear pain, what is the significance of vertigo?

Divers are highly subject to disorientation due to several factors. Spatial orientation in humans depends on three sensory signals: visual signs, limb proprioception, and the vestibular apparatus. Underwater, darkness may inhibit visual signals, and near-loss of gravity prevents proprioception. Orientation thus relies on the vestibular system, but this is at risk to fail. As water enters the external canals at different times, because of cerumen or tight hoods, the simple caloric stimulation can cause temporary physiologic vertigo. This disorder is worse if a unilateral eardrum perforation is present. Rapid pressure changes or failing to use the Valsalva maneuver during descent may cause a perilymphatic fistula, causing progressive vertigo. Some divers experience **alternobaric vertigo,** which is unequal pressures in the middle ears during ascent. The unequal pressure causes asymmetric stimulation of the vestibular apparatus.

In short, the differential diagnosis of vertigo in a diver includes simple disorientation, perilymphatic fistula, unequal plugging of the ears, perforated tympanic membrane, and alternobaric vertigo. Divers should know how to prevent vertigo and recognize its significance. Spatial disorientation underwater can be fatal. Divers know to observe their air bubbles whenever they become disoriented—air always goes up.

13. What is a perilymphatic fistula?

Rapid changes in relative pressure of the middle ear space produce implosive or explosive forces on the various membranes, i.e., the tympanic membrane, oval window, and round window. Any of these structures may rupture, causing vertigo and/or hearing loss. Rupture of the round or oval windows produces a fistula, allowing perilymph to leak into the middle ear space. The rupture damages the cochlea or vestibular apparatus, causing hearing loss or vertigo.

14. When a diver descends, what is the pathophysiology involved in explosive and implosive mechanisms causing oval and round window ruptures?

Explosive mechanism: On descent, inadequate ear clearing occurs, which causes a negative pressure, relative to the intralabyrinthine fluid pressure, to develop. As a result, the diver performs a Valsalva maneuver in an attempt to equalize the pressure. An increase in cerebrospinal fluid pressure is then transmitted to the inner ear through the cochlear duct, further increasing the pressure differential across the inner ear membranes. The differential pressure results in outward bulging of the round window and rupture.

Implosive mechanism: During descent, a relative negative pressure develops in the middle ear space, which causes the tympanic membrane to bulge inward. If a sudden forceful Valsalva maneuver is attempted, the eardrum suddenly approaches a neutral position, and the outward force is transmitted to the stapes. As a result, a relative negative pressure develops in the inner ear fluid, causing the round window to bulge inward and rupture.

15. What is a fistula test?

A fistula test involves applying positive pressure, via the pneumatic otoscope, to the middle ear. In the presence of a perilymphatic fistula, positive pressure will cause nystagmus. Unfortunately, the fistula test is neither very sensitive nor specific.

16. What is the significance of hemotympanum after flying or diving?

Hemotympanum presents as a purplish hue to the tympanic membrane and results from ruptured blood vessels in the middle ear space by barotrauma. Also known as **barotitis media,** this condition is usually self-limiting and clears itself. Treatment includes use of an oral and topical decongestant for a few days, and divers should abstain until the condition clears. Middle ear barotrauma is the most common disorder in divers. It is also common among skydivers.

17. How should the clinician manage an acute perforated eardrum secondary to barotrauma?

A simple perforation needs no treatment. Most holes spontaneously heal within 8 weeks. The patient should be careful to keep soapy and dirty water out of the ear. The patient should not dive.

If pus or drainage develops, antibiotic eardrops are indicated. If the perforation does not heal within 3 months, a paper patch can be applied in the office. The patch serves as a bridge under which epithelial cells migrate to repair the defect. If a paper patch fails, the patient should undergo formal tympanoplasty in the operating room. An audiogram should be performed. If there is a significant conductive hearing loss, there could also be ossicular dislocation.

18. Describe inner ear decompression sickness. What is the treatment of choice?

Inner ear decompression sickness involves the development of nitrogen bubbles in the microvasculature of the labyrinth and cochlea. These bubbles block the venous circulation in the stria vascularis, spiral ligament, and semicircular canals. The syndrome includes hemorrhage and the formation of protein exudates, as well as irritation of the endosteum of the bony semicircular canals. Symptoms include severe vertigo and/or sensorineural hearing loss, in addition to the joint pain typically seen in "the bends." The treatment of choice is hyperbaric oxygen.

19. Which types of hearing frequency losses have been associated with inner ear barotrauma?

The most common hearing losses are either high frequency or total frequency types. The high-frequency losses are usually in the 4000–8000 Hz range.

20. Is short-term use of decongestants contraindicated in diving?

No. Short-term use of decongestants is not contraindicated. Experienced divers report that they are better able to equalize if the medications are used immediately before diving. However, rebound from topical decongestants can occur, or topical decongestants may cause tachycardia or hypertension. If these drugs are to be used, they should be tested first on nondiving days. In addition, these drugs should not be used for patients with an upper respiratory infection. In these patients, there is a risk of severe ear squeeze.

CONTROVERSIES

21. Should children fly when they have a cold?

Flying requires adequate eustachian tube function for equilibration of middle ear pressure. Infants and young children have a poorly functioning tensor veli palatini as well as an already compromised eustachian tube during an upper respiratory infection. Therefore, some physicians recommend that they not fly if they have a cold. However, there is evidence that children with otitis media may fly safely, and, in fact, ears without effusion may be more at risk than ears with effusion. All children who fly should be encouraged to swallow repeatedly or chew gum (infants can be given a bottle) to maintain adequate operation of the eustachian tube to prevent severe pain and barotrauma.

22. What can be done for patients who have difficulty with otalgia while flying?

Many practitioners use sympathomimetics such as topical or oral pseudoephedrine before flying. Other techniques include having patients practice the Valsalva maneuver and use it during descent only. The Valsalva maneuver is a learned technique. There is some support for using oral decongestants in adults while flying. However, topical decongestants have been shown not to be effective. In addition, oral decongestants, topical decongestants, oral antihistamines, and combination drugs have all been shown not to be effective in children. Occasionally, myringotomy may be done just prior to flying.

25. How is a perilymphatic fistula diagnosed and treated?

Early surgical exploration: No noninvasive tests have proven effective in accurately diagnosing a perilymphatic fistula. By exploring acutely dizzy patients early, the clinician can both make the diagnosis and treat adequately in a timely fashion. Delay may result in permanent labyrinthine dysfunction and deafness. Surgery should not be delayed, especially in the patient with sudden hearing loss.

Noninvasive testing and observation: The diagnosis of perilymphatic fistula is difficult, even during surgery in some cases. The incidence of fistula due to indirect trauma is extremely low. Conservative therapy usually involves bedrest for 1–2 weeks with the head elevated. Many existing fistulas will heal spontaneously. Patients whose symptoms worsen should have surgery. A conservative approach will save many patients from surgery and the risk of complications.

———————

EUSTACHIAN TUBE DYSFUNCTION

During WWII, Allied pilots were often forced to fly with otitis media. To avoid barotitis, their eardrums were "lanced" before takeoff. It was reported that Japanese Zero pilots received similar treatment.

———————

BIBLIOGRAPHY

1. Benton PJ: Resumption of diving after illness or injury. J R Nav Med Serv 84:14–18, 1998.
2. Bettes TN, McKenas DK: Medical advice for commercial air travelers. Am Fam Phys 60:801–808, 1999.
3. Buchanan BJ, Hoagland J, Fischer PR: Pseudoephedrine and air travel-associated ear pain in children. Arch Pediatr Adolesc Med 153:466–468, 1999.
4. Desforges J: Medical problems associated with underwater diving. N Engl J Med 326:30–35, 1992.
5. Lacey JP, Amedee RG: The otologic manifestations of barotrauma. J LA State Med Soc 152:107–111, 2000.
6. Newbegin C, Ell S. Ear barotrauma after flying and diving. Practitioner 244:96–99, 101–102, 105, 2000.
7. Rubin BD: The basics of competitive diving and its injuries. Clin Sports Med 18:293–303, 1999.
8. Russi EW: Diving and the risk of barotrauma. Thorax 53 (Suppl 2):S20–4, 1998.
9. Spira A: Diving and marine medicine review part I: Diving physics and physiology. J Trav Med 6:180–198, 1999.
10. Spira A: Diving and marine medicine review part II: Diving diseases. J Trav Med 6:180–198, 1999.
11. Wall C III, Rauch SD: Perilymph fistula: Pathophysiology. Otolaryngol Head Neck Surg 112:145–153, 1995.
12. Woods DP: "Am I fit to fly?" Practitioner 242:384–387, 1998.

16 NEURO-OTOLOGY

Herman A. Jenkins, M.D., and Anne K. Stark, M.D.

1. Tumors of the ear may masquerade as what common otologic problem?

A neoplasm of the ear often presents with classic signs and symptoms of a **chronic ear infection**. The clinician should always consider neoplastic disease when evaluating patients with these signs and symptoms.

2. Name the three most common neoplasms of the auricle.

Basal cell carcinomas
Squamous cell carcinomas
Melanomas
Six percent of all skin cancers are auricular. Sebaceous cysts are a common benign neoplasm of the auricle.

3. Name the four most common true neoplasms of the temporal bone and external ear canal.

Fibrous dysplasia
Langerhans' cell histiocytosis
Leukemia
Sarcomas
These neoplasms are uncommon and account for $< 0.05\%$ of head and neck malignancies. Etiologic factors include a history of head and neck radiation or chronic ear inflammation. Osteomas/exostoses are very common benign lesions that generally need no treatment. Aural polyps are not uncommonly associated with perforations or cholesteatomas.

4. What percentage of leukemic patients eventually have leukemic involvement in the ear or temporal bone?

Twenty percent. Such involvement may present as mucosal ulceration or bleeding from the external auditory canal. The tympanic membrane and middle ear mucosa may become irregular and thickened. Leukemic patients may eventually exhibit deficits of cranial nerves VII and VIII.

5. What is the most common true neoplasm of the middle ear?

Glomus tumors, or paragangliomas. They are most often found in middle-aged Caucasians. Pulsatile tinnitus is the most common presenting symptom. On pneumatic otoscopy, positive pressure may cause blanching of the pulsating mass under the tympanic membrane (Brown's sign). Because of their appearance, these neoplasms may be mistaken for a high-riding jugular bulb or an aberrant carotid artery. Glomus tumors may grow to a significant size before becoming symptomatic with cranial nerve palsies. Although a conductive hearing loss may be an early sign of a glomus tumor, sensorineural hearing is often normal. These tumors are usually benign neoplasms and carry a $< 3\%$ malignancy rate. Also, $< 1\%$ of these tumors are associated with catecholamine secretion.

6. Which vascular anomalies may present as tumors of the middle ear?

A dehiscent jugular bulb or an aberrant internal carotid artery may appear as a tumor of the middle ear.

7. What other tumors affect the middle ear?

Cholesteatomas are the most common tumor growth in the middle ear and mastoid. Hemangiomas, squamous cell carcinomas, adenomas, and rhabdomyosarcomas may also affect the middle ear.

8. Name three tumors that affect the jugular foramen.
Paragangliomas
Nerve sheath tumors
Sarcomas

9. What is jugular foramen syndrome?
Jugular foramen syndrome may be due to lymphadenopathy, tumors, or skull fractures that involve the jugular foramen. This syndrome is associated with paralysis of cranial nerves (CN)IX, X, and XI. CN XII is spared because it runs through the hypoglossal canal.

10. What lesions affect the petrous apex?
Inflammatory: cholesterol granuloma, cholesteatoma, mucocele
Infectious: petrous apicitis or osteomyelitis
Neoplastic: schwannoma, meningioma, glomus tumor, chordoma, chondrosarcoma, nasopharyngeal carcinoma, or metastases from distant malignancies
Variants of normal: asymmetric bone marrow or air cell pattern
Aneurysm: aneurysm of the intrapetrous carotid artery

11. What is a cholesterol granuloma?
Acholesterol granuloma is an infrequently encountered temporal bone inflammatory lesion associated with a giant cell reaction. It may also be associated with otitis media, trauma, possibly barotrauma, or prior cholesteatoma. A cholesterol granuloma may present with pain and dysfunction of CN VII or VIII.

12. Are epidermoid cysts ever malignant?
In the temporal bone, an epidermoid cyst is an aggressive but benign lesion. It consists of stratified squamous epithelium and collagen and contains keratin debris and cholesterol crystals. This lesion may appear at the cerebellopontine angle or elsewhere intracranially. An epidermoid cyst is slow-growing and avascular and has little inflammatory effect. Rather, the lesion's progressive compression on neural structures leads to associated signs and symptoms.

13. Describe the common contemporary operations used to control balance disorders.
Vestibular nerve section: very high efficacy, spares hearing, and can be done best through middle fossa or retrolabyrinthine approaches; considered highly selectively destructive
Labyrinthectomy: high efficacy, always destroys hearing, less frequently performed currently; may be considered when intractable tinnitus is also an issue; considered a permanently destructive technique
Endolymphatic shunt: controversial; less efficacy, can also relieve inner ear symptoms of aural pressure and tinnitus associated with Ménière's disease; considered nondestructive
Chemical vestibular ablation: a recently popular, less demanding technique; in a variety of methods, various aminoglycoside antibiotics can be introduced to the round window; permanently destroys vestibular hair cells with some degree of selectivity while preserving cochlear hair cell function; considered destructive
Repair of oval or round window fistulas: controversial, but should be considered, especially when there is an antecedent history of ossicular surgery (especially stapes surgery), serious head trauma, or physical exertion; the predictive value of all preoperative and intraoperative testing for the existence of fistulas remains an enigma for neuro-otologists

14. Describe the six anatomic segments of the facial nerve.
Intracranial: from brainstem to internal auditory canal
Meatal: from fundus of internal auditory canal to meatal foramen (narrowest aperture of facial nerve's bony canaliculus)
Labyrinthine (narrowest segment of the facial nerve): from meatal foramen to geniculate

ganglion (which may be dehiscent). The nerve is surrounded by an extension of the subarachnoid space and cerebrospinal fluid. The geniculate ganglion is the "first genu" of the facial nerve, and here it gives off its first branch (superficial petrosal nerve).

Tympanic: after the geniculate ganglion, coursing adjacent to the oval window of the stapes, to the pyramidal eminence of the stapedius tendon ("second genu"); 15–30% of normal nerves may be dehiscent in this segment

Mastoid ("vertical segment"): from second genu to stylomastoid foramen

Extratemporal: from stylomastoid foramen to innervated facial mimetic muscles

15. Before operating on a patient with a facial nerve paralysis, how do you determine the site of the lesion ?

Depending on the cause of the paralysis, surgery is directed to the site of the lesion. For temporal bone or skull-base trauma, a high-resolution computed tomographic (CT) scan is obtained, and the site of the lesion is anatomically correlated. In transverse or longitudinal temporal bone fractures, a direct disruption may be identified with a CT scan. In longitudinal fractures of the temporal bone without direct facial nerve disruption, the most likely site of injury is the perigeniculate ganglion. For iatrogenic injury, the most common site is the tympanic segment; however, during mastoid surgery, the site may be the vertical segment. For Ramsay Hunt disease (herpes zoster oticus), or, less frequently, Bell's palsy, the site of the lesion is always the labyrinthine segment and meatal foramen.

16. How do you decide whether a paralyzed facial nerve should be explored for decompression or repair?

The Hilger facial nerve stimulator should be used for any paresis that is obvious. The threshold and maximum stimulation tests are performed and may easily be repeated on subsequent office visits. When there is no significant visible motion of the face or when the exact onset of the paralysis is unclear, a more precise method to quantify the residual activity of the paretic face should be employed, i.e., electroneuronography (ENOG). ENOG is an evoked electromyographic response of the facial muscles. This test can also be repeated periodically.

If and when the testing indicates progressive nerve weakness that is > 90%, the nerve is at high risk of incomplete recovery. Surgical intervention for facial nerve decompression (for severe Ramsay Hunt, Bell's palsy, or perigeniculate neural injury due to trauma) should be performed at the earliest convenience. For other discrete trauma to the nerve, the site of the lesion should be clarified by imaging (unless iatrogenic, in which case the site should be suspect from the history). In cases with unclear causes (including Bell's), the course of the nerve should be imaged with CT and/or magnetic resonance imaging (MRI) to clarify the diagnosis. Tumors or other temporal bone processes should be identified.

17. By which approaches are facial nerve injuries surgically treated?

Facial nerve decompression of the labyrinthine and meatal segments is best approached via the middle fossa technique. The transmastoid facial recess approach can be used to decompresss the tympanic segment, but this procedure can also be done via the middle fossa. In both cases, the incus must be removed and an ossiculoplasty performed to gain access to the tympanic segment. The mastoid segment is, of course, best visualized with a mastoidectomy. The parotid gland needs to be dissected for access to the extratemporal distal nerve pes and branches. Most proximally, the middle fossa approach, in which the dura is opened, can be used to gain access to the facial nerve as it exits the brainstem. Likewise, a retrolabyrinthine approach can show the brainstem exit of the facial nerve, but the exposure to the internal auditory canal (IAC) is lacking. For traumatic facial nerve paralysis with total deafness, a translabyrinthine approach may be indicated.

18. How are traumatized facial nerve injuries repaired?

No matter where the site of the lesion, end-to-end anastomosis for lacerations is appropriate if there is no residual tension on the nerve stumps across the anastomosis. Nerves that are physically damaged or have missing portions can be repaired with an interposition graft. Such a graft is taken from the greater auricular or sural nerves. Hypoglossal-facial nerve anastomosis can give acceptable results when the proximal facial nerve stump cannot be identified.

19. What is congenital aural atresia?

Congenital aural atresia ("congenital ear deformity") is embryonic failure or anomalous development of the middle ear, tympanic membrane, and external auditory canal. It usually manifests with some degree of external cosmetic auricular malformations, ranging from microtia to anotia.

20. What middle ear otologic anomalies are associated with congenital aural atresia?

The facial nerve tympanic segment and the vertical segments are often aberrant in location. The motor facial nerve rarely may be congenitally absent (Moebius syndrome) in association with congenital ear deformity. The chorda tympani nerve may contain motor fibers of the facial nerve. The stapedial artery may be persistent. The ossicular deformities range from malformation or absence of the stapes superstructure or crura, to fibrous unions of the ossicular linkages, to fusion of the malleus and incus into a single ossicle. The lateral ossicular component is usually fused to a plate of bone or soft tissue ("the atretic plate") that is located where the tympanic membrane would normally develop.

21. What are the significant findings and considerations for successful otologic surgery for congenital aural atresia?

On audiometry, there is usually a significant or maximal conductive component to the hearing loss, but there also may be a sensorineural component. CT scanning is used to decide whether the patient's anatomy is favorable or unfavorable for surgery. Favorable features include well-pneumatized mastoid with normal inner ear structures. Unilateral cases in children are usually operated on only when the child is old enough to participate in the decision to undergo surgery. A facial plastic and reconstructive surgeon (or general plastic surgeon) who has successful experience with reconstruction of the pinna should be consulted to coordinate any staged procedures. Finally, the family and patient must be committed to frequent (sometimes every 1 to 4 weeks) clinical follow-up for a period of months to a few years.

22. What are the features and landmarks for otologic surgery for congenital aural atresia?

With absence of the external auditory canal, the space for reconstruction is limited by retroposition of the mandible condyle, inferiorly positioned tegmen, anteriorly positioned sigmoid sinus, and, most importantly, the facial nerve. The facial nerve may be located anywhere. With absent or poor development of the mastoid tip, the facial nerve is often superficial, making it the limiting landmark both inferiorly and posteriorly, but it can limit the dissection in any direction.

23. What are the potential risks and complications of otologic surgery for congenital aural atresia?

Such operations are some of the most demanding for the otologic surgeon. Operative complications may include facial nerve paralysis; intraoperative monitoring is mandatory. Injury to the inner ear is possible as result of manipulation of the ossicles, and throughout the procedure an especially delicate touch is essential. When there is microtia or anotia, the design of the otologic approach incisions may be important to the successful auricular reconstruction of the pinna. Postoperative complications include infections and particularly stenosis of the newly made external auditory canal. This latter point is the reason why careful follow-up is so important for success.

24. What is the technique for cochlear implant surgery?

The selection for candidates for cochlear implant surgery is addressed in chapters 8 and 9. Briefly, a generous postauricular incision is made and a standard mastoidectomy is performed. The external cortex of the retromastoid cranial bone is carved to accommodate the implant components without violating the inner cortex of bone. A generous facial recess approach is used to visualize the middle ear through the mastoid cavity. The round window niche is drilled to reveal the membrane. A cochleostomy is drilled adjacent to the lateral aspect of the wound window membrane, so the electrode may be inserted into the scala tympani as fully as possible, and it is advantageous for intraoperative testing of the device. When preoperative CT scanning indicates membranous cochlear obliteration, the implant may be successful with even a partial insertion, but a complete "drill-out" of the cochlea at the promontory may be necessary to lay the device into the cochlea. The wound is closed.

25. What are the risks of cochlear implant surgery?

Infection, tissue breakdown at the incision or flap, implant stimulation of the facial nerve, vertigo, and device failure are potential postoperative complications. Aural rehabilitation often requires more than 50 hours and is crucial for successful implant use.

26. Name the structures contained in the internal auditory canal.

If the IAC is divided into four cross-sectional quadrants, each quadrant contains one major structure:

Anterior-superior quadrant: the facial nerve
Anterior-inferior quadrant: the cochlear nerve
Posterior-superior quadrant: the superior vestibular nerve
Posterior-inferior quadrant: the inferior vestibular nerve

27. What is an acoustic neuroma?

Acoustic neuromas, or schwannomas, account for approximately 6% of all intracranial neoplasms. These lesions, arising in the IAC, are benign encapsulated tumors of the 8th nerve sheath of Schwann. They tend to arise on the vestibular nerve twice as often as on the auditory nerve. Seventy percent of acoustic neuromas grow slowly (i.e., over years), whereas 30% remain stable. Although most of these tumors grow slowly, over time they may erode bone of the internal auditory meatus. Acoustic neuromas occur in a female to male ratio of 3:2. Asymptomatic, clinically silent acoustic neuromas occur in approximately 2% of the population.

28. How do acoustic neuromas present?

The most common presenting symptoms include **tinnitus** and a progressive, unilateral, high-frequency **hearing loss.** Patients are often unable to localize the tinnitus to a specific ear. About 50% of patients complain of **dysequilibrium.** Late manifestations develop as the tumor erodes into the internal canal and extends into the posterior cranial fossa. Facial nerve compression may lead to unilateral numbness and weakness. Cerebellar and brainstem symptoms, such as dysarthria and ataxia, may arise eventually. Very late disease may cause trigeminal symptoms.

29. What is Hitselberger's sign?

Numbness of the posterior aspect of the concha. This area is innervated by sensory fibers of the facial nerve. Numbness suggests facial nerve compression due to a neoplasm such as an acoustic neuroma.

30. Most acoustic neuromas arise on the vestibular nerve. Why don't patients present with vertigo more often?

Rarely do patients with an acoustic neuroma present with sudden-onset rotatory vertigo. Because these tumors grow slowly, the vestibular system adapts to their presence. More commonly, patients complain of mild dysequilibrium.

31. What do audiometric tests show in a patient with an acoustic neuroma?

Although 5% of patients with an acoustic neuroma will have a normal audiogram, most patients have characteristic audiometric abnormalities. These patients often exhibit a loss of discrimination that is disproportionate to the pure-tone results. Sixty-five percent of patients exhibit a high-frequency sensorineural hearing loss. Unilateral hearing loss is a suspicious finding. Any patient with a 20-dB asymmetry at one frequency or a 10-dB asymmetry at two or more frequencies should undergo further evaluation. In addition, almost 90% of patients have no stapedial reflex. Therefore, impedance audiometry should be done if a patient has a suspicious audiogram. Auditory brainstem response (ABR) is a valuable tool when evaluating patients for acoustic neuromas. The sensitivity of ABR in this setting approaches 95%, and it yields a false-positive rate of 10%. In the presence of an acoustic neuroma, wave V may be absent or prolonged.

32. What is the "gold standard" study for an acoustic neuroma?

Thin-section MRI with gadolinium enhancement can detect very small acoustic neuromas of only a few millimeters in size in the temporal bones. It is currently the best study, but generally is too expensive to use as a routine screening test.

33. Are acoustic neuromas associated with a genetic disease?

Although 95% of acoustic neuromas occur spontaneously without any genetic associations, 5% of patients have **neurofibromatosis** (NF), also known as **von Recklinghausen disease.** In contrast to the spontaneously occurring acoustic neuroma, NF-associated tumors are unencapsulated and may be multiple or bilateral. In addition, they are more aggressive and tend to invade surrounding axons. Rarely, such schwannomas in NF patients undergo malignant transformation.

34. What are the standard treatment options for a patient with an acoustic neuroma?

In general, acoustic neuromas are surgically excised. However, because these tumors are slow-growing, elderly patients or patients with serious medical problems may choose a more conservative approach, foregoing surgery and electing observation.

35. Describe the anatomy of the cerebellopontine angle (CPA).

The CPA is a potential space in the posterior fossa. Anteriorly, the CPA is bound by the temporal bone. Posteriorly, it is bound by the cerebellum. The cerebellar tonsil is located inferior to the CPA, and the pons and cerebellar peduncles are located superior to the CPA.

Cranial nerves also are anatomically associated with the CPA. CN VII and VIII travel superiorly and laterally through the CPA and into the IAC. CN V is located superior to the CPA. CN IX, X, and XI are located inferior to the CPA.

36. What is the differential diagnosis of tumors of the cerebellopontine angle?

Acoustic neuromas, or schwannomas, account for 80% of all angle lesions. Other lesions in this area (in decreasing order of frequency) include meningiomas, lipomas, epidermoids, cholesterol granulomas, cholesteatomas, arachnoid cysts, aneurysms, and metastatic malignant tumors.

37. Name four surgical approaches to the cerebellopontine angle.

Translabyrinthine
Retrolabyrinthine
Middle fossa
Suboccipital

38. What does a translabyrinthine approach involve?

It is used for CPA lesions that are < 3 cm. The approach is initiated in the postauricular area. The surgeon performs a mastoidectomy and labyrinthectomy, sparing the facial nerve. This provides direct access to the IAC. Bone overlying the posterior fossa, middle fossa, and sigmoid sinus is removed, exposing the dura. The IAC is opened, and the dura over the posterior fossa is incised and the tumor is removed. The dura is closed, and a fat graft taken from the abdomen is used to obliterate the space.

39. Outline the advantages and disadvantages of the translabyrinthine approach.

This approach is advantageous because it allows a direct approach to the IAC and preserves the 7th nerve. The approach also requires minimal cerebellar retraction.

Advantages: familiar approach for neurotologists, allowing access to contents of entire IAC. Variations include the transotic and transcochlear approaches which extend exposure anteriorly.

Disadvantages: complete hearing loss. However, "hearing-sparing" translabyrinthine techniques can be attempted, which, in some cases, may preserve hearing.

Exposure limits: sigmoid sinus, facial nerve, dura of middle fossa

40. What is the retrolabyrinthine approach?

The retrolabyrinthine approach to the IAC is an extension of a mastoidectomy. With this approach, the labyrinth remains intact. The CPA medial to the porus of the IAC may be visualized, and here, the vestibular nerve may be sectioned. If a tumor is small and does not extend into the IAC, it may be removed. The dura between the sigmoid sinus and labyrinth is opened, and the necessary surgery is performed.

Advantages: familiar approach for most neurotologists.

Disadvantages: no access to lateral intracanalicular IAC. As such, the indications for this approach are somewhat narrower.

Exposure limits: otic capsule, sigmoid sinus (a variant that transects the sigmoid sinus can expand the operative field significantly), dura and brain in middle fossa

41. What does the middle fossa approach involve?

The middle fossa, or transtemporal supralabyrinthine, approach is used for small intracanalicular tumors that are < 1 cm in size. An incision is made in the scalp above the auricle. A temporal craniotomy is performed, and the temporal lobe is minimally retracted extradurally. The superior aspect of the temporal bone is drilled, preserving the labyrinth. The facial nerve is identified in its meatal and labyrinthine segments. The bony canal is opened and the tumor is removed. Lastly, the wound is closed.

Advantages: may preserve hearing; can identify the entire course of the facial nerve in the IAC, meatal, labyrinthine, geniculate, and tympanic segments. As such, this approach is ideal for facial nerve decompression or repair, or vestibular nerve section. Any dural incision is limited.

Disadvantages: less familiar approach for many neurotologists, and more technically exacting; tumors must be smaller.

Exposure limits: the cochlea and superior semicircular canal are major landmarks that may be blue-lined but must be preserved; retraction of the middle fossa is less forgiving and must be done minimally.

42. Describe the suboccipital/retrosigmoid approach.

The suboccipital approach allows access to the CPA from a posterior approach and can be used for quite large tumors in the region (> 3 cm). A craniotomy behind the ear is made below the sigmoid sinus. The dura is opened, and the cerebellum is retracted. A large tumor is evident. The majority of the tumor is debulked to expose the posterior aspect of the temporal bone at the porus of the IAC. The posterior aspect of the temporal bone is drilled, preserving the contents of the IAC, and the posterior semicircular canal is the lateral limit of dissection to preserve the labyrinth. The tumor in the IAC is removed, preserving the facial nerve. Any remaining tumor medial and anterior to the IAC is removed as well. The wound is closed.

Advantages: can remove very large tumors with brainstem compression; can be used to attempt hearing preservation when appropriate

Disadvantages: less familiar approach for many neurotologists, great exposure of brain

Exposure limits: cerebellum and brainstem, blue-line of posterior semicircular canal (unless hearing cannot be preserved)

43. What are the potential postoperative sequelae of neuro-otologic skull-base surgery?

In general, the patient should know that surgery may result in sensorineural hearing loss, temporary (infrequently permanent) balance problems, temporary (infrequently permanent) facial nerve paralysis, CSF leak, and meningitis. Intracranial hemorrhage, air embolus, cerebellar ataxia, stroke, and death are very rare complications.

44. Of these complications, which are emergencies? How should they be handled?

Altered mental status (obtundation), asymmetric pupils, hemiplegia, seizures, or severe hypertension may be associated with postoperative emergencies. Intracranial hemorrhage, strokes, cerebrospinal fluid (CSF) leaks, meningitis, and pneumocephalus are emergencies. In the case of intracranial hemorrhage or stroke, the patient may require emergency return to the operating room to control hemorrhage. A CSF shunt may be necessary. Dressings should be removed and the wound opened to allow for decompression of the brainstem. The patient should be taken to the operating room to further control hemorrhage. If meningitis is suspected, a lumbar puncture should be obtained and sent for culture and sensitivities. Frank wound infections should be treated aggressively. Leaks that persist should be closed surgically. If an unstable patient has pneumocephalus, an emergency burr-hole may be necessary to remove air.

45. How is the integrity of salvageable cranial nerves maintained in neuro-otologic skull-base surgery?

Intraoperative cranial nerve monitoring and somatosensory monitoring have become essential tools and require specialized equipment. In any case with potential facial nerve exposure, the nerve may be monitored using EMG techniques. ABR or electrocochleography can monitor the cochlear nerve. Practically all of the remaining cranial nerves can be monitored with sophisticated techniques when appropriate.

CONTROVERSIES

46. Can an acoustic neuroma be cured with "radiosurgery"?

Stereotactic gamma-irradiation therapy ("gamma knife") or linear accelerator (LINAC) are recent treatment modalities used in selected patients. Considerable controversy exists around the efficacy of such radiosurgery. It is currently applied to tumors that are < 3 cm. In principle, a high dose of ionizing radiation is delivered to the target tissue, while the surrounding structures are spared. This technique claims a low rate of facial nerve damage and hearing loss. In the United States, long-term results are currently unknown.

47. Can glomus tumors be cured with radiosurgery or radiation therapy?

The main indication for radiation therapy of glomus tumors is contraindication to surgery. Such contraindications may be associated with a patient's poor medical health. If the extent of disease makes a surgical attempt at complete or near-total removal impossible, radiation therapy may also be recommended. Radiation may slow or halt the growth of the tumor, but this is controversial. In addition, radiation therapy is not without risks.

48. Is there a role for chemotherapy in the treatment of the benign tumors of the skull base or CPA?

No. Not with current chemotherapeutic agents.

49. What are the controversies surrounding otologic reconstructive surgery for congenital aural atresia?

The candidates for surgery are often children who may have mentally adjusted to a congenital imperfection such as unilateral atresia. It is sometimes debated whether such children should have elective surgery that entails the potential for serious risks. Furthermore, it is uncommon to achieve perfect closure of the hearing air-bone gap. More often, the hearing results, while improved, are not spectacular. Delayed postoperative stenosis of the ear canal may occur and necessitate reoperation of the canal to maintian patency.

50. What is the biggest controversy surrounding cochlear implant surgery?

Surprisingly, members of the deaf community are often against the use of cochlear implant surgery, particularly in children. Many members of this community feel that these devices are experimental and unproven, and threaten to diminish the population of the deaf community by giving an otherwise deaf person the ability to hear. History and experience have proved to most unbiased observers that cochlear implant surgery generally has significant potential benefits and may enrich the quality of life and increase the standard of living in selected patients.

—————

AMERICAN NEUROTOLOGY SOCIETY

By the early 1960s, otology was rapidly evolving beyond its early emphasis on infectious ear disease to encompass a much broader perspective. Practitioners and scientists alike began to focus increasing attention on disorders of the inner ear, 8th nerve, and central audiovestibular pathways. New diagnostic modalities such as site-of-lesion testing, electronystagmography, and polytomography provided clinicians with tools to investigate neuro-otologic disorders. These new-found capabilities engendered sufficient interest among otologists to stimulate the formation of an organization focused upon neuro-otologic concerns. Formed in 1963, the Society had its first meeting in 1965.

~*American Neurotology Society, 2000*

—————

BIBLIOGRAPHY

 1. Baloh RW: Advances in neuro-otology. Curr Opin Neurol 11:1–3, 1998.
 2. Baloh RW: Neurotology of migraine. Headache 37:615–621, 1997.
 3. Baloh RW, Jacobson KM: Neurotology. Neurol Clin 14:85–101, 1996.
 4. Baloh RW, Furman JM, Halmagyi GM, et al: Recent advances in clinical neurotology. J Vest Res 5:231–252, 1995.
 5. Battista RA, Wiet RJ: Stereotactic radiosurgery for acoustic neuromas: A survey of the American Neurotology Society. Am J Otol 21:371–381, 2000.
 6. Callanan V, O'Connor AF: Otolaryngology: Making the deaf hear and the dumb speak. Lancet 348 (Suppl 2): sII19, 1996.
 7. Coker NJ, Jenkins HA: Atlas of Otologic Surgery. Philadelphia, W.B. Saunders, 2001.
 8. Hart CW, Rubin AG: Medicolegal aspects of neurotology. Otolaryngol Clin North Am 29:503–520, 1996.
 9. Jackler RK, Brackmann DE (eds): Neurotology. St. Louis, Mosby, 1994.
10. Selesnick SH, Kacker A: Image-guided surgical navigation in otology and neurotology. Am J Otol 20:688–693; discussion 693–697, 1999.
11. Selesnick S, al-Rawi M: Adhesives in otology and neurotology. Am J Otol 18:81–89, 1997.
12. Wackym PA, Balaban CD: Molecules, motion, and man. Otolarygol Head Neck Surg 118(3 Pt 2):S16–24, 1998.

III. The Nose and Sinuses

17. ANATOMY AND PHYSIOLOGY OF THE NOSE

Bruce W. Jafek, M.D., FACS, FRSM

1. Developmentally, which structures form the external nose?

The nose forms from several mesenchymal processes around the primitive mouth, or **stomodeum.** The mesenchymal **frontonasal process** grows downward in the midline, above the roof of the stomodeum, to merge with the maxillary processes. The **maxillary processes** originate from the dorsal ends of the first visceral, or mandibular, arch and the lateral nasal processes. The **olfactory placode,** an ectodermal thickening, invaginates as a pit between the medial portion of the frontonasal process and the lateral nasal process. The frontonasal process then continues to elongate, forming the **median nasal process** and **fetal philtrum.** The lateral nasal processes form the lateral portion of the adult nose (e.g., lower lateral cartilage and lobule). The olfactory placode invaginates as the nasal pit and later as the nasal sac to rest high in the nose as the anlage of the olfactory epithelium.

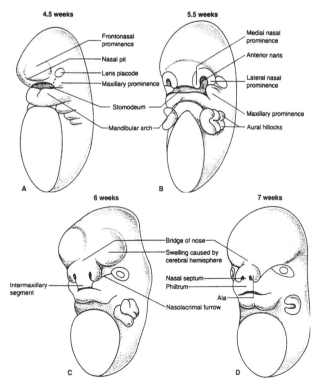

Nasal embryology. Development of the face. (From Fitzgerald MJT, Fitzgerald M: Human Embryology. London, Bailliere Tindall, 1994, pp 169–170, with permission.)

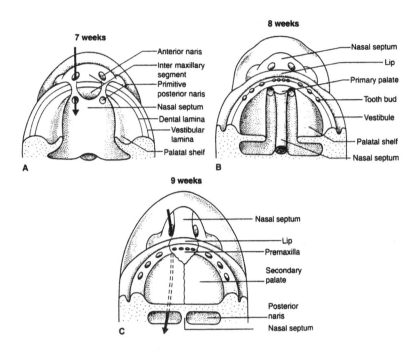

Nasal embryology. Head region, viewed from below, showing development of the palate. In (A) and (C), an arrow is passing along the nasal passage on one side. (From Fitzgerald MJT, Fitzgerald M: Human Embryology. London, Bailliere Tindall, 1994, pp 169–170, with permission.)

2. How does the internal nose form?

As the apices of the maxillary processes fuse with the median nasal process around the invaginating olfactory placode, **primitive anterior nares** form. This invagination leads posteriorly into an anterior (superior) nasal cavity. Posteriorly and inferiorly, a **posterior nasal cavity,** communicating with the anterior cavity superiorly, develops as the inner aspects of the **maxillary processes** form. These give rise to the **palatine processes,** which fuse in the midline to form the palate. Anteriorly, this fusion is completed first, as these processes fuse with the premaxilla from the median nasal process and then "zip" posteriorly. Premature arrest of this process may cause a cleft soft palate, submucous cleft palate, or bifid uvula. The **septum,** a divider between the two nasal cavities, is thought to arise because of the dual origin of the olfactory placodes. This division produces side-by-side nasal pits. In the midline, the mesenchyme grows downward from the roof of the nose, dividing the nasal cavity in half. The primitive openings of the nasal cavity, the **posterior choanae,** are initially closed by the **bucconasal membrane.** This plug of epithelial cells usually ruptures at the end of the fourth embryonic week. Failure to rupture, unilaterally or bilaterally, leads to choanal atresia.

2. Describe the nasal bones and cartilages.

Several bones and cartilages give the external nose its characteristic pyramidal shape. The **nasal bones** articulate with the nasal processes of the **frontal bone** superiorly and the nasal processes of the **maxilla** laterally. The nasal bones are attached inferiorly to the **upper (superior) lateral cartilages,** which then attach inferiorly to the **lower (inferior) lateral cartilages.** Medially, the superior and inferior lateral cartilages attach to the **cartilaginous septum.** Small rudimentary cartilages known as **sesamoid cartilages** or **alar cartilages,** give additional support to the lateral nasal ala, where the lower lateral cartilage extends to meet the cheek. The fibrofatty tissue of the lower lateral cartilage, which contains the sesamoid cartilages is known as the **lobule.**

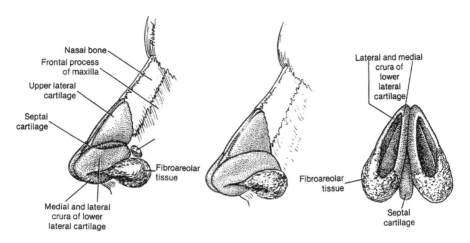

Nasal curtilages. (From Cummings CW, et al (eds): Otolaryngology–Head and Neck Surgery, 3rd ed. St. Louis, Mosby, 1998, with permission.)

4. The internal nose has five areas that are susceptible to nasal airflow obstruction. What are these five areas?

The internal nose, as described by Maurice Cottle, has five areas in which narrowing may lead to airflow obstruction. Each area of obstruction may be corrected differently.

- **Anterior nare,** or nostril. This structure may be constricted congenitally or traumatically. For example, burns may constrict the anterior nare.
- **Nasal valve.** This is the narrowest area in the entire respiratory tract and is identified as the nasal valve. This structure is limited medially by the septum, inferiorly by the floor of the nose, and by the junction between the cephalic lower lateral cartilage and caudal upper lateral cartilage. Further weakness, as might occur with injudicious resection of the lateral nasal cartilages in this area (e.g., unsuccessful rhinoplasty), produces collapse of the nose on inspiration and maximal "obstruction."
- **Upper and lower halves of the internal nasal vestibule.** Either may be obstructed by nasal septal deviation.
- **Posterior opening of the nasal vestibule,** or posterior choanae

5. What is the vascular supply to the nose?

The nose and sinuses are supplied by branches of the **external and internal carotid arteries.** The posterior inferior part of the internal nose is supplied by the external carotid artery and terminal branches of the **internal maxillary artery,** the **sphenopalatine** and **greater palatine arteries.** The anterior inferior nasal cavity is supplied by branches of the **facial artery.** The superior part of the nasal cavity is supplied by branches of the **ophthalmic artery** from the **internal carotid artery.** These branches include the **anterior** and **posterior ethmoid arteries.** Vascular distributions are important in the evaluation and treatment of nosebleeds.

The venous drainage of the nose does not parallel the arterial supply, but corresponds to regions, or arteriovenous units, such as the frontomedian area or orbitopalpebral area (see also Question 7). The nasal venous drainage nomenclature corresponds to arterial nomenclature, however. For example, venous drainage occurs through the sphenopalatine, ophthalmic, and anterior facial veins.

6. What is the "danger triangle?"

The danger triangle, also known as the danger area, is a triangle from the nasion, where the nose joins the forehead superiorly, to the lateral corners of the mouth, where the venous supply of the nose drains intracranially. From the angular vein, blood drains into the inferior ophthalmic vein and then into the cavernous sinus. This vascular supply provides cutaneous nasal infections, such as streptococcus, with a potential route to spread intracranially.

7. Discuss the various nasal functions.

Although the "nose" is really a paired structure, or two noses, functionally these act as a unit. In addition to smelling and breathing, it warms, humidifies, and cleanses the inspired air. The temperature of the inspired air increases to nearly body temperature by the time it reaches the pharynx. Similarly, the humidity increases to 100% by the time the inhaled air reaches the lung, regardless of the ambient humidity. Upon expiration, the nose removes water from the expired air, thus maintaining hydration, and removes heat, thus preventing hypothermia.

Larger particulate matter in inspired air (e.g. bugs) is removed anteriorly by the vibrissae. Progressively smaller particles are removed inside the nasal vestibule by direct impaction or electrostatic attraction with the nasal mucous blanket. The cilia move the mucus posteriorly, like a conveyor belt, causing the mucous blanket with inlaid particulate matter to empty into the stomach, where the gastric acid kills potential inspired pathogens.

8. How is the nose innervated?

The muscles of the nose are innervated by the **facial** (7th cranial) nerve but are almost of vestigial importance. The external skin is innervated by the first and second branches of the **trigeminal** (5th cranial) nerve. The trigeminal nerve also supplies general sensory innervation, or touch, to the internal nose and general chemosensation (e.g., irritation from acrid odors). **Olfactory** (1st cranial) fibers are located in the superior portion of the internal nose on both the septum and superior and superior middle turbinates and serve the sense of smell.

The **sympathetic** innervation originates from the hypothalamus, passes through the thoracolumbar region of the spinal cord, and synapses in the superior cervical ganglion in the neck. Postganglionic fibers then extend through the sphenopalatine ganglion to reach the nose. Additional fibers that run along blood vessels also extend from the carotid plexus to the nose.

The **parasympathetic** supply originates in the facial nucleus of the brain, is relayed to the sphenopalatine ganglion, and finally reaches the nose via the posterior nasal nerve. The posterior nasal nerve also carries most of the postganglionic sympathetics. Nitric oxide, previously thought to be a poison, appears to be one of the mediators of nasal reflexes.

9 What is the name of the muscle with the longest name and what does it do?

The muscle with the longest name of any of those of the body, the **levator labii superioris alaeque nasii,** attaches to the nose. It provides minimal depressor activity to the lateral nasal lobule, along with elevator motor action to the lateral corner of the mouth.

10. What is the nasal reflex?

Clinical observations suggest the existence of poorly characterized reflex pathways between the upper and lower respiratory passages. Strong stimuli produce profound and widespread cardiopulmonary responses, including breathing cessation and bradycardia. Such responses may be the basis for some characteristics of sleep apnea syndrome. Milder stimuli may produce expulsion of the noxious stimulus with sneezing. A finger under the nose may actually abort a sneeze by triggering the nasal reflex!

11. What is the electro-olfactogram?

Recorded by an electrode placed on the olfactory epithelium, an electro-olfactogram (EOG) is a slow, negative, purely monophasic potential in response to odorants. Analogous to an electroretinogram of the eye, an EOG is thought to represent a generator potential from the olfactory epithelium.

12. What is the electrovomerogram?

The electrovomerogram, or EVG, was characterized by Grosser and Monti-Bloch and appears to represent a unique electrical current arising from the vomeronasal organ (of Jacobson) in response to certain steroidal stimulants such as androstadienone. Whether this current represents "smell," however, is open to question.

13. Where do the lymphatics of the nose and paranasal sinuses form and drain?

The lymphatics of the nose and paranasal sinuses arise from the superficial portion of the mucous membrane and travel posteriorly to the retropharyngeal lymph nodes. Anteriorly, the lymphatics drain into the submandibular (submental) lymph nodes or the upper deep cervical nodes.

14. Describe the epithelial lining of the nose.

The respiratory tract, with the exception of the pharynx, is generally lined by specialized respiratory epithelium (pseudostratified, columnar, ciliated epithelium with interspersed goblet cells). The same epithelium lines the paranasal sinuses and eustachian tubes, but here the epithelium is somewhat flattened. In contrast, the nares are lined with **stratified squamous epithelium,** and the superior aspect of the internal nose is lined with **olfactory epithelium.** Beneath this surface epithelium on the lateral aspect of the nose are both **racemose** and **tubular glands** that provide serous and mucous secretions for the surface mucous blanket. Deeper yet, there is a specialized **vascular plexus,** consisting of arterioles, capillaries, vascular sinusoids, venous plexuses, and venules. This plexus forms erectile tissue, most prominently over the inferior turbinates, adjacent septum, and posterior middle turbinates, which assists the nose in its physiologic function.

15. How do the cilia function?

In mammals, cilia beat 10–20 times per second at room temperature. This beat has a characteristic biphasic motion, with a rapid effective stroke and a slower recovery stroke. During the effective stroke, the extended cilium reaches a superficial, viscous mucous layer. During the recovery stroke, the cilium bends to travel in the other direction through the thinner periciliary layer. Thus, the mucous layer is conveyed in the direction of the effective stroke.

16. What is Kartagener's syndrome?

Kartagener's syndrome, or immotile cilia syndrome, is due to absence of the dynein arm on the peripheral ciliary microtubules. The cilia are unable to beat effectively. This syndrome produces a characteristic triad of chronic rhinosinusitis, bronchiectasis, and situs inversus. Clinically, nasal examination shows mucus or mucous accumulation.

17. What factors inhibit normal ciliary activity?

Normally, cilia beat 10–20 times per second. Drying (possibly produced by localized deflections or turbulence within the nasal cavity), drugs (e.g., cocaine, adrenaline, benzalkonium chloride), excessive heat or cold, hypertonic or hypotonic solutions, smoking (nicotine), infections (viral or bacterial), and noxious fumes (e.g., sulfur dioxide, carbon monoxide) all inhibit the normal ciliary beat.

18. What is the mucous blanket?

The goblet cells and submucosal glands of the nose produce mucus that forms a continuous blanket throughout the nose and sinuses. This blanket is composed of a superficial, thick, mucous layer and a deep, thin, periciliary layer. Dust, bacteria, viruses, and pollens impact on and stick to this layer. Ciliary action then carries the blanket to the pharynx, where it is swallowed into the stomach and digested. About 1–1.5 pints of mucus are produced each day. Lysozyme, an important enzyme of the mucus, initiates bacterial destruction. Both ciliary and lysozyme activity are optimal at pH 7.0. Anything that interferes with pH (e.g., medication, infection) interferes with nasal function.

19. Describe the function of the nasal submucosal vascular plexus.

Many of the mechanisms that control the nasal vasculature are not fully understood. It is clear, however, that the blood vessel system resembles that of the erectile tissue of the genitalia. It is therefore possible to vary the flow of blood through the nasal mucosal surfaces independent of the variations in submucosal vascular engorgement. This deeper vasculature is under the control of the autonomic nervous system, but the precise receptor-reflex arcs have not yet been fully identified. Stimulation of sympathetic nerves causes noradrenaline release and vasoconstriction, whereas parasympathetic stimulation releases acetylcholine, resulting in vasodilatation and a watery nasal discharge. Mild mechanical or chemical stimulation of the internal nose produces sneezing, while stronger stimulation may result in apnea or bradycardia. Variations in nasal airflow are measured by rhinomanometry.

21. What is rhinomanometry?

Rhinomanometry is a measure of transnasal pressure and resultant airflow. Initially measured with water columns and mechanical devices, this pressure is now measured with electronic techniques and computers. Widely used in research, it has not yet achieved the clinical status of audiometric or vestibular function assessment.

21. Clinically, how is mucociliary flow measured?

Mucous transport can be measured clinically with the indigo carmine/saccharin sodium test. The test can be performed easily, without sophisticated equipment. A drop of indigo carmine (8 mg/ml), or, alternatively, methylene blue, and a drop of saccharin sodium (3 mg/ml) are placed in the anterior nasal cavity, at the bottom of the inferior nasal meatus on the mucosa just behind the internal ostium. After 3 minutes, the patient is instructed to swallow every 30 seconds and to report any perception of sweet taste. The posterior pharynx is also inspected at these intervals for the presence of the blue dye. In general, the lag between the perception of a sweet taste and the appearance of the blue dye in the pharynx may be minimal or it may be several minutes. The lag, or mucous transport time (MTT), is normally 12–15 minutes. This normal MTT tends to correlate with a ciliary beat frequency of 10/second and a transit time of 6 mm/minute. An MTT of > 30 minutes is considered significantly abnormal.

Ciliary beat frequency can also be measured with a photoelectric-registration device, as well as by other methods. The MTT may also be measured by radioactive particle transit observed by gamma camera or multicollimator detectors. These latter methods, however, require sophisticated equipment and are not generally available.

22. What is the nasal cycle?

The nasal cycle was first described by Kayser in 1895 and has been studied with a variety of techniques, most notably by rhinomanometry. The total resistance to nasal airflow remains relatively constant because of the reciprocal relationship between the resistance of each nasal passage. It is observed in up to 80% of normal subjects, most of whom are unaware of the alteration in airflow since the total resistance remains constant. The alternating cycles of congestion and decongestion on each side of the nose are thought to be under the control of the autonomic innervation of the nose, possibly primarily the adrenergic innervation, through action on the specialized vascular plexus described previously. It is also observed in children and animals.

23. Name the standard x-ray views of the nose and sinuses.

Previously, four standard views were used:

The **Waters view** tips the occiput down so that the maxillary and frontal sinuses are well seen.

The **Caldwell view,** or posteroanterior view, offers a superior view of the frontal and ethmoid sinuses.

The **lateral view** provides superior visualization of the sphenoid sinus and posterior frontal sinus wall.

The **submentovertex view** provides a superior view of the sphenoid sinuses.

Because of the difficulty in visualizing the sinuses through the overlying bone, the most currently and most frequently used study is the limited computed tomography of the ethmoid sinuses. In this study, 3- to 5-mm cuts, without contrast, are obtained of the ethmoid sinuses in the coronal view. This technique allows visualization of all sinuses, especially the osteomeatal complex.

CONTROVERSIES

24. What is the function of the organ of Jacobson?
The **vomeronasal organ** (VNO), or organ of Jacobson, is an accessory concentration of olfactory tissue. In animals, the VNO primarily functions in mating behavior. Thought to be vestigial in humans, its existence in the adult has been described recently. Located in a 1- to 3-mm tubule with an oval orifice, this structure is approximately 1 cm posterior from the caudal septum and 2–4 mm off the floor of the nose. Its pale yellowish mucosa distinguishes it from the surrounding pinkish respiratory mucosa. An electrovomerogram has recently been recorded from the vomeronasal region in response to specific odorants. Whether the VNO has a similar function in human mating is a subject of ongoing research, but as yet the function of this organ in humans remains unknown.

25. How do you measure nasal obstruction?
Rhinometry, a measurement of nasal airflow, would seemingly provide an inverse measurement of obstruction. However, airflow measurements correlate poorly with the patient's perception of "obstruction." Acoustic rhinometry is a new way of performing rhinometry and appears quite promising. But maybe you'll be stimulated to do the research that will eventually provide a simple, reproducible, reliable method of measuring and quantifying nasal breathing.

GEORGE CATLIN (1796–1872)

Catlin was trained as a lawyer but devoted his career to painting Indians in their native land, and he spent his life championing their cause. He was internationally recognized for his work in this area, and his paintings hang in the Library of Congress. He was a friend of William Clark, the noted western explorer. He was also a rhinologic pioneer who was the first in America to call attention to mouth breathing. His article, published in 1862, entitled "Breath of Life, Malrespiration and its Effects on the Life of Man" was later published under the less formal title, "Shut Your Mouth and Save Your Life." His observations on sleep physiology were also widely respected.

BIBLIOGRAPHY

1. Cole P: Biophysics of nasal airflow: A review. Am J Rhinol 14:245–249, 2000.
2. Dahl R, Mygind N: Anatomy, physiology and function of the nasal cavities in health and disease. Adv Drug Deliv Rev 29(1–2):3–12, 1998.
3. Djupesland PG, Qian W, Furlott H, et al: Acoustic rhinometry: A study of transient and continuous noise techniques with nasal models. Am J Rhinol 13:323–329, 1999.
4. Drake-Lee A: The physiology of the nose and paranasal sinuses. In Gleeson M (ed): Basic Sciences, Vol. 1 of Kerr AG (ed): Scott-Brown's Otolaryngology, 6th ed. Oxford, Butterworth-Heinemann, 1997.
5. Durland WF Jr, Lane AP, et al: Nitric oxide is a mediator of the late-phase response in an animal model of nasal allergy. Otolaryngol Head Neck Surg 122:706–711, 2000.
6. Grosser BI, Monti-Bloch L, Jennings-White C, Berliner DL: Behavioral and electrophysiological effects of androstadienone, a human pheromone. Psychoneuroendocrinology 25:289–299, 2000.
7. Jafek, BW, Johnson EW, Eller PM, et al: Olfactory mucosal biopsy and related histology. In Seiden, A (ed): Smell and Taste Disorders. New York, Thieme, 1997.
8. Lund VJ: Anatomy of the nose and paranasal sinuses. In Gleeson M (ed): Basic Sciences, Vol. 1 of Kerr AG (ed.): Scott-Brown's Otolaryngology, 6th ed. Oxford, Butterworth-Heinemann, 1997.
9. Stocks J: Respiratory physiology during early life. Monaldi Arch Chest Dis 54:358–364, 1999.
10. Watelet JB, Van Cauwenberge P: Applied anatomy and physiology of the nose and paranasal sinuses. Allergy 54 (Supp 57) 14–25, 1999.
11. Watson L: Jacobson's Organ and the Remarkable Sense of Smell. New York, W.W. Norton, 2000.

18. NASAL SEPTAL ABNORMALITIES

Michael Leo Lepore, M.D., FACS

1. Describe the anatomy of the nasal septum.

The nasal septum is made up of the nasal septal cartilage, or quadrangular septal cartilage, anteriorly; of the vomer and the perpendicular plate of the ethmoid posteriorly; and of the maxillary crest anteroinferiorly. The anterior portion is flexible, whereas the posterior portion is bony and fixed.

2. What is the most common deformity of the nasal septum resulting from trauma?

Caudal deformity involving the anterior cartilaginous septum. Usually, the cartilage is displaced off the maxillary crest, lying either in the left or right nasal cavity, contralateral to the direction of the force. The caudal septum, or the anterior-most part of the cartilaginous septum, can project into the nasal cavity causing obstructive symptoms.

3. What complications commonly result from trauma to the nasal septum?

Epistaxis, hematomas, and dislocations of the quadrangular septal cartilage are the most common complications. Epistaxis usually involves the anterior septum at **Kiesselbach's plexus** (or **Little's area**). Hematomas result from disruption of the vascular supply within the perichondrial layer with subsequent bleeding into the soft tissue. The hematoma will appear as a fluctuant swelling of the septum covered by reddish-purple mucosa. Hematomas are uncommon in children, but when they occur spontaneously, a blood dyscrasia needs to be excluded. Septal hematomas should be drained.

4. What characteristic deformity results from untreated septal hematomas?

Septal hematomas that are not surgically drained may become infected, leading to destruction of the cartilage. Alternatively, bilateral elevation of the septal mucoperichondrium may, itself, lead to necrosis of the cartilage. This destruction of cartilage causes a loss of dorsal nasal support with a resultant cosmetic deformity termed a **saddle-nose deformity.**

5. What is a septal abscess?

A septal abscess is a collection of purulent material beneath the perichondrial layer of the quadrangular septal cartilage, which may be unilateral or bilateral. Patients with this condition normally complain of severe pain, with an elevated temperature and nasal obstruction. The cause is usually trauma, with the formation of a septal hematoma that becomes infected. It may also result from surgery on the nasal septum. The most common organism isolated is *Staphylococcus aureus*.

6. What is the treatment of a septal abscess?

Under normal conditions, the patient is admitted to the hospital and treatment is initiated with intravenous antibiotics targeted at *Staphyoloccus aureus*. Incision and drainage is done as soon as possible and cultures are obtained, along with a Gram stain, to guide the initial antimicrobial therapy.

7. What are the complications of untreated septal abscess?

Both cosmetic and functional sequelae may result if this condition is untreated. These include **saddle nose deformity, nasal airway obstruction, nasal septal perforation,** and **extension of the infection** to the paranasal sinuses or even intracranial cavity through the venous system.

8. What is the significance of granulation tissue attached to the nasal septum?

Granulation tissue is a response to nasal infections or a history of foreign body. The granulation tissue must be biopsied to rule out sarcoidosis, tuberculosis, malignant lethal midline granuloma (Wegener's disease), and neoplasms. The differential diagnosis of a nasal granuloma is a classic Board question and includes rhinosporidiosis, yaws, and infection by *Leishmaniasis, Histoplasmosis,* and *Sporotrichosis.* Any history of foreign travel should be evaluated.

9. How is nasal biopsy used in detecting Wegener's granulomatosis?

Wegener's granulomatosis is a potentially lethal systemic disease that affects the upper respiratory tract, including the nasal mucosa and the kidneys. It is characterized histologically by granulomatous inflammation, focal necrosis, fibrinoid degeneration, and multinucleated giant cells. Nasal mucosal biopsy may be diagnostic, but several biopsies may be required to obtain histologic proof of Wegener's disease. It is essential to differentiate this disease from other nasal processes, such as infections, connective tissue disorders, Goodpasture's syndrome, and hypersensitive vasculitis. Biopsy specimens > 5 mm in diameter from ulcerated areas, especially on the edge of the involvement, are recommended for better yield.

10. What are inverted papillomas?

Inverted nasal papilloma is a histologically benign but clinically malignant neoplasm. The papilloma usually affects the lateral wall, with the most common site of occurrence in the area of the ethmoid sinus and the opening of the maxillary antrum. Occasionally, a biopsy of the nasal septum will reveal this entity. A nasal papilloma is usually unilateral and causes nasal obstruction. Physical examination reveals a fleshy papillary exophytic growth in either one or both nasal passages. Treatment involves complete resection, since inverted nasal papilloma is associated with a 13% transformation into squamous cell carcinoma.

11. List the causes of a septal perforation.

Perforations of the anterior nasal septum may be caused by trauma, digital manipulation (nose-picking), and surgery (submucous resection). Chrome workers are susceptible to a septal perichondritis causing a perforation. Cocaine abuse may also lead to septal perforation, either secondary to infection or to the use of "cut" contaminated cocaine, or directly, due to severe bilateral vasoconstriction by the cocaine itself. Posterior perforations involving the vomer and perpendicular plate of the ethmoid bone may be the result of gumma formation secondary to tertiary syphilis.

12. Describe the effects of cocaine inhalation on the septum.

Chronic cocaine inhalation can result in symptoms of nasal stuffiness, anosmia, rhinorrhea, sinusitis, and bleeding. In addition, its use often results in crusting and nasal septum perforation. Furthermore, chronic inflammation might lead to the use of prescription intranasal sprays, which further exacerbate the problem and contribute to the formation of a septal perforation. Vasoconstriction from cocaine leads to inflammation, infection, chondritis, and nasal septal perforations with chronic rhinitis. Long-term abuse of cocaine may lead to total loss of the nasal mucosal lining with nasal septal collapse and total nasal obstruction.

13. How should you treat nasal septal defects?

Conservative treatment for mild symptoms includes saline irrigation, emollients (mineral oil), and ointments such as Bactroban. Some physicians recommend "nasal rest" by occluding the nasal airflow with an ointment-impregnated cotton for several hours a day. Surgical repair is usually considered in symptomatic patients who fail to respond to conservative care. Perforations > 2 cm in diameter are seldomly closed successfully, and repair is contraindicated in perforations caused by continuing cocaine abuse, infection, neoplasm, granulomatous disease, or vascular diseases.

14. How does nasal septal deviation affect nasal physiology?

Nasal septal obstruction is the most common symptom of septal deviation. Where mucosa are closely approximated, dryness occurs secondary to a **Bernoulli effect** of airflow, causing mucus formation and impairing ciliary mobility. This obstruction, in time, may lead to inflammatory disease, termed **bacterial rhinitis.** Septal deviation may also impair the normal flow of sinus secretions, producing symptoms and signs of sinusitis, such as infection, purulent drainage, pain, tenderness, and fever.

15. Which organism is most commonly found in bacterial rhinitis? How is it treated?

Alterations of airflow cause an inflammatory response with associated mucosal drying, crusting with retained secretions, and bacterial rhinitis, which further aggravate the inflammatory response. Frequently, *Staphylococcus aureus* is found on nasal cultures. Treatment consists of the following:

- Saline douches—mix 1 cup of water with 1/2 tsp of salt and a pinch of baking soda
- Saline nasal sprays
- Topical applications of mupirocin (Bactroban) ointment twice daily for 1 week and once daily at bedtime for another week.

16. Describe the presentation and treatment of primary squamous cell carcinoma arising from the nasal septum.

These tumors are extremely rare. The usual presentation is nasal obstruction, bleeding, and crusting of the nasal septum. The clinical picture often depends on the direction of extension. Local and distant metastases are very rare, and the treatment of choice is wide surgical excision with postoperative radiation.

17. What are the otolaryngologic manifestations and diagnostic criteria for polychondritis?

Polychondritis is probably of autoimmune origin and is characterized by inflammation of cartilage with its consequent destruction. It is often associated with Hashimoto's thyroiditis, Sjögren's syndrome, scleroderma, and collagen III antibodies. Otolaryngologic manifestations are common, with 70–80% of cases exhibiting septal involvement, commonly presenting as rhinitis and epistaxis with progression to saddle-nose deformities. For diagnosis, patients must meet three out of six criteria:

Bilateral, recurrent ear chondritis
Noneroding polyarthritis
Nasal chondritis
Ocular inflammation
Laryngotracheal chondritis
Cochlear or vestibular lesions

18. Postoperative nasal adhesions can be seen following septal and/or turbinate surgery. How often do nasal adhesions occur, and how are they managed?

Studies cite an incidence of up to 14% following nasal surgery. Turbinate resection is associated with one of the highest complication rates for adhesions, up to 36%. Adhesions may lead to nasal obstruction requiring a second surgery, and up to 80% of patients who develop postoperative adhesions may require this second operation.

CONTROVERSIES

19. Intranasal splints have been recommended for the prevention of postoperative nasal adhesions. What is their efficacy? Are they associated with comorbidity?

Although intranasal splints have been advocated as a preventive measure for postoperative nasal adhesion formation, recent studies have found that splints do not decrease the rate of adhesion formation. Many patients find them very uncomfortable and significantly painful. In addition, intranasal splints may contribute to septal perforations. Adequate nasal toilet and attentive postoperative care have been proposed as alternative strategies to reduce nasal adhesion formation.

20. Does surgery on the nasal septum affect midfacial growth in children?

This subject has been argued among otolaryngologists for quite some time. Some surgeons are conservative in their approach, only operating on children after their last growth spurt. Although controversial, recent literature suggests that although septal cartilage appears to be a factor in midfacial growth in the human fetus, it does not appear to be a factor in midfacial growth postnatally. Therefore, septoplasty and rhinoplasty in childhood failed to demonstrate any significant effect in retarding midfacial growth by anthropometric studies. On the other hand, elective nasal surgery is generally deferred until "full facial and nasal growth have been achieved," generally approximately age 16–18.

21. You are called to the neonatal unit to examine a full-term infant with respiratory distress. What is your initial diagnosis?

Septal deformities in infants are not uncommon. They may be found in 4% of infants born of normal vaginal delivery and in 13% of difficult births (e.g., occipitoposterior presentations). Infants at birth are obligate nasal breathers. Since the nasal cartilage is extremely soft and easily mobile, the cartilage may be manually manipulated without too much difficulty relieving the obstructive symptoms. Rapid passage of a soft rubber catheter (e.g., 16 French red Robinson catheter) through both nares should also be done to rule out possible **choanal atresia.**

BERNARD RUDOLPH KONRAD VON LANGENBECK (1810–1887)

Von Langenbeck is generally regarded as the "Father of Septal Surgery," as he described a method of shaving down acute spurs and angulations of the nasal septum. Most of these early procedures exchanged a septal deflection for a septal perforation, however.

~Weir N, Otolaryngology: An Illustrated History, 1990

BIBLIOGRAPHY

1. Anonymous: What's a deviated nasal septum? Does it need to be corrected? Mayo Clin Health Lett 18:8, 2000.
2. Bizri AR, al-Ajam M, Zaytoun G, et al: Direct carotid cavernous fistula after submucous resection of the nasal septum. J Otorhinolaryngol Rel Spec 62:49–52, 2000.
3. Cogswell LK, Goodacre TE: The management of nasoseptal perforation. Br J Plast Surg 53:117–120, 2000.
4. Grymer LF, Bosch C: The nasal septum and the development of the midface. A longitudinal study of a pair of monozygotic twins. Rhinology 35:6–10, 1997.
5. Isaksson M, Bruze M, Wihl JA: Contact allergy to budesonide and perforation of the nasal septum. Contact Dermatitis 37:133, 1997.
6. Lopatin AS: Do laws of biomechanics work in reconstruction of the cartilaginous nasal septum? Eur Arch Otorhinolaryngol 253:309–312, 1996.
7. Newman MH: Surgery of the nasal septum. Clin Plast Surg 23:271–279, 1996.
8. Passali D, Ferri R, Becchini G, et al: Alterations of nasal mucociliary transport in patients with hypertrophy of the inferior turbinates, deviations of the nasal septum and chronic sinusitis. Eur Arch Otorhinolaryngol 256:335–337, 1999.
9. Urquhart AC, Bersalona FB, Ejercito VS: Nasal septum after sublabial transseptal transsphenoidal pituitary surgery. Otolaryngol Head Neck Surg 115:64–69, 1996.
10. Van Loosen J, Van Zanten GA, Howard CV, et al: Growth characteristics of the human nasal septum. Rhinology 34:78–82, 1996.
11. Williams N: What are the causes of a perforated nasal septum? Occup Med (Oxford) 50(2):135–136, 2000.

19. RHINITIS

Bruce Murrow, M.D., Ph.D.

1. Define rhinitis.

Rhinitis is nasal **hyperfunction** and **tissue inflammation** that leads to nasal congestion, rhinorrhea, nasal obstruction, pruritus, and/or sneezing. Although rhinitis is generally not life-threatening, it is associated with significant loss of productivity and decreased quality of life.

2. What pathophysiology underlies rhinitis?

Nasal congestion arises from engorgement of blood vessels due to the effects of **vasoactive mediators** and **neural stimuli. Rhinorrhea** is due to hypersecretion of the nasal glands, leading to tissue transudate. The autonomic nervous system mediates both vascular tone and secretions. Sympathetic innervation constricts the vessels, decreasing secretions, while the parasympathetic innervation vasodilates the vessels, enhancing nasal secretions. **Pruritus** occurs in association with histamine release from mast cells and basophils secondary to antigenic stimulation

3. How is rhinitis categorized?

Rhinitis can be divided into *allergic* and *nonallergic* types.

ALLERGIC RHINITIS

4. Describe the allergic response in allergic rhinitis.

The *primary phase* involves a type 1 Gell and Coomb's type of hypersensitivity with the antigen binding to IgE receptors, causing mast cells and basophils to release mediators such as histamine, serotonin, leukotrienes, and prostaglandins. This phase occurs within 5 minutes of antigen exposure. The *late phase* (secondary phase) occurs 4–6 hours after antigen exposure and involves migration of inflammatory cells (neutrophils and eosinophils) and basophil release of mediators.

5. Which types of antigens cause allergic rhinitis?

In general, inhalants, foods, and chemicals cause allergic rhinitis. **Inhalants** usually produce an immediate response upon exposure and include pollens, animal dander, mold spores, and dust. Food allergies can be more difficult to diagnose. A **fixed food allergy** causes symptoms each time the food is ingested, whereas a **cyclic food allergy** is based on the amount and frequency of the allergen consumed.

6. What are the "allergic salute" and "allergic shiners"?

Patients (particularly children) with persistent rhinorrhea often wipe the nose in a upward direction with the palm of the hand, which has been referred to as the "allergic salute." Consequently, these patients may have a horizontal crease in the skin of the lower nose by the tip. Also, patients with allergic rhinitis can have darkened areas under their eyes, which are referred to as "allergic shiners."

7. Describe the treatment of allergic rhinitis.

Treatment includes avoidance of the stimulus, pharmacologic agents, and immunotherapy. **Avoidance** of the offending antigen is most applicable with food allergies and chemical allergies. **Pharmacotherapy** includes antihistamines (block the effects of released histamine), topical or systemic sympathomimetics (decongest the nasal tissue), cromolyn sodium (stabilize mast cell membranes), and topical or systemic corticosteroids (reduce inflammation). **Immunotherapy** involves injecting the offending antigen into the patient. This therapy is thought to decrease the serum levels of IgE, increase IgG antibody ("blocking antibody"), decrease sensitivity of hista-mine-releasing cells, and decrease responsiveness of lymphocytes. However, the specific mech-anism behind the relief of immunotherapy is unknown.

8. What complications are associated with allergic rhinitis?

Poorly controlled symptoms of allergic rhinitis can lead to a surprising amount of disability, with reported 3.5 million workdays lost and 2 million school days missed. Consequences include sleep loss with daytime somnolence, significant cognitive disability, and reduced quality of life. Children in particular can suffer psychosocial detriment and learning difficulties. Subsequent pathologies can evolve, including sinusitis, otitis media with hearing loss, abnormal craniofacial abnormalities, and/or aggravation of asthma. Some treatments for allergic rhinitis may also indirectly contribute to lack of productivity, such as first-generation H_1 antihistamines that unfortunately are sedating.

9. Describe the natural history of allergic rhinitis.

Allergic rhinitis symptoms often begin in childhood and adolescence. With increasing age, in general, symptoms and skin reactivity decrease. There also is a trend toward a greater chance of improvement with a younger age of onset.

NONALLERGIC RHINITIS

10. What are the causes of nonallergic rhinitis?.

Pharmacologic (rhinitis medicamentosa)
Hormonal
Irritative
Atrophic
Structural
Infectious
Substance abuse (cocaine, alcohol, nicotine).
Emotions
Temperature
Exercise
Recumbency
Trauma
Foreign bodies
Decreased nasal airflo states (post-laryngectomy or tracheostomy)
Systemic diseases (Wegener's granulomatosis, sarcoid, superior vena cava syndrome, and
  Horner's syndrome)
Idiopathic (vasomotor rhinitis, eosinophilic or basophilic nonallergic rhinitis)

11. How does the effect of irritants in nonallergic rhinitis differ from an allergic response?

Dust, gases (formaldehyde), chemicals, and air pollution (smoke, sulfur dioxide) can cause nasal congestion and rhinorrhea via direct irritative effects on the mucosa. In contrast, an allergic response is due to interaction with IgE antibodies and histamine-releasing cells.

12. Describe the endocrine or hormonal causes of nonallergic rhinitis.

Pregnancy, menstruation, and oral contraceptive use can all cause nasal congestion. The in-creased estrogen levels associated with these states inhibit acetylcholinesterase, leading to in-creased parasympathetic tone and tissue edema. Hypothyroidism is also associated with rhinitis. In this state, parasympathetic activity predominates over the hypoactive sympathetic state, caus-ing vasodilation of the nasal mucosa.

13. Name some structural abnormalities that can cause rhinitis.

Deviated nasal septums
Nasal valve collapse
Polyps
Neoplasms (e.g., papilloma, angiofibroma, malignancy)
Intranasal and extranasal deformities

14. What is atrophic rhinitis?

Atrophic rhinitis, or **ozena,** is associated with atrophy of the nasal mucosa and turbinates in association with excessive crusting and mucopurulent discharge. This socially debilitating condition is marked by an extremely foul odor that can be easily detected by others. Patients often complain of epistaxis, nasal obstruction, headaches, and the foul smell. Although the cause is unknown, hereditary, infectious, developmental, nutritional, and endocrine factors have been implicated. Atrophic rhinitis may also be iatrogenic, as it may be associated with excessive turbinate resection. Although no cure exists, treatment revolves around frequent saline irrigation and topical antibiotics. Surgical options have been aimed at narrowing the nasal cavity and nostril.

15. What is vasomotor rhinitis?

Vasomotor rhinitis is idiopathic nasal congestion and rhinorrhea that is not associated with sneezing or pruritus. After other causes of the rhinitis are ruled out, it becomes a diagnosis of exclusion. In this disorder, autonomic imbalance with parasympathetic predominance causes vasodilation and hyperresponsive glands.

16. What is rhinitis medicamentosa?

Rhinitis medicamentosa is drug-induced rhinitis that is due to rebound nasal congestion. It is most often associated with prolonged use of topical decongestants. It is thought that a semi-ischemic state is induced by the strong vasoconstrictive effect of topical decongestants. With time, this effect leads to the metabolic accumulation of vasodilators that are responsible for the rebound vasodilation. The condition can become irreversible with the development of vascular atony. Also, benzylalkonian chloride, a preservative in some vasoconstrictor preparations, can cause mucosal irritation, decreased mucoilliary clearance via ciliostasis, and exasperate rhinitis medicamentosa.

17. How long should topical decongestants be continuously used for symptomatic relief of rhinitis?

Because of the risk of rhinitis medicamentosa, topical decongestants should not be used for more than 3–5 days.

18. How is rhinitis medicamentosa treated?

Topical decongestants should be completely discontinued. Systemic decongestants and nasal saline spray can be substituted for symptomatic relief. The cause of the nasal congestion should be specifically treated (i.e., allergy, structural problem, infection). Topical steroids can be use to lessen the congestion of withdrawl of the vasoconstrictor. Care should be taken in restarting topical vasoconstrictors because rebound problems can recur faster.

19. Describe the medical treatment of nonallergic rhinitis.

In general, treatment should be directed toward the specific cause of the rhinitis (e.g., removal of the offending agent, correction of the hormonal problem, treatment of infection). Symptomatic treatment includes the use of antihistamines, sympathomimetic agents (topical or systemic), anticholinergics, and steroids as appropriate.

20. How do antihistamines aid in the treatment of chronic rhinitis?

Antihistamines act by blocking H1 receptor sites, thereby interfering with basophil and mast cell histamine release. Although the first-generation antihistamines are associated with drowsiness, the newer antihistamines are nonsedating.

21. How do sympathomimetics aid in the treatment of chronic rhinitis?

Sympathomimetics are decongestants that can be orally administered (e.g., ephedrine, pseudoephedrine, phenylpropanolamine) or topically administered (e.g., oxymetazoline, phenylephrine). Side effects of oral decongestants include nervousness, insomnia, irritability, and difficulty urinating. They should be avoided in patients with hypertension, cardiac arrhythmias, or glaucoma. Although topical decongestants are potent, their duration of use must be limited secondary to rebound decongestion.

22. What is the role of ipratropium bromide in the treatment of rhinitis?

Ipratropium bromide is a topical anticholinergic agent that antagonizes the effect of acetylcholine at parasympathetically innervated submucosal glands. It is effective in reducing mucosal gland hypersecretion that causes rhinorrhea. Systemic side effects are limited because of poor absorption topically. Unlike topical vasoconstrictors, ipratropium bromide does not exhibit rebound effects.

23. How do steroids aid in treating chronic rhinitis?

Corticosteroids can be given topically or orally, but oral agents are limited by suppression of the hypothalamic-pituitary-adrenal axis. Topical steroids decrease local inflammation caused by vasoactive mediators, decrease rhinorrhea by reducing the reactivity of acetylcholine receptors, decrease basophil and eosinophil counts, and decrease sneezing by desensitizing irritant receptors. Allergic and nonallergic rhinitis (including vasomotor rhinitis, hypothyroid-related rhinitis, and polyposis) are effectively treated with topical corticosteroids. Short-duration systemic steroids are useful as initial decongestants in cases of severe obstruction or polyposis.

24. What are the side effects of corticosteroids when they are used to treat rhinitis?

Systemic corticosteroids can suppress the hypothalamic-pituitary-adrenal axis. The newer topical steroids, in general, are thought to be free of this problem at their recommended dosages. However, nasal steroids can cause mucosal edema, mild erythema, burning, drying, and epistaxis.

25. Is treatment of rhinosinusitus and nasal polyps different in aspirin-sensitive patients?

Aspirin sensitivity in conjunction with rhinosinusitus and nasal polyps is referred to as triad asthma, aspirin triad, or Samter's syndrome. Overall, the treatment of this condition follows that for rhinosinusitus and nasal polyps with some important points. The severity of the disease is worse in patients with aspirin sensitivity. Topical steroids are particularly useful. Patients should avoid aspirin and nonsteroidal anti-inflammatory drugs. However, newer approaches have included the use of oral or nasal topical preparations of aspirin *after* desensitization has been undertaken, reportedly with improvement of chronic rhinosinusitus and decreased nasal polyps.

26. If chronic rhinitis is refractory to the usual medical modalities, what disorders should be further considered in the differential diagnosis?

Uncommon chronic conditions are likely to be referred to an otolaryngologist. Chronic infectious processes, such as tuberculosis, syphilis, and fungal rhinosinusitis, may lead to granulomas, ulceration, masses, or necrosis in the nose. In these cases, it is important to rule out neoplasia histologically. Tissue should also be stained and cultured for mycobacteria and fungi.

27. How is surgery useful in treating rhinitis?

Most surgical procedures are directed toward mechanical-obstructive issues to decrease nasal congestion and improve the penetration of topically applied medication. Surgeries include septoplasty for the repair of deviated septums, polypectomies, out-fracture of the inferior turbinates, and total or partial inferior turbinectomies. The inferior turbinates may also be treated with electrical/chemical cautery or cryosurgery. Cryosurgery of the inferior turbinates with vidian nerve sectioning has also provided relief from the secretory aspect of vasomotor rhinitis.

CONTROVERSIES

28. How should you approach treating allergic rhinitis in a pregnant patient?

In general, you should discuss with an obstetrician the safety of various treatments for pregnant patients. Many labels of over-the-counter medications for rhinitis warn of a potential risk, mostly because of the lack of studies and unknown safety profiles of the medications on the fetus. One review of the literature suggests that the first line of treatment include immunosuppresion, cromolyn, and beclomethasone; first-generation antihistamines are favored over second-generation ones because less is known of the safety profile on fetuses of the latter. Second line treatment may be considered to include oral/topical decongestants. In contrast, some practitioners do not recommend using immunotherapy (risk to the fetus in cases of rare anaphylaxis) or decongestants (possible effects on blood flow to the fetus). At the conservative extreme, some do not recommend any treatment beyond antigen avoidance and good nasal hygiene, including saline rinses.

29. What role may leukotrienes and their antagonists play in allergic rhinitis?

Although the literature is in its early infancy with respect to leukotriene involvement in allergic rhinitis, it appears that they may contribute with a primary effect on nasal vascularity, inducing nasal congestion and plasma exudates. Leukotriene antagonists may add to the treatment arsenal for allergic rhinitis, but further research is needed.

30. What is the role of corticosteroid turbinate injections in the treatment of rhinitis?

Injection of the inferior turbinate with a small-particle corticosteroid, such as triamcinolone (Kenalog), provides relief from chronic hypertrophy of the turbinates that is refractory to medical treatment. Opponents argue that turbinate injection, if intravascular, can lead to embolization/vasospasm of the orbital vessels and possible blindness. In addition, some patients do not experience long-term relief.

31. Should an inferior turbinectomy be utilized for treatment of rhinitis?

Some practitioners advocate a **total inferior turbinectomy,** because this procedure may provide relief of nasal congestion. Others argue that the relief is often not permanent. In addition, normal humidification and warming of inspired air is compromised. Postoperative bleeding can be problematic. This group argues that most patients have extensive nasal crusting, which is debilitating, and atrophic rhinitis can ensue. However, there are reports of minimal crusting complications and no atrophic rhinitis following **partial inferior turbinectomies** (anterior aspect).

32. What role does vidian neurectomy play in rhinitis?

The vidian nerve carries sympathetic and parasympathetic supply to the nasal mucosa. In medically refractory cases of vasomotor rhinitis, sectioning of this nerve can relieve hypersecretion in $> 90\%$ of cases. Other practitioners argue that serious risks of this procedure include ophthalmoplegia, decreased lacrimation, and paresthesias.

NITRIC OXIDE

Nitric oxide (NO), a substance with many important physiologic functions, including bacteriostasis and stimulating ciliary beat rate, is produced in remarkably large quantities from epithelial cells in the maxillary sinuses. NO is reported to be locally increased in allergic rhinitis but decreased in chronic sinusitis and Kartagener's syndrome, indicating an important role as a regulator of mucociliary function. High levels of NO increase ciliary beat frequency, wheras low levels are correlated to ciliary dysfunction.

~Kennedy, Diseases of the Sinuses, 2001

―――――▷●◁―――――

BIBLIOGRAPHY

1. Bernstein L: Is the use of benzalkonium chloride as a preservative for nasal formulations a safety concern? A cautionary note based on compromised mucociliary transport. J Allerg Clin Immunol 105(1 pt 1): 39–44, 2000.
2. Blaiss MS: Cognitive, social, and economic costs of allergic rhinitis. Allergy Asthma Proc 21(1):7–13, 2000.
3. Corren J: Allergic rhinitis: Treating the adult. J Allergy Clin Immunol 105(6 pt 2): S610–615. 2000.
4. Cummings CW, Frederickson JM, Harker LA (eds.): Otolaryngology: Head & Neck Surgery, 3rd ed. St. Louis, Mosby-Year Book 1998.
5. Fireman P: Therapeutic approaches to allergic rhinitis: Treating the child. J Allergy Clin Immunol 105(6 Pt 2):S616–621, 2000.
6. Howarth PH: Leukotrienes in rhinitis. Am J Resp Crit Care Med 161(2 Pt 2):S133–136, 2000.
7. Kowalski ML: Rhinosinusitis and nasal polyposis in aspirin sensitive and aspirin tolerant patients: Are they different? Thorax 55 (Suppl 2):S84–86, 2000.
8. Mazzotta P, et al: Treating allergic rhinitis in pregnancy. Safety considerations. Drug Saf 20(4): 361–375, 1999.
9. Mygind N, Dahl R, Bisgaard H: Leukotrienes, leukotriene receptor antagonists, and rhinitis. Allergy 55(5):421–424, 2000.
10. Pasha R: Otolaryngology Head and Neck Surgery. Clinical Reference Guide, Canada, Singular, 2000.
11. Schoenwetter WF: Allergic rhinitis: Epidemiology and natural history. Allergy Asthma Proc 21(1):1–6, 2000.
12. Settipane RA: Complications of allergic rhinitis. Allergy Asthma Proc 20(4):209–213. 1999.

20. SINUS ANATOMY AND FUNCTION

Lynnette C. Telck, M.S. III and Kent E. Gardner, M.D.

1. Name the paranasal sinuses and describe their location.

There are four pairs of paranasal sinuses: the frontal, maxillary, ethmoid, and sphenoid sinuses.

The **frontal sinuses** are located in the vertical portion of the frontal bone. They are pyramidal, with their base formed by the floor of the sinus. The apex of each sinus projects superiorly.

The **maxillary sinuses** occupy the body of the maxilla. They are bound medially by the lateral nasal wall, superiorly by the orbital floor, anteriorly by the canine fossa, and inferiorly by the alveolar process of the maxilla.

The **ethmoid sinuses** are located in the superior half of the lateral nasal wall. They are bound superiorly by the skull base in the region of the cribriform plate and laterally by the lamina papyracea, forming the medial wall of the orbit.

The **sphenoid sinuses** lie in the body of the sphenoid bone. They are surrounded posteriorly, superiorly, and laterally by important structures, including the pons, pituitary gland, carotid artery, optic nerve, and cavernous sinus. Anteroinferiorly, the sinus wall is exposed to the choanae and nasal cavity.

2. Describe the microanatomy of the paranasal sinuses.

The normally sterile paranasal sinuses are lined by ciliated pseudostratified columnar epithelium covered by a double-layered mucous blanket. The deep layer lubricates the cilia whereas the superficial layer captures foreign particles, which are transported by the cilia to the sinus ostium. Ciliary dysfunction or alterations in mucus composition can contribute to mucus stasis and subsequent sinusitis.

3. What are the uncinate process, hiatus semilunaris, and ethmoid infundibulum?

The **uncinate process** is a small thin piece of bone, covered by mucoperiosteum, that runs parallel and medial to the lateral nasal wall in the anterior middle meatus. Anteriorly and inferiorly, the bone is attached to the lateral nasal wall. The posterosuperior margin ends freely without attachment to other structures. This posterior margin is concave and runs parallel to the anterior surface of the ethmoid bulla. The two-dimensional trough formed by the gap between the ethmoid bulla and uncinate is known as the **hiatus semilunaris.** The hiatus semilunaris is the opening to the three-dimensional space bound medially by the uncinate process and laterally by the lateral nasal wall. This three-dimensional space is known as the **ethmoid infundibulum.** The frontal, anterior ethmoid, and maxillary sinuses all usually drain into the infundibulum and then out through the hiatus semilunaris.

4. What is the osteomeatal complex?

The osteomeatal complex is a term used to describe the region made up of the uncinate process, maxillary ostium, middle turbinate, bulla ethmoidalis, and ethmoid infundibulum. The frontal, ethmoid, and maxillary sinuses all drain through this area, which contains very narrow clefts. Any mucosal thickening or congenital variation is likely to produce obstruction, stasis, and recurrent infection of the "upstream" sinuses. Functional endoscopic sinus surgery (FESS) is based on the concept that the osteomeatal complex, also known as the osteomeatal unit, must be cleaned to restore and enhance normal sinus drainage.

5. Where do each of the sinuses drain into the nasal cavity?

Each paranasal sinus communicates with the nasal cavity through an opening known as an **ostium.** The ostium of the frontal sinus opens into the frontal recess in the anterior portion of the middle meatus. It may drain directly into the ethmoid infundibulum lateral to the uncinate process, or medial to the uncinate if the uncinate process inserts into the lamina papyracea. The ostium of the maxillary sinus is located in the ethmoid infundibulum of the middle meatus. The ostia of the ethmoid sinuses are inconsistent in location. Anterior ethmoid cells generally drain into the ethmoid infundibulum or in the region of the ethmoid bulla. Posterior ethmoid cells drain into the superior meatus. The ostium of the sphenoid sinus opens into the sphenoethmoidal recess above the superior concha.

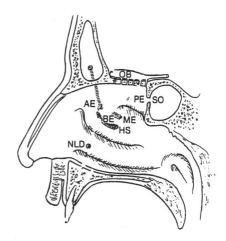

Sagittal section of the head illustrating position of ostia of paranasal sinuses. *OB,* olfactory bulb; *SO,* sphenoid ostium; *PE,* posterior ethmoidal ostium; *ME,* middle ethmoidal ostium; *BE,* ethmoidal bulla; *HS,* hiatus semilunaris; *AE,* anterior ethmoidal ostium; *NLD,* nasolacrimal duct (From Cummings CW, et al (eds): Otolaryngology–Head and Neck Surgery, 3rd ed. St. Louis. Mosby, 1998, with permission.)

6. Describe the development of the maxillary sinuses.

The maxillary sinus is the first to develop in the human fetus. Initial pneumatization is seen during the 65–70th day of fetal life. At birth, this sinus is 4–7 mm in diameter. Further growth of the maxillary sinus is biphasic. The first growth spurt occurs from birth until 3 years of age. At the end of this growth spurt, the floor of the sinus lies approximately 4–5 mm above the nasal floor. The second spurt occurs from 7 years of age until adolescence. By adolescence, the sinus lies 3–4 mm below the level of the nasal floor. Later in adult life, the sinus floor may be 5–10 mm below the nasal floor, and the roots of the second maxillary premolar and first and second maxillary molars may break through into the sinus cavity. The average volume of the adult maxillary sinus is 14.75 ml.

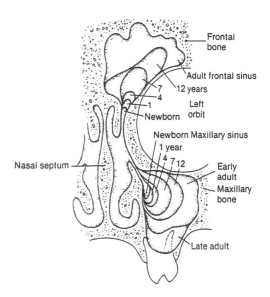

Developmental stages of maxillary frontal sinuses. (From Cummings CW, et al (eds): Otolaryngology–Head and Neck Surgery, 3rd ed. St. Louis, Mosby, 1998, with permission.)

7. Describe the development of the frontal sinuses.

Frontal sinus pneumatization begins during the 4th month of fetal life as an upward extension in the region of the frontal recess. At birth, it is not clinically significant and cannot be distinguished from the anterior ethmoid cells. At about 2–4 years of age, the sinus begins to invade the vertical portion of the frontal bone. At 6 years of age, it is visible radiographically. At 12 years, the sinus is quite large. During the teens, the sinus becomes fully developed, with a volume of 6–7 ml. Frontal sinus development is extremely variable, and approximately 5% of the population has at least one undeveloped frontal sinus.

8. Describe the development of the ethmoid sinuses.

Ethmoid sinus development begins during the 3rd or 4th month of fetal development. Ethmoid cells are classified into anterior and posterior divisions based on the cells' location relative to the ground lamella of the middle turbinate. Anterior ethmoid cells develop from the lateral nasal wall in the region of the middle meatus. Posterior ethmoid cells begin as evaginations of the lateral nasal wall in the region of the superior meatus. At birth, three or four cells are usually present. The ethmoid and maxillary sinuses are the only sinuses at birth that are large enough to be of clinical significance. Through childhood, the sinuses continue to grow until age 12 when they reach adult size. An average adult ethmoid sinus has 10–15 cells with a total volume of 15 ml.

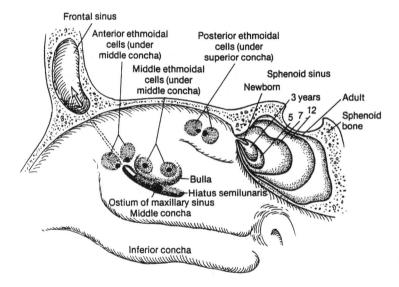

Developmental stages of the ethmiod and sphenoid sinuses. (From Cummings CW, et al (eds): Otolaryngology–Head and Neck Surgery, 3rd ed. St. Louis, Mosby, 1998, with permission.)

9. How does the sphenoid sinus develop?

Sphenoid sinus development begins in the 4th month of fetal development as an evagination of the nasal mucosa in the posterior nasal cavity. At birth, there is no clinically significant sphenoid sinus. Significant further development begins after the 5th year of life. By age 7, the sinus has extended posteriorly to the sella turcica. Its final volume of 7.5 ml is usually attained by 12–15 years of life.

10. Which arteries supply each of the paranasal sinuses?

The frontal sinus is supplied by the supraorbital and supratrochlear arteries. The maxillary sinus is supplied predominantly by branches of the maxillary artery, with some contribution from the facial artery. The ethmoid sinus receives contributions from the sphenopalatine artery and anterior and posterior ethmoid arteries. The sphenoid sinus receives input predominantly from the sphenopalatine and posterior ethmoid arteries.

11. Describe the course of the sphenopalatine artery.

The sphenopalatine artery is a branch of the internal maxillary artery. It enters the nasal cavity through the sphenopalatine foramen just posterior to the middle turbinate in the sphenoethmoidal recess. It then divides into two main branches. The first branch passes across the inferior aspect of the face of the sphenoid sinus to supply the septum. It can cause significant hemorrhage if violated during sphenoidotomy. The second branch supplies the lateral wall of the nose.

12. Where are the anterior and posterior ethmoid arteries located?

These arteries are branches of the ophthalmic artery in the orbital cavity. They leave the orbital cavity through the anterior and posterior ethmoid foramina. These foramina occur on the medial wall of the orbit at or just superior to the frontoethmoid suture line. The anterior ethmoid foramen is usually located 14–22 mm posterior to the maxillolacrimal suture line. The location of the posterior ethmoid foramen is more variable, but it is usually 3–13 mm posterior to the anterior ethmoid foramen. The anterior and posterior arteries lie at the level of the ethmoid sinus roof and are helpful landmarks during external ethmoidectomy.

13. What is the innervation of each of the paranasal sinuses?

The paranasal sinuses are predominantly innervated by the sensory branches of the trigeminal nerve. Sensory innervation of the frontal sinus mucosa is via the supraorbital and supratrochlear nerves. Sensory innervation of the maxillary sinus is via multiple branches of the maxillary nerve, including the greater palatine, posterolateral nasal, and superior alveolar branches of the infraorbital nerve. Postganglionic parasympathetic secretomotor fibers from the pterygopalatine ganglion also supply the mucosa of the maxillary sinus. The ethmoid sinuses receive innervation from both the ophthalmic and the maxillary divisions of the trigeminal nerve. The anterior cells are supplied by the anterior ethmoid nerve. The posterior cells are supplied by the posterior ethmoid nerve and the sphenopalatine nerve. The sphenoid sinus is supplied by the posterior ethmoid nerve and the sphenopalatine nerve.

14. What is the functional significance of the sinuses?

Many theories exist about the possible functional significance of the sinuses, including humidification and warming of inspired air, lightening of the weight of the skull, improving vocal resonance, absorption of shock to the face or skull, increasing the area of the olfactory membrane, regulation of intranasal pressure, and secretion of mucus to keep the nasal chambers moist. However, all of these theories have flaws. The real functional significance of the sinuses is unknown.

15. What type of cells form the lining of the paranasal sinuses?

The paranasal sinuses are lined with **ciliated, pseudostratified, columnar epithelial** cells. Also, numerous mucoserous glands and goblet cells produce the mucous blanket that lines the sinuses. This lining consists of two layers. The first layer is the inner serous layer, or sol phase, in which the cilia beat. The second layer is a more viscous layer, or gel phase. The gel phase is transported by the beat of the cilia toward the sinus ostia.

16. Discuss the pattern of mucous clearance or secretion from the maxillary sinus.

In the maxillary sinus, secretion transport starts from the floor of the sinus in a **stellate pattern.** The mucus is transported along the anterior, medial, posterior, and lateral walls of the sinuses as well as along the roof. All of the secretions converge at the natural ostium of the maxillary sinus. After secretions leave the sinus ostium, they flow out the middle meatus over the medial aspect of the posterior inferior turbinate and into the nasopharynx.

17. How is the mucus cleared or secreted from the frontal sinus?

The frontal sinus has a flow of secretions both into and out of the sinus. Inward flow begins on the medial aspect of the sinus ostium. This flow continues superiorly and then laterally along the roof of the frontal sinus. Next, secretions are transported back toward the ostium along the floor of the sinus as well as along the inferior aspect of the anterior and posterior sinus walls. Secretions then flow out the nasofrontal duct and into the ethmoid infundibulum. These secretions then merge with the secretions of the maxillary sinuses and are transported out through the nasopharynx.

18. What factors can lead to inadequate drainage of sinus secretions?

Normal clearance of sinus secretions requires normal secretion and transport mechanisms. The secretion mechanism involves the amount and consistency of the mucus produced. A normal transport mechanism requires normal mucosal cilia, normal ciliary beat, and a patent sinus ostia or drainage opening. Factors that influence the secretion and transport mechanisms include environmental pollution, humidity, other airborne external irritants, parasympathetic nerve fibers, and neuromediators.

19. Where do you find agger nasi cells? What is their significance?

Agger nasi cells are the most anterior of the anterior ethmoid cells. These cells are located at the agger ridge, just anterior to the anterosuperior attachment of the middle turbinate. They are in close proximity to the frontal recess. The surgeon often opens the agger nasi cells during endoscopic sinus surgery to get a better view of the nasofrontal duct. They also can occasionally obstruct outflow from the frontal sinus.

20. What are Haller cells?

Haller cells are ethmoid cells that have extended into the maxillary sinus and are adherent to the roof of the maxillary sinus in the region of the maxillary sinus ostium. Haller cells occur in 10% of the population. They can be asymptomatic or can have a negative influence on maxillary sinus ventilation and drainage, leading to recurrent or chronic sinusitis.

21. What is an Onodi cell? What structure can lie within an Onodi cell?

Onodi cells are posterior ethmoid cells that extend posteriorly, either laterally or superiorly, along the sphenoid sinus. The optic nerve can lie *within* an Onodi cell. These cells should be recognized prior to endoscopic sinus surgery to avoid injury to the optic nerve on posterior dissection of the ethmoids.

22. What is the clinical significance of a concha bullosa?

The term concha bullosa refers to the pneumatization of the middle turbinate. Approximately 30% of the population have concha bullosa, and in most circumstances, these are asymptomatic. If the drainage system of the concha bullosa itself becomes obstructed, it can become symptomatic and require surgical drainage. Also, the concha bullosa is associated with enlargement of the middle turbinate. This enlarged turbinate is felt to have a negative effect on paranasal sinus ventilation and mucociliary clearance in the osteomeatal complex. To relieve the obstruction, either one wall of the concha or the entire concha bullosa must be removed surgically.

23. Where is the grand (basal) lamella?

The grand lamella is the bony insertion of the middle turbinate into the skull base and lateral nasal wall. This landmark is used to differentiate anterior from posterior ethmoid cells. The grand lamella can be divided into thirds. The anterior third inserts directly into the lamina cribosa. The middle third inserts into the lamina papyracea and runs in an oblique anterosuperior to posteroinferior course. The posterior third inserts into the lateral nasal wall and runs in a horizontal direction.

24. What is the relationship of the face of the sphenoid sinus to the nasal sill?

The face of the sphenoid sinus lies 7 cm from the nasal sill at a 30-degree angle with the floor of the nasal cavity.

25. What anatomic computed tomographic (CT) landmarks do you look for in the frontal sinuses?

Make sure the air cells are pneumatized and well aerated bilaterally, the interfrontal septum is intact, the frontoethmoidal recesses is patent, and the fovea ethmoidalis is normal.

26. What anatomic CT landmarks do you look for in the ethmoidal sinuses?

Make sure the air cells are pneumatized and well aerated bilaterally, and pay specific attention to the agger nasi and the bulla ethmoidalis.

27. What anatomic CT landmarks do you look for in the maxillary sinuses?

Make sure the antra is pneumatized and well aerated bilaterally and that the anterior ostiomeatal units are patent.

28. What anatomic CT landmarks do you look for in the sphenoidal sinuses?

Make sure the air cells are pneumatized and well aerated bilaterally, the posterior ostiomeatal units are patent, and the intersphenoidal septum is intact.

29. What anatomic CT landmarks do you look for in the perisinus anatomy?

The posterior nasal septum should be midline. The nasal mucosa should be normal, and the crista galli and cribriform plate should be intact. Look for any thickening or erosion of the osseous structures.

30. When imaging the sinuses, why is high-resolution computed tomography preferred to plain radiographs?

The plain radiographs, unlike the CT scan, do not allow adequate evaluation of the ostiomeatal complex or of the sphenoid and ethmoid sinuses due to overlapping anatomic structures.

CONTROVERSIES

31. What is an accessory ostium? Is it an effective drain of the maxillary sinus?

In addition to the natural maxillary sinus ostium, one or more accessory sinus ostia can be located in the lateral nasal wall. There is some controversy as to whether these accessory ostia are effective drainage sites for sinus secretions. Accessory ostia can be quite large. However, studies have shown that the mucous blanket tends to bypass the accessory ostium and leave through the natural ostium. This is thought to occur secondary to the natural beat of all cilia in the maxillary sinus toward the natural ostium. For the same reason, nasoantral windows surgically placed in the inferior meatus tend to be less effective at improving sinus drainage than nasoantral windows made at the natural ostium, assuming that the ciliary beat is still effective.

32. Is the correct term "osteomeatal" or "ostiomeatal"?

Actually, either spelling is correct. Some use *osteo-*, referring to the bone. Others argue that *ostio-* is the proper prefix, referring to the ostium, or meatal opening.

PARANASAL SINUS ANATOMY

The anatomy of the paranasal sinuses is complex and varies widely from patient to patient. Understanding this anatomy and resultant function is, however, essential for otolaryngologists who wish to achieve optimal surgical (and medical) results and to avoid surgical complications.

~Kennedy, Diseases of the Sinuses, 2001

BIBLIOGRAPHY

1. Chong VF, Fan YF, Lau D, et al: Functional endoscopic sinus surgery (FESS): What radiologists need to know, Clin Radiol 53:650–658, 1998.
2. Cole P: Physiology of the nose and paranasal sinuses. Clin Rev Allergy Immunol 16:25–54, 1998.
3. Graney DO, Rice DH: Paranasal sinuses: Anatomy. In Cummings CW (ed): Otolaryngology—Head and Neck Surgery, 3rd ed. St. Louis, Mosby, 1998.
4. Illum L: Transport of drugs from the nasal cavity to the central nervous system. Eur J Pharmaceut Sci 11:1–18, 2000.
5. Jorissen M, Hermans R, Bertrand B, et al: Anatomical variations and sinusitis. Acta Otorhinolaryngol Belg 51:219–226, 1997.
6. Krouse JH: Introduction to sinus disease: I. Anatomy and physiology. Otorhinolaryngol Head Neck Nurs 17:7–12, 1999.
7. Nayak S: Radiologic anatomy of the paranasal air sinuses. Semin Ultrasound CT MR 20:354–378, 1999.
8. Rao VM, el-Noueam KI: Sinonasal imaging: Anatomy and pathology. Radiol Clin North Am 36:921–939, vi, 1998.
9. Watelet JB, Van Cauwenberge P: Applied anatomy and physiology of the nose and paranasal sinuses. Allergy 54 (Suppl 57):14–25, 1999.
10. Yanagisawa E, Christmas DA: The value of computer-aided (image-guided) systems for endoscopic sinus surgery, Ear Nose Throat J 78:822–824, 826, 1999.
11. Zeifer B: Update on sinonasal imaging: Anatomy and inflammatory disease. Neuroimag Clin North Am 8:607–630, 1998.
12. Zeifer B: Pediatric sinonasal imaging: Normal anatomy and inflammatory disease. Neuroimag Clin North Am 10:137–159, ix, 2000.

21. SINUSITIS

Gresham Richter, M.D., Bruce W. Jafek, M.D., FACS, FRSM,
and Tyler M. Lewark, M.D.

1. Define sinusitis.

Sinusitis is inflammation of the mucosal lining of the paranasal sinuses secondary to both infectious and allergic mechanisms. The term *rhinosinusitis* is probably more correct and stresses the importance of nasal mucosal pathology on the overall disease process.

2. What is the epidemiology of sinusitis?

Sinusitis accounts for nearly 5% of physician visits and affects more than 31 million people annually. It is the fifth most common diagnosis for which antibiotics are prescribed, accounting for 7–12% of all antibiotic prescriptions written. This primary diagnosis leads to an annual expenditure of almost $3.39 billion in the United States and accounts for 11.6 million office visits per year.

3. What is the pathophysiology of sinusitis?

The retention of sinus secretions is the single most important event in the development of sinusitis. This creates a favorable milieu for the growth of infectious agents (most often bacteria) and may be caused by the following:

Obstruction or narrowing of sinus ostia. Mucosal edema (secondary to viral upper respiratory tract infection [URI] or allergic inflammation) and anatomic variants contribute to the majority of narrowed ostia. Bacterial growth is further favored by lowered oxygen tension and decreased pH created in obstructed sinuses.

Mucociliary dysfunction. Mucus hypersecretion and the release of inflammatory mediators in response to allergens, viruses, or bacteria can impair ciliary motility and mucus drainage. This leads to mucosal edema, ostia obstruction, further loss of ciliary function, and subsequent mucus retention. Specific ciliary and mucosal insults include cold air, viral and bacterial ciliotoxins, cytokines, irritants, pollutants, and surgery.

Changes in mucus composition. Increased viscosity and/or decreased elasticity of sinus mucus inhibits normal clearing of these secretions and aids bacterial accumulation.

Recently, mucus recirculation and osteitis have been proposed to contribute to the pathophysiology of chronic sinusitis. In **mucus recirculation,** secretions can re-enter the maxillary sinus by commonly present accessory sinus ostia (20% of cases) and lead to mucous accumulation. **Osteitis** has been described in the ethmoid bone of patients with chronic sinusitis with changes that resemble osteomyelitis. This suggests that residual bone infection may account for sinusitis recurrence.

4. Which sinus is most often involved in sinusitis and why?

Ninety percent of sinus infections involve the **maxillary sinus.** The narrow ostiomeatal complex and its association with frontal and ethmoid sinus ostia contribute to easy obstruction and spread of infection into the maxillary sinuses.

5. What are the predisposing factors of sinusitis?

The most common cause of acute bacterial sinusitis is recurrent viral URIs. Extension of apical dental infections can also cause sinusitis. Nonetheless, predisposing factors of acute or chronic sinusitis are related to events leading to retained secretions.

Obstruction of sinus ostia. Mucosal edema (due to URI, allergy, pregnancy, or barotrauma) and anatomic abnormalities can impede sinus drainage. Anatomic abnormalities include nasal polyps, septal deviation, paradoxically curved middle turbinate, uncinate process deviation, Haller's cells, and overhanging ethmoidal bulla. Midface trauma (altering the osteomeatal complex), foreign bodies, nasal packing, nasal tubes, nasal tumors, and choanal atresia are also associated with impaired sinus outflow and subsequent sinusitis.

Mucociliary dysfunction. Medications, drugs, infectious toxins, inflammatory mediators, environmental pollutants, chronic disease, malnutrition, and surgery can lead to ciliated epithelial cell loss or decreased ciliary beat frequency and coordination. Primary ciliary dyskinesia may also be congenital, as in Kartagener's and Young's syndromes.

Changes in mucus composition. Cystic fibrosis, dehydration, chronic disease, pollutants, and irritants can affect mucus composition by altering water and electrolyte transport.

Factors predisposing to **fungal sinusitis** may be related to **immune deficiency,** but a more common type is now described, often accompanied by allergic mucin, containing a preponderance of eosinophils. Fungal sinusitis in the immunologically incompetent patient is often life threatening.

Iatrogenic factors have become increasingly important due to mechanical ventilation, nasogastric tubes, nasotracheal tubes, and nasal packing.

Other predisposing factors include allergy, foreign body, dental procedures, and barotrauma. Less common causes of sinusitis include trauma and mucosal edema associated with pregnancy.

6. What systemic factors predispose patients to sinusitis?

Systemic factors that cause metabolic depletion predispose patients to sinusitis. These include uncontrolled diabetes, malnutrition, long-term steroid use, chemotherapy, and blood dyscrasias. Patients with abnormal antibody production to bacteria are also predisposed to sinus infections and include those with selective IgA deficiency and common variable hypogammaglobinemia (IgG deficiency). Human immunodeficiency virus (HIV) patients have an increased incidence of acute sinusitis.

7. What percentages of acquired immunodeficiency syndrome (AIDS) patients develop sinusitis?

HIV-positive patients are susceptible to bacterial infection due to deficits in cell-mediated and humoral immunity. Thus, this leads to impaired mucociliary function and chronic sinusitis in approximately 80% of patients with AIDS. Causative pathogens are similar to those for immunocompetent patients. However, *Cryptococcus neoformans,* cytomegalovirus, *Pseudomonas aeruginosa* , and fungal species also are found. Sinusitis is difficult to manage in these patients.

8. How do allergies predispose a patient to sinusitis?

Mucus hypersecretion caused by cytokines released during upper respiratory allergic reactions contribute to mucosal edema, nasal polyp formation, and turbinate hypertrophy. This inflammation likely leads to ostia obstruction and mucous stasis in acute sinusitis. However, the relationship between allergies and sinusitis is still unclear.

9. How is sinusitis classified?

Sinusitis is classified by duration of symptoms, anatomic site, infectious agent, and presence of extrasinus involvement (complicated or uncomplicated). *Acute, subacute,* and *chronic* sinusitis refer to symptom duration lasting < 4 weeks, 4 weeks to 3 months, and > 3 months, respectively.

10. Describe the symptoms of acute bacterial sinusitis.

The early symptoms of acute sinusitis may be difficult to distinguish from those of the common cold or allergic rhinitis. However, pain (headache, nasal, or facial), nasal obstruction, mucopurulent nasal discharge (if ostia patent), history of previous URI, poor response to decongestants, tachycardia, fever, malaise, and lethargy are common to acute sinusitis. The location of pain is related to the sinus involved: ethmoid→medial nose or retro-orbital pain; sphenoid→occipital, vertex, or parietal headaches, maxillary→suborbital tenderness; and frontal→frontal headaches and tenderness. Dental pain is common in maxillary sinusitis.

In children, symptoms are less specific. Persistent nasal congestion and cough ($>$ 7 days), high fever, purulent nasal discharge, halitosis, low-grade fever, and mild periorbital edema probably indicate sinusitis. Pain is not a common feature in childhood disease.

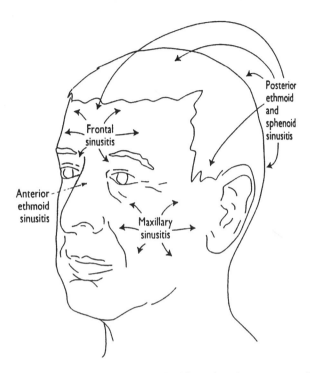

Sites of referred pain from the sinuses. (From Evans KL: Diagnosis and management of sinusitis. BMJ 309:1416, 1994, with permission.)

11. How do the symptoms of chronic bacterial sinusitis differ from those of acute sinusitis?

In both children and adults, systemic symptoms and pain are often absent whereas mucopurulent discharge and mild nasal obstruction occur in chronic sinusitis. Patients may also complain of persistent cough, foul taste, wheezing, and laryngitis due to postnasal secretions. Severe morning headaches can affect half of the patients with chronic sinusitis. Many children also have an associated chronic or recurrent otitis media.

12. What are the signs of acute and chronic bacterial sinusitis?

Nasal mucosal edema and erythema, sinus or tooth tenderness to palpation, malodorous breath, postnasal discharge, and periorbital edema are often present in patients with sinusitis. The middle turbinate may be red and swollen, and the uncinate process prominent. Pus emerging from middle meatus is often diagnostic. Signs of an infected posterior sinus include superior nasal hyperemia and pus near the posterior end of the middle turbinate or descending from the sphenoethmoid recess. Nasal anatomic abnormalities may also be present in cases of chronic sinusitis.

13. How does the clinician differentiate allergy-related (noninfectious) sinusitis from chronic sinusitis?

The typical patient with allergy-associated sinusitis reports a history of inhalant allergies. In this case, allergic skin testing is conducted after resolution of symptoms. However, predominant sinus signs and symptoms of allergic (noninfectious) sinusitis are bilateral nasal congestion, facial pressure, lack of sinus pain, postnasal drainage, hyposmia, bilateral musosal thickening and nasal polyps. Many allergic patients have associated asthma (50%) and aspirin sensitivity (30–40%). Sinus contents predominately reveal eosinophils and not neutrophils, as seen in chronic bacterial sinusitis.

14. What is Samter's triad?

Approximately 10% of patients with nasal polyposis have aspirin intolerance. This sensitivity generally applies to all nonsteroidal anitinflammatory drugs. This is more common in women and in adults. Different types of aspirin sensitivity have been observed, but the most frequent is the most dangerous: potentially fatal bronchospasm. Skin tests do not usually show reactions to seasonal or perennial allergens. There is currently no in vitro test for this sensitivity, and in vivo tests are complicated and may be fatal. Desensitization is being developed but is tedious and expensive. And it must be reversed for elective surgery; emergency surgery is, of course, much more risky because of increased bleeding. When the aspirin intolerance is associated with bronchial asthma and nasal polyposis, the syndrome is called **Samter's triad.** The associated chronic sinusitis is especially difficult to control.

15. What organisms are responsible for acute bacterial sinusitis?

Streptococcus pneumoniae, Haemophilus influenzae, and (in 20% of children) *Moraxella catarrhalis* cause the majority of community-acquired cases of acute sinusitis. β-lactamase-producing strains of these organisms has increased, with recent reports as high as 52% for *H. influenzae*. Anaerobic organisms, often from dental infections, also account for approximately 6–10% of cases and include *Fusobacterium, Peptostreptococcus,* and *Bacteroides.*

16. Which organisms are associated with chronic bacterial sinusitis?

The most common organisms found in chronic sinusitis are *Staphylococcus aureus,* coagulase-negative *Staphylococcus, Streptococcus* species, and anaerobic organisms (*Bacteroides, Fusobacterium,* and anaerobic cocci). In children with long-standing symptoms, both anaerobic and *Staphylococcus* species should be suspected. *Pseudomonas aeruginosa* commonly affects patients with nosocomial disease, imunocompromised patients, and cystic fibrosis patients.

17. Describe the categories of fungal sinusitis.

Fungal sinusitis includes both invasive and noninvasive categories. Mycetoma (a fungal ball) and allergic fungal sinusitis are noninvasive fungal diseases. Fulminant fungal sinusitis and indolent fungal sinusitis can invade through sinus walls but have different prognoses. Fulminant fungal sinusitis affects immunocompromised patients and is often fatal, whereas indolent fungal sinusitis is primarily a chronic disease of immunocompetent patients.

18. What organisms cause fungal sinusitis?

Aspergillus species are the most common cause of both noninvasive and invasive fungal sinusitis. Other organisms implicated in noninvasive cases include *Pseudallescheria boydii, Schizophyllum commune,* and *Alternaria* species.

19. What is allergic fungal sinusitis?

Allergic fungal sinusitis is an allergic and eosinophilic inflammatory response to a sinus fungal species and "represents an upper airway equivalent of allergic bronchopulmonary aspergillosis." Patients complain of chronic nasal obstruction, sinus pain, rhinnorhea, orbital symptoms, anosmia, and exacerbation of asthma. Nearly all patients have unilateral disease, nasal polyps, and evidence of "allergic mucin," a thick, green to brown mucous of butter-like quality laced with eosinophils and fungal hyphae. Diagnostic criteria include fungal atopy, nasal polyposis, computed tomographic (CT) scan with evidence of hyperdense sinus infiltrate, allergic mucin with eosinophils, and fungal identification. Allergic fungal sinusitis can erode sinus cavity walls but is noninvasive.

20. Discuss the differential diagnosis of sinusitis.

Nasal obstruction and discharge due to allergic, viral, or vasomotor rhinitis is often mistaken for sinusitis. Pain associated with sinusitis may be difficult to distinguish from that associated with dental disease, migraine or stress headaches, temporal arteritis, and trigeminal neuralgia. Pressure symptoms seen in sinusitis may also be caused by advancing cancer in nasal or paranasal cavities.

21. What techniques are used in diagnosing sinusitis? Discuss their significance.

Diagnosis of sinusitis is based largely on history and physical examination findings. However, frontal and maxillary sinus transillumination, nasal cultures, nasal endoscopy, plain film radiographs, ultrasonography, CT scans, magnetic resonance imaging (MRI), and direct sinus aspiration have all been used in the diagnosis of sinusitis. **Transillumination** and **nasal cultures** have mostly been abandoned because of questions about their reliability and clinical significance. **Nasal endoscopy** (rigid or flexible) is easily and commonly employed in the clinical setting because it can provide important information about the presence of purulent secretions, patency of sinus outflow tracts, nasal anatomy, and the extent of mucosal damage and edema. **Sinus aspiration** is the gold standard in evaluating sinus disease but this technique is often too invasive and impractical. **Radiography, ultrasonography, CT scans,** and **MRI** are useful imaging techniques for describing sinus anatomy, confirming sinusitis and following the resolution of disease. However, the predictive value of these techniques used alone in the diagnosis of sinusitis has been debated.

22. Are plain film radiographs helpful in evaluating sinusitis?

Yes. Plain films aid in confirming the diagnosis of acute sinusitis in patients with limited signs and symptoms. Air-fluid levels and sinus opacification are highly suggestive of sinus involvement, whereas a clear radiograph makes sinus pathology unlikely. However, the results of plain film radiography rarely change management and should not be used when history and physical examination clearly suggests sinus disease. Plain films are not useful in chronic disease.

23. Which views are employed in plain film radiography in evaluating sinusitis?

Waters (occipitomental), Caldwell (occipitofrontal), and lateral sinus films are most often used in evaluating acute sinusitis. However, some authors suggest that a single Waters view is sufficient for diagnosing acute sinusitis in cases involving the maxillary sinus (90% of cases with 87% positive predictive value).

24. When is a CT scan indicated in the evaluation of sinusitis?

The CT scan is the most sensitive technique in evaluating sinus disease. It is especially useful in defining bony landmarks and sinus abnormalities within the sphenoid and ethmoid sinuses where plain radiographs are less effective. However, because of cost and poor specificity (40% of normal subjects show some mucosal abnormality), CT scans should not be used routinely to diagnose acute sinusitis. Indications for CT evaluation include cases of chronic refractory sinusitis, suspected complicated disease (extrasinus involvement) and suspected malignancy. CT scans are also used to assess sinus anatomy before surgery.

25. Describe the advantages and disadvantages of MRI for evaluating sinusitis.

Advantages: MRI has superior soft-tissue resolution, as different signal intensities aid in distinguishing fungal sinusitis, sinus neoplasia, and intracranial extension from uncomplicated sinusitis. MRI also avoids the use of radiation and can therefore be used in children and pregnant patients.

Disadvantages: The ethmoid mucosa has a natural cycle of edema and shrinkage. During the edematous phase, the signal intensity of normal mucosa is indistinguishable from that of inflammatory disease and leads to false-positive results. Moreover, MRI resolution of bony landmarks is poor and prevents its use in planning endoscopic sinus surgery. High cost and poor patient tolerance of the procedure also limit its use.

26. Should your management of the immunocompromised patient with possible sinusitis differ from that for the immunocompetent patient?

Yes. The clinician needs to have a high index of suspicion when evaluating the immuno-compromised patient with possible sinusitis. Headache, facial pain, fever of unknown origin, and nasal crusting should prompt urgent evaluation of the sinuses. In addition, hospital admission with prompt initiation of treatment is indicated in patients with suspected sinusitis.

27. In a patient with very poor dentition and persistent sinusitis, what should be considered?

Sinusitis can result from periapical or periodontal disease. An oroantral fistula, often sec-ondary to molar extraction, may also lead to sinusitis. Symptoms of dental sinusitis include facial pain, swelling, tooth tenderness, and nasal or oral fistula discharge. The maxillary sinus may ap-pear opaque on plain films or CT scan. Antibiotic treatment should cover anaerobic organisms.

28. What are the potential complications of sinusitis? Which complication is most common and why?

Complications include disease extension into orbit or intracranial structures, osteomyelitis, oroantral fistula, visual changes, and mucocele formation. Each complication requires aggressive surgical and medical management. Orbital complications are most common, owing to easy ex-tension of infection along the thin sinus bone surrounding the orbit on three sides.

29. How are orbital complications classified?

Orbital complications are classified into five categories based on extent of invasion and in-jury of the orbit. The higher the classification the greater proptosis and impairment of extraocu-lar movement and visual acuity will occur.

Inflammatory Orbital Involvement by Sinusitis

Group 1	Inflammatory edema	Most common type. Upper eyelid is swollen without evidence of orbital infection. No visual acuity loss or limitation of extraocular movement.
Group 2	Orbital cellulitis	Inflammatory cells and bacteria diffusely invade orbit without forming abscess. Proptosis of globe results from inflammatory edema. Extraocular movement impaired. Chemosis present.
Group 3	Subperiosteal abscess	Pus collection at medial aspect of orbit between periorbital and bone. Globe displaced downward and laterally. Extraocular movement impaired. Visual acuity may be affected.
Group 4	Orbital abscess	Abscess formation within orbit. Severe proptosis and complete ophthalmoplegia. Visual acuity usually impaired, leading to possible irreversible blindness.
Group 5	Cavernous sinus thrombosis	Sepsis, chemosis, proptosis, orbital pain, ophthalmoplegia. Opposite eye may be affected through spread of infection through cavernous sinus.

30. Describe the intracranial complications of sinusitis.

Meningitis is usually regarded as the most common intracranial complication of sinusitis and arises from the sphenoid and/or ethmoid sinuses. Although now rare owing to early treatment, **epidural** and **subdural abscesses** are associated with frontal sinusitis. Fever and meningeal signs may be present with associated tenderness and swelling along the frontal sinus. A **brain abscess**

may also occur in the setting of sinusitis (approximately 15% of cases), carries a high mortality rate (20–30%), and is associated with frontal or ethmoid disease. Symptoms include headache and mild behavioral changes. **Venous sinus thrombosis** may occur during sinusitis. Valveless veins of the face, orbit, and sinuses allow for retrograde extension of infection. Both cavernous and sagittal sinus infiltrations may occur. Most patients recover with appropriate treatment; however, in advanced cases, the outcome is almost always fatal.

31. What is a mucocele?

A mucocele is an expanding mass of mucoid secretions lined by cuboidal epithelium as the result of obstructed sinus ostia secondary to inflammation and scarring. They are potentially dangerous if they invade surrounding structures, including the orbit and brain. A secondary infection, or mucopyocele, facilitates the expansion of these lesions. They can rupture intracranially with catastrophic results. The most commonly affected sinuses are the posterior ethmoid, sphenoid, and frontal. CT scans or MRI aid in the diagnosis.

32. What is a Pott's puffy tumor?

Originally described by Sir Percivall Pott in 1760, Pott's puffy tumor is a doughy swelling on the forehead caused by erosion of the anterior sinus wall secondary to frontal sinus osteomyelitis. Infection of the bone and bone marrow can occur via direct extension or, more commonly, by thrombophlebitis of the diploic veins. This complication is often seen in young adults, possibly because of the more extensive system of diploic veins in this group. The most common offending organism is *Staphylococcus aureus*. The characteristic radiographic pattern is a "motheaten" pattern of the bone.

CONTROVERSIES

33. How common is sinusitis in the intensive care unit (ICU) population?

ICU hospitalization is a known risk factor for the development of sinusitis and is thought to result from direct mechanical obstruction of the sinus ostia by nasal tubes as well as mucosal edema caused by disruption of normal nasal airflow by mechanical ventilation. Early studies suggested that sinusitis occurred in 2–17% of nasally cannulated ICU patients. However, more recent investigations indicate that sinusitis may occur in 100% of nasaotracheally intubated patients as well as nearly 80% of patients with nasogastric tubes. The presence of purulence at the middle meatus along with CT evidence of sinus disease warrants antral lavage in >90% of ICU patients.

34. What is hospital-acquired sinusitis called? Why is it different?

Nosocomial. The clinician, therefore, must maintain a high index of suspicion of this source of infection in any patient with fever of unknown origin. Radiologic studies, including plain sinus radiographs, or, preferably, a CT scan, will usually show the presence of fluid or inflammation. Lavage of the maxillary sinus is helpful to verify the presence of infection, obtain culture material, and provide therapeutic benefit. These infections tend to be polymicrobial and often display a predominance of gram-negative organisms, particularly *Pseudomonas aeruginosa*. The treatment includes removal of all nasal tubes and institution of appropriate antibiotics, along with decongestant therapy. In some cases, surgical drainage will be necessary. For patients who are immunocompromised, or requiring intubation for > 7 days, the nasotracheal route is best avoided.

35. What is the relationship between asthma and sinusitis?

Recently, evidence suggesting a link between sinusitis and asthma has emerged. Radiographic sinus abnormalities have been illustrated in the majority of patients with asthma (40–60%). However, the relationship between sinusitis and asthma is still unclear. Common inflammatory mechanisms are thought to exist among paranasal sinusitis and bronchial hyperreactivity. Fluid draining from infected sinuses contains large amounts of eosinophils and cytokines known to induce bronchial spacicity. This relationship is further illustrated by reduced bronchial spacicity with topical nasal corticosteroids, animal evidence of inflammatory mediators leaking from upper to lower airways, and improved asthma symptoms with adequate treatment of sinusitis. Reduced nitric oxide in upper airways during sinusitis has also been implicated in modulating bronchial tone in asthmatic patients.

36. When diagnosing a patient as having "sinusitis," do you risk missing the diagnosis of sinonasal malignancy?

Compared with sinusitis, malignancy in the paranasal sinuses is very rare. It is seldom picked up at an early stage, and symptoms and signs relate to expansion of the sinus wall or local extension. Local symptoms include epistaxis, proptosis, trismus, fullness of the cheek or palate, cranial nerve palsy, facial numbness, and loosening of the upper teeth. Nodal metastases are rare and usually indicate a poor prognosis.

37. Is "holistic treatment" of any value in the management of sinusitis?

Dr. Robert Ivker's book, *Sinus Survival,* is of particular value in assisting the patient with chronic sinus disease.

38. Is there any genetic basis for sinusitis?

The genetic mutation that causes cystic fibrosis may be responsible for chronic sinus infections in some people who carry the gene but do not suffer from the disease. Recent research suggests that 7% of 147 patients who sought treatment for repeated bouts of sinusitis had a copy of the mutated gene responsible for cystic fibrosis (CF). Follow-up sweat testing and nasal potential difference testing of these patients and a comparison group of control subjects showed no clinical or laboratory evidence of CF. The controls (123 sinusitis-free patients) also lacked clinical or laboratory signs of CF and were sinusitis-free.

The report did not recommend that everyone with chronic sinus problems undergo genetic testing, saying that the research is still at an early stage. But it did say that mutations in the gene responsible for CF may be associated with the develovment of chronic rhinosinusitis in the general population and that this knowledge may eventually prove useful therapeutically, since some sinusitis patients might be helped by treatments developed for CF. It was already known that CF patients often presented with nasal polyps and that this even suggested the diagnosis of CF in pediatric patients, and also that CF patients had chronic rhinosinusitis. Further, patients with immotile cilia syndrome, also apparently on a genetic basis, have recurrent and chronic sinusitis.

39. How is sinusitis staged?

Outcomes assessment for disease management depends upon pretreatment staging (e.g., cancer). To determine outcome indicators for the treatment of sinusitis, several staging systems have been suggested over the past 15 years, most incorporating the concept of obstruction with retrograde involvement of additional sinus cavities. The ideal staging system should depend on factors of the patient's disease and facilitate uniform reporting and comparisons between patient groups. It should be easy to use and minimize interobserver variability. Finding objective, quantifiable parameters for the evaluation of sinusitis has, however, proved to be very difficult. Although the endoscope has revolutionized thinking about basic sinus disease, CT evaluation has facilitated assessment of the extent of mucosal involvement, and additional information on the molecular basis of sinusitis has accumulated, a uniform staging system has not yet been agreed upon.

BIBLIOGRAPHY

1. Benninger MS: The impact of cigarette smoking and environmental tobacco smoke on nasal and sinus disease: A review of the literature. Am J Rhinol 13:435–438, 1999.
2. Biel MA, Brown CA, Levinson RM, Garvis GE, Paisner HM, Sigel ME, Tedford TM: Evaluation of the microbiology of chronic maxillary sinusitis. Ann Otol Rhinol Laryngol 107:942–945, 1998.
3. de Benedicts FM, Bush A: Rhinosinusitis and asthma: Epiphenomenon or causal association? Chest 115: 550–556, 1999

4. Evans KL: Recognition and management of sinusitis. Drugs 56:59–71, 1998.
5. Ferguson BJ: Definition of fungal rhinosinusitis. Otolaryngol Clin North Am 33:227–235, 2000.
6. Hamilos DL: Chronic sinusitis. J Allergy Clin Immunol 106:213–227, 2000.
7. Eustis HS, Mafee MF, Walton C, Mondonca J: MR imaging and CT of orbital infections and complications in acute rhinosinusitis. Radiol Clin North Am 36:1165–1183, xi, 1998.
8. Isaacson G, Yanagisawa E: Cystic fibrosis and sinusitis. Ear Nose Throat J 77:886–888, 1998.
9. Ivker R: Sinus Survival, 4th ed. New York, Putnam, 2000.
10. Kennedy DW, Bolger WE, Zinreich SJ: Diseases of the Sinuses: Diagnosis and Treatment. London, B.C. Decker, 2001.
11. Lebeda MD, Haller JR, Graham SM, Hoffman HT: Evaluation of maxillary sinus aspiration in patients with fever of unknown origin. Laryngoscope 105:683–685, 1995.
12. Low DE, Desrosiers M, McSherry J, Garber G, Williams JW Jr, Remy H, Fenton RS, Forte V, Balter M, Rotstein C, Craft C, Dubois J, Harding G, Schloss M, Miller M, McIvor RA, Davidson RJ: A practical guide for the diagnosis and treatment of acute sinusitis. Can Med Assoc J 156(6 suppl): S1–S12, 1997.
13. Pinheiro AD, Facer GW, Kern EB: Sinusitis: Current concepts and managment. In Baily B, Calhoun K (eds): Head and Neck Surgery—Otolaryngology. Philadelphia, Lippincott-Raven Publishers, 1998, pp 441–454.
14. Sinus & Allergy Partnership: Antimicrobial Treatment Guidelines for Acute Bacterial Rhinosinusitis. Otolaryngol Head Neck Surg 123(Supp 1, Pt 2):S1-S32, 2000.
15. Wang X, Moylan B, Leopold DA: Mutation in the gene responsible for cystic fibrosis and predisposition to chronic rhinosinusitis in the general population. JAMA 284:1814–1819, 2000.

22. MEDICAL MANAGEMENT OF SINUSITIS

Wendy M. Ahlbrandt, M.S. IV, Bruce W. Jafek, M.D., and Tyler M. Lewark, M.D.

1. What therapeutic agents can be used to manage sinusitis?

Many therapeutic agents are available to the clinician for the management of sinusitis. However, in successfully managing this condition, one must understand and treat all the contributory factors in each individual case (see Chapter 21). The primary therapeutic agents include antibiotics, decongestants, mucolytics, nasal sprays or irrigation, humidification, and corticosteroids.

2. What percentage of cases of acute bacterial sinusitis spontaneously resolve? Should antibiotics still be used?

An estimated 40% of cases of acute bacterial sinusitis will spontaneously resolve. Antibiotics may still be used, as they are felt to facilitate recovery from the acute episode, prevent complications, and prevent progressive mucosal changes that may result in chronic sinusitis.

3. What factors should be considered when choosing an antibiotic?

Severity of disease, rate of progression of disease, prior antibiotic use and failures, history of drug allergies, cost, and the incidence of β-lactamase-producing strains of bacteria.

4. Describe the goals of management of acute sinusitis.

Arrest the acute infection; reduce tissue edema; re-establish sinus drainage and ventilation of the sinus; avoid permanent mucosal damage; and prevent complications, sequellae, or progression to chronic sinusitis.

5. Which antibiotics should be used in adults with acute sinusitis?

Many clinicians empirically employ ampicillin or amoxicillin as first-line antimicrobials in the treatment of sinusitis. However, recent guidelines offer a more comprehensive approach. Acute bacterial rhinosinusitis (ABRS) is first divided into "mild" and "moderate" cases relative to the clinical severity of the disease present. Prior antibiotic use (previous 4–6 weeks) is also incorporated into patient stratification within the treatment algorithm.

See table next page.

Recommended Antibiotic Therapy for Adults with Acute Bacterial Rhinosinusitis

SEVERITY	PRIOR ANTIBIOTICS (PAST 4–6 WEEKS)	INITIAL THERAPY	CALCULATED BACTERIOLOGIC EFFICACY (%)	PERCENTAGE NONSUSCEPTIBLE S PNEUMONIAE	PERCENTAGE NONSUSCEPTIBLE H INFLUENZAE	SWITCH THERAPY OPTIONS (NO IMPROVEMENT OR WORSENING AFTER 72 HOURS)
Mild	No	Amoxicillin/clavulanate	93.3±1.1	6	0.4	Gatifloxacin/Levofloxacin/Moxifloxacin; Re-evaluate patient
		Amoxicillin	88.8±0.6	6	39	Amoxicillin/clavulanate; Gatifloxacin/Levofloxacin/Moxifloxacin; Cefpodoxime or Cefixime; Amoxicillin
		Cefpodoxime	86.7±2.1	37	0.1	Clindamycin; Gatifloxacin/Levofloxacin/Moxifloxacin
		Cefuroxime	84.4±2.5	35	20	Amoxicillin/clavulanate
		Beta-lactam Allergic:				
		TMP/SMX	81.4±2.5	30	25	
		Doxycycline	79.9±2.5	22	80	Gatifloxacin/Levofloxacin/Moxifloxacin or combination
		Azithromycin, clarithromycin, erythromycin	74.8±2.5	33	99	
Mild or Moderate	Yes / No	Amoxicillin/clavulanate	93.3±1.1	6	0.4	Gatifloxacin/Levofloxacin/Moxifloxacin; Re-evaluate patient
		Amoxicillin	88.8±0.6	6	39	Amoxicillin/clavulanate; Gatifloxacin/Levofloxacin/Moxifloxacin; Cefpodoxime or Cefixime; Amoxicillin
		Cefpodoxime	86.7±2.1	37	0.1	Clindamycin; Gatifloxacin/Levofloxacin/Moxifloxacin
		Cefuroxime	84.4±2.5	35	20	Amoxicillin/clavulanate; Gatifloxacin/Levofloxacin/Moxifloxacin; Combination
		Beta-lactam Allergic:				
		Gatifloxacin, Levofloxacin, Moxifloxacin	95.4±0	3	0	Re-evaluate patient
Moderate	Yes	Gatifloxacin, Levofloxacin, Moxifloxacin	95.1±0.4	3	0	Re-evaluate patient
		Amoxicillin/clavulanate	94.4±0.6	6	0.4	Gatifloxacin/Levofloxacin/Moxifloxacin
		Combination		6/11	0.1	Re-evaluate patient

Adapted from Sinus & Allergy Partnership: Antimicrobial Treatment Guidelines for Acute Bacterial Rhinosinusitis. Otolaryngol Head Neck Surg 123 (Supp 1, Pt 2):S1–S32, 2000.

6. How would you sum up this treatment algorithm for a clinician?

According to the Partnership, recommendations for the initial therapy for adults with mild ABRS, who have not received antibiotics in the previous 4–6 weeks, include the following choices: amoxicillin/clavulonate, amoxicillin (1.5–3.5 g/day), cefpodoxime proxetil, or cefuroxime axetil. Cefprozil may have a 25% bacterial failure rate. For those with mild ABRS who have received antibiotics in the previous 4–6 weeks, *or* adults with moderate disease who have not received antibiotics in the previous 4–6 weeks, initial choices include amoxicillin/clavulanate, amoxicillin (3–3.5 g/day), cefpodoxime proxetil, or cefuroxime axetil. The recommendations for initial therapy for adults with moderate disease who have received antibiotics in the previous 4–6 weeks include amoxicillin/clavulonate, gatifloxacin, levofloxacin, moxifloxacin, or combination therapy (amoxicillin or clindamycin [gram-positive coverage] plus cefpodoxime proxetil or cefixime [gram-negative coverage]).

7. Why is prior antibiotic usage a consideration?

Recent antimicrobial exposure increases the risk of carriage of and infection with resistant organisms and therefore subsequent antibiotic therapy should be based on this recent antibiotic use. "Prior antibiotic exposure" is arbitrarily defined as the use of antibiotics within the previous 4–6 weeks, and the type of antibiotic should be taken into consideration in prescribing subsequent therapy.

8. What are the "second-line" antibiotics?

Lack of response to therapy (or worsening) at >72 hours is an arbitrary time established to define treatment failures. When a change in antibiotic therapy ("switch" therapy) is made, the clinician needs to take into account the limitations in coverage of the initial antibiotic and the organism likely to be producing the clinical failure.

For example, amoxicillin lacks complete *Haemophilus influenzae* coverage; cefuroxime and cefpodoxime do not cover penicillin-resistant *Streptococcus pneumoniae*. Erythromycin, doxycycline, and trimethoprim/sulfamethoxazole (TMP/SMX) have limited coverage for both *H. influenzae* and *S. pneumoniae*. Amoxicillin/clavulanate, gatifloxacin, levofloxacin, and moxifloxacin currently have the best coverage for both *H. influenzae* and *S. pneumoniae*. Although cefpodoxime and cefixime have excellent activity against *H. influenzae,* they are not active against penicillin-resistant *S. pneumoniae*. Clindamycin provides excellent coverage for *S. pneumoniae* but has no activity against *H. influenzae*.

Patients who have received effective antibiotics may also need further evaluation. A computed tomographic (CT) scan, fiberoptic (or rigid) endoscopy, or sinus aspiration with culture and sensitivities, especially in the immunocompromised patient, may be indicated.

9. Which antibiotics should be used in β-lactam-allergic patients?

For β-lactam-allergic patients with mild ABRS, alternatives include TMP/SMX, doxycycline, azithromycin, clarithromycin, and erythromycin. The effectiveness of these antibiotics against the major pathogens of ABRS is limited, however, and bacterial failure of 20–25% is possible. Also, life-threatening toxic epidermal necrolysis has been associated with the use of TMP/SMX. For moderate ABRS in β-lactam-allergic patients, gatifloxacin, levofloxacin, and moxifloxacin should be considered initially. A fluoroquinolone is recommended for patients who have allergies or intolerance to β-lactams, or who have recently not responded to other regimens of therapy.

10. Which antibiotics should be used in children with acute sinusitis?

As for adults, you must consider the patient's drug allergy history, previous antibiotic failures, potential side effects, and prevalence of β-lactamase-producing bacteria in the population. The Partership recommends, for initial therapy in children with mild disease who have not received antibiotics in the previous 4–6 weeks, amoxicillin/clavulanate, amoxicillin (45–90 mg/kg/day), cefpodoxime proxetil, or cefuroxime axetil. Azithromycin, clarithromycin, erythromycin, or TMP/SMX is recommended if the patient has a history of immediate type I hypersensitivity to β-lactams. These antibiotics have limited effectiveness against the major pathogens of ABRS, and a bacterial failure rate of 20–25% is reported. Again, the use of TMP/SMX has been associated with increases in the risk of life-threatening toxic epidermal necrolysis. Children with immediate hypersensitivity reactions to β-lactams may need desensitization, sinus cultures, or other ancillary procedures and studies. Children with other types of reactions and side effects may tolerate one specific β-lactam but not another.

For the initial therapy in children with mild disease who have received antibiotics in the previous 4–6 weeks or with moderate ABRS, who have not received antibiotics in the previous 4–6 weeks, recommendations include amoxicillin/clavulanate, amoxicillin (80–90 mg/kg/d), cefpodoxime proxetil, or cefuroxime axetil. Azithromycin, clarithromycin, erythromycin, or TMP/SMX is recommended if the patient is allergic to β-lactams. Clindamycin is appropriate if *S. pneumoniae* is identified as the pathogen.

With moderate disease in children who have received antibiotics in the previous 4–6 weeks, treatment choices include amoxicillin/clavulanate or combination therapy (amoxicillin or clindamycin [gram-positive coverage] plus cefpodoxime proxetil or cefixime [gram-negative coverage]).

11. What do you do if the child doesn't respond to initial treatment?

As with adults (see Question 8), "switch," or "second-line," therapy in children who show no improvement or worsening at >72 hours depends on the organism likely to be producing the infection. Children who have received effective antibiotic therapy who continue to be symptomatic may require further evaluation. A CT scan, endoscopy, or sinus aspiration with culture may be necessary. This need is heightened, of course, in immunocompromised children.

12. How long is antimicrobial therapy continued in uncomplicated acute sinusitis?

In uncomplicated maxillary sinusitis, treatment with the above-indicated antibiotic for 10–14 days is usually adequate. Clinical improvement usually occurs within 48–72 hours of initiation of antimicrobial therapy. However, antibiotic therapy should be continued for a minimum 7 days after the disappearance of symptoms. Because of the increased prevalence of β-lactamase-producing bacteria in the pediatric population, lack of clinical improvement after 48–72 hours should prompt an antibiotic change to cover these pathogens. Lack of symptom resolution after 10–14 days requires additional evaluation, and antibiotics be continued until all symptoms are resolved. The rationale for this approach to acute sinusitis is discussed in much greater detail in the Partnership reference for the interested reader.

13. What are the efficacy rates for the above regimen?

For *adults,* bacterial efficacy rates are >90% for gatifloxacin, levofloxacin, moxifloxacin, and amoxicillin/clavulanate; 80–90% for high-dose amoxicillin, cefpodoxime proxetil, cefixime (based on *H. influenzae* and *Moraxella catarrhalis* coverage only); 70–80% for clindamycin (based on gram-positive coverage only), doxycycline, cefprozil, azithromycin, clarithromycin, and erythromycin; and 50–60% for cefaclor and loracarbef. The predicted spontaneous resolution rate in adults with ARBS is 46.6%.

In *children* with ARBS, the predicted efficacy rates are >90% for amoxicillin/clavulanate and high-dose amoxicillin; 80–90% for cefpodoxime proxetil, cefixime (based on *H. influenzae* and *M. catarrhalis* coverage only), cefuroxime axetil, clindamycin (based on gram-positive coverage only), azithromycin, clarithromycin, erythromycin, and TMP/SMX; 70–80% for cefprozil; and 60–70% for cefaclor and loracarbef. The predicted spontaneous resolution rate in untreated children with ABRS is 49.6%.

14. How are these efficacy rates determined?

The bacterial efficacy, or microbiologic adequacy, is the mean and range of three sets of calculations from the Poole Therapeutic Outcome Model using three susceptibility data bases: the US component of the 1998 Alexander Project, 1998 Sentry surveillance, and the 1998 CDC Active Bacterial Core Surveillance Report. The qualifying statement is that "these values do not guarantee clinical success or failure."

15. What is the Poole Therapeutic Outcome Model?

Actually, it's way over my head! And no student should be held responsible for this, at least not on the basis of memory alone. Basically, in the past, the choice of antibiotic treatment may have been based almost exclusively on the susceptibiliity of the pathogen in an in vitro system (i.e., minimal inhibitory concentration [MIC]). But obviously the clinical efficacy of antibiotic treatment depends on many other parameters. In addition to in vitro susceptibility data of antibiotics from pharmacokinetic and pharmacodynamic measurements, the prevalence of culture-positive aspirates from clinically diagnosed patients, the distribution of pathogens in culture, the spontaneous resolution rate of each pathogen and the clinical resolution of disease in culture-negative patients all play a role in the clinical efficacy of the antibiotic.

The Poole Therapeutic Outcome Model takes these variables into account, on a local, updated basis, and is designed to be a dynamic interactive mathematical model for evaluating treatment effectiveness in ABRS. The model was developed by Michael D. Poole, MD, PhD (a really bright and committed student of antimicrobial activity), of the University of Texas Medical School at Houston, with JAVA programming by Michael Poole, Jr., BS (obviously a relative!). This program takes into account the significant variables that are known to affect the outcome of treatment of ABRS. By inserting values for the estimated antibacterial efficacy of any considered therapy (antibiotic), one can model the expected outcome as other parameters change. It has been adapted to run as a JAVA self-calculating Web applet. Although the most recent and best data were used for this model, it is recognized that resistance rates will change over time and vary from community to community.

The JAVA applet is available at the Sinus and Allergy website (http://www.allergysinus.org) and allows interested clinicians to input their own local resistance rates and to obtain their own optimal treatment recommendations. It is recommended that local resistance data be based on PK/PD (pharmacokinetic/pharmacodynamic) breakpoints, not NCCLS (National Committee for Clinical Laboratory Standards) breakpoints, as discussed in the Partnership citation.

16. What factor must be addressed for the successful treatment of recurrent or chronic sinusitis?

Back to basics! The most important factor contributing to the development of sinusitis is obstruction of the sinus ostia. Accordingly, the key to effective management of recurrent or chronic sinusitis is early correction of osteomeatal complex obstruction. Medical management of this condition is necessary if the obstruction is due to, or affected by, physiologic abnormalities. If the obstruction is anatomic, surgery is usually required, especially in the recalcitrant case (see Chapter 23).

17. Does antimicrobial treatment differ in chronic sinusitis?

When compared with treatment for acute sinusitis, medical management in chronic sinusitis treatment has a limited role. Antibiotic therapy differs both in choice of agent and duration of treatment. Because anaerobes or a combination of aerobes and anaerobes are often implicated in chronic cases, antibiotic choice should include anaerobic coverage. Penicillin VK is useful, but as many as 44% of anaerobic isolates may be β-lactamase-positive, and so amoxicillin–clavulanic acid or clindamycin may be necessary. Some success in these patients has been seen with the prolonged use of doxycycline. Antibiotic therapy should be administered for a minimum of 4 weeks. Treatment of chronic sinusitis in children is similar to treatment for adults. Special care should be given to the choice of antibiotic because of the increased prevalence of β-lactamase-producing bacteria in this population.

18. Describe the goals of management of chronic sinusitis.

Eradicate infection, relieve osteomeatal obstuction, normalize mucociliary clearance, and prevent complications.

19. What is the Mecca position? When is it used?

Topical nasal decongestants are more effective when given in the Mecca position. It should be maintained for 2–3 minutes after decongestants are administered.

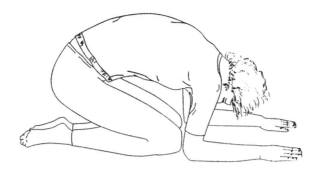

The "Mecca position" for adequate distribution of topical nasal medications. (From Evans KL: Diagnosis and management of sinusitis. BMJ 309:1418, 1994, with permission.)

20. Describe the role of mucolytics in the treatment of sinusitis.

Mucolytic agents are used in sinusitis to decrease the tenacity of mucus. Home remedies include horseradish, chicken soup, and increased fluid intake. Although less well established in cases of sinusitis, organic iodide preparations have been shown to be effective in treating patients with bronchitis. The most widely used mucolytic agent in the treatment of sinusitis is guaifenesin. Because effective doses approach levels that cause emesis, guaifenesin may cause gastrointestinal side effects.

21. Should corticosteroids be used in the treatment of sinusitis? When? What type?

Because of the significant potential for undesirable side effects on multiple organ systems, systemic corticosteroids have largely been supplanted by topical preparations. Nasal steroids reduce edema of the osteomeatal complex. Because they may decrease inflammation necessary for combating infection, appropriate antibiotic therapy should be initiated prior to topical steroids. Thus, they may be helpful when treating chronic sinusitis or when used prophylactically in recurrent sinusitis.

To be beneficial, the medication must contact the affected mucosa. Topical steroids are less effective if the airway is obstructed by septal deviation, turbinate hypertrophy, polyps, or anterior nasal edema. Maximal benefit will not be seen for 1–2 weeks, and further therapy depends on therapeutic response and other treatment employed. Potential side effects of topical preparations include nasal irritation, crusting, bleeding, and even septal perforation. Local candidiasis and some systemic absorption may result from prolonged use.

22. Are any nonpharmacologic treatments effective in sinusitis?

Great benefit is derived from **regular saline nasal irrigations** in many patients with sinusitis. Delivered with a bulb syringe or nasal irrigator, this treatment helps to move secretions through the nasal cavity. Saline solutions of roughly physiologic proportions can be prepared by patients or may be purchased as a commercially prepared, sterile physiologic solution. Self-prepared solutions are easily delivered with the use of an empty conventional squeeze-spray or pump-spray bottle. Irrigations must be thorough and performed several times a day. For patients with bothersome thick postnasal secretions, powered, pulsating devices that deliver warm saline into the nasal cavity are available. Moist heat to the face and the inhalation of steam may give some relief to the patient with facial pressure. This can be accomplished with a hot shower, sauna, or hot towel.

23. What types of alternative or complementary therapies do patients with sinusitis use?

Air filters, dietary supplements, herbal therapy, biofeedback, and acupuncture, among others.

24. How is fungal sinusitis treated? Is medical management effective?

Fungal sinusitis may be invasive or noninvasive, and medical management alone rarely eradicates the disease. Acute noninvasive fungal sinusitis most commonly involves the maxillary sinus and is treated surgically. Antifungal therapy is usually not indicated. Invasive fungal sinusitis can be life-threatening and requires surgical débridement and prompt fungal chemotherapy, usually with intravenous amphotericin B.

25. Does the medical management of sinusitis differ for the patient with allergy?

Repeated or severe allergic reactions lead to osteomeatal complex obstruction and stasis of secretions within the sinus. Therefore, it is important either to prevent or to rapidly and effectively treat acute reactions. If possible, the patient should avoid inciting allergens. Antibiotics, decongestants, mucolytics, corticosteroids, and nasal irrigation should be employed as for acute and chronic sinusitis. Because histamine is the major product released during an anaphylactic or immediate allergic reaction, antihistamines are usually employed in the treatment of allergy-associated sinusitis. Potential side effects of antihistamines include sedation and excessive dryness and crusting within the nose. The newer second-generation antihistamines (e.g., terfenadine, loratadine) are less sedating because they are lipophobic and do not cross the blood-brain barrier. Unlike first-generation antihistamines, these newer agents do not cause dryness and crusting.

Cromolyn sodium, a mast cell stabilizer, may also be administered to the allergic patient with sinusitis. Because this agent acts on acute and late-phase allergic reactions, its use is limited to prevention and treatment of sinusitis caused by allergic flares.

26. When is immunotherapy indicated in the treatment of sinusitis?

Immunotherapy is the administration of carefully determined allergen doses over a period of years. IgG-blocking antibodies prevent the allergic event by disrupting the IgE–allergen–mast cell interaction. This therapy should be considered in patients with allergen-induced sinusitis whose symptoms are not controlled by simple pharmacologic measures. It should also be used when the offending allergens are unavoidable.

27. How does the medical management of sinusitis differ for the immunocompromised patient?

Fungal infections are prevalent in the immunocompromised population, especially in those patients with lymphoproliferative neoplasms. The clinician's threshold for administration of antibacterial and antifungal agents in this population should be quite low. Because acquired immunodeficiency syndrome (AIDS) patients have deficits in both cell-mediated and humoral immunity, they are more susceptible to bacterial infection. Treatment is often very difficult, especially when the patient's CD4 count is $< 200 \times 10^6$/liter. Antral aspiration may be necessary for organism identification and antibiotic sensitivity determination. Uncomplicated cases may respond to oral antibiotics. However, when patients appear systemically affected, hospital admission may be required for antral lavage (see Chapter 23) and intravenous therapy.

28. How are orbital complications of sinusitis managed?

Early preseptal infections may be managed on an outpatient basis with oral antibiotics active against β-lactamase-producing strains of bacteria. However, the clinician must have a low threshold for hospital admission and aggressive treatment, because unrecognized orbital infection may have catastrophic consequences. Advanced cases of orbital infection require intravenous antibiotics. Strict visual acuity monitoring, CT scan evaluation, and ophthalmology consultation are also necessary. Surgical intervention is indicated if the patient experiences visual loss, progression of symptoms over 24 hours, or no improvement after 48–72 hours.

29. How are the intracranial complications of sinusitis treated?

Despite the reduced frequency of these complications, they are life-threatening and require immediate attention. In all cases, the underlying sinus disease should be treated and usually requires a drainage procedure of the involved sinuses. High-dose intravenous antibiotic therapy is the primary medical treatment. Sinusitis-induced meningitis requires antibiotics with good cerebrospinal penetration. Surgery is required for the treatment of epidural, subdural, and brain abscesses and for venous sinus thrombosis. Concurrent high-dose intravenous antibiotics should be administered. Some clinicians advocate the use of heparin for the treatment of cavernous venous thrombosis. In cases of superior sagittal sinus thrombosis, aggressive medical management may be lifesaving.

30. Can sinusitis-induced mucocele be treated medically?

If infection is suspected, broad-spectrum antibiotics should be instituted. Otherwise, mucoceles are primarily treated surgically (see Chapter 23).

31. How is sinusitis-induced osteomyelitis managed? How long should you follow the patient after resolution of the infection?

The mainstay of treatment of sinusitis-induced osteomyelitis is prolonged antibiotic therapy with wide surgical débridement of necrotic bone. Although ineffective when used alone, antibiotics should be continued for at least 6 weeks. The patient should be followed on a long-term basis due to the tendency for the condition to recur many years after resolution of the infection.

32. When should the primary care physician refer a patient with sinusitis to an otolaryngologist?

• If there is no response to a first-line course of antibiotics, a course of a second-line medication may be administered. If there is no response to the second course, the patient should be referred to an otolaryngologist.

• Any symptom suggestive of incipient complications should prompt immediate referral.

• Patients who have at least three attacks per year for 2 years or four or more attacks in 1 year warrant referral. Specialist care is necessary to investigate a possible correctable local anatomic factor or predisposing systemic condition, such as immunosuppression.

CONTROVERSIES

33. When is a case considered a medical failure? When is surgical management indicated?

This question has both medical and financial considerations. Although some third-party payers have guidelines for the management of sinusitis, no set criteria are generally accepted. Some clinicians do not easily abandon medical therapy and favor long-term antimicrobial treatment. Some argue that surgery is indicated only in cases of proven mechanical obstruction. Others argue that surgery is indicated with either evidence of mechanical obstruction or residual infection following adequate medical management. Further concerns revolve around medical and surgical management in the pediatric patient. Cost-effectiveness of the various modalities is also disputed. Consideration should be given to the cost of sinus surgery versus the cost of long-term second-line antimicrobial treatment.

34. The intensive care unit (ICU) team consults you on a patient who is intubated, obtunded, and has a fever of unknown origin. CT scan of the patient's sinuses indicate the patient has sinusitis. Should maxillary sinus aspiration be performed to identify possible sinus pathogens contributing to the patient's fever?

The controversy concerns how often sinusitis causes a fever of unknown origin in the ICU patient. Some investigators have found sinusitis to be an often overlooked cause of occult fever and sepsis in the ICU patient. These authors advocate more aggressive search for and treatment of sinusitis in these patients, including maxillary sinus aspiration. In contrast, others argue that although radiographic evidence of sinusitis is very common in the nasally cannulated ICU patient, this condition is rarely the cause of occult fever. These authors also argue that maxillary sinus aspiration for identification of possible inciting pathogens is often not necessary and that medical management, including decongestants and antibiotics, often eliminates the need for this procedure.

BIBLIOGRAPHY

1. Borman KR, Brown PM, Mezera KK, et al: Occult fever in surgical intensive care unit patients is seldom caused by sinusitis. Am J Surg 164:412–416, 1992.
2. Evans KL: Diagnosis and management of sinusitis. Br Med J 309:1415–1422, 1994.
3. Goh YH, Goode RL: Current status of topical nasal antimicrobial agents. Laryngoscope 110:875–880, 2000.
4. Gwaltney JM Jr: Acute community acquired bacterial sinusitis: To treat or not to treat. Can Resp J 6 (Suppl A):46A–50A, 1999.
5. Mabry RL, Mabry CS: Allergic fungal sinusitis: The role of immunotherapy. Otolaryngol Clin North Am 33:433–440, 2000.
6. Marple BF, Mabry RL: Allergic fungal sinusitis: Learning from our failures. Am J Rhinol 14:223–226, 2000.
7. Scadding G: The effect of medical treatment of sinusitis upon concomitant asthma. Allergy 54 (Suppl 57):136–140, 1999.
8. Sinus & Allergy Partnership: Antimicrobial Treatment Guidelines for Acute Bacterial Rhinosinusitis. Otolaryngol Head Neck Surg 123 (Supp 1, Pt 2):S1–S32, 2000.
9. Stankiewicz JA, Newell DJ, Park AH: Complications of inflammatory disease of the sinuses. Otolaryngol Clin North Am 26:639–655, 1993.
10. Temple ME, Nahata MC: Pharmacotherapy of acute sinusitis in children. Am J Health Syst Pharm 57:663–668, 2000.
11. Thomas MG, Arroll B: "Just say no"—reducing the use of antibiotics for colds, bronchitis and sinusitis. N Z Med J 113:287–289, 2000.

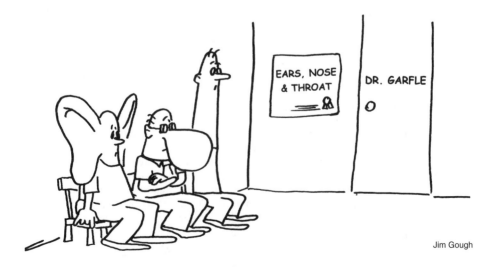

Jim Gough

23. SURGICAL MANAGEMENT OF SINUSITIS

Bruce W. Jafek, M.D., FACS, FRSM, and Nicolas G. Slenkovich, M.D.

1. What is the aim of surgical intervention for sinus infections?

The goal for any treatment of sinusitis is to clear infection rapidly and to prevent serious complications from orbital or intracranial spread. The aim of surgery, when medical treatment has failed, or when complications dictate a surgical approach, is to establish effective sinus drainage, either through minimal techniques to restore physiologic mucociliary drainage or through more aggressive techniques involving sinus ventilation or sinus obliteration. Except in the case of sinus obliteration, these techniques are said to be *mucosal-sparing,* in which removal of irreversibly diseased mucosa facilitates re-establishment of a healthy mucosal blanket by regeneration from the adjacent normal mucosa.

Although initially it was felt that drainage/ventilation of involved sinuses was sufficient to induce disease resolution, it now appears that this is suitable primarily for children and early and mild disease, which might even respond to more aggressive medical, rather than surgical management. Simply draining involved cells or sinuses may be insufficient in chronic disease. Based on additional studies by Kennedy, which suggest that the underlying bone may become osteitic in the face of overlying mucosal infection, more complete removal of the underlying bony partitions is now advocated, while preserving the adjacent normal mucosa to facilitate regeneration.

2. What knowledge is needed to understand the surgical management of sinusitis?

Sinus anatomy and physiology. Observing an endoscopic sinus procedure can be a humbling experience to the neophyte. Surgical landmarks such as the uncinate process, ethmoid bulla, and ground lamella are foreign concepts. How they relate to the pathology may not be initially understood from the endoscopic view. Before attempting to decipher the complex surgical anatomy, it is important to study the relatively simple anatomic and physiologic basis of sinusitis.

3. Describe the details of sinus drainage via the osteomeatal complex into the infundibulum and semilunar hiatus.

The anterior sinuses normally drain into the middle meatus. Drainage from the frontal, anterior ethmoid, and maxillary sinuses transits the **osteomeatal complex** into the middle meatus via an initial anatomic collecting space referred to as the infundibulum and exits into the middle meatus via the semilunar hiatus. The **infundibulum,** which is Latin for *funnel,* refers to an inverted funnel that originates at the frontonasal duct superiorly, where it receives the frontal sinus effluent, and next receives drainage from the small anterior ethmoid ostia and the maxillary ostium through its lateral wall. The **semilunar hiatus,** which translates as "a curved aperture," refers to the slot-like aperture in the lateral nasal wall that curves from the frontonasal duct inferiorly and posteriorly to just below the maxillary ostium. Through the semilunar hiatus, the anterior sinus drainage exits the infundibulum into the middle meatus. The posterior ethmoids drain via small ostia directly into the middle meatus. (See figure next page.)

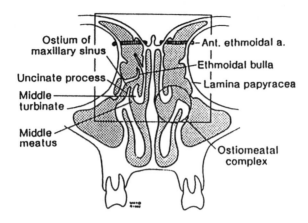

Anatomy of the midportion of the nasal cavity. The box identifies the boundaries of ethmoid bone, and the circle identifies the osteomeatal complex. (From McCaffrey TV: Functional endoscopic sinus surgery: An overview. Mayo Clin Proc 68:572, 1993, with permission.)

4. What is functional endoscopic sinus surgery (FESS)?

FESS describes endoscopic techniques that have revolutionized the approach to sinus disease. These techniques were initially developed in Europe by Messerklinger and Stammberger and were popularized in the United States in the mid-1980s by Kennedy and others. The procedure is aimed at restoring the functional physiology of sinus aeration and drainage via the expanded osteomeatal complex while minimizing surgical alteration of the normal anatomic pathways. Accurate coronal computed tomographic (CT) images, together with advances in endoscopic instrumentation and techniques, and an improved understanding of mucociliary flow patterns, led to the development of FESS.

5. What are the principles behind FESS?

Detailed CT scans led to our current understanding that anterior ethmoid sinusitis, with resultant obstruction of the osteomeatal complex, plays a major role in promoting retrograde sinus disease. FESS directs the surgeon to initiate dissection in the anterior ethmoids and limit surgical intervention to the diseased anatomy to restore normal sinus drainage. FESS techniques have reduced the length of hospitalization and discomfort associated with traditional sinus surgery. In the past, many patients with anterior ethmoidal disease may have escaped diagnosis. The disease can now be diagnosed accurately and treated successfully.

6. How are patients selected for FESS?

Surgery is indicated for patients with refractory sinusitis or complicated cases of sinusitis. The highest success rates have been achieved in patients with chronic or recurrent acute episodes of sinusitis despite maximal medical therapy. Patients with recurrent polyps, severe allergies, a history of previous external procedures, or an immunocompromised state may undergo endoscopic sinus surgery, but with lower success rates. From a symptom standpoint, pressure, discharge, and obstruction are most likely to respond to FESS surgery, with pain being somewhat less responsive. Additional indications include expansive mucoceles, invasive fungal sinusitis, and suspected or actual neoplasms.

7. Describe the physical examination and surgical work-up performed in evaluating patients for sinus surgery.

After a complete head and neck examination, nasal endoscopy using rigid or flexible scopes should be performed to evaluate for mucosal inflammation and a source of purulence or obstruction. Nasal cultures are not routinely indicated unless a source of purulence is visualized, as results correlate poorly with cultures of actual sinus aspirates. With the price of CT scans decreasing, CT is increasingly being utilized to image the sinuses because of its superior definition of bone and mucosal changes.

8. Which FESS techniques are used to gain access to the anterior ethmoid area?

Coronal sinus CT scans are consulted both preoperatively and in the operating room to assist in identifying landmarks and areas of diseased mucosa. Following inward fracturing of the middle turbinate, an incision is made over the infundibulum to remove the uncinate process and enter the infundibulum; this technique provides access to the anterior ethmoid area. Many surgeons will perform a middle turbinate reduction together with FESS techniques to provide additional anatomic relief. Generally, the anterior two-thirds of the inferior portion of the middle turbinate is removed, taking care to avoid a major sphenopalatine artery branch posteriorly.

9. Describe the FESS techniques used for anterior ethmoid sinus drainage and frontal duct identification.

The surgeon drains the anterior ethmoids, or exteriorizes them, by entering the sinuses via the semilunar hiatus. Working posteriorly, the surgeon enters the middle ethmoids through the ethmoid bulla, taking care to identify the roof of the ethmoid, the lamina papyracea, and the anterior ethmoid artery. From the anterior ethmoid area, a 70- or 120-degree endoscope should allow the surgeon to look backward up into the infundibulum and view the frontal recess and frontonasal duct anterosuperiorly. The frontonasal duct may be *gently* probed to ensure its patency, but this is controversial, as some feel it may lead to scarring and subsequent stenosis.

10. How is FESS used to re-establish maxillary sinus drainage?

The surgeon identifies the maxillary ostium using the 30-degree endoscope or by palpating the area. If the ostium is small or obstructed, it can be enlarged anteriorly and inferiorly with the backbiter, preserving the posterior ostia intact to enhance mucosal regeneration. The surgeon should take care not to damage the nasolacrimal duct during this procedure; this duct is encased in thicker bone anteriorly—*but not much thicker!* The reason that the backbiter is not heavier or stronger is that that would encourage removal of the thicker bone that surrounds the area of the lacrimal duct. (The surgeon should always look at an instrument and try to understand what the designer intended to accomplish by designing it in exactly that way. Why does each bend and curve exist, and what anatomic problem was it designed to overcome? This facilitates correct instrument selection and use and makes the surgeon a better surgeon.)

If needed, the surgeon can use instruments to remove diseased mucosa within the maxillary sinus, or to biopsy this tissue, by entering the anterior maxillary wall from an oral approach, above the superior gum line at the canine fossa. In this situation, mucosa can be removed via the anterior puncture under direct endoscopic visualization through the maxillary ostium. Some surgeons feel that creating an additional nasoantral window under the inferior turbinate may improve maxillary drainage and ventilation by more favorably utilizing gravity as well as the "beer-can" effect of creating two patent openings. This second hole is generally reserved for cases of irreversibly diseased maxillary sinus mucosa in which there is no hope of regeneration of the mucosa and restoration of the normal mucociliary flow pattern. Some "small hole" surgeons believe that simple removal of the uncinate process (and possibly surrounding edematous mucosa) will allow the maxillary sinus ostia to regain function. With this conservative approach, however, there appears to be an increased incidence of stenosis and early recurrence of symptoms.

11. Describe FESS techniques for dissection of the posterior sinuses.

Surgery proceeds posteriorly as needed to address disease. To enter the posterior ethmoids, the basal lamella is taken down. The basal lamella is somewhat thicker than the rest of the eggshell septae in the ethmoids and represents the intersinus lateral projection ("lamella") of the middle turbinate. If necessary, the sphenoid sinus can be identified posteriorly and opened under direct vision. The goal of this surgery is to proceed one stage or space beyond the diseased mucosa, to facilitate normalization of mucociliary clearance and healing.

12. What postoperative care is needed in patients having endoscopic sinus surgery?

Endoscopic sinus surgery is commonly performed on an outpatient basis. Nasal packing, if placed, is usually removed before discharge. Prophylactic oral antibiotics may be given. Careful postoperative care and nasal hygiene with rinses are important in preventing recurrence and adhesions. Some advocate early nasal steroids to decrease inflammation and the potential for adhesions.

13. What types of complications result from endoscopic sinus surgery?

Recurrence of disease is a frustrating complication that tends to occur more readily in immunocompromised patients and patients with severe allergies or polyps. Other complications are generally either orbital or intracranial and have decreased in frequency with improvements in technique and experience. A large retrospective comparison study of endoscopic versus traditional nonendoscopic intranasal sinus surgery found no statistical difference in the overall incidence of complications. Major complications occurred in < 1% of patients and minor complications in < 7% of patients. The most common "minor" complication is the occurrence of synechiae between the lateral wall of the nose (ethmoid wall) and middle turbinate. This "complication" is obviated by the resection of the inferior portion of the middle turbinate (see Question 15).

14. What minor complications may result from FESS?

Minor complications most commonly result from middle turbinate adhesions or lamina papyracea penetration. Other minor complications include sinus infection, which was often the indication for the operation and cannot really be considered a "complication"; transient periorbital edema or ecchymosis, generally due to the penetration of the lamina papyracea; epistaxis; bronchospasm; and loss of smell. Retrobulbar orbital hematomas are thought to occur more often in traditional intranasal techniques, probably owing to a lack of direct visualization. Middle turbinate adhesions occur in endoscopic surgery and not in traditional techniques, as the middle turbinate is routinely removed in the latter. Even with turbinate reduction in conjunction with endoscopic techniques, some authors still report infrequent adhesions.

15. What are the major complications of FESS?

Major complications include cerebrospinal fluid (CSF) leak, orbital hematoma, hemorrhage requiring transfusion, and symptomatic lacrimal duct obstruction requiring surgical intervention. Rarer major complications include diplopia, loss of vision, meningitis, brain abscess, intracranial hemorrhage, stroke, carotid artery injury, and death.

16. How can you minimize complications of endoscopic sinus surgery and manage complications when they occur?

Orbital complications generally occur from penetration of the lamina papyracea along the lateral wall of the ethmoid labyrinth. Orbital fat may be visible through the lamina papyracea and will float if placed in a specimen cup filled with saline. Pressing on the eye may reveal transmitted movement of the suspected area. Retrobulbar accumulation of blood in the orbit is suspected in the presence of proptosis, pupillary dilation with decreased light reactivity, and pain around the eye. When visual impairment is present, it is imperative to decompress the orbit immediately, as blindness can result. Traumatic injury of the optic nerve, medial rectus, or superior oblique muscle is often irreversible and requires immediate ophthalmologic consultation. CSF leaks and other intracranial complications are minimized by meticulous attention to detail. In particular, all instruments should be placed under direct vision, and the mucosa along the roof of the ethmoid should be left intact. The procedure should be terminated if landmarks or surgical relationships are unclear.

17. What is the traditional approach to chronic maxillary sinusitis?

With the proliferation of endoscopic sinus surgery, traditional techniques are less commonly employed, in part due to our current understanding that ethmoiditis typically serves as the impetus for maxillary sinusitis. The traditional approach to refractory chronic sinusitis begins with weekly puncture and lavage of the maxillary sinus. If three or more antral lavages fail to clear maxillary sinusitis, a large antrostomy is created to remove diseased mucosa.

18. What is a Caldwell-Luc procedure?

The Caldwell-Luc procedure is an external approach to the anterior maxillary wall through the canine fossa above the gum line. Alternatively, an intranasal approach can be used to create an inferior meatal antrostomy. The Caldwell-Luc procedure provides excellent sinus visualization and subsequent creation of a large nasoantral window in the inferior meatus for permanent sinus drainage. The Caldwell-Luc procedure has the potential for more complications, and care must be taken to protect the infraorbital nerve superiorly and the tooth roots inferiorly. When performing an inferior meatal antrostomy, care must be taken to avoid damage to the nasolacrimal duct anteriorly and the greater palatine artery and branches of the sphenopalatine artery posteriorly.

19. Are there traditional surgical approaches that address ethmoid sinusitis?

Yes. External ethmoidectomy, transantral ethmoidectomy, and intranasal ethmoidectomy without endoscopic visualization all predate current endoscopic techniques. In cases of sinusitis complications, sinus mucoceles, or sinus neoplasms, the external and transantral approaches are commonly employed.

20. How are external ethmoidectomy and transantral ethmoidectomy performed?

External ethmoidectomy provides exposure of the orbit and excellent visualization of the ethmoid labyrinth. From the Lynch incision at the medial orbital rim, external ethmoidectomy proceeds posteriorly with exposure of the ethmoids via removal of the medial orbital wall (the lamina papyracea). This approach also provides access to the frontal sinuses superiorly and sphenoid posteriorly. Important landmarks include the suture line between the frontal bone and lamina papyracea, which identifies the plane of the cribriform plate, and the anterior and posterior ethmoid arteries. The optic nerve lies 0.5 cm behind the posterior ethmoid artery.

Transantral ethmoidectomy is performed through a large Caldwell-Luc antrostomy and allows an inferior approach to the ethmoids. The procedure can be combined with intranasal ethmoidectomy, allowing nasal instrumentation under direct vision through the maxillary sinus.

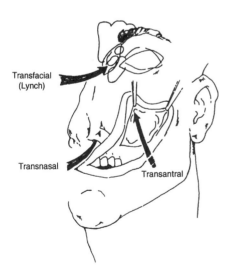

Three approaches to ethmoidectomy: transfacial (Lynch), transantral, and transnasal. (From Osguthorpe DJ, Hochman M: Inflamatory sinus diseases affecting the orbit. Otolaryngol Clin North Am 26:657–671, 1993, with permission.)

21. What are the surgical approaches to the frontal sinus?

The internal approach to the frontal sinus in FESS allows identification of the frontal recess and cannulation of the frontonasal duct. However, removal of diseased frontal mucosa is better accomplished via external approaches. The frontal sinus can be approached externally from the Lynch incision as used in external ethmoidectomy or by elevating a large bicoronal tissue flap forward from within the hairline to the orbital rims.

22. Compare the Lynch approach to the bicoronal osteoplastic approach to the frontal sinuses.

A Lynch incision at the medial orbital rim provides access to the anterior table of the frontal sinus and can be used in combination with ethmoidectomy, allowing a combined frontoethmoidectomy with removal of the frontal sinus floor and establishment of a widely patent frontonasal duct. The Lynch incision can also be used to perform a frontal trephination, in which the frontal sinus is entered and drained externally, without dissection to the nasal passage. In either case, external frontal sinus approaches permit access to the intersinus septum, which can be taken down to facilitate drainage of both sinuses through either frontonasal duct.

The bicoronal flap is used in osteoplastic frontal sinus obliteration for chronic recurrent frontal sinusitis. A scalp flap is raised in the subperiosteal plane and elevated anteriorly to expose the frontal bone over the sinuses. Using a template made from a cutout of a plain film radiograph, bone incisions are planned and created, raising the anterior table of the frontal sinuses in a single bony flap. Then the sinus mucosa is removed, and the sinus is obliterated using a fat graft and packing of the frontal ducts with bone and muscle.

23. What are the surgical approaches to the sphenoid sinus?

The sphenoid sinus is approached through its anterior wall. This can be accomplished alone or in combination with external ethmoidectomy or intranasal ethmoidectomy. Resection of the pituitary is commonly performed using a transphenoidal approach.

CONTROVERSIES

24. When should pediatric sinusitis be treated surgically?

Although a technically feasible procedure, endoscopic sinus surgery in young children is controversial. There is general agreement that surgical techniques can be indicated in children with orbital or intracranial complications of sinusitis or in patients with mucoceles or nasal polyps. However, some authors argue against pediatric sinus surgery in all but extreme refractory cases. This group argues that pediatric sinusitis is generally a self-limited disease, rarely persisting past 7–8 years of age, and complications are rare. Minimum criteria for consideration of surgery should include the following:
- Persistent or recurrent symptoms, most often unabated rhinorrhea
- Failure of maximal medical therapy
- Abnormal mucosal changes on CT scan.

25. What is minimally invasive sinus therapy?

Advocates of "transition space" or minimally invasive surgical therapy recommend removing only sufficient tissue to provide sinus ventilation and mucociliary clearance. It appears, however, that this may be suitable only for mild disease, as it is dependent on reversibility of the entire disease process and restoration of normal mucociliary clearance. While this may be a laudable goal, recent studies on mucosal regeneration, as well as the genetic basis for chronic sinusitis, suggest that the "older techniques" of gravity drainage and obliteration may still be applicable in selected cases.

26. Do residency training programs experience increased complications in endoscopic sinus surgery?

This is a question that goes to the heart of the surgical educational system. Stankiewicz reported that there is a learning curve in developing expertise in endoscopic sinus procedures and that formal training should be mandatory for the endoscopic sinus surgeon. However, a recent study reported that while there was some increase in minor complications in training programs, residents in a carefully structured and supervised training program can safely perform endoscopic sinus surgery.

HARRIS P. MOSHER (1872–1954)

In 1929, Mosher wrote, "if (the ethmoid) were placed in any other part of the body it would be an insignificant and harmless collection of bony cells. In the place where nature has put it, it has major relationships so that diseases and surgery of the labyrinth often lead to tragedy. Any surgery in this region should be simple but it has proven one of the easiest ways to kill a patient." We've come a long way since Mosher's time!

~Kennedy DW, Otolaryngol Clin North Am 30:313, 1997

BIBLIOGRAPHY

1. Gross CW: Surgical treatments for symptomatic chronic frontal sinusitis [comment]. Arch Otolaryngol Head Neck Surg 126:101–102, 2000.
2. Hoseman WG, Weber RK, Keerl RE, et al: Minimally Invasive Endonasal Sinus Surgery. New York, Thieme, 2000.
3. Keerl R, Stankiewicz J, Weber R, et al: Surgical experience and complications during endonasal sinus surgery. Laryngoscope 109:546–550, 1999.
4. Kennedy DW, Bolger WE, Zinreich SJ: Diseases of the Sinuses: Diagnosis and Management. London, B.C. Decker, 2001.
5. Kinsella JB, Calhoun KH, Bradfield JJ, et al: Complications of endoscopic sinus surgery in a residency training program. Laryngoscope 105:1029–1032, 1995.
6. Kuhn FA, Javer AR, Nagpaz K, et al: The frontal sinus rescue procedure: Early experience and three-year follow-up. Am J Rhinol 14:211–216, 2000.
7. Metson R, Gliklich RE, Stankiewicz JA, et al: Comparison of sinus computed tomography staging systems. Otolaryngol Head Neck Surg 117:372–379, 1997.
8. Park AH, Lau J, Stankiewicz J, et al: The role of functional endoscopic sinus surgery in asthmatic patients. J Otolaryngol 27:275–280, 1998.
9. Park AH, Stankiewicz JA, Chow J, et al: A protocol for management of a catastrophic complication of functional endoscopic sinus surgery: Internal carotid artery injury. Am J Rhinol 12:153–158, 1998.
10. Poole MD: Pediatric sinusitis is not a surgical disease. Ear Nose Throat J 71:622–623, 1992.
11. Seiden AM, Stankiewicz JA: Frontal sinus surgery: The state of the art. Am J Otol 19:183–193, 1998.
12. Setleff RC III: The small-hole technique in endoscopic sinus surgery. Otolaryngol Clin North Am 30:341–354, 1997.
13. Stankiewicz JA: Blindness and intranasal endoscopic ethmoidectomy: Prevention and management. Otolaryngol Head Neck Surg 101:320–329, 1989.

IV. General Otolaryngology

24. TEMPOROMANDIBULAR JOINT DISEASE

Steven B. Aragon, M.D., D.D.S.

1. Are the terms *temporomandibular disorder* and *temporomandibular joint disease* synonymous?

No. Temporomandibular disorders (TMD), also called craniomandibular disorders, encompass a variety of disorders affecting not only the temporomandibular joint (TMJ) but also areas extrinsic to the joint. TMD has traditionally been described as a constellation of related pathologic changes that produce musculoskeletal symptoms. These may present as pain associated with jaw function, limited range of mandibular motion, masticatory muscle tenderness, and TMJ tenderness. TMD has a very broad interpretation and describes a general population of patients suffering from abnormal and usually painful function of the jaw muscle and joints. This is not a homogeneous group of patients, as many different causes and mechanisms of pain are responsible for similar presentations.

It is imperative to definitively diagnose the specific causal factor to treat the patient effectively. TMJ conditions are not "cured" but are managed instead. The basic goal is to allow the muscles and joints to heal through rest and care. Often damage to the joint itself cannot be reversed, but the body can heal it enough to return to function without pain. The basic philosophy of treatment is to do the conservative and reversible treatments first. Irreversible treatments , such as surgery or orthodontics, are considered only if conservative steps have failed to bring lasting relief. This condition can often recur later on but early care can minimize the severity.

2. Describe the anatomy of the temporomandibular joint.

The TMJ is a diarthrodial (freely movable) joint with articulation between the condyle of the mandible and the glenoid fossa of the temporal bone. It is a true synovial joint with gliding and hinging motions. Avascular fibrocartilage lines both the condyle and glenoid fossa. A meniscus made of fibrocartilage lies between the condyle and temporal bone, producing a superior and inferior joint space.

3. Describe the normal relationship of the disc within the temporomandibular joint.

The disc is composed of a posterior band, an intermediate zone, and an anterior band. The posterior band is usually thicker (about 3 mm) than both the anterior band (about 2 mm) and the central zone (about 1 mm thick). The upper band conforms to the depth of the glenoid fossa, whereas the central and anterior bands conform to the articular eminence anteriorly. The inferior surface adapts to the contour of the mandibular condyle. Posteriorly, the disc is contiguous with the posterior attachment tissue, which is attached to the tympanic plate of the temporal bone superiorly and the neck of the condyle inferiorly. Anteriorly, the disc is contiguous with the superior head of the lateral pterygoid muscle.

4. What are the common signs and symptoms of temporomandibular disorder?

Preauricular (TMJ) pain	Deviation in mandibular motion
Limited mandibular range of motion	Pain in the muscles of mastication
Clicking and/or crepitus within the TMJ	Locking of the jaw in open or closed position

5. What is the differential diagnosis in these disorders?

TMJ disorders
Arthralgia (capsulitis)
Disc displacement
Disc dysfunction
Disc perforation
Masticatory muscle disorders (myogenic disorders)
Muscle trismus or splinting
Chronic mandibular hypomobilities
Fibrosis of muscular tissue (contracture)
Capsular fibrosis
Ankylosis (bony ankylosis, bony fusion)
Adhesions (intracapsular fibrosis, fibrous ankylosis)
Coronoid process elongation
Chronic mandibular hypermobilities
Subluxation
Dislocation

Fractures
Mandible
Maxilla
Inflammatory disorders
Synovitis, capsulitis
Traumatic arthritis
Degenerative arthritis
Infectious arthritis
Rheumatoid arthritis
Hyperuricemia
Disorders of maxillomandibular growth
Masticatory muscle hypertrophy or atrophy
Maxillomandibular or condylar hypoplasiaor hyperplasia
Neoplasia

6. Explain the etiology of myogenic disorders.

Myogenic disorders were previously classified as myofunctional pain dysfunction, but this term is outdated and not generally used today. Most patients with myogenic pain have normal TMJs. They present with limitation of the normal mandibular movement secondary to muscle pain and stiffness. Pain usually develops without a specific history of significant trauma. Myogenic pain is usually considered to be the result of hyperactivity or hyperfunction.

Many of these patients will have a history of nocturnal or diurnal bruxism (grinding or clenching), which may become more exaggerated during periods of physical or emotional stress. This stress results in hyperactivity, which leads to muscle fatigue and spasm, resulting in pain and limitation. This disorder is usually classified as a strain due to overuse or improper use and is treated as such. This category of disorders includes myalgias (myofascial pain, fibrositis), muscle splinting (trismus), spasm, myositis (muscle swelling), contracture, hypertrophy, dyskinesia, and bruxism.

7. How are muscle disorders diagnosed?

The most common sign of myogenic disorders is diffuse facial pain. The pain of muscular origin is poorly localized and diffuse, as opposed to the well-localized pain associated with internal derangement of the TMJ. Although muscle disorders may occur with true internal derangement of the TMJ, they must be diagnosed separately from internal derangement. There is usually no clinical or radiographic evidence of internal derangement.

8. Which muscles are usually affected in temporomandibular disorders?

The **masseter muscle** is the most common muscle involved, producing what is described as "jaw pain."

The **temporalis muscle** is the second most common site, producing "headache."

Involvement of the **lateral pterygoid muscle** produces otalgia or retrobulbar pain.

Involvement of the **medial pterygoid** may result in odynophagia or the sensation of a painful swollen gland beneath the angle of the mandible.

9. How is myogenic pain treated?

Muscle hyperactivity is treated as most strains are—by reducing the functional load and stress. Patients are placed on a soft diet and utilize heat or ice to reduce the pain and inflammation. The most commonly prescribed medications include nonsteroidal anti-inflammatory drugs (NSAIDs) and muscle relaxants. Other useful medications include anxiolytics, antidepressants, and, less commonly, narcotics such as codeine or hydrocodone. Orthotic (splint) therapy may be useful to prevent or alter excessive muscle contraction and tight intercuspation (wearing of the dentition). Physical therapy, behavioral training, and stress management are also effective modalities of treatment.

10. What is internal derangement of the temporomandibular joint?

Internal derangement has been traditionally accepted to be synonymous with disc displacement. However, the strict orthopedic use of the term includes all abnormal processes that occur within the confines of the TMJ, including not only disc displacements, but also osteoarthrosis, inflammatory arthritides, congenital deformities, adhesive disease, and traumatic, neoplastic, and developmental abnormalities

11. Explain the pathophysiology of disc displacement.

Disc displacement is usually in the anteromedial direction, probably due to the orientation of the lateral pterygoid muscle and its attachment to the capsule of the TMJ. Disruption of the ligamentous attachment of the disc to the condyle and subsequent pull by the lateral pterygoid muscle result in such displacement. While it is easy to understand how a significant external force may result in such a derangement, the exact cause often remains a mystery. Any cause of ligamentous rupture or tear can lead to displacement. This trauma may be due to a purely structural weakness or to hyperextension due to prolonged dental visits or forceful extraction of teeth, difficult anesthetic intubation, or use of retraction during a tonsillectomy.

12. What is the significance of meniscal displacement?

Although osteoarthritis has been documented in $> 50\%$ of patients with disc displacement, it is unclear whether disc displacement is a cause or a result of osteoarthritis. Several animal studies have shown osteoarthritis after producing disc displacement, but osteoarthritis has been seen in joints with normal disc–condyle relationships. Pain is often associated with disc displacement. As the disc becomes displaced, the condyle may function on the innervated posterior attachment resulting in marked discomfort. However, not all disc displacements lead to pain nor do all disc displacements require treatment. As much as 20% of the random population may have some form of disc displacement without pain or dysfunction. Temporomandibular joint mobility may be more important than meniscal displacement in the overall health of the TMJ.

13. Describe the nonsurgical treatment of disc displacement of the temporomandibular joint.

Initial therapy includes NSAIDs to reduce inflammation and provide analgesia. Limitation of function with restricted opening and soft diet help reduce painful loads on the inflamed joint. Often a concomitant muscular disorder is present that requires simultaneous treatment. Splint therapy may reduce the symptoms of both TMJ and muscular pain. Physical therapy may provide relief of symptoms. If pain and dysfunction persist despite therapy, surgical correction is indicated.

14. What imaging studies are available for the temporomandibular joint?

Plain radiographs, such as the **panoramic view,** are capable of screening gross disease, destruction, and general joint configuration. Panoramic films may be useful for bony alterations, such as degenerative joint disease, ankylosis, or other gross deformities. However, if fine detail is required, **computed tomography** (CT) is far superior to the panoramic or plain radiographs for fine osseous or fibrous evaluation.

Disc position can be evaluated by **arthrography**. A contrast material is placed into the superior and inferior joint space and outlines the disc and its position. Although this modality is an effective tool for evaluating disc position and even perforation, it is an invasive study, and there may be a fair amount of discomfort associated with its use. **Magnetic resonance imaging** (MRI) is an excellent technique for evaluating disc morphology and position as well as a sensitive indicator of early degenerative bone changes. In addition, MRI is a noninvasive technique and requires no injection of a contrast material.

15. When is a bite appliance used?

An appliance is a device worn on the teeth to relieve acute muscle and TMJ pain. The bite appliance is also known as an interocclusal appliance, orthopedic appliance, night guard, orthotic, and occlusal appliance. Many types of splints are available with different purposes. These appliances are used to stabilize an occlusion when a bruxing disorder is present. They may also decrease the load on a compromised joint when it is acutely inflamed. These devices are considered conservative and reversible. Keep in mind, however, that close follow-up is in order when these splints are worn for long periods to prevent permanent occlusal changes from occurring.

16. Are narcotics useful in the management of temporomandibular disorders?

The pharmacologic management of TMJ disorders is very similar to the treatment of arthralgias of other joints. Careful narcotic therapy has become more popular in recent years, especially for the chronic pain patient. The clinicain should be cautious, however, in administering any long-term narcotic therapy to prevent habituation.

17. What is the role of nonsteroidal anti-inflammatory drugs in the treatment of temporomandibular disorder?

NSAIDs inhibit cyclo-oxygenase and the production of prostaglandins. Recent evidence suggests they may also have a central analgesic effect. Individual response to NSAIDs is highly variable, and when response to a particular NSAID is poor, a different one should be prescribed rather than turning to narcotics.

Generic Name	Brand Name	Usual Dose
Ibuprofen	Motrin	900–2400 mg/day in divided doses
Naproxen	Anaprox	275–550 mg/day
Meclofenmate	Meclomen	50 mg q4–6h
Etodolac	Lodine	200–400 mg q8h
Piroxicam	Feldene	20 mg/d
Celecoxib	Celebrex	100–200 mg bid or 200 mg qd
Diclofenac	Voltaren, Cataflam	50 mg bid or tid

18. What is the role of muscle relaxants in the treatment of temporomandibular disorder?

Muscle relaxants can be divided into centrally acting or peripherally acting agents. The centrally acting agents relax skeletal muscle via their generally sedating effect on the central nervous system (CNS) and are more commonly prescribed.

Generic Name	Brand Name	Usual Dose
Carisoprodol	Soma	100–1400 mg/d in divided doses
Methocarbamol	Robaxin	1500–3000 mg/d in divided doses
Cyclobenzaprine	Flexeril	5–30 mg/d

19. When are benzodiazepines used in the management of temporomandibular disorders?

Benzodiazepines bind to gamma-aminobutyric acid type A receptors in the CNS. These are indicated for reduction of anxiety and muscle hyperactivity. Sedation is the most common side effect.

Generic Name	Brand Name	Usual Dose
Diazepam	Valium	2–10 mg 1–4 times a day
Clonazepam	Clonopin	0.52–1 mg 1–4 times a day
Alprazolam	Xanax	0.5 mg 1–3 times a day

20. When are antidepressants called for in the management of temporomandibular disorder?

Recent evidence suggests that antidepressant medication is often useful for chronic pain management in patients without symptoms of depression. Antidepressants have been used to manage chronic pain, headaches, sleep disorders, panic disorders, and neurologic and sympathetically mediated pain. Tricyclic and serotonin-reuptake inhibitors are most commonly used.

Generic Name	Brand Name	Initial Dose
Amitriptyline	Elavil	10–25 mg/d
Imipramine	Tofranil	10–25 mg/d
Nortriptyline	Pamelor	10–25 mg/d
Fluoxetine	Prozac	5 mg/d
Sertraline	Zoloft	50 mg/d
Celexa	Citalopram	20 mg/d
Paroxetine	Paxil	20 mg/d
Venlafaxine	Effexor	75 mg/d
Bupropion	Wellbutrin	100 mg bid

21. When is surgery indicated for temporomandibular disorder?

Surgery is indicated when nonsurgical therapy has been ineffective and when pain and/or dysfunction is moderate to severe in nature. Surgery is not indicated for asymptomatic or minimally symptomatic patients. It is not indicated for masticatory muscle disorders without internal derangement. Surgery also is not indicated for preventive reasons in patients without pain and with satisfactory function.

22. What are the surgical therapies available for temporomandibular joint disorders?

Arthrocentesis is lavaging the TMJ with saline and placing medications such as steroids, local anesthetics, and analgesics directly into the superior joint space. This may be done with local anesthesia, intravenous medication, or general anesthesia. Mandibular manipulation is also usually accomplished.

Arthroscopy enables the surgeon to treat the TMJ via a closed technique. An arthroscope is placed into the superior joint space. The articular surfaces are evaluated for synovitis, osteoarthritis, and articular dysfunction. Adhesions can be lysed to achieve improved mobility and function. Small shavers are now available to remove degenerated fibrocartilage, create smooth articulating surfaces, and remove fibrillated cartilage.

Arthrotomy is the more traditional surgical approach to the TMJ. It is an external approach utilizing a preauricular incision for access. Arthrotomy is indicated when the surgical treatment is beyond the scope of arthroscopy. The internal derangement may be so severe as to require a menisectomy or even joint reconstruction. Disc repositioning (plication), disc replacement, and grafting can be accomplished with the greater access of open joint surgery. Furthermore, TMJ reconstruction with autologous or alloplastic materials can be achieved with the open technique.

23. What is the effectiveness of arthrocentesis and arthroscopy?

Recent studies have revealed a success rate of 70–89% for arthrocentesis when measuring for decreased pain and increased opening postoperatively. Arthroscopy has been reported to be successful in 79–91% of patients postoperatively when using the same measures noted above. A recent prospective study randomized patients unresponsive to nonsurgical therapy into arthroscopy and arthrocentesis groups. They reported 75% success with arthrocentesis and 82% success with arthroscopy. Arthroscopy has also been noted to give similar results to those patients undergoing arthroplasty (79% and 76% respectively).

CONTROVERSY

24. How is occlusion related to temporomandibular disorder?

Dental occlusion has been a central theme in the etiology and treatment of TMD for decades. Proponents argued that malocclusion leads to abnormal function and proprioceptive alterations in occlusal function, resulting in clenching and grinding, inappropriate muscle use, and myogenic pain. Others believed that occlusion has little to do with TMJ disorders and that these parafunctional habits are the result of stress, leading to clenching, grinding, muscle hyperactivity, and eventually myogenic pain. Today, a multifactorial etiology is believed to be responsible, which may include portions of both theories.

25. Do menisectomies require interpositional replacements?

Controversy continues on the need for meniscal replacement following removal. Autogenous tissues used for implants include dermis, fascia, temporalis muscle, and conchal cartilage, all reporting equivalent success. Historically, alloplastic interpositional implants have included silastic and proplast. Proplast, which was removed from the market in 1990, was noted to cause a severe giant cell foreign body granulation response, which proved to be very destructive to both the glenoid fossa and condyle. Long-term success of discectomy is also possible without replacement. The success of discectomy may be attributable to the formation of new tissue between the condyle and fossa, which acts as a pseudodisc.

BIBLIOGRAPHY

1. Baker GI: Surgical considerations in the management of temporomandibular joint and masticatory muscle disorders. J Orofac Pain 13:307–312, 1999.
2. Carvajal WA, Laskin DM: The long-evaluation of arthrocentesis for the treatment of internal derangements of the temporomandibular joint. J Oral Maxillofac Surg 58:852–855, 2000.
3. Cascone P, Vetrano S, Nicolai G, et al: Temporomandibular joint biomechanical restrictions: the fluid and synovial membrane. J Craniofac Surg 10:301–7, 1999.
4. Clark GT, Kim YJ: A logical approach to the treatment of temporomandibular disorders. Oral Maxillofac Surg Clin, North Am 7:149–166, 1995.
5. Goldberg MB: Posttraumatic temporomandibular disorders. J Orofac Pain 13:291–294, 1999.
6. Goldstein BH: Medical legal considerations in temporomandibular disorders. Oral Surg Oral Med Oral Pathol Oral Radiol Endod 88:395–399, 1999.
7. Israel HA: The use of arthroscopic surgery for treatment of temporomandibular joint disorders. J Oral Maxillofac Surg 57:579–582, 1999.
8. Kopp S: The influence of neuropeptides, serotonin, and interleukin 1beta on temporomandibular joint pain and inflammation. J Oral Maxillofac Surg 56:189–191, 1998.
9. Quinn P: Pain management in the multiply operated temporomandibular joint patient. J Oral Maxillofac Surg 58(Suppl 2):12–14, 2000.
10. Ryan DE: Management of failed alloplastic implants: immunologic considerations. In Fonseca RJ (ed): Oral and Maxillofacial Surgery. Philadelphia, W.B. Saunders, 2000.
11. Scarfe WC: A common sense approach to TMJ and implant imaging. Ann R Austr Coll Dent Surg 14:48–61, 1998.
12. Takaku S, Sano T, Yoshida M: Long-term magnetic resonance imaging after temporomandibular joint discectomy without replacement. J Oral Maxillofac Surg 58:739–745, 2000.
13. Woda A, Pionchon P: A unified concept of idiopathic orofacial pain: clinical features. J Orofac Pain 13:172–184; discussion 185–195, 1999.

25. ORAL LESIONS

Michael L. Lepore, M.D., FACS

1. What is the most common cause of xerostomia?

Medications are the most common cause of oral dryness, or xerostomia, especially in older persons. In fact, the increased medication use in the geriatric population may explain the widely believed myth that salivary gland dysfunction is a part of the normal aging process.

2. How do medications cause xerostomia?

Numerous mechanisms are responsible for the xerostomia: salivary gland hypofunction, mucosal dehydration, total body dehydration, altered sensory function, and cognitive disorders. Medications that frequently cause decreased salivary flow rates by blocking cholinergic activity include tricyclic antidepressants; antipsychotics; centrally acting antihypertensives, such as clonidine and diphenhydramine; and the belladonna alkaloids such as atropine, scopolamine, and hyoscyamine.

3. Which medical conditions are commonly associated with xerostomia?

Two of the most common are **Sjögren's syndrome** and **radiation-induced salivary gland dysfunction**. In its primary form, Sjögren's syndrome is characterized by lymphocytic infiltration of the salivary and lacrimal glands, which leads to dry mouth and dry eyes. Xerostomia may also occur in association with another major rheumatologic disease, such as rheumatoid arthritis, systemic lupus erythematosus, primary biliary cirrhosis, or scleroderma. The vast majority of patients with radiation-induced salivary gland dysfunction have received ionizing radiation for head and neck carcinoma. This type of salivary dysfunction is usually more severe during the active radiation, but return to normal salivation almost never occurs. Several other disorders also can lead to dysfunction of one or more of the major salivary glands (parotid, submandibular, and sublingual), but patients are rarely symptomatic because salivary flow must decrease by approximately 50% before xerostomia develops.

4. Are there complications of salivary gland hypofunction?

Saliva contains a variety of polypeptides and glycoproteins that have antimicrobial activity. In the absence of these elements, the most common complications are recurrent **oral candidiasis** and **dental caries**.

5. Name the three types of aphthous ulcers.

Minor, major, and herpetiform.

6. How do the various types of aphthous ulcers differ?

Minor: Prior to the appearance of the ulceration, the patient usually notices a tingling or burning sensation. The ulcerations usually measure < 1.0 cm and are localized to the freely moveable keratinized gingiva. They are white in the center surrounded by a red border. They are extremely painful and usually resolve in approximately 7–10 days.

Major: These can occur on the moveable mucosa, soft palate, tongue, and tonsillar pillars. They are much more painful than the minor ulcers and are also much larger, measuring 1–3 cm. Anywhere from 1–10 ulcers may be present.

Herpetiform: These ulcers are similar to herpetic lesions. There are usually 10–100 ulcers present, measuring 1–3 mm in diameter. These small ulcers may coalesce to form larger ulcers.

The minor and major types generally do not leave a scar, whereas the herpetiform variety may leave a scar if the ulcerations coalesce.

7. What causes aphthous ulcers?

The cause of these lesions is still unknown. However, the following have been implicated:
   Viral agents (herpes simplex virus)
   Bacteria (*Streptococcus sanguis*)
   Nutritional deficiencies (B_{12}, folate, iron)
   Hormonal alterations
   Stress
   Trauma
   Food allergies (nuts, chocolate, gluten)
   Immunologic abnormalities

8. A 27-year-old woman comes to your office with painful mouth sores that began 24 hours ago. On examination, you find several white lesions on her pharynx, soft palate, and tongue. She had similar lesions 3 years ago, which resolved over a week. What is the most likely diagnosis?

Most likely, **recurrent aphthous stomatitis**. Aphthous ulcers are the most common type of nontraumatic ulcers. In the general population, the incidence is 10–20%. For reasons that we do not understand, the incidence in professionals and upper socioeconomic groups is higher.

9. What is the current treatment for aphthous stomatitis?

Treatment includes both medical management and cauterization. Cauterization of the ulcer bed can be done either chemically or electrically. Silver nitrate is commonly used for chemical cauterization. After the application of silver nitrate, the area should be swabbed with a cotton-tip applicator impregnated with sodium chloride. This agent converts the silver nitrate to silver chloride, preventing a deep burn. When using electrical cauterization, care must be taken not to produce a deep burn.

Medical treatment includes oral antibiotics, anti-inflammatory agents, or immunosuppressants. Treatment with yogurt, cultured buttermilk, and *Lactobacillus* capsules has also been recommended. Local measures include the use of an oral suspension of tetracycline or topical steroids, such as 0.5% fluocinonide ointment or betamethasone solution.

10. A 30-year-old, otherwise healthy man presents with small, creamy white, curdlike lesions on his tongue and buccal mucosa of several weeks' duration. What is your diagnosis?

This presentation is consistent with the diagnosis of thrush, or **oral candidiasis.** *Candida* species are present in normal oral flora in 40–60% of the population. In certain immunocompromised states, overgrowth of the candida can occur, leading to thrush. The lesions represent patches of *Candida albicans* with leukocytes and desquamated epithelial cells.

11. How is the diagnosis of thrush made?

Scraping the lesions (they are easy to remove and have an erythematous base) and then examining the scrapings in potassium hydroxide under the microscope can easily make the diagnosis. Characteristic hyphae and blastospores are easily recognized.

12. When thrush is suspected, what should your diagnostic work-up include?

Common conditions that lead to thrush include inhaled corticosteroid use for reactive airways disease, debilitating systemic illnesses such as cancer, and other immunocompromised states such as acquired immunodeficiency syndrome (AIDS) and neutropenia. Less common causes include diabetes, pregnancy, adrenal insufficiency, systemic antibiotic and systemic steroid use, nutritional deficiencies, and poor oral hygiene; the differential diagnosis includes leukoplakia and hyperkeratosis. Patients who have thrush for no obvious reason, such as the patient presented above, should be evaluated for human immunodeficiency virus (HIV) infection.

13. A 60-year-old woman seen in your office complains of ulcerations involving the free and attached gingiva. She noted some raised areas and a diffuse redness and peeling of the mucous membrane prior to the appearance of the ulcerations. What is the most likely diagnosis?

Desquamative gingivitis affects females after the age of 30. It is characterized by a diffuse erythematous desquamation, ulceration, and, at times, bullae formation involving the free and attached gingiva. Associated conditions include lichen planus, cicatricial pemphigoid, bullous pemphigoid, pemphigus vulgaris, dermatitis herpetiformis, and drug reactions. Incisional biopsy is frequently necessary for diagnosis. Immunofluorescent studies may aid in differentiating the various entities.

14. How often are white oral lesions malignant?

Acutely, lesions of the oral cavity may be erythematous. However, during the course of the disease, white elements may appear and predominate. White lesions of the mouth are often benign. However, 5–10% of oral malignancies present as white lesions. Thus, the examining physician must always be concerned that the lesion in question is a possible malignancy.

15. What are the two broad clinical categories of white lesions?

Keratotic and nonkeratotic. The most important clinical feature distinguishing the two groups is the lesion's ability to adhere to the surface epithelium. The more common lesions can therefore be categorized into one of these two groups.

Keratotic	**Nonkeratotic**
Firmly adherent	Removed relatively easily
Usually of long duration	Usually of short duration
Usually change slowly	Frequently change rapidly
Surface is usually elevated and may be smooth, roughened, or even verrucous	Usually erosive or ulcerative

In some cases, the pathologic process causing the oral lesions also involves the skin. If a diagnosis cannot be made clinically by observation or association with a cutaneous counterpart, a biopsy with immunofluorescent staining will be of value in establishing a diagnosis.

16. Which disease states can lead to keratotic and nonkeratotic white lesions?

Keratotic

Clinical leukoplakia	Chronic candidiasis
Stomatitis nicotina of the palate	Interstitial glossitis (tertiary syphilis)
Carcinoma in situ	Hereditary and nevoid white lesions
Squamous cell carcinoma	Primary skin lesions
Florid oral papillomatosis	Lichen planus
Verruca	Lupus erythematosus
Squamous papilloma	Psoriasis

Nonkeratotic

Acute candidiasis	Erythema multiforme
Aphthous stomatitis	Trauma
Vesiculobulbous diseases	Mechanical
Viral infection	Chemical
Contact dermatitis	Thermal
Drug reaction	Desquamative gingivitis
Pemphigus vulgaris	Acute lupus erythematosus
Benign mucous-membrane pemphigus	Secondary syphilis
Bullous pemphigoid	Psoriasis

17. A 45-year-old man who drinks and smokes heavily has a white plaque lesion on the undersurface of his tongue. He noticed the area when brushing his teeth and could not rub it off with the brush. What is the most likely diagnosis?

Clinical leukoplakia is the most likely diagnosis. **Leukoplakia** refers to any white patch or plaque of the mouth that cannot be removed by rubbing and cannot be ascribed to other diseases, such as lichen planus. A biopsy is necessary because 30% of these lesions are malignant. Asymptomatic, velvety red lesions of the mouth may be even more suspicious for carcinoma in situ and should be biopsied.

18. What is a "geographic" tongue?

Loss and regrowth of papillae lead to red patches on the tongue. This map-like appearance is asymptomatic and results from an idiopathic inflammatory condition.

19. Where does squamous cell carcinoma most often occur in the mouth?

The lower lip, floor of the mouth, and tongue. Painless ulcers that do not heal in 1–2 weeks are highly suspect and should be biopsied.

20. What is the differential diagnosis of an oral pigmented lesion?

The most worrisome diagnosis is malignant melanoma, but other possibilities include nevi and benign maccules, lesions of Peutz-Jeghers disease, or Addison's disease. Any new suspicious lesion should be biopsied early.

21. Who develops hairy leukoplakia?

White, painless lesions that appear "hairy" are often found in patients with AIDS, usually on the lateral aspects of the tongue. These lesions are caused by the Epstein-Barr virus and may temporarily respond to high-dose acyclovir.

22. What is torus mandibulae? Torus palatinus?

Both torus mandibulae and torus palatinus are usually an incidental finding on routine examination of the oral cavity.

Torus mandibulae consists of an enlargement of bone, usually on the lingual surface of the mandible. The enlargement is found above the insertion of the mylohyoid muscle. It is covered by normal mucosa of the oral cavity. The mass may consist of one single bony formation or multiple bony ridges. These bony abnormalities are thought to be autosomal dominantly inherited with variable penetration.

Torus palatinus is a slow-growing enlargement located on the hard palate at its midportion. It may be single or multiple and is covered by normal-appearing oral mucosa. This bony growth is more frequent in females; however, in the American Indian population, males predominate. Torus palatinus is thought to be inherited in an autosomal dominant pattern, but X-linked dominance may be a factor.

23. How is torus mandibulae managed? Torus palatinus?

Neither of these lesions should be surgically removed unless they interfere with denture placement or normal function. However, a torus palatinus may become excessively large, altering speech and thus necessitating its removal. Occasionally, both can ulcerate, causing persistent discomfort and pain and again necessitating surgical removal.

24. What is trench mouth?

Acute necrotizing ulcerative gingivitis (ANUG), or Vincent's gingivitis, is a synergistic infection involving multiple oral anaerobic bacteria found in adolescents and young adults. Numerous factors increase the susceptibility to bacterial destruction and include debilitating disease, nutritional deficiencies, psychogenic factors, and degenerative disease. ANUG spares the edentulous patient.

Patients usually complain of ulcerations on the gingival margin. On physical examination, the typical lesions are punched-out, crater-like depressions in the interdental papillae and along the gingival margins. A gray pseudomembrane containing a meshwork of fibrin, necrotic epithelial cells, and various bacterial organisms covers the lesions. During the acute phase, the patient may have malaise, fever, regional lymphadenitis, fetor oris, increased salivation, and spontaneous gingival hemorrhage. Treatment consists of local measures (e.g., vigorous oral hygiene and removal of callus formation) and antibiotics to cover predominantly anaerobic organisms.

25. What are Fordyce spots?

Fordyce spots are very small, yellowish, granular lesions consistent with sebaceous glands on histologic examination. They are normally located in the mucosa lateral to the anterior pillar but also can be found in the upper lip, along the distal portion of the lower lip, and on the buccal mucosa at the angle of the mouth. To see them, the clinician must spread the oral mucosa by placing it under tension. Removal of these structures is unnecessary unless the lesions are increasing in size, denoting an underlying pathologic condition.

26. During a routine physical examination, a 32-year-old man is noted to have a papillary lesion involving the uvula and anterior tonsillar pillar on the left. What is the significance of this finding?

Squamous papillomas are the most common benign tumors of the oral cavity and pharynx. Like their laryngeal counterparts, these papillary growths are locally noninvasive. Malignant degeneration of this benign tumor is rare. Polymerase chain reaction studies of the DNA of the oral papillomas fail to demonstrate any human papillomavirus type 6a or 11a, which is normally associated with the more aggressive types found in laryngeal papillomas of children.

27. What are mucoceles of the oral cavity?

A **mucous retention cyst,** or mucocele, is a lesion of the lower lip or buccal mucosa. Chiefly of cosmetic concern, this benign nodule is either translucent or bluish in color and ranges from 1–2 cm in diameter. These cysts result from the retention of saliva and are commonly caused by trauma to the lower lip. The lesions are usually superficial and very thin-walled, transparent in nature, and true cysts. If a thin wall is not present with mucoid material, this type of lesion is commonly referred to as a mucous retention cyst. Mucoceles located deep in the lip tissue may appear as ill-defined discrete masses.

CONTROVERSIES

28. How are mucoceles treated?

These lesions can be surgically excised in their entirety or they can be **marsupialized** (the cyst is incised and the mucoid material allowed to drain). The recurrence rate after removal of these lesions is high because there are numerous minor salivary glands present in the lip and other areas of the oral mucosa. The treatment may also involve repeated needle aspiration. The injection of sclerosing material may be helpful only in very superficial mucoceles. Recurrence is particularly frequent in the **plunging ranula**, where the salivary duct ectasia extends down below the myelohyoid of the floor of the mouth. Marsupialization is usually unsuccessful and the treatment requires excision of the gland and usually the adjacent submandibular and sublingual glands.

ORAL CANCER

The incidence of both oral and pharyngeal cancer among men is highest in northern France, southern India, a few areas of central and eastern Europe, and Latin America. Among women, the highest incidence is observed in India. The ratio of oral to pharyngeal cancer everywhere is systematically lower in men compared with women. Recent trends for oral cancer are more favorable than those for pharyngeal cancer in developing countries. In developed countries, trends in oral cancer appears to be more closely correlated to changes in alcohol consumption than those of pharyngeal cancer.

~Franceschi S, et al, Oral Oncology 36:106, 2000

———»●«———

BIBLIOGRAPHY

1. Allen CM, Blozis GG: Oral mucosal lesions. In Cummings CW, Frederickson JM, Harker LA (eds): Otolaryngology: Head & Neck Surgery, 3rd ed. St. Louis, Mosby-Year Book, 1998.
2. Aragon SB, Jafek BW: Stomatitis. In Bailey BJ, Calhoun KH (ed): Head & Neck Surgery—Otolaryngology, 2nd ed. Philadelphia, Lippincott Williams & Wilkins, 1998.
3. Atkinson JC, O'Connell A, Aframian D: Oral manifestations of primary immunological diseases. J Am Dent Assoc 131:345–356, 2000.
4. Cannon RD, Chaffin WL: Oral colonization by *Candida albicans*. Crit Rev Oral Biol Med 10:359–383, 1999.
5. Mandell GL, Bennett JE, Dolin R (eds): Principles and Practice of Infectious Disease. New York, Churchill Livingstone, 2000.
6. Martin W: Oral health and the older diabetic. Clin Geriatr Med 15:339–350, 1999.
7. McBride DR: Management of aphthous ulcers. Am Fam Physician 62:149–154, 160, 2000.
8. Mulliken RA, Casner MJ: Oral manifestations of systemic disease. Emerg Med Clin North Am 18:565–575, 2000.
9. Popovsky JL, Camisa C: New and emerging therapies for diseases of the oral cavity. Dermatol Clin 18:113–125, 2000.
10. Raber-Durlacher JE: Current practices for management of oral mucositis in cancer patients. Supp Care Cancer 7:71–74, 1999.
11. Rosenthal C, Karthaus M, Ganser A: New strategies in the treatment and prophylaxis of chemo- and radiotherapy-induced oral mucositis. Antibiot Chemother 50:115–132, 2000.
12. Scully C, Porter S: ABC of oral health. Swellings and red, white, and pigmented lesions. Br Med J 321:225–228, 2000.
13. Sykes L: Oral management of irradiated head and neck cancer patients. SADJ. 54:59–62, 1999.
14. Triantos D, Porter SR, Scully C, Teo CG: Oral hairy leukoplakia: Clinicopatholgic features, pathogenesis, diagnosis, and clinical significance. Clin Infect Dis 25:1392–1396, 1997.
15. Walsh PM, Epstein JB: The oral effects of smokeless tobacco. J Can Dent Assoc 66:22–25, 2000.

26. FACIAL NERVE DISORDERS

Richard D. Thrasher, M.D., and Stephen P. Cass, M.D., MPH

1. With which branchial arch is the facial nerve associated? Name the types of fibers, both motor and sensory, carried by the facial nerve.

The second branchial arch:

Special visceral efferent—to the muscles of facial expression, stylohyoid, stapedius, and posterior belly of digastricus

General visceral efferent—to lacrimal, nasal, sublingual, and submandibular salivary glands

Special sensory afferent—taste from the anterior two-thirds of the tongue

Somatic sensory afferent—sensation from the posterior ear canal and concha

General visceral afferent sensory—sensation from the nose, palate, and pharynx

2. What is significantly different between the neonatal and adult extratemporal facial nerve anatomy?

The stylomastoid foramen is not protected by the mastoid tip until at least 18 months of age. This has obvious implications for the surgical anatomy of the neck in neonates.

3. Name the five segments of the facial nerve, their course, and their length.

Meatal: from brainstem to internal auditory canal; 23–24 mm

Labyrinthine: from meatal foramen to the geniculate ganglion; represents the narrowest portion of the fallopian canal at 3–5 mm

Tympanic: from geniculate ganglion to pyramidal eminence; 8–11 mm. The facial nerve is frequently (70%) dehiscent in this segment.

Mastoid: from pyramidal process to stylomastoid foramen; 10–14 mm

Extratemporal: from the stylomastoid foramen to the muscles of facial expression and posterior belly of digastric, stylohyoid, and postauricular; 15–20 mm

4. Name the five major branches of the extratemporal segment of cranial nerve VII. What do they innervate?

Cervical: platysma

Marginal mandibular: lower orbicularis oris, depressor anguli oris, depressor labii inferioris, and mentalis; it travels superficial to the facial vein at the inferior border of the mandible

Buccal: zygomaticus major and minor, levator anguli oris, buccinator, and upper orbicularis oris; it courses in close relation to the parotid duct

Zygomatic: lower orbicularis oculi; it anastomoses with the buccal branch

Temporal: frontalis, corrugator supercilii, procerus, and upper orbicularis oculi

5. Name the site of the first major branching of the extratemporal facial nerve.

The pes anserinus.

6. What is the blood supply to the 7th nerve and what is its clinical importance?

Labyrinthine branches of the anterior inferior cerebellar artery (AICA) supply the meatal segment within the internal auditory canal. The petrosal branch of the middle meningeal artery supplies the nerve in the perigeniculate region. There are few anastomotic connections between these two vascular supplies in the region of the meatal foramen. This may be of significance in Bell's palsy because edema in the area can lead to ischemic injury of the nerve. The stylomastoid branch of the postauricular artery feeds the mastoid and tympanic segments.

7. During parotid surgery, what are the landmarks for identifying the facial nerve?
There are a number of methods to find the main trunk:
- Identify the tragal pointer which is a triangular extension of the tragal cartilage. Aptly named, this structure "points" toward the main trunk of cranial nerve (CN) VII, which typically lies 10 mm inferior and 10 mm deep to it.
- Follow the posterior belly of the digastric muscle to the styloid process. The stylomastoid foramen lies deep to this structure and is the outlet for the nerve from the skull. Typically it is 25 mm deep to the skin's surface. An important clinical note is that in children under the age of 2, the mastoid is not well developed, and the facial nerve lies much closer to the surface of the skin than would otherwise be expected.
- Find the tympanomastoid fissure; the nerve can be found 6–8 mm below the inferior drop-off of the fissure.
- Follow the marginal mandibular nerve proximally.
- In parotid dissections that are complicated (e.g., by prior surgery or neoplasm), it may only be possible to find the trunk by following a peripheral branch in the face proximally.

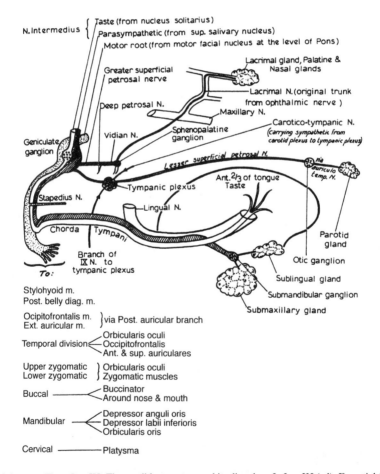

The facial nerve. (From Lee KJ: The vestibluar system and its disorders. In Lee KJ (ed): Essential Otolaryngology–Head and Heck Surgery. Norwalk, CT, Appleton & Lange, 1995, p 194; with permission.)

8. **Discuss the pathophysiology of nerve injury.**

Nerve injury is classically described in terms of neuropraxia, axonotmesis, or neurotmesis.

Neuropraxia results when a lesion blocks the flow of axoplasm from the somata to the distal axons. In this case, the nerve is viable and returns to normal function when the blockade is corrected. Electrophysiologic testing reveals normal function, except that the electromyogram fails to show voluntary motor action potentials because they are not conducted across the blockade.

Axonotmesis is a state of wallerian degeneration distal to the lesion with preservation of the motor axon endoneural sheaths. Electrically, the nerve shows rapid and complete degeneration, with loss of voluntary motor units. Regeneration to the motor end plates will occur, as long as the endoneural tubules are intact.

Neurotmesis is characterized by both wallerian degeneration and loss of endoneural tubules. Electrophysiologic studies yield evidence of complete nerve degeneration. Regeneration is dependent on many factors, including the integrity of the endoneurium, perineurium, and epineurium and the extent of ischemia and scarring around the lesion.

9. **List some common categories and a few of the associated causes of facial paralysis.**

Idiopathic: Recurrent facial palsy

Congenital: Möbius syndrome, congenital unilateral lower lip paralysis, Melkersson-Rosenthal syndrome, dystrophic myotonia

Traumatic: temporal bone fractures, intrauterine compression, birth trauma/forceps delivery, facial contusions or lacerations, penetrating wounds to face or ear, iatrogenic injury (parotid/ear/cranial surgery, embolization for epistaxis, mandibular block anesthesia)

Infection: Bell's palsy, herpes zoster oticus, otitis media with effusion, acute mastoiditis, malignant otitis externa, tuberculosis, Lyme disease, acquired immunodeficiency syndrome, mononucleosis, influenza, encephalitis, malaria, syphilis, botulism

Neoplasia: cholesteatoma, carcinoma, acoustic neuroma, meningioma, facial neuroma, glomus jugulare or tympanicum, leukemia, hemangioblastoma, osteopetrosis, histiocytosis, rhabdomyosarcoma

Metabolic/systemic: diabetes, hyperthyroidism, pregnancy, autoimmune disorders, sarcoidosis, hypertension

Neurologic: Guillain-Barré syndrome, multiple sclerosis, Millard-Gubler syndrome

10. **What is the House-Brackmann Facial Nerve Grading System?**

House-Brackmann Facial Nerve Grading System

GRADE	GROSS CHARACTERISTICS	MOTION CHARACTERISTICS
I. Normal	Normal facial appearance in all areas	Normal facial function in all areas
II. Mild dysfunction	Slight weakness noticeable only on close inspection. Normal symmetry and tone at rest	Forehead: moderate to good function Eye: complete closure with minimal effort Mouth: slight asymmetry
III. Moderate dysfunction	Obvious but not disfiguring asymmetry Normal symmetry and tone at rest	Forehead: slight to moderate movement Eye: complete closure with effort Mouth: slightly weak with maximum effort
IV. Moderately severe dysfunction	Obvious weakness with possible disfiguring asymmetry, but normal symmetry and tone at rest	Forehead: none Eye: incomplete closure Mouth: asymmetric with maximum effort
V. Severe dysfunction	Only minimally perceptible motion Asymmetry at rest	Forehead: none Eye: incomplete closure Mouth: slight movement
VI. Total paralysis	No movement and obvious asymmetry at rest	No movement at any level

11. What elements of the history and physical examination are important in evaluating a facial paralysis?

The history allows the long differential diagnosis listed above to be narrowed significantly. Any palsy with progression beyond a 3-week period or with lack of improvement should be considered a neoplasm until proven otherwise. Signs of possible tumor involvement include facial twitching, other cranial nerve involvement, sensorineural hearing loss, recurrent episodes of facial paralysis, facial weakness in the presence of a conductive hearing loss or a mass behind the tympanic membrane, and/or prolonged ear pain.

Bell's palsy and herpes zoster oticus may also have associated with them numbness in the middle and lower face, otalgia, hyperacusis, decreased tearing, or altered taste sensation. Obviously, a pertinent medical history to ascertain the risk factors for systemic and/or infectious causes is mandatory.

A pertinent clinical reminder for the physical examination is that upper eyelid motion is not indicative of an intact facial nerve, since the levator palpebrae muscle is innervated by the oculomotor nerve. The physical examination should also attempt to ascertain whether the lesion is peripheral or central. A unilateral central lesion will often spare the upper face, since these muscles receive both crossed and uncrossed fibers. Lesions of the peripheral system involve both the upper and the lower face. A central lesion is also suggested by the lack of emotional facial movement as well as decreased lacrimation, taste, and salivation on the ipsilateral side.

12. How can you evaluate the five branches of the extratemporal segment of the facial nerve during physical examination?

It is important to test each of the five branches of the nerve to exclude isolated branch paralysis or central lesions. To ensure that contraction of the masseter or temporalis muscle is not mistaken for facial nerve function, you should make each of the following assessments while jaw movements are minimized.

    Cervical—contract the neck muscles
    Marginal mandibular—whistle or pucker the lips
    Buccal—smile or show teeth
    Zygomatic—squeeze eyes shut tightly
    Temporal—raise eyebrows

13. What is Schirmer's test?

Schirmer's test is a method to assess parasympathetic innervation to the lacrimal gland via the greater superficial petrosal nerve. The procedure entails placing 5-mm paper strips in the conjunctival fornix of each eye and measuring lacrimation by comparing the length of paper moistened by tear flow over a 5-minute period. An abnormal Schirmer's test involves a 25% reduction of the ipsilateral eye as compared to normal lacrimation, a 30% reduction of the involved side versus total lacrimation, or < 25 mm bilateral lacrimation.

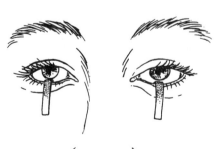

Schirmer's test. (From Pender DJ: Practical Otology. Philadelphia, J.B. Lippincott Company, 1992, p 118, with permission.)

14. Which radiologic studies should be part of the diagnostic work-up for a patient with a facial paralysis?

Radiologic tests are not indicated for the assessment of every patient presenting with a facial nerve paralysis. The need for such studies is based on both the clinical history and the course of the paralysis (i.e., if a neoplasm is suspected). If radiologic imaging is deemed necessary, high-resolution computed tomography (CT) or magnetic resonance imaging (MRI) is the study of choice. MRI scans are superior to CT in imaging the nerve at the cerebellopontine angle and internal auditory canal. Gadolinium-enhanced MRI is the test of choice for facial nerve paralysis secondary to inflammatory and other nontraumatic etiologies. CT, on the other hand, is preferred for the evaluation of traumatic 7th nerve paralysis.

15. Which electrophysiologic tests are important in evaluating a patient with a facial paralysis?

Nerve Excitability Test (NET): In this study, a $1/sec^2$ wave pulse, which is 1 msec in duration, is applied over both the affected and the unaffected facial nerves. Thresholds for minimal facial muscle response are recorded and compared. A 3- to 4 mA or greater difference is considered significant, suggesting denervation. This test is not accurate druing the first 72 hours after onset of paralysis, since it takes 3 days for wallerian degeneration to occur.

Maximal Stimulation Test (MST): A variation of the NET, the MST stimulates the ipsilateral and contralateral facial muscles at a level sufficient to depolarize all motor axons underlying the stimulator. Therefore, it utilizes maximal as opposed to minimal stimulation to evaluate muscular response. The results of the test are recorded as a subjective account of the difference in facial muscle movement between the normal and involved sides. Generally, it is thought that the MST becomes abnormal before the NET and is therefore a better prognostic indicator. However, the MST is limited by its lack of objectivity.

Electroneuronography (ENoG): ENoG measures and compares the amplitudes of the muscle summation potentials that are elicited when a supramaximal level of current is applied over the main trunk of the facial nerve on the affected and unaffected sides. The peak-to-peak amplitude is directly proportional to the number of intact motor axons, thus providing a gauge to assess neuronal degeneration. For example, an evoked summation potential of = 10% indicates 90% degeneration. To accurately predict which patients may benefit from surgical decompression, ENoG must be performed within 2 weeks of the onset of symptoms.

Electromyography (EMG): EMG is complementary in the evaluation of acute facial paralysis, helping to eliminate false-positive results obtained by NET, MST, and ENoG. The EMG determines the activity of the muscle rather than the activity of the nerve. This test can (1) provide information regarding intact motor units in the acute phase and (2) confirm the integrity of intact axons in the recovery phase, detecting reinnervation potentials 6–12 weeks before the return of facial muscle function is clinically evident. However, unlike NET, MST, and ENoG, an EMG cannot assess the degree of degeneration or prognosis for recovery.

Audiometry: Audiometry should be performed to evaluate the potential for conductive and sensorineural hearing losses, which can be coexistent in patients with facial nerve palsies. Conductive hearing losses are most consistent with middle ear tumors, cholesteatomas, and other middle ear processes involving the horizontal segment of the facial nerve. Sensorineural deficits, on the other hand, indicate conditions such as acoustic neuroma, meningioma, congenital cholesteatoma, and dermoid and facial nerve neuromas, which affect the nerve in the cerebellopontine angle or internal auditory canal.

16. What is Bell's palsy?

Bell's palsy formerly was thought of as an idiopathic facial paralysis, but is now shown to be a viral neuropathy with the following minimal diagnostic criteria:

- Paralysis or paresis of all facial muscle groups on one side of the face
- Sudden onset
- Absence of signs of central nervous system (CNS) diasease, ear disease, or cerebellopontine angle disease

It often follows a viral prodrome with a typical 3- to 5-day duration and a peak in symptoms at 48 hours. The patient may have a widened palpebral fissure, diminished taste, difficulty chewing, hypesthesia in one or more branches of the fifth cranial nerve, and hyperacusis. In 14% of patients with Bell's palsy, family history will be positive. Some 12% of patients may have recurrent facial paralysis, either ipsilateral or contralateral.

Recent evidence has been published that documents via polymerase chain reaction the presence, in statistically significant numbers, of herpes simplex virus (HSV) within the facial nerve of patients affected by Bell's palsy. A comparison of the geniculate ganglion in affected versus nonaffected individuals has demonstrated the near absence of any detectable virus in the unaffected population. The conclusion being drawn now is that the most common cause of Bell's palsy is HSV reactivation in the geniculate ganglion and that it is not an idiopathic disease.

17. How common is Bell's palsy?

Bell's palsy has an estimated incidence of 15–40 per 100,000 people. It is most prevalent in the 3rd decade of life, although it can be seen at any age. Bell's palsy accounts for over 50% of acute facial palsies. However, it is important to realize that this is a diagnosis of exclusion. A diagnosis of Bell's palsy is less probable if any of the following signs and symptoms are present:

> History of known trauma along the course of the nerve
> Multiple cranial nerve involvement
> Bilateral paralysis
> Slowly progressive paresis evolving for > 3 weeks
> Signs of neoplasia
> Vesicles on the head or neck
> Evidence of a temporal bone infection
> Palsy at birth
> Signs of a CNS lesion
> Failure to have onset of recovery within 6 months after onset of palsy

18. What are the most common complications following the onset of facial paralysis?

Exposure keratitis secondary to (1) paralysis with inability to close the eyelid completely, (2) diminished tearing, and (3) loss of corneal sensitivity with trigeminal nerve involvement. Evidence for corneal irritation includes redness, itching, foreign-body sensation, and visual blurring. Treatment involves using artificial tears 4–5 times/day. Ophthalmic lubricant should be followed by patching or taping the eye shut at night. The eye should be protected from wind, foreign bodies, and drying with glasses and/or moisture chambers. Ophthalmology consult should be obtained for these patients.

19. What are crocodile tears?

Injuries to the facial nerve may be associated with aberrant nerve regeneration. Fibers that normally innervate the alivary glands may regenerate to innervate the lacrimal gland. This leads to "crying" when the patient eats (gustatory tearing).

20. How do you treat facial nerve paralysis medically?

The medical management of facial nerve paralysis employs several philosophies:

- If infectious processes are ascertained, appropriate treatment with antimicrobial and/or antiviral agents, in addition to eradication of the infectious nidus (i.e., mastoidectomy/myringotomy), should be instituted.
- Previously a more controversial issue, a 7- to 10-day course of oral steroids, if initiated within the first 48 hours after onset of symptoms, may improve recovery via decreased inflammation.
- Electrophysiologic assessment of the extent of nerve damage provides valuable information, particularly in cases in which surgical decompression may be a treatment option.

- Prophylactic eye care to protect against exposure keratitis should be initiated in all patients with a facial nerve paralysis.
- For Bell's palsy, specifically, the current recommendation for treatment is (1) prednisone 1 mg/kg/day for 10 days, tapering over the next 4–7 days, (2) acyclovir 800 mg 5 times/day or valacyclovir 500 mg 2 times/day, and (3) eye care.

21. When is surgical treatment indicated?

Surgery is advocated for decompression when total paralysis is present with evidence of extensive nerve degeneration. Serial studies with ENoG have shown that when the number of motor fibers falls to less than 10% of normal (tested prior to day 14 post-onset), the recovery rate is substantially decreased. The exact approach, whether middle cranial fossa or translabyrinthine, depends on the presence of hearing. When absent, the latter will allow for greater decompression. However, surgical intervention remains controversial, since medical therapy, as described above, has proven to be an effective treatment.

Clinical Scenario	Surgical Intervention
Facial paralysis due to trauma	Nerve decompression, anastomosis
Paralysis secondary to acute OM	Myringotomy
Nerve paralysis due to chronic OM	Decompression, mastoidectomy
Iatrogenic injury to facial nerve	Decompression, anastomosis
Complete idiopathic paralysis	Decompression

OM = otitis media

22. If the nerve is cut during surgery, can it be fixed?

Yes. Several techniques have been employed for repairing a transected or partially transected nerve.

Direct anastomosis involves nerve anastamosis via perineural repair performed by exact end-to-end approximation under the illumination and magnification of the operating microscope. A 9.0 or 10.0 monofilament suture is used to tie the nerve ends together without putting tension on the anastomosis.

Grafting, most often from the greater auricular or sural nerves, can enhance nerve-end apposition if the direct anastamosis would create tension. Jump grafts from other cranial nerves (such as CN XII) have also been used successfully to reanimate the facial muscles in cases in which the facial nerve is lost.

23. What is the Möbius syndrome?

This congenital condition is characterized by facial paralysis that can be either unilateral or bilateral, complete or incomplete, in association with bilateral abducens nerve palsies. Concomitant findings include tongue weakness and talipes equinovarus (clubfoot) in one-third of patients. Abnormal development of the 7th nerve itself, of the facial musculature, or of the facial motor nucleus has been postulated as a cause of the syndrome, although the cause may also be a destructive process secondary to in utero hypoxia.

24. What is the association between facial nerve paralysis and otitis media? Mastoiditis? Cholesteatoma?

In otitis media (OM), facial palsy can present as a complication of acute suppurative OM, OM with effusion, and chronic OM. The palsy results from an inflammatory reaction within the narrow fallopian canal. Recent evidence suggests that bacterial toxins may inhibit neurotransmission directly. In both mastoiditis and cholesteatoma, direct mass compression, in addition to the inflammatory response, results in a facial nerve palsy.

The mainstay of treatment, particularly if the palsy is a complication of OM, is to eradicate the infection with a combination of aggressive antibiotic therapy and surgical drainage via myringotomy or tympanomastoid surgery. Facial palsy secondary to coalescent mastoiditis can be managed surgically with myringotomy followed by a mastoidectomy. The presence of cholesteatoma requires surgical management.

25. Describe the most common traumatic injuries to the facial nerve.

Traumatic injuries to the facial nerve generally fall within two categories, penetrating wounds and temporal bone fractures.

Penetrating wounds of the cheek, face, or parotid gland may lacerate the facial nerve trunk or one of its branches. Seventh nerve lacerations such as these are repaired surgically by approximating the two ends of the cut nerve using 10.0 monofilament nylon suture. Generally, the results of facial nerve repairs are excellent. However, if the main facial nerve trunk has been divided by the laceration, synkinesis results during the regenerative process.

Temporal bone fractures involve the facial nerve via laceration or contusion injury within its bony fallopian canal. Eighty to ninety percent of temporal bone fractures are longitudinal. They will have an associated CN VII injury only 20% of the time, however. Transverse temporal bone fractures, by contrast, account for 15% of cases, but they have an associated CN VII injury about 50% of the time. Immediate facial paralysis following nonpenetrating head trauma is caused by shearing and tearing of facial nerve axons where the fractures cross the bony fallopian canal. Hematoma formation and bony impingment frequently occur and can lead to endoneurial fibrosis that impairs facial nerve regeneration. In these instances, surgical repair may be required. If, following a closed head injury, a delayed facial paralysis develops over a period of 1–7 days, medical management with steroidal anti-inflammatory agents and electrophysiologic monitoring to map the course of recovery are instituted.

26. What conditions suggest the possibility of a neoplastic cause for facial paralysis?

Slowly progressive facial paralysis
Coexistence of facial twitching with an evolving paresis
Development of chronic unilateral eustachian tube dysfunction in a patient with no prior
    history of chronic middle ear disease
Presence of multiple cranial nerve deficits
No recovery of facial function
Recurrent palsy on the same side
Presence of neck or parotid mass
History of cancer

27. What are the most common facial nerve tumors?

Although previously facial schwannomas were considered the most common primary tumor, osseous hemangiomas of the geniculate ganglion have been recognized as possibly even more common. Osseous hemangiomas are not tumors of the nerve itself, but arise from the vascular plexus surrounding the geniculate ganglion.

28. A patient presents to the ENT clinic complaining of involuntary, annoying facial movements. What are the most common types of facial "tics"?

Essential blepharospasm is a neurologic disease of unknown origin that results in rapid blinking of the eyes bilaterally, indicating that the lesion is central rather than peripheral. Some patients suffering from essential blepharospasm are declared legally blind because their eyelids close so frequently and so tightly. Medical treatment consists of injections of modified botulinum toxin into the orbicularis oris muscle. Surgically, the nerve branches and/or the orbicularis oculi muscle can be resected.

Hemifacial spasm, a spastic disease that is most often unilateral, is thought to be the result of an idiopathic demyelination of the peripheral facial nerve. It is characterized by severe, grotesque contraction of the muscles of facial expression. Treatment with botulinum toxin injections often provides effective relief, but microvascular decompression of the facial nerve in the posterior fossa is also effective.

Facial myokymia, usually associated with multiple sclerosis or a malignant neoplasm of the brainstem, is a peculiar wormlike motion in the midfacial muscles.

Segmental fasciculation, consisting of barely perceptible twitches of one or two facial muscles, is often a precursor to a facial nerve neuroma. Clinically, this disorder begins with slight twitches around the eye or in the cheek, followed by enlargement of the involved area with concomitant paralysis. Surgical removal is the only treatment of a facial nerve tumor.

29. What are herpes zoster oticus and Ramsay Hunt syndrome?

Herpes zoster oticus, in its simplest form, is characterized by intense ear pain and vesicles on the external auditory canal and concha, thus indicating that the dormant herpes zoster (chickenpox) virus has reactivated to affect sensory afferent neurons. If viral involvement progresses to involve the efferent motor axons of the facial nerve, then Ramsay Hunt syndrome has developed. This syndrome is characterized by the coexistence of (1) a facial nerve palsy and (2) vesicular eruptions on the head and neck in the distribution of the affected cranial nerve or cervical plexus. Hearing loss and vertigo may also occur. Treatment includes narcotic analgesics for pain relief, tapering doses of oral steroids to decrease inflammation, and acyclovir to inhibit viral DNA replication. If a secondary bacterial otitis externa develops, a topical otic antibiotic-hydrocortisone solution may be employed.

CONTROVERSIES

29. What role do corticosteroids play in the treatment of Bell's palsy?

The use of corticosteroids in the treatment of idiopathic facial nerve paralysis is indeed an area of controversy. Although some protocols recommend steroids to treat all patients with Bell's palsy, others indicate steroid therapy only in cases with total facial palsy. Still others advocate no role whatsoever for corticosteroid treatment. A study published in 1998 by De Diego et al. reports, in a prospective series of 101 Bell's palsy patients randomized to either receive prednisone or acyclovir, that those in the prednisone group had less neural degeneration and had a statistically significantly improved recovery time. Furthermore, a large meta-analysis of 47 papers on treatment with corticosteroids published by Ramsey et al. in 2000 reports clinically and statistically significant improvement with corticosteroid therapy.

FACIAL PARALYSIS

In most cases, the cause of facial paralysis can be determined on the basis of the clinical evaluation, and expensive diagnostic tests can be avoided. Because Bell's palsy is not always the cause, physicians need to be able to identify critical findings on history and physical examination that indicate an alternative diagnosis. Once identified, these findings can lead to a specific and directed evaluation.

~*Marenda SA, Otolaryngol Clin North Am 30:669–682, 1997*

BIBLIOGRAPHY

1. Carrasco VN, Zdanski CJ, Logan TC, Lee KJ: Facial nerve paralysis. In Lee KJ, et al: Essential Otolaryngology Head and Neck Surgery, 7th ed. Stamford, Appleton & Lange, 1999, pp 171–194.

2. Chang CY, Cass SP: Management of facial nerve injury due to temporal bone trauma. Am J Otol 20:96–114, 1999.
3. De Diego JI, Prim MP, De Sarria MJ, Madero R, Gavilan J: Idiopathic facial paralysis: A randomized, prospective, and controlled study using single-dose prednisone bersus acyclovir three times daily. Laryngoscope 108(4 Pt l):573–575, 1998.
4. Dulguerov P, Marchal F, Wang D, et al: Review of objective topographic facial nerve evaluation methods. Am J Otol 20:672–678, 1999.
5. Gidley PW, Gantz BJ, Rubinstein JT: Facial nerve grafts: From cerebellopontine angle and beyond. Am J Otol 20:781–788, 1999.
6. Jackson CG, von Doersten PG: The facial nerve. Current trends in diagnosis, treatment, and rehabilitation. Med Clin North Am 83:179–195, x, 1999.
7. Knox GW: Treatment controversies in Bell palsy. Arch Otolaryngol Head Neck Surg 124:821–823, 1998.
8. Marenda SA, Olsson JE: The evaluation of facial paralysis. Otolaryngol Clin North Am 30:669–682, 1997.
9. Ramsey MJ, DerSimonian R, Holtel MR, Burgess LP: Corticosteroid treatment for idiopathic facial nerve paralysis: A meta-analysis. Laryngoscope 110(3 Pt 1):335–341, 2000.
10. Roob G, Fazekas F, Hartung HP: Peripheral facial palsy: Etiology, diagnosis and treatment. Eur Neurol 41:3–9, 1999.
11. Ruckenstein MJ: Evaluating facial paralysis. Expensive diagnostic tests are often unnecessary. Postgrad Med 103:187–188, 191–192, 1998.
12. Salinas RA, Alvarez G, Alvarez, et al: Corticosteroids for treating Bell's palsy (idiopathic facial paralysis). [Protocol] Cochrane Neuromuscular Disease Group.
13. Schirm J, Mulkens PS: Bell's palsy and herpes simplex virus. APMIS 105(11):815–823, 1997.
14. Sipe J, Dunn L: Aciclovir for Bell's palsy (idiopathic facial paralysis). [Protocol] Cochrane Neuromuscular Disease Group.
15. Shindo M: Management of facial nerve paralysis. Otolaryngol Clin North Am 32:945–964, 1999.

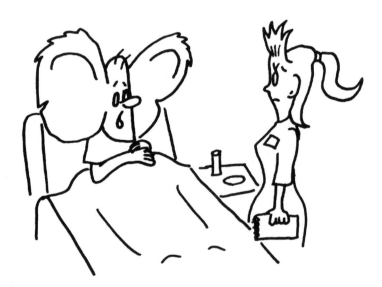

"So the doctor said, it's just like lasik surgery–
a little operation to fix your hearing."

Jim Gough

27. ESOPHAGEAL DISORDERS

Bruce W. Jafek, M.D., FACS, FRSM, and Michael F. Spafford, M.D.

1. Describe the anatomy of the esophagus.

The esophagus is a 25-cm neuromuscular tube extending from the mouth to the stomach. The outer musculature layer is composed of **outer longitudinal** and **inner circular fibers** of striated muscle in the upper third of the esophagus and nonstriated muscle in the lower third of the esophagus. Between the two muscle layers is the **myenteric (Auerbach's) parasympathetic plexus** and the **submucous (Meissner's) plexus**. The submucosa contains mucous glands, blood vessels, and lymphatics. The esophageal mucosa is lined by stratified squamous epithelium. The arterial supply and venous drainage systems of the esophagus are segmental. The lymphatic drainage of the cervical esophagus is via paraesophageal cervical and lower jugular nodes. The thoracic esophagus drains via mediastinal, hilar, and paraesophageal nodes, and the abdominal portion of the esophagus drains into gastric and celiac nodes. The esophagus receives both sympathetic and parasympathetic innervation from cranial nerves IX and X.

2. What is the function of the esophagus?

The esophagus transports nutrients from the mouth to the stomach and prevents regurgitation. The former is accomplished by involuntary peristalsis initiated by delivery of a food bolus from the oropharynx, supplemented by the force of gravity. The latter is accomplished by tonic closure of the lower esophageal sphincter.

3. Describe the embryology of the esophagus.

The esophagus is derived from the embryonic foregut of the primitive gut tube. The foregut is separated by the tracheoesophageal septum into the dorsal esophagus and the more ventral trachea. The shortened esophagus lengthens as it descends with the heart and lungs to reach its full length in the 7th embryonic week. The stratified squamous epithelium and glands of the esophagus are derived from endoderm, whereas the striated and smooth muscle are derived from mesenchyme. During development, epithelial proliferation initially obliterates the lumen of the esophagus, which recanalizes by the 8th week.

4. How do congenital esophageal atresia, esophageal stenosis, and tracheoesophageal fistula occur?

Esophageal atresia occurs as a result of dorsal deviation of the tracheoesophageal septum and subsequent blind closure of the esophagus. Because the fetus is then unable to swallow amniotic fluid, this condition is frequently associated with polyhydramnios.

Esophageal stenosis, or congenital webbing, usually occurs in the distal third of the esophagus and results from incomplete recanalization of the lumen after epithelial proliferation.

Tracheoesophageal fistula (TEF), usually associated with esophageal atresia, occurs in about 1 in 2500 births. As the name implies, this disorder is an abnormal communication between the trachea and esophagus and results from a developmental failure of the tracheoesophageal septum between weeks 4 and 8 and/or failure of recannulation of the esophagus between weeks 3 and 8.

5. What are the four major types of tracheoesophageal fistula?

- Most commonly, the superior portion of the esophagus ends blindly, and the inferior portion joins the trachea directly.
- The inferior portion of the esophagus ends blindly, and the superior portion joins the esophagus directly.

- Both superior and inferior portions join the trachea directly without joining each other.
- The esophagus is a continuous tube with a side-to-side communication with the trachea ("H-type").

6. How is a tracheoesophageal fistula diagnosed?

Esophageal atresia (EA) is the most common congenital anomaly affecting the esophagus, with an incidence of 1 in 3000. Variations are classified anatomically by whether a fistula is present and by its location relative to the atresia. The most common variation (86%) is esophageal atresia with a distal TEF, followed by isolated EA (7.7%), and then isolated TEF or H-type anomaly (4.2%). When EA is present, fluids will be quickly regurgitated during and after feeding. A small **isolated TEF** (H-type anomaly) may remain asymptomatic until recurrent or refractory pneumonia presents. When a **distal TEF** is present, the stomach becomes distended with inspired air. Repeated aspiration of stomach contents will manifest itself as recurrent pneumonia. With a **proximal TEF**, feeding results in immediate choking and gagging, and if the distal segment is not connected to the airway, no gas will appear in the gastrointestinal tract. Diagnosis can be made by the inability to pass a soft rubber catheter into the stomach or by the absence of gas on abdominal plain radiograph, and is confirmed with a barium contrast study.

7. In the complex neuromuscular sequence of swallowing, which step is most important for airway protection?

Laryngeal elevation. As the swallowing reflex begins, the suprahyoid muscles contract, as well as the thyrohyoid muscle. The resulting elevation brings the laryngeal inlet into a protected position under the tongue base. It also passively deflects the epiglottis to a position 60 degrees below the horizontal, thereby shielding the airway and directing food laterally. Finally, laryngeal elevation serves to dilate the upper esophageal sphincter, allowing food passage into the esophagus. **Dysphagia** is the name of the symptom of abnormal swallowing.

8. What are the most common causes of dysphagia?

Swallowing disorders can be divided into oropharyngeal dysphagia and esophageal dysphagia. The most common cause of oropharyngeal dysphagia is cerebrovascular accidents; other causes may include oropharyngeal structural lesions, systematic and local muscular diseases, and diverse neurologic disorders. Esophageal dysphagia may result from neuromuscular disorders, mortality abnormalities, and intrinsic or extrinsic obstructive lesions. Clinical history taking helps define the type of dysphagia and can guide diagnostic testing. Important questions to ask patients with the disorder include specific features of the dysphagia, its onset and progression, accompanying problems, and eating habits adopted to relieve symptoms.

9. What are the most common causes of gastroesophageal reflux disease (GERD)?

The most common causes of GERD are factors that decrease lower esophageal sphincter pressure and include hiatal hernia and a variety of substances such as dietary fat, chocolate, mints, tobacco, ethanol, and many drugs. Other less common causes include abnormal esophageal motility, delayed gastric emptying, increased intra-abdominal pressure, and gastric hypersecretion.

10. What are the most common otolaryngologic manifestations of GERD?

The most common symptoms are hoarseness (71%), cough (51%), globus pharyngeus (47%), throat–clearing (42%), and difficulty swallowing (35%). Only 43% of patients had gastrointestinal symptoms such as heartburn or acid regurgitation. On physical examination, these patients often have laryngoscopic findings of chronic laryngitis, including vocal cord granulomas. The inflammation may be localized to the posterior larynx, with thickened, edematous interarytenoid tissue. The clinical presentation of GERD is commonly characterized by chronic intermittent symptoms.

11. How is GERD treated?

The treatment has three phases:

- Lifestyle modification, including raising the head of the bed 6–8 inches, losing weight, and avoiding overeating and eating before bedtime. Tobacco, alcohol, and caffeine should be eliminated.
- Pharmacologic therapy, including H_2 blockers (i.e., ranitidine) or proton–pump inhibitors (i.e., omeprazole).
- If these therapies fail, surgery may be considered (Nissen fundoplication).

12. Name the types of hiatal hernia.

Type I, or **sliding hiatal hernia,** features a phrenoesophageal membrane that is intact. Although a portion of the stomach can "slide" into the thorax, its size is limited, and no peritoneum actually enters the thorax.

In **type II hiatal hernia,** the membrane is defective, allowing a peritoneal sac to enter the thorax, which can progressively increase in size.

13. Are any systemic diseases associated with esophageal motility disorders?

Polymyositis, characterized by systemic degenerative and inflammatory changes of the skin and striated muscle, is associated with esophageal dysmotility in 30% of cases. The affected portion is the pharynx and striated upper one-third of the esophageal musculature.

Scleroderma and other **connective tissue disorders** such as systemic lupus erythematosus, dermatomyositis, and Raynaud's disease produce a distinct pattern of esophageal dysmotility. Scleroderma, the most common of these disorders, produces a 52% rate of dysphagia and a 74% rate of histologic involvement. Small vessel arteritis and collagen deposition in the region of esophageal smooth muscle produce a dilated and aperistaltic lower two-thirds of the esophagus. This, combined with decreased function of the lower esophageal sphincter, leads to unremitting reflux with a high rate of esophagitis. This may lead to dysphagia, bleeding, and stricture.

Other systemic diseases that can affect esophageal motility include **diabetes mellitus** and **alcoholism**, causing a peripheral neuropathy. The degenerative and demyelinating central nervous system (CNS) diseases also can decrease motility. **Chagas' disease** is a systemic parasitic infection that destroys the ganglion cells of Auerbach's plexus and produces a picture similar to **achalasia**.

14. What is globus pharyngeus?

Globus pharyngeus is a foreign-body sensation, or "lump," in the throat. First described by Hippocrates, the sensation is familiar to many. This sensation localizes in the midline between the suprasternal notch and thyroid cartilage and occurs during strong emotion. The persistent sensation is estimated to account for 3–4% of otolaryngology referrals, and a work-up is indicated to exclude serious underlying disease. Globus pharyngeus is considered a diagnosis of exclusion. Although controversial, several authors have recently reported a high incidence of GERD in patients with globus pharyngeus.

15. Where do you find a Schatzki's ring?

Schatzki's ring is a concentric or weblike narrowing that appears at the junction of the esophageal and gastric mucosa in 6–14% of barium swallows. It is symptomatic only one-third of the time, when the esophageal lumen is reduced to < 13 mm. Intermittent solid food dysphagia is the most common symptom.

16. Are the terms *esophageal web* and *esophageal ring* interchangeable?

No. An esophageal web is a thin membrane that projects into the esophageal lumen and is covered with squamous epithelium. Webs can occur anywhere in the esophagus and may be single or multiple, concentric or eccentric. Esophageal rings, on the other hand, occur at the gastroesophageal junction and are covered with squamous epithelium on the upper surface and columnar epithelium on the lower surface.

17. Describe the characteristic radiographic finding associated with diffuse esophageal spasm.

The barium esophagogram in this condition has been described to demonstrate a **corkscrew esophagus,** with curling or beading of the barium column. This curling develops because non-peristaltic simultaneous contraction of the lower two-thirds of the esophagus occurs. The symptoms are intermittent and consist of dysphagia, odynophagia, and chest pain that often forces a cardiac evaluation. Treatment includes reassurance and pharmacologic relaxation of the smooth muscle with nitrates, calcium channel blockers, and anticholinergic agents. Underlying GERD is also treated. Dilatation and myotomy are reserved for incapacitating cases.

18. What is dysphagia lusoria?

Dysphagia lusoria is caused by extrinsic esophageal compression by an anomalous right sub-clavian artery. Arising from the descending aorta, it must cross posteriorly behind the esophagus to reach the right arm. In 15% of cases, it passes between the trachea and esophagus. It is a fourth branchial arch anomaly.

19. What sort of swallowing complaints can be expected in the elderly population?

Presbyesophagus is a term for the abnormalities of esophageal motility seen in the elderly. Histologically, partial denervation (a decrease in the number of ganglion cells in Auerbach's plexus) has been documented with aging. Although some degree of reduced peristalsis and occasional failure of lower esophageal relaxation can be seen in the elderly, most of these patients remain asymptomatic. When dysphasia does occur in this group, its location is most often oropharyngeal or hypopharyngeal, and its etiology is neuropathologic. Intubation no longer remains the only solution to feeding problems of the elderly patient with dysphagia. Dysphagic disorders result from neurogenic, myogenic, psychogenic, or mechanical causes. Thus numerous hospitalized or institutionalized elderly patients may have dysphagic symptoms. The consequences of this disorder are significant, and aspiration pneumonia is often the outcome.

20. What are the three manometric findings in achalasia?

The three manometric findings that distinguish achalasia from other esophageal motility disorders are
- Increase in lower esophageal sphincter (LES) pressure
- Absence of LES relaxation
- Absence of esophageal peristalsis

In its primary form, achalasia is associated with an idiopathic degeneration of the ganglion cells of Auerbach's plexus. The above forces produce esophageal dilatation or "megaesophagus."

21. How is achalasia treated?

Usually, achalasia can be managed on an outpatient basis by serial dilatation. Sometimes, forceful acute controlled dilatation under general anesthesia or (preferable in most cases) intravenous sedation is required.

22. How can cardiac pain be distinguished from esophageal pain?

It is thought that Galen (130–200 AD) coined the term *cardia* for the gastroesophageal region because pain arising there can closely mimic cardiac pain. The absence of an exertional component, temporal relationship to swallowing, and concomitant complaints of dysphagia or odynophagia may help identify an esophageal source of pain, but the more common and serious cardiac etiology must always be first ruled out.

23. What is nutcracker esophagus?

Nutcracker esophagus is the most common esophageal motility disorder in patients evaluated for noncardiac chest pain. It resembles diffuse esophageal spasm with substernal chest pain and dysphagia; however, the esophageal contractions remain peristaltic. Its cause is also unknown. Calcium-channel blockers are the initial medical therapy.

CONTROVERSIES

24. What is the best way of evaluating dysphagia?

Barium-contrast swallow should be the initial test in evaluating dysphagia. This test identifies most anatomic causes of dysphagia and some motor disorders and is better than endoscopy at identifying extrinsic esophageal compression and intramural lesions not involving the esophageal mucosa. **Modified barium swallow** (MBS) (cinefluoroscopy) may provide clues to a possible esophageal motor disorder causing dysphagia. As the "gold standard," MBS examines the oral, pharyngeal, laryngeal, and cervical physiology, along with the actual dynamic swallow before, during, and after the event. The test uses three consistencies of materials in specific amounts: liquid barium, barium paste, and substances that require mastication such as a barium-coated cookie.

Alternatively, **fiberendoscopic evaluation of swallowing** (FEES) may be employed. This can be done at the bedside and allows the clinician to directly observe the larynx for anatomical changes along with the actual swallow. Unlimited time may be taken, and radiation exposure is avoided. It is less risky in terms of aspiration but requires a trained endoscopist. In view of cognitive and other issues present in the population with brain injury, the use of fiberoptic endoscopy to address dysphagia assessment is preferred in this group of patients. Endoscopy is the test of choice if obstruction or gastroesophageal reflux disease is suspected, because biopsies can confirm the presence of esophagitis and provide specific pathologic identification of the obstructive lesion. In addition, therapeutic dilatation of a stricture and removal of foreign bodies can be accomplished as part of the evaluation procedure. When no obvious source of dysphagia is apparent after radiologic and endoscopic assessment, **manometry** for possible motility disorder should be considered.

Thus, the final selection of the method of evaluation is dependent upon the "working diagnosis," or condition to be evaluated, and the clinical status of the patient at the time of the evaluation and several evaluations may be necessary to make the final diagnosis.

25. How do you approach dysphagia or odynophagia in the immunocompromised patient?

In the immunocompromised patient, one must have a high index of suspicion for esophageal infection. In human immunodeficiency virus (HIV)-infected patients, the esophagus may be the site of the first acquired immunodeficiency syndrome (AIDS)-defining opportunistic illness. Candida esophagitis is the most common cause of new-onset esophageal symptoms in these patients. Initial empiric treatment with oral antifungal therapy (fluconazole or ketaconazole) is indicated. Opportunistic disorders such as cytomegalovirus, herpes simplex virus of the esophagus (HSEV), and idiopathic esophageal ulceration rarely present until the CD4 lymphocyte count falls below $100/mm^3$. Endoscopy is the most valuable tool for evaluating esophageal complaints in AIDS.

HSVE is characterized by acute onset, systemic manifestations, and extensive erosive-ulcerative involvement of the mid-distal esophagus. Histopathologic examination alone may miss the diagnosis; adding tissue-viral culture optimizes the diagnostic sensitivity. Almost all esophageal infections in patients with AIDS are treatable; therefore, a thorough work-up is indicated. With the widespread use of more effective antiretroviral therapy, including the protease inhibitors, there is a general consensus that the incidence of many opportunistic diseases appears to be decreasing. HSVE is usually self-limiting, and whether antiviral therapy is beneficial remains unknown.

In contrast, esophageal symptoms in non–HIV-infected immunocompromised patients, such as transplant recipients, are likely to represent infection with viral disease such as herpes or cytomegalovirus, and, less often, candida and fungal diseases. Therefore, these patients are more commonly taken initially for endoscopy and biopsy to help establish a diagnosis.

DYSPHAGIA

Familiar medical problems, including cerebrovascular accidents, gastroesophageal reflux disease, and medication-related side effects, often lead to complaints of dysphagia. Stroke patients are at particular risk of aspiration because of dysphagia. Classifying dysphagia as oropharyngeal, esophageal and obstructive, or neuromuscular symptom complexes leads to a successful diagnosis in 80 to 85% of patients. Based on the patient history and physical examination, barium esophagram and/or gastroesophageal endoscopy can confirm the diagnosis. Special studies and consultation with subspecialists can confirm difficult diagnoses and help guide treatment strategies.

~Spieker MR, Am Fam Phys 61:3639, 2000

BIBLIOGRAPHY

1. Couturier D, Samama J: Clinical aspects and manometric criteria in achalasia. Hepatogastroenterology 38:481–487, 1991.
2. Ergon GA, Miskovitz PF: Aging and the esophagus: Common pathologic conditions and their effect upon swallowing in the geriatric population. Dysphagia 7(2):58–63, 1992.
3. Hoogerwerf WA, Pasricha PJ: Achalasia: Treatment options revisited. Can J Gastroent 14:406–409, 2000.
4. Koufman JA: The otolaryngologic manifestations of gastroesophageal reflux disease (GERD): A clinical investigation of 225 patients using ambulatory 24-hour pH monitoring and an experimental investigation of the role of acid and pepsin in the development of laryngeal injury. Laryngoscope 101(4 pt 2/ suppl 53):1–78, 1991. (*A classic*)
5. Kuo WH, Kalloo AN: Reflux strictures of the esophagus. Gastrointest Endosc Clin North Am 8:273–281, 1998.
6. Lautner D, Gray R, Reid D: Esophageal strictures: A radiologic approach to diagnosis and management. Gastrointest Endosc Clin North Am 8:283–313, 1998.
7. Massey BT: Management of idiopathic achalasia: Short-term and long-term outcomes. Curr Gastroenterol Rpts 2:196–200, 2000.
8. Mujica VR, Conklin J: When it's hard to swallow: What to look for in patients with dysphagia. Postgrad Med 105:131–134, 141–142, 145, 1999.
9. Peracchia A, Bonavina L: Achalasia: Dilation, injection or surgery? Can J Gastroent 14:441–3, 2000.
10. Timon C, O'Dwyer T, Cagney D, Walsh M: Globus pharyngeus: Long-term follow-up and prognostic factors. Ann Otol Rhinol Laryngol 100(5 pt 1):351–354, 1991.
11. Ulualp SO, Toohill RJ: Laryngopharyngeal reflux: State of the art diagnosis and treatment. Otolaryngol Clin North Am 33:785–802, 2000.
12. Wilcox CM, Monkemuller KE: Diagnosis and management of esophageal disease in the acquired immunodeficiency syndrome. South Med J 91:1002–1008, 1998.

28. THE THYROID AND PARATHYROID GLANDS

Catherine Winslow, M.D.

1. What does thyroid hormone do?

Thyroxine (T_4) and triiodothyronine (T_3) increase cellular metabolism, influence genomic expression, and alter the transcellular flux of substrates. The production is dependent on iodine, of which the normal adult requires 80 g/day.

2. A patient presents with a mass at the base of his tongue. A colleague suspects a lingual thyroid. What is this and how would you evaluate it?

The thyroid originates from the foramen cecum on the posterior tongue. It descends during development to its usual location in front of the second tracheal ring. If the thyroid gland fails to descend during development, lingual thyroid tissue may persist. A mass at the base of the tongue may be such a remnant or it may be an oral cancer. A good history and physical examination are of utmost importance. Evaluate the patient for oral cancer risk factors, such as smoking and alcohol intake. Feel the mass for irregularities, and palpate the neck for a normally located thyroid gland. If there is doubt, a thyroid scan that includes the base of the tongue should be obtained.

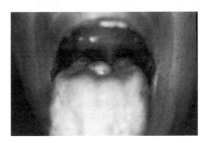

3. Does the lingual thyroid function normally in patients with no other thyroid tissue?

Most lingual thyroids are asymptomatic. They are the only functioning thyroid tissue in 70–80% of patients with lingual thyroids. About 15% of these patients are hypothyroid. Intervention is warranted if the mass is symptomatic, as evidenced by airway obstruction, dysphagia, or dysphonia. Excision should be performed if the symptoms are refractory to suppression therapy.

4. Would the treatment of this condition necessitate surgery?

Not necessarily. If the patient is asymptomatic, suppression therapy with thyroxine should suffice. However, occasionally a patient will have airway obstruction or significant swallowing difficulties, and surgery might be indicated.

5. How is thyroid replacement performed clinically?

Synthetic thyroid hormone is available for daily replacement. It is available as triiodothyroxine (Cytomel) or levothyroxine (Synthroid). Thyroxine is less expensive and has a longer half-life. It is used for treatment of hypothyroidism.

6. The patient indeed has a lingual thyroid and no thyroid tissue in the neck. Where are the parathyroids expected to be?

In the normal anatomic location.

7. How does the embryology of the thyroid and parathyroid glands differ?
The thyroid gland arises from pharyngeal endoderm in the region of the base of the tongue. It descends during development, staying in the midline and in close proximity to the hyoid bone. The parathyroid glands originate from the third (inferior) and fourth (superior) branchial pouches. The inferior parathyroid descends in concert with the thymus, while the superior parathyroid remains posterior at about the level of the cricothyroid junction.

8. What tests are available to determine whether a patient is hypo-, hyper-, or euthyroid?
The levels of T_3 and T_4 can be determined by assays. The level of thyroglobulin will assist in determining whether the disturbance is central or peripheral. A T_3 resin uptake will assist in evaluating the impact of binding.

9. What is the most common cause of hyperthyroidism?
Grave's disease, or diffuse toxic goiter, is the most common cause of hyperthyroidism. Usually affecting women aged 20–50, this autoimmune disease leads to enlargement of the thyroid gland. **Plummer's disease**, or nodular toxic goiter, is a less common cause of hyperthyroidism and affects elderly individuals. Rarer causes of hyperthyroidism include subacute thyroiditis, pituitary tumors, and struma ovarii, and inappropriate injestion of thyroid replacement hormone.

10. Is the management of Grave's disease medical or surgical?
The treatment is generally medical. Surgical indications include nodules suspicious for carcinoma, inability to tolerate medical suppression, excessive thyroid size resulting in airway or esophageal compromise, cosmetic disturbances that do not respond to suppression, and patient choice. Hypothyroidism requiring lifelong replacement is common following surgery or iodine ablation.

11. What is the blood supply to the parathyroids?
The **inferior thyroid artery**, a branch of the thyrocervical trunk, supplies the parathyroids. The **superior parathyroid artery**, a branch of the external carotid, may also give branches. With vascular compromise, the parathyroids darken from tan to black.

12. What tests can be performed to diagnose parathyroid disorders?
A parathyroid hormone assay will allow identification of parathyroid excess or deficiency. A calcium and magnesium level should also be assessed. A creatinine level will assist in determining adequacy of renal function. An alkaline phosphatase level will detect active bone resorption. A serum chloride level should be obtained to differentiate hyperparathyroidism from pseudohyperparathyroidism.

13. What is the most common cause of hyperparathyroidism?
Adenoma is the cause in 80% of hyperparathyroidism cases. **Diffuse hyperplasia** is the cause in 20% of cases. Carcinoma is rare (1–3%).

14. How frequently is hypercalcemia associated with hyperparathyroidism?
Hyperparathyroidism accounts for 20% of hypercalcemia cases. More than half of cases of hypercalcemia are due to bone metastases.

15. How does hypercalcemia manifest clinically?
"Stones, bones, moans, and abdominal groans" will help you remember the symptoms. Patients suffer from renal stones, frequently multiple and recurrent. Long bone fractures without trauma can occur, and resorption can sometimes be seen on radiographic imaging. Psychological manifestions such as depression may occur, and peptic ulcers are common. Severe hypercalcemia can lead to electrocardiographic changes and cardiac arrhythmias.

16. What predisposing factors are associated with hyperparathyroidism?

Although most cases arise spontaneously without a known cause, > 10% of patients have a history of **radiation** to the neck. Familial parathyroid hyperplasia and multiple endocrine neoplasia syndromes suggest that **genetic factors** also may play an important role.

17. What is the difference between primary, secondary, and tertiary hyperparathyroidism?

Primary hyperparathyroidism occurs when the parathyroid glands manufacture an excess of parathyroid hormone (PTH), thus leading to hypercalcemia. **Secondary hyperparathyroidism** is a result of renal failure. Hypocalcemia and hyperphospatemia are caused by renal insufficiency. Continued hypersecretion of PTH to correct the electrolyte imbalance leads to a relative resistance of the bones to PTH. Increasing amounts of PTH are required to combat this effect. Secondary hyperparathyroidism is remedied by dialysis or transplant. **Tertiary hyperparathyroidism** results when chronic hyperactivity of the parathyroid glands leads to autonomous functioning. Correction of the renal failure (such as by transplant) would not reverse this process, and surgery may be indicated.

18. What is the management of hyperparathyroidism?

Surgery is generally indicated. An exploration of the neck is made to identify and remove the adenoma. At least one normal-appearing gland is evaluated with frozen section to identify hyperplasia. Temporary or permanent hypocalcemia may occur postoperatively, and calcium replacement may be necessary.

CONTROVERSIES

19. Is preoperative imaging necessary prior to parathyroid removal?

Most surgeons agree that it is ideal to determine where an adenoma is located preoperatively. Several tests are available. The sesta-MIBI scan is currently favored to identify a hyperfunctioning gland. Magnetic resonance imaging, computed tomography, ultrasonography, and invasive tests such as venous PTH sampling have all been performed as well. The argument against preoperative localization is made by surgeons who routinely identify all four glands regardless of the results of tests, in which case preoperative testing is expensive and does not change management.

20. How many glands should be removed for adequate assurance that hyperplasia is not present?

Opinion varies widely on this subject. Many surgeons do not feel comfortable sampling just one normal gland and prefer to have identified at least two histologically normal parathyroids before closing the neck. Arguments for sampling all four glands include absolute assurance of an adenoma (not hyperplasia) and the need to violate both necks anyway to sample a total of three glands. Proponents of sampling three or fewer glands cite the up to 15% incidence of patients who have fewer or greater than four glands. Additionally, searching for a greater number of glands may cause an increased incidence of postoperative hypocalcemia and increase the risk to the recurrent laryngeal nerves.

THYROID NODULES

In non–iodine-deficient areas, 4% to 7% of the population are reported to have thyroid abnormalities. Prophylactic operations of these nodules in the thyroid are not indicated and not cost-effective, as at least four of five nodules are colloid goiter and only a few are malignant. The need for a reliable preoperative diagnosis is great, and fine-needle aspiration (FNA) is now considered the first choice during work-up for thyroid nodules. The problem of differentiating follicular adenoma from follicular carcinoma remains a significant problem. It is now well established that FNA biopsy and cytology is the best modality available for the work-up of thyroid nodules, and this is widely utilized in endocrine surgical centers worldwide.

~Werga P, World J Surg 24:907, 2000

BIBLIOGRAPHY

1. Arthur JR, Beckett GJ: Thyroid function. Br Med Bull 55:658–668, 1999.
2. Barraclough BM, Barraclough BH: Ultrasound of the thyroid and parathyroid glands. World J Surg 24:158–165, 2000.
3. Bliss RD, Gauger PG, Delbridge LW: Surgeon's approach to the thyroid gland: Surgical anatomy and the importance of technique. World J Surg 24:891–897, 2000.
4. Dackiw AP, Sussman JJ, Fritsche HA Jr, et al: Relative contributions of technetium Tc 99m sestamibi scintigraphy, intraoperative gamma probe detection, and the rapid parathyroid hormone assay to the surgical management of hyperparathyroidism. Arch Surg 135:550–555; discussion 555–557, 2000.
5. D'Avanzo A, Parangi S, Morita E, et al: Hyperparathyroidism after thyroid surgery and autotransplantation of histologically normal parathyroid glands. J Am Coll Surg 190:546–552, 2000.
6. Fraker DL: Update on the management of parathyroid tumors. Curr Opin Oncol 12:41–48, 2000.
7. Fukagawa M, Tominaga Y, Kitaoka M, et al: Medical and surgical aspects of parathyroidectomy. Kidney Int Suppl. 73:S65–69, 1999.
8. Goretzki PE, Simon D, Dotzenrath C, et al: Growth regulation of thyroid and thyroid tumors in humans. World J Surg 24:913–922, 2000.
9. Gotway MB, Higgins CB: MR imaging of the thyroid and parathyroid glands. Mag Res Imag Clin North Am 8:163–182, ix, 2000.
10. Hellman P, Liu W, Westin G, et al: Vitamin D and retinoids in parathyroid glands. Int J Molec Med 3:355–361, 1999.
11. Nishiyama RH: Overview of surgical pathology of the thyroid gland. World J Surg 24:898–906, 2000.
12. Phelps E, Wu P, Bretz J, et al: Thyroid cell apoptosis: A new understanding of thyroid autoimmunity. Endocrinol Metab Clin North Am 29:375–388, viii, 2000.
13. Spitzweg C, Heufelder AE, Morris JC: Thyroid iodine transport. Thyroid 10:321–330, 2000.
14. Werga P, Wallin G, Skoog L, et al: Expanding role of fine-needle aspiration cytology in thyroid diagnosis and management. World J Surg 24:907–912, 2000.

29. SALIVARY GLAND DISORDERS

Bruce W. Jafek, M.D., FACS, FRSM

1. What is the embryonic origin of the salivary glands?

The salivary glands arise as epithelial outpouchings from the primitive oral cavity, or stomodeum, beginning in the 4th week. The parotids usually arise first (4th week), followed by the submandibular glands (6th week), and the sublingual glands (9th week).

2. What is Stenson's duct?

The mature parotid gland is the largest of the salivary glands and lies on the side of the face, just anterior and inferior to the ear, and is in contact with the posterior surface of the ascending ramus of the mandible. Stenson's duct, which drains the parotid gland, arises at the anterior border of the gland, travels forward over the masseter muscle, and passes through the buccinator muscle to enter the oral cavity in proximity to the second upper molar.3

3. Where do you find Wharton's duct?

The submandibular gland lies under the horizontal ramus of the mandible just superficial to the hyoglossus muscle. Its duct, called Wharton's duct, opens anteriorly in the floor of the mouth, just lateral to the base of the frenulum of the tongue.

4. What is the plica sublingualis?

The smallest named salivary glands are the sublingual glands, which lie along a fold under the tongue called the plica sublingualis. This fold originates anteriorly at the frenulum of the tongue and travels posteriorly and laterally toward the angle of the mandible. The sublingual glands have 8–15 excretory ducts with their minute orifices along the plica.

5. How do the submandibular and submaxillary glands differ?

These two terms are interchangeable. Both are descriptive terms, based on the location of the gland. The gland, after all, lies beneath both the maxilla and the mandible. Because the gland lies closer to the mandible, many authors prefer the term "submandibular."

6. What are the superficial and deep lobes of the parotid gland?

Although not having true "lobes," the parotid gland does have superficial and deep portions. The facial nerve (CN VIII) runs between these portions of the gland and defines them. This nerve exits the skull via the stylomastoid foramen, enters the substance of the parotid gland between its superficial and deep portions, and divides into five terminal branches. These branches leave the gland anteriorly to supply the mimetic musculature of the face.

7. Describe the branches of the facial nerve.

Following its exit from the stylomastoid foramen, the facial nerve divides into an upper and lower division at the pes anserinus ("foot of the goose"). The upper division divides into the **temporal branch**, which supplies the frontalis and orbicularis oculi, and the **zygomatic branch**, which also supplies the orbicularis oculi. The lower division divides into the **mandibular branch**, which supplies the muscles of the lower lip and chin, and the **cervical branch**, which supplies the platysma. A middle branch, the **buccal branch**, supplies the buccinator. The buccal branch may receive contributions from the upper and lower divisions, or it may arise separately at the pes. Other variations occur, making careful identification of the facial nerve and its branches critical.

8. Which nerves are at risk when the submandibular gland is resected?
During removal of the submandibular gland, for any reason, the lingual, marginal mandibular, and hypoglossal nerves are at risk. The marginal mandibular nerve is usually superior to the gland, while the hypoglossal nerve is inferior and deep to the gland. The lingual nerve is deep to the gland in the resection bed. These branches should be identified and preserved.

9. What common problems, besides tumors, cause salivary gland enlargement?
Parotitis
Salivary calculi or duct stricture
Benign lymphoepithelial disease (e.g., Sjögren's syndrome, Mikulicz' disease, Heerfordt's syndrome, Melkersson's syndrome)
Granulomatous parotitis (e.g., tuberculosis)
Bulimia
Lead or mercury intoxication
Chronic fatty infiltration (e.g., secondary to alcoholism, hypovitaminoses)

10. What causes viral parotitis?
Inflammation of the parotid gland, or parotitis, may be nonsuppurative or suppurative. The most common example of nonsuppurative viral parotitis is mumps, a once-common childhood disease. Mumps, caused by a paramyxovirus, is associated with bilateral painful parotid swelling, malaise, and trismus. Treatment is conservative (e.g., bedrest, heat, fluids, pain medications), as the condition is usually self-limited.

11. How is recurrent, nonsuppurative sialadenitis treated?
Recurrent, nonsuppurative enlargement of the submandibular or parotid salivary gland may occur due to obstruction of the draining duct by mucous plugs or stones. Mucolytic agents, massage, hydration, and secretagogues (e.g., lemon wedges) may be helpful.

12. What is suppurative sialadenitis?
Suppurative sialadenitis may be acute or chronic. **Acute** suppurative sialadenitis is characterized by swelling of the involved gland, pain, fever, and purulent discharge that may be expressed from the affected duct. It is often a complication of chronic dehydration in a debilitated patient such as a diabetic. Acute suppurative sialadenitis may also follow immunosuppression, radiation therapy, or chemotherapy. Classically, *Staphylococcus* is involved. Treatment revolves around hydration and antibiotics, but surgical drainage may be required in unresponsive cases. **Chronic** or **recurrent** suppurative sialadenitis may also require removal of the gland. Removal of these glands is more surgically complex than removal of a tumor because extensive fibrosis and bleeding are often present.

13. What is the pathogenesis of suppurative sialadenitis?
There are two primary contributors: retrograde contamination of the ductile system by bacteria inhabiting the oral cavity and stasis of salivary flow. Thus, the usual bacterial contaminants of the mouth (e.g., *Staphylococcus aureus* and *Streptococcus* spp., along with *Haemophilus influenzae*) are the most common organisms responsible.

14. What medical conditions predispose patients to acute sialadenitis?
Hepatic or renal failure, diabetes mellitus, hypothyroidism, malnutrition, human immunodeficiency virus (HIV) or actual acquired immunodeficiency syndrome (AIDS), Sjögren's syndrome, depression, anorexia or bulimia, hyperuricemia, hyperlipoproteinemia, cystic fibrosis, lead intoxication, and Cushing's syndrome. In addition, medications that tend to dehydrate patients also predispose them to acute sialadenitis, because of increased stasis of saliva: diuretics, certain antibiotics, tricyclic antidepressants, phenothiazines, β-blockers, barbiturates, and anticholinergics.

15. Which gland is most commonly affected by sialolithiasis?

Sialolithiasis, the formation of calculi or "stones" within the ductal system of a salivary gland, is characterized by pain and swelling of the affected gland, and symptoms may worsen when the patient eats. The **submandibular gland** is affected in about 80% of cases, followed by the **sublingual** and finally **parotid gland**. The stones are most commonly composed of hydroxyapatite.

16. Why are these glands most commonly affected?

First of all, the ductal system of the submangibular gland is the most "gravity dependent." Thus, it is most dependent on muscular activity, rather than simple gravity drainage, to convey the secretions to the oral cavity. Second (and probably the most important), the submandibular (and sublingual) gland secretions are richer in mucin than those of the parotid (which are, of course, more serous, and therefore thinner in character). The mucin makes the saliva thicker and therefore more subject to stasis (see Questions 13).

17. How are salivary gland calculi managed?

Calculi are usually apparent on intraoral inspection or bimanual palpation. Sometimes they can be expressed bimanually. If this is impossible, an intraoral incision made over the stones facilitates their removal. Often, the duct eventually fistulizes into the oral cavity in this area, relieving the retrograde obstruction. If a stricture of the duct results, the duct can be reconstructed with a procedure termed *sialodochoplasty*. It may be necessary to remove the involved gland if the stones are recurrent and symptomatic or if the two described maneuvers are unsuccessful.

18. What is benign lymphoepithelial disease of the salivary glands?

Benign lymphoepithelial disease is an autoimmune disease commonly known as **Sjögren's syndrome**. The main salivary manifestations are xerostomia, recurrent infections, and glandular hypertrophy. Sialectasis, or dilatation of the ducts may be demonstrated on sialography. The diagnosis is confirmed with a minor salivary gland biopsy from the lip. Cholinergic drugs tend to produce significant side effects, and artificial saliva is poorly tolerated. Therefore, these patient often must carry a small bottle of water at all times. Infections are managed as necessary. Steroids may be beneficial. A parotidectomy may be indicated for cosmetic reasons.

19. How are parotid cysts managed? Why are special precautions needed?

Prior to the HIV era, cystic lesions of the parotid were thought to occur rarely. However, over the past decade, the reported incidence of these lesions has increased substantially. The classic management for any parotid mass includes a superficial parotidectomy as well as biopsy. However, because elective surgery on HIV patients poses additional risks for patients and health-care workers, and because surgical management does not affect the underlying disease, nonsurgical management of parotid cysts in these patients is now gaining favor.

Computed tomographic (CT) scanning is recommended to confirm the cystic nature of the parotid mass, followed by a fine needle aspiration (FNA) in patients at high risk for HIV infection. If the lesion is cystic on CT scan and benign on FNA, then watchful waiting and a nonsurgical approach are recommended, with repeat FNA for palliation. Although patients may request surgery for cosmetic or other unpleasant symptoms, Huang et al. do not recommend this procedure. Surgery should be reserved for suspicious solid lesions, especially with findings such as abnormal cells or a uniform lymphoid population on cytologic examination. In these cases, further pathologic diagnosis is warranted. They also feel that an elevated amylase level in the parotid FNA specimen is suggestive of benign cystic disease. Finally, they suggest that any patient who presents with a parotid cyst should be investigated for possible HIV infection. Injection of the cyst with a sclerosing agent, such as tetracycline, has recently been shown to be helpful in treating these cysts.

20. What is a ranula?

Ranula is a nonspecific term for a cystic mass in the floor of the mouth. A localized form is limited to the oral cavity and is usually cured by excision or by marsupialization. A "plunging" form, characterized histologically by extravasated mucus, is more extensive and extends along muscle planes. It requires a more extensive procedure, often including excision of the submandibular gland.

21. How is trauma to the salivary glands managed?

For practical purposes, significant trauma to the salivary glands most commonly affects the parotid and submandibular glands, primarily the former. For **submandibular gland trauma**, the wound can be closed and observed, or the gland can be removed. A superficial salivary fistula is exceedingly rare in these cases; the gland usually undergoes atrophy if the saliva is unable to enter the oral cavity, either via the duct or via a new fistula. Where the duct is identified, it can be stented over a small silastic cannula. Trauma to the adjacent nerves (marginal mandibular, lingual, or hypoglossal) is managed by microsurgical approximation of the divided segments, with sharp freshening of the edges if necessary.

With **parotid trauma**, the facial nerve is managed similarly. After presurgical evaluation, the divided ends are microscopically approximated with 8-0 to 10-0 monofilament sutures. The duct is stented, if possible, or ligated. Subsequent external salivary fistulas can be managed by observation, elimination of parotid function (e.g., denervation or radiation therapy), or re-establishment of flow to the oral cavity. A sialocele can be managed by eliminating parotid function or re-establishing flow to the oral cavity, possibly by an intraoral incision and placement of a long-term drain.

CONTROVERSIES

22. How is drooling managed?

A normal person produces 1–1.5 pints of saliva a day. This saliva is important in initiating digestion, lubricating the teeth, and so on. In neuromuscular problems such as cerebral palsy, drooling may occur, even though saliva production is normal. Treatment with anticholinergics is rarely successful, but salivary duct rerouting is often curative. In this procedure, the parotid duct is mobilized and the orifice is sutured to a new, more posterior location in the mouth. This surgery facilitates swallowing and eliminates drooling. Alternatively, ligation of one or two major salivary gland ducts may be required.

23. How can chronic, recurrent parotid sialadenitis be managed?

Excision of the gland is probably the first choice. In cases in which this has been unsuccessful, or is contraindicated, radiation of the gland is considered. Usually 35 cGy is sufficient to eliminate salivation and prevent recurrence. Alternatively, denervation by Jacobsen's neurectomy (resection of the nerve where it crosses the promontory of the ear) has been described as efficacious. The problem is that the nerve may divide high on the promontory or branches may remain in a "canal" as it crosses the promontory, preventing total ablation. But re-resection of acute and chronically inflamed salivary gland remnants is a very difficult procedure.

BIBLIOGRAPHY

1. Almadori G, Ottaviani F, Del Ninno M, et al: Monolateral aplasia of the parotid gland. Ann Otol Rhinol Laryngol 106:522–525, 1997.
2. Bodner L: Parotid sialolithiasis. J Laryngol Otol 113:266–267, 1999.
3. Carlson GW: The salivary glands: Embryology, anatomy, and surgical applications. Surg Clin North Am 80:261–273, xii, 2000.
4. Caruso D, Klein H: Diagnosis and treatment of bulimia nervosa. Semin Gastrointest Dis 9:176–182, 1998.
5. Daud AS, Pahor AL: Tympanic neurectomy in the management of parotidsialectasis. J Laryngol Otol 109:1155–1158, 1995.
6. Holland AJ, Baron-Hay GS, Brennan BA: Parotid lipomatosis. J Pediatr Surg 31:1422–1423, 1997.
7. Hussein I, Kershaw AE, Tahmassebi JF, et al: The management of drooling in children and patients with mental and physical disabilities: A literature review. Int J Paediatr Dent 8:3–11, 1998.
8. Mandel L: Ranula, or, what's in a name? N Y State Dent J 62:37–39, 1996.

9. Mandel L, Hamele-Bena D: Alcoholic parotid sialadenosis. J Am Dent Assoc 128:1411–1415, 1997.
10. McQuone SJ: Acute viral and bacterial infections of the salivary glands. Otolaryngol Clin North Am 32:793–811, 1999.
11. Rice DH: Noninflammatory, non-neoplastic disorders of the salivary glands. Otolaryngol Clin North Am 32:835–843, 1999.
12. Seifert G: Aetiological and histological classification of sialadenitis. Pathologica 89:7–17, 1997.
13. Sood S, Quraishi MS, Bradley PJ: Frey's syndrome and parotid surgery. Clin Otol Allied Sci 23:291–301, 1998.
14. Tandler B, Nagato T, Toyoshima K, et al: Comparative ultrastructure of intercalated ducts in major salivary glands: A review. Anat Rec 252:64–91, 1998.
15. Teague A, Akhtar S, Phillips J: Frey's syndrome following submandibular gland excision: An unusual postoperative complication. Otolrhinolaryngol Rel Spec 60:346–348, 1998.

30. DEEP SPACE NECK INFECTIONS

Arvin K. Rao, M.S. IV, and John Campana, M.D.

1. What are deep space neck infections (DSNIs)?
These are dangerous and potentially lethal infections of the deep tissues of the neck that can cause death if they are not appropriately treated.

2. How is the cervical fascia important in DSNIs?
The cervical fascia is fibrous connective tissue that dictates the presentation, spread, and treatment of DSNIs. These fascial layers have two main components, the superficial and deep cervical fascia, which envelop structures and separate the neck into potential spaces. The deep cervical fascia is further divided into the external, middle, and internal layers.

- **Superficial cervical fascia**—Envelops the platysma and muscles of facial expression.
- **Deep cervical fascia:**
  External or investing fascia—Envelops the trapezius, sternocleidomastoid (SCM), submandibular and parotid glands, and muscles of mastication.
  Middle or visceral fascia—Envelops the pharynx, larynx, trachea, and esophagus, thyroid, parathyroids, buccinator, constrictor muscles, and strap muscles. In the posterior midline, this layer forms a midline raphe that adheres to the prevertebral fascia.
  Internal or prevertebral fascia—Envelops the paraspinous muscles and cervical vertebrae. It has two layers. The true *prevertebral* layer is just anterior to the vertebrae and goes from the base of skull to the coccyx. The *alar layer* lies between the prevertebral and visceral fascia (see Question 4).
  Carotid space—has components of all three layers.

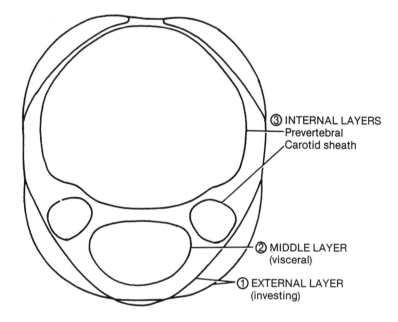

Divisions of deep cervical fascia: transverse section at level of CN VII. (From Graney DO: Anatomy. In Cummings CW, et al (eds): Otolaryngology—Head and Neck Surgery, 3rd ed. St. Louis, Mosby, 1998; with permission.)

3. What are the deep neck spaces?

The deep neck spaces can be divided into three types according to where they're located in relation to the hyoid bone. The hyoid bone is a critical landmark that divides the neck into three different general areas and limits the spread of infection.

- **Above the hyoid bone**
  Submandibular (sublingual, submaxillary)
  Pharyngomaxillary (lateral pharyngeal, multiple infection sources)
  Peritonsillar
  Masticator (gets infected from molar teeth)
  Parotid
- **Below the hyoid bone**
  Visceral
- **Involving the entire length of the neck**
  Vascular (carotid sheath)
  Prevertebral (dense connective tissue, can spread to coccyx)
  Danger space or alar space (spreads to superior mediastinum)
  Retropharyngeal (spreads to danger space)

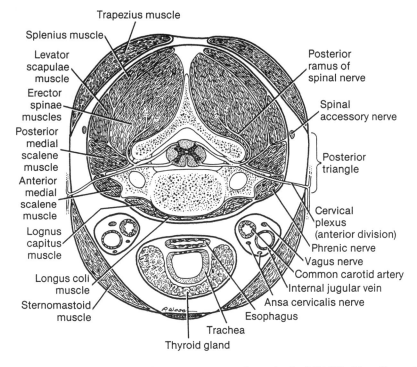

Structures contained by deep cervical fascia: transverse section at level of CN VII. (From Graney DO: Anatomy. In Cummings CW, et al (eds): Otolaryngology—Head and Neck Surgery, 3rd ed. St. Louis, Mosby, 1998; with permission.)

4. Why are all these spaces at the back of the throat so confusing? What is the "danger space"?

They are confusing *and* controversial. The retropharyngeal space contains lymph nodes, so occult metastases may occur here. It lies just anterior to the alar layer and posterior to the esophagus and pharynx. Just posterior to this is a potential space known as the *danger space,* which lies between the alar fascia anteriorly and the prevertebral space posteriorly. This potential space goes from the skull base to the mediastinum. It has only loose connective tissue and is an easy route of spread into the mediastinum, causing mediastinitis. This may be a point of anatomic minutia. During surgical drainage of these areas, a dissecting finger is used to disrupt and drain the retropharynx and danger space as one unit.

5. How do DSNIs present?

Fever, chills, sore throat, pain at the central focus of infection, referred ear pain, neck swelling with or without overt fluctuance, dysphagia, trismus, and decreased appetite. It is often difficult to differentiate between true abscess and cellulitis or adenitis on physical examination.

6. What organisms typically cause DSNIs?

Most DSNIs are polymicrobial. β-Lactamase production by aerobic pathogens is common. Infections of dental origin generally involve anaerobes, especially *Bacteroides*. In 10–20% of cases, "no growth" occurs in cultures. Common organisms include:

> *Staphylococcus aureus*
> Beta-hemolytic *Streptococcus*
> Alpha-hemolytic *Streptococcus*
> *Streptococcus pyogenes*
> *Bacteroides*
> *Peptostreptococcus*
> *Fusobacterium*

7. What is *Actinomyces israelii* and why is it different from other infectious agents?

It is normal flora that usually resides in the tonsils and periodontal space. It can cause deep neck infections that cross fascial planes. It is a gram-positive anaerobic bacillus that forms filaments, chronic granulomas, and "sulfur granules" (actually the bacterium and its waste) on histologic examination. The bacillus is hard to culture. For many years, this was thought to be a fungus. *Actinomyces* infection is usually treated with penicillin for 6 to 12 months. It tends to recur repeatedly if not treated for long enough.

8. Where do most DSNIs originate?

Most DNSIs are the result of **pharyngeal** and **tonsillar** infections that spread to the peritonsillar and pharyngomaxillary (lateral pharyngeal) space or **odontogenic** (dental) in origin. In addition, **salivary gland** infections are a common source and involve the submaxillary or parotid space. Intravenous drug abusers are prone to DSNI of the **vascular region,** as they may inject this area.

9. After a good history and physical examination, how do you work up a DNSI?

A complete blood cell count (CBC) and electrolytes are often ordered. Cultures of the throat, blood, sputum, and needle aspirations of possible abscesses are obtained. If appropriate, anteroposterior and lateral neck radiographs, Panorex and dental radiographs, and chest radiographs are frequently used. If a DSNI is suspected, a computed tomography (CT) scan is often the examination of choice to help differentiate cellulitis from abscess and to delineate which structures are involved. Ultrasonography is useful for guiding needle aspiration and can help diagnose abscess in many cases. Magnetic resonance imaging (MRI) can also provide excellent visualization but is not ordered as frequently.

10. What is the initial step in managing a DSNI?

Airway, airway, and airway. Most patients require only humidified oxygen. But, trismus and soft tissue swelling can make these patients very difficult to intubate. If an airway is needed, and the patient cannot be intubated, tracheotomy or cricothyrotomy may be necessary.

11. What are good, empiric antibiotics to use for DSNIs?

Broad-spectrum beta-lactamase stable agents that are effective against the most gram-positive, gram-negative, and anaerobic bacteria possible in these polymicrobial infections. Ampicillin/sulbactam and clindamycin/cefuroxime are common initial choices. If good cultures and sensitivities are obtained, the antibiotics can be adjusted appropriately.

12. When is surgical intervention indicated?

If the airway is in danger and intubation is difficult or impossible, a surgical airway should be emergently obtained. If the patient has had an appropriate work-up and the presumptive diagnosis is cellulitis or adenitis, observation with hydration and antibiotics is appropriate. If there is a high index of suspicion, clinically or radiographically, that there is a purulent collection, surgical drainage is appropriate. Wide drainage of the involved space and spaces around the involved space is the usual course of action. Penrose drains are used by most surgeons and advanced slowly from the postoperative sites over the course of a week or more.

13. When, if ever, are steroids indicated?

Rarely, steroids can be appropriate to help temporize a borderline airway while waiting to go to the operating room. But they should not be used in a prolonged fashion. They can mask a worsening infection. The patient may look better and feel better while progressing to a disaster, such as mediastinitis. Also, steroids demarginate white blood cells (WBC) and artificially elevate the patient's WBC count. This important test then can no longer be followed with confidence to help gauge clinical response to treatment.

14. In addition to airway compromise, what other major complications are associated with DSNI?

Mediastinitis, septic shock, septic thrombosis of the internal jugular vein, and carotid artery rupture can occur.

15. If a DSNI spreads to the coccyx, which space did it spread in?

The **prevertebral space** extends the length of the vertebral column to the level of the coccyx. Such infection is relatively rare, but can lead to vertebral osteomyelitis. These infections can also occur with penetrating trauma. **Pott's abscess** is a tuberculosis infection of the spine. Often these patients are chronically ill with low-grade fevers.

16. What three critical structures are contained in the vascular space?

The carotid artery, internal jugular vein, and vagus nerve. These structures are contained in the carotid sheath, a structure formed by all three layers of the deep cervical fascia.

17. A patient with a suspected DSNI develops bleeding from the nose, mouth, or external auditory canal. What is the cause?

In this case, the infection has likely spread to the vascular space, eroding the carotid artery and resulting in major bleeding. The mortality rate is 20–40%. It is usually accompanied by an ipsilateral Horner's syndrome (ptosis, miosis, anhydrosis from the cervical sympathetic chain) and palsies of cranial nerves IX, X, and XII from pressure or infection of these structures. Ligation of the carotid artery is usually required. Internal jugular infection usually causes thrombosis instead of major hemorrhage. Ligation of the internal jugular vein is not recommended. Resection of the vein and heparinization is controversial. Septic emboli, most often to the lungs, are possible.

18. A patient has suffered a stab wound to the face and develops a DSNI. What are you most concerned about?

The parotid space has the potential to become infected. In cases of parotitis, you should be concerned about spread to the pharyngomaxillary space and subsequent spread to the danger space.

19. Who is most prone to develop an infection in the spaces involving the entire length of the neck?

Patients who have sustained esophageal trauma, have a foreign body that pierces the posterior esophageal wall, or have vertebral fractures. In addition, infections of the ears, nose, and throat can lead to infections of this area. The characteristic infection of this space is the **midline retropharyngeal abscess,** which is most common in infants and young children after suppurative breakdown of retropharyngeal lymph nodes. The onset can be slow, often following an upper respiratory tract infection. Frequently, a feverish child will have difficulty swallowing or breathing. Trismus is generally not present. On inspection, the posterior pharyngeal wall is bulging. Transoral drainage can often be effective. Mediastinal extension is characterized by its widening on chest radiograph, chest pain, dyspnea, and fever.

20. A patient presents with trismus, uvular deviation, bulging of the soft palate, "hot potato" voice, dysphagia, drooling, and a fever. What diagnosis should you consider?

Peritonsillar abscess. Intraoral drainage is indicated. In adults, this can generally be performed in the clinic or emergency department with local anesthesia. Children usually go to the operating room. Immediate drainage options include needle aspiration, incisional drainage, and primary tonsillectomy. Aspiration and incisional drainage are equivalent treatments in most series. The majority of surgeons avoid primary tonsillectomy in the face of an abscess because of increased inflammation and bleeding at the time of surgery.

21. What is Ludwig's angina?

Ludwig's angina is a bilateral infection of the sublingual and submandibular spaces, usually from a dental source. The myelohyoid divides this potential space into a superior and an inferior portion. It is an emergency situation, in which the patient presents with firmness of the floor of the mouth and a swollen tongue, sometimes so bad that it causes airway difficulties. Intubation is often difficult and tracheotomy may be necessary. The patient may experience severe pain, difficulty swallowing, drooling, and trismus. Often, there is no overt abscess with little or no frank pus at the time of surgery. The infection can spread via the styloglossus muscle back into the pharyngomaxillary space, resulting in possible seeding of the retropharyngeal space and superior mediastinum. Intravenous antibiotics may be curative if started early. However, rapid surgical intervention is crucial because of potential airway compromise.

The relationship of the teeth to the myelohyoid muscle and the myelohyoid line determines the route by which dental infections spread. If there is an apical infection of the teeth anterior to the second molar, a sublingual infection that can progress to Ludwig's angina results. If the infection involves the second or third molars, the space involved is usually the submandibular and/or the lateral pharyngeal.

22. What neck infections may occur in an immunocompromised patient?

In the immunocompromised patient, fungal infections, scrofula (tuberculosis), and atypical mycobacterial infection should be considered. Diagnosis can be confirmed with fungal stains, acid fast bacilli stains, appropriate culture, and biopsy. Treatment generally consists of surgical débridement and antifungal chemotherapy if there is a fungal infection. Scrofula and atypical mycobacterial infection are not surgical diseases unless there is skin breakdown, necrosis, and fistulization. Medical therapy is usually appropriate.

23. A patient with a DSNI presents with severe dyspnea, chest pain, and fever. What is the diagnosis, and how is it confirmed?

This picture is characteristic of **mediastinitis.** This diagnosis can be confirmed with a chest radiograph that shows characteristic mediastinal widening. CT scans are usually used to help confirm the diagnosis. A thoracic surgeon should be involved if mediastinitis is suspected. Treatment consists of aggressive drainage and intravenous antibiotics. Mediastinitis has a mortality rate of 14–40%.

BIBLIOGRAPHY

1. Chan CH, McGurk M: Cervical necrotising fasciitis—a rare complication of periodontal disease. Br Dent J 183:293–296, 1997.
2. Clark LA, Moon RE: Hyperbaric oxygen in the treatment of life-threatening soft-tissue infections. Respir Care Clin North Am 5:203–219, 1999.
3. File TM Jr, Tan JS: Group A streptococcus necrotizing fasciitis. Compr Ther 26:73–81, 2000.
4. Johnson JT: Abscesses and deep space infections of the head and neck. Infect Dis Clin North Am 6:705–717, 1992.
5. Kaplan HT, Eichel BS: Deep neck infections. In English GM (ed): Otolaryngology. Philadelphia, J.B. Lippincott, 3(30):1–35, 2000.
6. Kiernan PD, Hernandez A, et al: Descending cervical mediastinitis. Ann Thorac Surg 65:1483–1488, 1998.
7. Leitch HA, Palepu A, Fernandes CM: Necrotizing fasciitis secondary to group A streptococcus: Morbidity and mortality still high. Can Fam Physician 46:1460–6, 2000.
8. Levitt GW: Cervical fascia and deep neck infections. Otolaryngol Clin North Am 9:703–728, 1976. (*A classic*)
9. Mortimore S, Thorp M: Cervical necrotizing fasciitis and radiotherapy: A report of two cases. J Laryngol Otol 112:298–300, 1998.
10. Neal MS: Necrotising fasciitis. J Wnd Care 8:18–19, 1999.
11. Sancho LM, Minamoto H, et al: Descending necrotizing mediastinitis: A retrospective surgical experience. Eur J Cardiothorac Surg 16:200–205, 1999.
12. Stevens DL: Streptococcal toxic shock syndrome associated with necrotizing fasciitis. Annu Rev Med 51:271–288, 2000.
13. Stevens DL: The flesh-eating bacterium: What's next? J Infect Dis 179(Suppl 2):S366–374, 1999.
14. Urschel JD: Necrotizing soft tissue infections. Postgrad Med J 75:645–649, 1999.
15. Wall DB, Klein SR, Black S, et al: A simple model to help distinguish necrotizing fasciitis from nonnecrotizing soft tissue infection. J Am Coll Surg 191:227–231, 2000.
16. Zerr DM, Rubens CE: NSAIDS and necrotizing fasciitis. Pediatr Infect Dis J 18:724–725, 1999.

31. SNORING AND OBSTRUCTIVE SLEEP APNEA

John P. Campana, M.D.

1. What is snoring and how is it different from obstructive sleep apnea?
Snoring is simply noisy breathing during sleep. It can be socially disabling. Patients tell dramatic stories. One woman reported that her "significant other" sleeps in the van in the garage to try and get some sleep. Another man was asked to leave a campground in the middle of the night by a forest ranger because of numerous enthusiastic complaints from other campers. There are even occasional stories in the media about sleep-deprived bed-partners shooting snorers in frustration and desperation. If your spouse does not shoot you, simple snoring is otherwise not dangerous. However, obstructive sleep apnea (OSA) *is* dangerous, in and of itself.

2. Who snores?
At age 30, 20% of men and 5% of women snore. This increases to 60% and 40%, respectively, at age 60. With increasing age, the mucosa of the palate, oropharynx, and hypopharynx becomes less elastic and more collapsible with inspiration. Snoring is three times more common in obese persons. Obesity often contributes to OSA because of the weight of the neck, increased fat in the parapharyngeal space that narrows the pharynx, redundancy in the soft palate, and fullness in the tongue base.

3. How loud can snoring get?
Snores by Käre Walkert of Kumla, Sweden, who suffered from OSA, were recorded at 93 dBA at the Örebro regional hospital on May 24, 1993. This noise level is similar to the noise of a screaming child, a passing motorcycle, or a passing subway train (all about 90dB).

4. Who has OSA?
Sleep occupies approximately one-third of our lives. Data suggest that sleep plays a restorative role in physiologic mechanisms and that long-term disruption of sleep may contribute to the development of disease. However, sleep and the disorders of sleep are not widely understood. Nearly a third of the adult population is chronically afflicted by sleep disorders, and substantial economic loss is attributable to these disorders in terms of lost time, inefficiency, and accidents. Of the sleep disorders, OSA is one of the more common, clinically affecting up to 5% of the adult population. Although most patients are overweight and have a short, thick neck, some are of normal weight but have a small, receding jaw. OSA is defined as a disorder of intermittent cessation of airflow during sleep that lasts 10 seconds or longer. This cessation in airflow is usually measured at the nose and lips. Sleep apnea is divided into three classes: central, obstructive, and mixed.

All snoring and apnea is abnormal in children. Their "pathology" may be simple, such as a common cold causing nasal obstruction and adenotonsillar enlargement. Or, it can be more complex, such as "adenoid facies"(chronic nasal obstruction yielding mouth breathing, a narrow midface with crowded teeth, a high-arched palate, and a retrognathic mandible from the downward and medial pull of the muscles of mastication) or a craniofacial abnormality (Pierre Robin syndrome). Other causes include nasopharyngeal cysts, encephaloceles, choanal atresia, and deviated nasal septum. Complications include neurocognitive deficits, growth failure, and pulmonary hypertension. Nevertheless, sleep-disordered breathing is often unrecognized in children. New syndromes, such as the upper airway resistance syndrome, have recently been described.

Twenty-five percent of patients with hypertension have OSA. And 50% of apnea patients have systemic hypertension. Obesity plays a significant role in adult OSA, but children with apnea tend to be underweight and short in stature.

5. What questions should you ask when evaluating a patient with suspected OSA?
Does your snoring ever awaken you from sleep?
Do you ever awaken suddenly, gasping for air?

Do family members complain about your snoring?

Does your spouse notice periods in which breathing temporarily stops?

Do you feel rested after a night's sleep?

Do you feel drowsy at work, or do you fall asleep at inappropriate times (such as at work, while driving, or while on the telephone)?

Do you have morning headaches?

6. What should you look for on the physical examination of a patient with suspected OSA?

A complete head and neck examination should be performed, as well as further examination if problems such as cor pulmonale or hypertension are suspected. The nose should be examined for signs of obstruction due to a deviated septum, hypertrophic turbinates, allergic rhinitis, etc. Examination of the oral cavity may reveal potential obstruction due to large tonsils, redundant soft palate and uvula, redundant lateral pharyngeal walls, and/or a full base of the tongue. Retrognathia and/or macroglossia can also contribute to OSA. Full, thick necks may also predispose patients to OSA, especially in the setting of an overall "pickwickian" patient. Laryngeal examination should be performed to rule out any obstructing lesion.

7. What is the pathophysiology of OSA?

OSA can be caused by an obstruction at any level of the upper airway (i.e., above the true vocal cords or glottis). Respiratory physiology dictates that during inspiration, there is a negative pressure within the upper airway. Sleep physiology reveals that during the deeper stages of sleep (stages III, IV, and REM), there is muscle relaxation of the entire body, including the muscles of the upper airway. Most patients with OSA have redundant tissue or an abnormally small air passage. In the presence of these anatomic variants, these two physiologic events combine to result in collapse of the upper airway, with resulting obstruction to airflow. Oxyhemoglobin desaturation eventually leads to an arousal to a lighter level of sleep, and the airway is re-established with the characteristic loud snoring respiration. Any factor that adds to upper airway obstruction can cause or exacerbate OSA, including adenotonsillar hypertrophy, obstructive laryngeal masses, bulky soft palate or uvula, fullness in the base of the tongue, a low-lying hyoid bone, or nasal obstruction.

8. Are there special tests to evaluate for OSA?

Epworth Sleepiness Scale is a sensitive screening tool for OSA. It is a series of questions about daytime somnolence. A numerical score is assigned that correlates well to the eventual diagnosis of OSA.

Polysomnography is the most sensitive and specific test in the evaluation of OSA. This test measures brain activity (electroencephalography), leg muscle movements (electromyography), cardiac rhythm (electrocardiography), eye movements (electrooculography), oxygen saturation, respiratory effort, and air movement at the nose and mouth. Polysomnography can differentiate between snoring without OSA, pure OSA, and central sleep apnea and can characterize the severity of the apnea. This test, however, is very expensive and requires the patient to spend a night in a formal sleep laboratory. This study generates an apnea index (AI), respiratory disturbance index (RDI), and a summary of oxygen desaturations (see Question #9).

Home sleep studies have recently been implemented in an effort to reduce cost. These studies range from simple continuous pulse oximetry recordings to multichannel recordings using devices similar to those used in a formal sleep laboratory. Although these tests are gaining popularity, none is as sensitive or specific as a formal sleep laboratory study.

The **multiple sleep latency test** is also performed in a sleep laboratory, but it is done during the day. The subject is given the chance to take naps, and this test assesses the time it takes for the subject to fall asleep. An average sleep onset of < 5 minutes is generally considered pathologic and suggests excessive daytime sleepiness.

Müller's maneuver is performed as part of an extensive physical examination and involves passing the flexible fiberoptic scope into the hypopharynx to obtain a view of the entire hypopharynx and larynx. The examiner then pinches the nostrils closed, and the patient closes his or her lips while attempting to inhale. If the hypopharynx and/or larynx collapse, then the test is positive. A positive test means that the site of upper airway obstruction is very likely below the level of the soft palate, and the patient will probably not benefit from a uvulopalatopharyngoplasty alone. Tongue base procedures may be necessary.

Sleep endoscopy is occasionally performed at the time of other surgical procedures for apnea. A flexible fiberoptic scope is passed into the hypopharynx to watch the patient breathe while under a light general anesthetic. This can help evaluate the site of obstruction and may encourage the physician to do some type of tongue base procedure.

In children, formal sleep studies are not done as often. Some physicians use 24-hour pulse oximetry or sleep sonography, which is recording of nocturnal breathing sounds. Usually a history and physical (usually large tonsils and adenoids) consistent with OSA are enough to make a surgical decision for a child. Other causes include nasopharyngeal cysts, encephaloceles, choanal atresia, a deviated nasal septum, and craniofacial or orthodontic malformations.

When in doubt, a formal sleep study is still indicated.

9. What are the polysomnographic characteristics of OSA?

Apnea means "want of breath" in Greek. OSA is repetitive, temporary cessation of air exchange due to obstruction of the upper airway while normal or extraordinary respiratory efforts are being made. Significant apnea events are longer than 10 seconds. Fewer than five apnea events an hour is normal. Other important definitions are as follows:

- **Central sleep apnea** — the cessation in airflow is due to a transient lack of respiratory effort. The phrenic nerve and diaphragm are temporarily inactive due to intermittent failure in the respiratory drive centers of the central nervous system (CNS). Rarely, this may be the result of primary medullary brainstem injury from polio or tumors of the posterior fossa. **Ondine's curse** is an idiopathic failure of brainstem respiratory drive. Patients with this disorder breath insufficiently, or not at all, unless fully awake. Neurologists and pulmonary sleep specialists generally treat true central apnea.
- **Hypopnea** — a reduction of air exchange associated with oxygen desaturation. It can be obstructive or central.
- **Mixed sleep apnea** — Exhibits components of both central and obstructive apnea but is considered a variant of OSA. Treatment is similar to treatment for OSA.
- **Apnea Index** (AI) — number of apnea events per hour.
- **Respiratory Disturbance Index** (RDI) — number of apnea events plus number of hypopnea events per hour.
- **"Pickwickian"** — Charles Dickens, in *The Posthumous Papers of the Pickwick Club* (1837), described the obese and somnolent Joe who "goes on errands fast asleep and snores as he waits at a table." Pickwickian syndrome is characterized by obesity and hypersomnolence.

10. Describe the classic sleep pattern seen in OSA.

Typically, OSA patients exhibit a quick onset of sleep and multiple arousals. The patient maintains relatively more stage I and II sleep and less stage III, IV, and REM sleep. This lack of deep sleep results in the symptoms of sleep deprivation.

11. How are mild, moderate, and severe OSA defined?

Several parameters can be used to classify the severity of OSA, the most common of which is the RDI. This is the sum of the number of apnea events (cessation of air flow for > 10 seconds) and hypopneas events (reduction of airflow by 50%) per hour. The degree of oxyhemoglobin desaturation can also be useful.

12. During which stage of sleep do most obstructive events occur?

Most obstructive events occur during the deeper stages of sleep, including stages III, IV, and REM sleep. It is during these stages that muscles are most relaxed, and thus pharyngeal wall collapse is most likely. OSA patients are therefore being deprived of deep sleep. This explains the restless sleep patterns and daytime somnolence. In fact, the hallmark of successful treatment of OSA is REM rebound, or a significant increase in REM sleep (clinical increase in dreaming) due to correction of previous sleep deprivation.

13. Should everyone who snores undergo a sleep study?

When the snoring is accompanied by symptoms of OSA, such as hypersomnolence, morning headache, and restless sleep, a thorough examination and sleep study are probably indicated. When snoring is socially disruptive but not accompanied by symptoms of sleep apnea, the picture is not so clear. Unfortunately, even "apneas" witnessed by bed-partners are not predictive of OSA. The only reasonably accurate method of detecting OSA remains the formal sleep study. Therefore, current recommendations suggest obtaining a sleep study prior to any surgery for sleep apnea or snoring.

14. What are the complications of OSA?

Left untreated, chronic OSA is definitely associated with significant morbidity and mortality. An increased rate of nocturnal death has been reported, presumably due to lethal cardiac arrhythmias. Cor pulmonale and chronic heart failure have also been well documented and improve dramatically after successful treatment. Idiopathic hypertension has also been associated with OSA, although the precise mechanism has not yet been elucidated. Again, this hypertension often reverses after successful treatment of the apnea, reducing the need for antihypertensive medication. There is also a higher rate of mortality in OSA patients due to automobile accidents, presumably due to excessive daytime somnolence. The physician who recognizes OSA should also recognize the dangers associated with excessive somnolence and driving or operating dangerous equipment. It appears that the natural history of OSA tends to worsen with age and with weight gain. Often, a vicious cycle develops in which daytime somnolence leads to less exercise, more weight gain, and more severe sleep apnea. Therefore, once it is identified, OSA should be treated promptly and aggressively.

15. What are the nonsurgical treatments of snoring and OSA?

- Hundreds of patents for snoring and apnea devices, such as antisnoring pillows and aversion devices that shock people when they snore, have been granted. Most are useless. There are numerous herbal treatments that are marketed. Again, none have been studied and shown to help.
- Improvement of nasal airway obstruction with "BreatheRight" external nasal dilator strips or allergy treatment can sometimes improve snoring and OSA to a modest degree. Allergy treatment with nasal steroids, nonsedating antihistamines, and occasionally immunotherapy can be helpful.
- Avoidance of alcohol and sedatives may reduce OSA. A physician should be aware that even mild sedatives, such as cough suppressants, may be dangerous if administered to a patient with OSA.
- Weight loss can help if a patient is obese.
- Sleeping position manipulation, such as sewing a tennis ball into the back of a patient's pajamas to discourage sleeping on the back, can help an occasional person.
- Tongue-retaining devices and mandibular advancement appliances can be very effective in some patients. Average AHI decreases from 47 to 19. These devices open the airway by holding the tongue and/or mandible forward during sleep. However, for mandibular advancement devices, 40% of users reported jaw/facial muscle pain, 40% had occlusal changes, 38% reported tooth pain, 30% reported jaw joint pain, and 30% experienced xerostomia. Compliance is about 50% at 3 years.
- Nasal continuous positive airway pressure (CPAP) is the most effective nonsurgical treatment of OSA. An airtight mask is held over the nose by a strap wrapped around the patient's head. CPAP is maintained by a machine that is similar to a ventilator. Although

nasal CPAP is nearly 100% effective in relieving OSA, compliance is a problem. The masks and positive pressure are uncomfortable for many people. Long-term compliance is 50% to 75%, depending on the level of support the patients are given by the medical staff. Bilevel positive airway pressure (BiPAP) is often tolerated better by decreasing the expiratory pressure.

16. What are the surgical treatments of snoring and OSA?

The operative management varies according to the surgeon's judgment of the site or sites of obstruction, the age of the patient, and the standards of care in the local community. Anatomic sites will be addressed individually:

Nose—Nasal obstruction can be treated by septoplasty, or submucosal resection of the septum, and turbinate reduction. Turbinate reduction is achieved by partial and submucosal resection, cautery, cryotherapy, laser, and submucosal radiofrequency devices (low-temperature heat that causes necrosis and resorption of tissue). Ninety to 98% of patients who undergo surgery to improve their nasal airway subjectively have improved nasal breathing. Thirty to 50% have elimination of simple snoring. Occasionally, a patient will have a significant decrease in OSA after nasal surgery alone, but this is rare. More aggressive surgery is usually required. In the pediatric population, medical treatment of nasal obstruction is more common. Many people do the Nasal Spray Test. Oxymetazolone or neosynephrine are sprayed in the nose before sleep. If improvement in snoring or apnea is encountered, it is a reasonable assumption that nasal surgery will give similar improvement.

Adenoids—Adenoidectomy in children is often done. It is 80% to 90% effective, often in conjunction with tonsillectomy, for improving nasal airway, snoring, and apnea in children. This operation is rarely necessary in adults.

Tonsils—Tonsil obstruction is treated with a variety of techniques: Tonsillar enlargement can be managed by debulking tonsil with a laser or submucosal radiofrequency device. Traditional tonsillectomy, done by a variety of techniques, is still the standard of care. In adults with OSA, tonsillectomy is often done as part of a uvulopalatopharyngoplasty. As mentioned above, it is 80–90% effective in children, often in association with adenoidectomy, for improving snoring and apnea. Children who have had an adenotonsillectomy actually have been shown to have a half letter grade improvement in school 1 year after the procedure. The children who did not have surgery did not improve.

Palate—Palate reduction can be achieved by laser-assisted uvulopalatoplasty (LAUP), submucosal radiofrequency device, electrocautery (termed Bovie-assisted uvulopalatoplasty or BAUP), or uvulopalatopharyngoplasty (UPPP or "U-triple-P").

For snoring, LAUP, BAUP, and the radiofrequency procedures are usually performed. For each of these procedures, as healing occurs the soft palate elevates, shortens, and stiffens, reducing the tendency to vibrate. Electrocautery is less expensive and more widely available. These procedures are performed in a doctor's office or in an outpatient setting under local anesthesia. They often require two to four stages, each separated by about 1 month, titrating the procedures to resolve the snoring without causing velopharyngeal insufficiency. Radiofrequency procedures usually help about 80% of the patients achieve significant improvement in their snoring. It is only minimally uncomfortable for the patients. LAUP, BAUP, and UPPP improve snoring in 90% of patients but cause severe pain for 10–14 days. LAUP and radiofrequency palate procedures for the treatment of true OSA have not been widely accepted, although they appear to have some positive effect in mild to moderate OSA.

For OSA, the standard of care for treating the palate is a UPPP. It is the most common procedure performed for OSA. In this procedure, the tonsils are removed (if they have not been removed previously), along with the posterior edge of the soft palate, including the uvula. The tonsillar pillars are then sewn together and the mucosa on the nasal side and oral side of the cut edge of the soft palate are sewn together. This procedure enlarges the oropharyngeal airway in an anterior-superior and lateral dimension. UPPP is a not a technically difficult operation, but it generally requires a 1- or 2-day stay in the hospital. Most surgeons require their patients to stay overnight in a monitored setting or intensive care unit (ICU) after apnea surgery. These patients depend on their ability to startle themselves awake to stay alive. Anesthetic agents and narcotics inhibit this and postoperative arrests can occur.

Tongue base—Radiofrequency tongue base reduction, lag screw and suture suspension of the tongue and hyoid, advancement genioplasty combined with a hyoid suspension, distraction osteogenesis, partial midline glossectomy, and maxillomandibular advancement are used to reduce obstruction at the tongue base.

- **Radiofrequency tongue base reduction** can obtain a 17% reduction in tongue base volume and has been shown to decrease RDI from 40 to 18, but it can require four to eight staged procedures, with a month between each one. Patients should be in a monitored setting for the night after the procedure. Between the use of multiple, expensive hand-pieces and 4 to 8 nights of inpatient monitoring, the insurance industry has been less than enthusiastic about this procedure.
- **Lag screw and suture suspension of the tongue and hyoid** are procedures that pull the tongue forward. Lag screws with preloaded sutures are driven into the inner cortex of the anterior mandible below the level of the teeth. A floor-of-mouth incision is made for the tongue suture. Submental incisions are made for the hyoid suspension. Sutures are then passed around the hyoid and through the tongue base to pull the tongue forward. The best data presented showed a 60% average decrease in RDI from 74 to about 30. Although this is a painful procedure, it is less morbid than some of the other options.
- **Advancement genioplasty and hyoid suspension** also pull the tongue forward. Rare tooth loss and pathologic fracture of the mandible can occur as complications. If these procedures are done in conjunction with nasal, palate, and tonsil surgery, the overall chance of reducing a patient's RDI by half is 70%.
- **Distraction osteogenesis** is a mechanical screw and gear device that slowly lengthens the mandible after an osteotomy is made. About 20 mm of new bone can be generated. This is a useful technique in cases of retrognathia and micrognathia such as Pierre Robin or Treacher-Collins syndrome. Significant facial scars can occur because many of these devices are lengthened by drive shafts that penetrate the facial skin.
- **Partial midline glossectomy,** using either a laser or electrocautery, can be performed. It requires a tracheotomy because significant bleeding and swelling can occur. It is highly effective, with average decreases in RDI from 59 to 8. Because of the tracheotomy and severe pain, this procedure has not gained wide acceptance.
- **Maxillomandibular advancement** is highly effective in a select group of relatively young, healthy, thin patients with retrusive midfaces and retrognathic mandibles. Success in this select group of patients is essentially 100%. This is a much larger operation than the UPPP, but it does successfully alter the anatomic anomalies that cause OSA. Maxillomandibular advancement is achieved using **bilateral sagittal split osteotomies** in the mandible and **LeFort I osteotomies** in the midface.

17. What are the surgical options for treatment of snoring without OSA?

As described in Question 16, an outpatient procedure has been devised in which a Bovie (BAUP) or laser (LAUP; usually CO_2) is used to amputate the uvula and to create 1-cm trenches in the soft palate on either side of the uvula. The procedure is performed in stages, titrating the resection to resolve the snoring without causing velopharyngeal insufficiency. The superiority of the laser over the Bovie has not been established, although both appear to be effective treatments for snoring. The Bovie is less expensive and more widely available, but the laser may prevent deep tissue damage.

18. How effective is using UPPP to treat OSA or snoring without OSA?

UPPP is very successful in treating snoring alone but is not as successful in treating OSA. Approximately 90% of patients stop snoring after a UPPP, regardless of whether they have sleep apnea. However, significant improvement in OSA occurs in only about 50% of patients. In addition, significant improvement may mean a reduction in the RDI of 50% or more, but the patient still may have significant OSA, especially if their RDI was very high at the start. Overall, studies have not shown a reduction in the rate of mortality associated with OSA following UPPP alone. Studies have shown dramatically improved mortality rates following treatment with tracheostomy or CPAP, however. Therefore, the decision to proceed with UPPP must be individualized to each patient, and the patient must be aware of the possible need for additional procedures if the UPPP fails.

19. Describe the potential complications of a UPPP.

UPPP has been described as a "radical tonsillectomy," and therefore the potential complications are similar to those of a tonsillectomy. Bleeding is by far the most common postoperative complication, occasionally requiring another visit to the operating room for control. Transient velopharyngeal insufficiency occurs in 5–10% of patients but is rarely permanent. Nasopharyngeal stenosis is a very rare but devastating complication in which the nasopharynx scars down completely. Patients may complain of a dry mouth, tightness in the throat, an increased gag reflex, and/or a change in taste; however, these are usually transient.

CONTROVERSIES

20. What is the role of laser-assisted uvulopalatoplasty (LAUP) in OSA and snoring?

LAUP is highly effective in the treatment of snoring, with resolution of snoring occurring in 85–90% of patients. However, the effectiveness of LAUP in the treatment of OSA has not been established. Snoring and OSA probably represent a continuum of a similar pathology, but along this continuum, it is hard to differentiate where LAUP is effective and where it is not effective. In addition, a patient's symptoms, including snoring or daytime somnolence, cannot be used as predictors of OSA nor as indicators for successful treatment of OSA. Therefore, the current recommendation is that all patients undergo a sleep study prior to surgery for snoring or OSA and that OSA of any degree is a contraindication to LAUP. It should be noted, however, that there is ongoing research in this area, and LAUP may well prove to be effective for the treatment of mild or moderate OSA. These observations also hold for BAUP, in which the bovie is used in place of the laser to perform the surgery.

21. What is the most effective surgical treatment for OSA?

Tracheotomy remains the gold standard in the treatment of OSA. It bypasses the upper airway entirely and is effective in almost all patients, including those with severe disease. In patients with very severe disease, those who are markedly obese, or those who are debilitated, it is probably the initial procedure of choice. Effectiveness in this group of patients is in the high 90% range. The other methods that have been described realistically have little chance of benefit. However, the patient must live with and care for the tracheotomy on a daily basis, which is undesirable to most patients. For children with craniofacial abnormalities, such as Pierre Robin syndrome, a tracheotomy is a good intervention until the child grows enough to undergo mandibular advancement procedures.

22. What does the future hold?

Improvement in weight control may be available in the near future with advances in behavioral, pharmacologic, nutritional, and possibly genetic treatments. Continued improvement of CPAP and BiPAP machines is likely. Surgical advances, such as radiofrequency reduction of parapharyngeal fat pads, are being investigated. Phrenic nerve to hypoglossal nerve pacing has been studied in animal models. When a breath is taken, the phrenic nerve would stimulate the hypoglossal nerve to move the tongue forward.

—➤●◄—

BRAHMS' LULLABY

Johannes Brahms, composer of history's most famous lullaby, apparently suffered from obstructive sleep apnea. Described as an irritable, ill-tempered, intermittently depressed man who suffered from daytime somnolence (all symptoms of sleep deprivation), Brahms was overweight and a "horrible snorer." His famous lullaby was reportedly written to comfort the newborn daughter of a friend, but might it also have been an attempt to lull himself off to a better night's sleep?

~Gugliotta G, Washington Post, January 29, 2001

—➤●◄—

BIBLIOGRAPHY

1. Alwani A, Rubinstein I: The nose and obstructive sleep apnea. Curr Opin Pulm Med 4:361–362, 1998.
2. Ayas NT, Epstein LJ: Oral appliances in the treatment of obstructive sleep apnea and snoring. Curr Opin Pulm Med 4:355–360, 1998.
3. Bennett LS: Adult obstructive sleep apnoea syndrome. J R Coll Phys London 33:439–444, 1999.
4. Braver HM: Treatment for snoring: Combined weight loss, sleeping on side, and nasal spray. Chest 107:1283–1288, 1995.
5. Bridgman SA, Dunn KM: Surgery for obstructive sleep apnoea. Cochrane Database Syst Revs [computer file] 2:CD001004, 2000.
6. Clark GT, Sohn JW, Hong CN: Treating obstructive sleep apnea and snoring: Assessment of an anterior mandibular positioning device. J Am Dent Assoc 131(6):765–771, 2000.
7. Fairbanks DN: Snoring—An overview with historical perspectives. In Fairbanks DN, Fujita S (eds): Snoring and Obstructive Sleep Apnea, 2nd ed. Philadelphia, Raven Press, 1994, pp. 1–16.
8. Foresman BH: Sleep and breathing disorders: The genesis of obstructive sleep apnea. J Am Osteopath Assoc 100(8 Suppl):S1–8, 2000.
9. Lindberg E, Janson C, Svardsudd K, et al: Increased mortality among sleepy snorers: A prospective population based study. Thorax 53:631–637, 1998.
10. Littner M: Polysomnography in the diagnosis of the obstructive sleep apnea-hypopnea syndrome: Where do we draw the line? Chest 118:286–288, 2000.
11. Messner AH, Pelayo R: Pediatric sleep-related breathing disorders. Am J Otol 21:98–107, 2000.
12. Phillips BG, Somers VK: Neural and humoral mechanisms mediating cardiovascular responses to obstructive sleep apnea. Resp Phys 119:181–187, 2000.
13. Powell NB, Riley RW, et al: Radiofrequency volumetric tissue reduction of the palate in subjects with sleep-disordered breathing. Chest 113:1163–1174, 1998.
14. Victor LD: Obstructive sleep apnea. Am Fam Phys 60:2279–2286, 1999.
15. Wright J, White J: Continuous positive airways pressure for obstructive sleep apnoea. Cochrane Database Syst Revs [computer file] 2:CD001106, 2000.

32. THE HOARSE PATIENT

Bozena Wrobel, M.D., and Mona Abaza, M.D.

1. What is hoarseness?

Hoarseness is a vague term that patients often use to describe a change in voice quality, ranging from voice harshness to voice weakness. However, the term can reflect abnormalities anywhere along the vocal tract, from the oral cavity to lungs. Ideally, the term hoarseness refers to laryngeal dysfunction caused by abnormal vocal cord vibration.

2. How is speech produced?

There are three phases in speech: pulmonary, laryngeal, and supraglottis/oral. The **pulmonary phase** creates the energy flow with inflation and expulsion of air. This activity provides the larynx with a column of air for the laryngeal phase. In the laryngeal phase, vocal folds vibrate at certain frequencies to create sound that then is modified in the **supraglottic/oral phase** to the sound that is unique to the individual. Words are formed by the action of the pharynx, tongue, lips, and teeth. Dysfunction in any of these stages can lead to voice changes, which may be interpreted as hoarseness by the patient.

3. What clinical signs in voice quality and frequency may help to localize the speech abnormality?

When the speech abnormality is limited to the lungs or tracheobronchial tree, the patient exhibits a weak, damped voice. The lungs may be restricted in movement, making the voice barely perceptible. On the other hand, if the patient has difficulty articulating words or if the voice resonates as if coming from the nose, the problem probably originates in the oral stage. Oral-stage abnormalities may also lead to a muffled or "hot potato" voice. Abnormalities originating in either the lung or oral cavity are not considered to be true hoarseness. True hoarseness from a laryngeal origin usually results in a rough, raspy voice.

4. What produces the frequency of a given sound?

Different frequencies are produced by expiratory pulmonary force in conjunction with changes in the length, breadth, elasticity, and extension of the vocal folds. The adductor laryngeal muscle modifies length of the vocal folds. Vocal folds are approximated, and the pressure of moving air causes vibration of the elastic fold. It is important to note that vocal fold vibration is not an active process caused by laryngeal muscles.

5. What terms are useful in characterizing hoarseness or voice change?

Dysphonia—describes a general alteration in voice quality.

Diplophonia—describes a sound made by vibrating cords at two different frequencies. It indicates that the vocal folds are being affected differently.

Aphonia—occurs when no sound is emanated from the vocal folds. It often occurs secondary to a lack of air passing through the vocal folds or a deficiency in vocal fold approximation.

Stridor—indicates noise emanating from the upper airway during inspiration and/or expiration due to an obstruction.

Stridor is a medical emergency; it is not considered hoarseness. It may coexist with hoarseness when the obstruction occurs at the level of the vocal folds.

6. How is hoarseness categorized?

Hoarseness can be broken down into two broad categories, acute onset and chronic onset. Acute onset is more common and is often caused by local inflammation of the larynx, such as seen with acute laryngitis. In most cases it is self-limited process. Voice rest, increased fluid intake, and humidification are recommended. If secondary bacterial infection is suspected, antibiotics are prescribed. Most common pathogens are *Moraxella, Haemophilus, Pneumococcus, Streptococcus, Staphyloccocus,* and *Mycoplasma.* In the absence of infection, acute laryngitis may result from chemical or environmental irritants or brief periods of vocal overuse. Chronic hoarseness, on the other hand, may be caused by pharyngeal reflux, benign polyps, vocal folds nodules, laryngeal papillomatosis, tumor, functional dysphonia, neurologic involvement, or chronic inflammation secondary to smoking or voice abuse. Note that acute hoarseness is unlikely to have a malignant etiology. A malignant process should always be considered if hoarseness has been progressive and present for several months.

7. What are the most common causes of hoarseness?

Acute viral laryngitis	Laryngeal cancer
Vocal fold nodules, polyps, cysts, papillomas	Postnasal drip
Vocal fold paralysis	Laryngopharyngeal reflux
Hypothyroidism	Recent intubation
Rhinosinusitis	Allergies

8. What systemic diseases can affect the voice and cause hoarseness?

Hypothyroidism	Wegener's granulomatosis
Multiple sclerosis	Myasthenia gravis
Rheumatoid arthritis	Sarcoidosis
Parkinson's disease	Tremor disorders
Systemic lupus	Amyloidosis
Amyotrophic lateral sclerosis (ALS)	

9. How is chronic laryngitis treated?

Chronic laryngitis is general inflammation of the larynx often caused by smoking, voice abuse, or laryngopharyngeal reflux. The voice usually improves if the irritating factors are discontinued. This may involve smoking cessation or voice rest. Patients with reflux laryngitis present with symptoms of chronic hoarseness, chronic cough, throat irritation, frequent throat clearing, and globus sensation. All these symptoms are attributed to gastroesophageal and laryngopharyngeal reflux. Fifty percent of patients with reflux laryngitis do not complain of heartburn. H_2 blockers and proton pump inhibitors are highly effective in treatment. In addition, patients with reflux may benefit from resting their voice, sleeping with the head of their bed elevated, and waiting 3–4 hours after eating before going to bed.

10. What are the most common findings associated with laryngopharyngeal reflux on flexible nasopharyngoscopy?

Posterior glottic edema, interarytenoid edema and erythema, vocal folds edema, mucosal thickening, vocal process ulceration, and vocal process granuloma.

11. How do you define Reinke's edema?

Reinke's edema, also known as chronic hypertrophic laryngitis, is characterized by chronic edematous changes involving the full length of the vocal fold. It is an inflammatory process secondary to chronic vocal abuse and cigarette smoking. Patients, usually female, present with a hoarse, breathy, harsh, low-pitched voice. Treatment includes smoking cessation, voice therapy, and, in advanced cases, surgery.

12. An elderly person with rheumatoid arthritis presents with symptoms of hoarseness, dyspnea, difficulty swallowing pills, and a sensation of throat fullness. What will be the characteristic findings on flexible scope examination of the larynx in this patient?

This patient's symptoms are most likely secondary to inflammatory arthritic changes in the cricoarytenoid joint. On flexible scope examination, the following pathology can be visualized:

acute inflammation or edema overlying arytenoid cartilage, decreased mobility with fixed vocal fold in adducted position, arytenoid process tenderness on palpation, and "bamboo lesions" on vocal folds corresponding to rheumatoid nodule–like deposits. Computed tomographic (CT) scan may demonstrate subluxation of the cricoarytenoid joint.

13. Which infections are likely to cause hoarseness?

Viral infections are most commonly responsible for laryngitis, causing diffuse erythema of the vocal folds and an increase in vocal folds mass. In children, **subglottic edema** also may cause croup (barking cough). In contrast, epiglottitis does not typically present with hoarseness but instead causes a muffled "hot potato" voice due to supraglottic swelling. **Bacterial infections** of the endolarynx are not common, but they can occur. **Laryngeal papillomatosis** is a relatively common infectious cause of hoarseness. It results from human papilloma virus infection, inducing wart-like growths on the vocal folds. Because laryngeal papillomatosis is more common in children, examination of the larynx should be considered if this disorder is suspected.

14. What questions should be included in the history when evaluating a patient with hoarseness?

What is the duration of symptoms, and is there any progression? Such questions determine whether the process is acute or chronic.

Is there a coexistent sore throat or otalgia?

Is there dysphagia or odynophagia? If present, these symptoms may indicate a problem with the pharynx, esophagus, or larynx.

Is there a cough? Although cough may be associated with an infection, cancer of the lung with vocal fold paralysis (secondary to recurrent laryngeal nerve involvement) often presents with hoarseness and cough.

Is there hemoptysis? This potentially serious symptom may indicate malignancy.

What are the occupation and habits of patient? Singers,teachers, sports fanatics (shouting), and some people who eat spicy food are more likely to suffer from benign hoarseness.

Is there heartburn or symptoms of reflux?

What is the timing of the hoarseness (e.g. AM, PM)?

Is there previous surgery (on the neck or resulting in intubation)?

15. Which parts of the physical examination are vital when evaluating a patient with hoarseness?

Patients presenting with hoarseness lasting longer than 2 weeks require a complete head and neck evaluation with laryngeal examination to rule out malignancy. In the head and neck examination, pneumatic otoscopy, nasal examination, oral examination, and neck palpation, indirect laryngoscopy are extremely important. For better visualization of the glottis and evaluation of the vocal folds function, flexible nasopharyngoscopy and videostroboscopy might be necessary.

16. A 38-year-old woman presents to you with a history of hoarseness persisting for several months. On flexible scope examination, unilateral vocal fold paralysis is diagnosed. Results of the rest of the ENT examination are normal. What studies will be helpful to establish the diagnosis?

Chest radiography, CT with contrast (fine 1-mm cuts, from the skull base to the aortic arch), thyroid stimulating hormone level, erythrocyte sedimentation rate, CHEM 7, complete blood cell count, and RA. Magnetic resonance imaging of the head should also be considered.

17. What is the most common cause of hoarseness in the elderly?

Presbylaryngeus is the most common cause of hoarseness in the elderly. With aging, the vocalis muscle loses its tone, which results in a bowed appearance when the vocal folds adduct. Women are more affected by the changes.

18. What innervates voice production?

The motor neurons that innervate the larynx are found in the nucleus ambiguous of the medulla. Fibers travel from the nucleus ambiguous with the vagus nerve to exit through the jugular foramen within the carotid sheath. Superiorly, the vagus nerve gives rise to the superior laryngeal nerve, which innervates the cricothyroid muscle of the larynx and provides sensory innervation to the endolarynx. The vagus continues traveling inferiorly. In the thorax, it gives rise to the recurrent laryngeal nerve. The recurrent laryngeal nerve loops around the arch of the aorta on the left and around the subclavian artery on the right to innervate the larynx inferiorly.

19. Which neurologic abnormalities may cause hoarseness?

If a neoplasm is present, **nerve compression** may lead to hoarseness. This compression can occur anywhere from the brainstem to the aortic arch. For example, vocal fold paralysis can be secondary to tumors of the jugular foramen (glomus jugulare), neck, thyroid, bronchus, lung, or esophagus. Thyroid tumors are the most common cause of bilateral vocal fold paralysis, whereas bronchogenic carcinoma and malignant esophageal tumors are common causes of unilateral vocal fold paralysis. **Nerve injury** should also be suspected if a patient is hoarse after any surgical procedure on the neck. Injury may be due to transection, cricothyroid joint injury, or compression from an overinflated endotracheal cuff. Hoarseness could be a part of presentation of **central neurologic** disorders, such as: stroke (Wallenberg's syndrome), Parkinson's disease, myasthenia gravis, multiple sclerosis, amyotrophic lateral sclerosis.

20. How do you treat unilateral vocal fold paralysis?

The goal of treatment of unilateral vocal fold paralysis is to improve the quality of voice and prevent aspiration. Voice therapy is recommended before and after surgical treatment. Surgical methods of treatment are injection laryngoplasty (fat, gelfoam, collagen), medialization laryngoplasty, and arytenoid adduction procedures.

21. What is spasmodic dysphonia? How is it treated?

Spasmodic dysphonia is a focal dystonia affecting the control of laryngeal muscles during speech. Patients present with a breathy voice, intermittent voice breaks, and complaints of voice tension, spasms, tremor that worsens particularly during period of excessive stress, speech performance, and upper respiratory infection. There are two types of spasmodic dysphonia (SD): adductor SD (voice breaks in vowels) and abductor SD (prolonged voiceless consonants). The treatment of choice for adductor dysphonia (more common type of SD) is percutaneous botulinum toxin injection into the thyroarytenoid muscle under electromyography (EMG) monitoring.

22. What are the neoplastic disorders of the vocal folds?

The true vocal folds are most commonly affected by **squamous cell carcinoma**. Such a malignancy is exophytic in appearance and, if treated early, has a high cure rate and excellent possibility of voice preservation. Therefore, laryngeal examination of the hoarse patient is vital for early diagnosis and intervention.

23. Can nonorganic disorders present as hoarseness?

A **conversion disorder**, a psychiatric condition, may present as hoarseness. One of the most common nonorganic causes of hoarseness is **functional dysphonia**. Patients exhibit paradoxical motion of the vocal folds during speech. During quiet respiration or sleep, laughing, or coughing, the vocal folds work normally. During speech, the vocal folds abduct and fail to vibrate adequately to produce sound. The diagnosis can be made if a normal cough is present. The laryngoscopic examination will reveal normal-appearing vocal folds in the face of dramatic voice manifestations.

24. How do you differentiate vocal cord polyps, nodules, cysts, and contact granulomas?

Polyps are asymmetrical and appear soft and smooth. Polyps may occur on one or both vocal folds. In contrast, **vocal nodules** are easily identified because they are usually paired. Nodules are small and discrete and are usually located in the middle of the membranous vocal fold, often at the junction of the anterior one-third of the cord with the posterior two-thirds. **Contact gran-**

ulomas are not actually found on the vocal fold itself. Contact granulomas are found on the vocal processes of the arytenoid cartilage. **Vocal fold cysts** are mucous retention or epidermoid cysts located in the superficial layer of lamina propria, usually at the middle third of the vocal fold in the medial and superior aspect. A vocal fold cyst requires surgical excision.

CONTROVERSIES

25. What are the treatment options for vocal fold nodules?
Vocal fold nodules often arise as a result of excessive laryngeal use. Voice therapy is a highly effective method of treatment. In rare cases in which voice therapy does not give satisfactory results, surgical removal of nodules may improve the voice. Generally, surgery will not resolve the hoarseness completely, and it is rarely indicated, since vocal coaching is usually curative.

26. How is a laryngeal polyp treated?
A laryngeal polyp is a single benign lesion of the larynx. Voice therapy is recommended prior to and after surgery and could be the only required treatment. Laryngeal polyps can be removed with a standard cold knife, which is preferable, or with CO_2 laser. Microflap technique is used to preserve the mucosal cover and underlying vocal ligament when possible. Normal voice usually returns after treatment.

27. How are laryngeal papillomas treated?
Laryngeal papillomas are recurrent benign lesions caused by infection with human papilloma virus types 6 and 11. They tend to recur despite surgery because the virus remains in the cord tissue. Multiple surgical resection, often with a laser, is required. Normal baseline voice does not usually return. Adjuvant medical treatments using cidofovir (intraoperative injections), indole 3-carbinol/diindolymethane, acyclovir, and alpha-interferon are under investigation.

BIBLIOGRAPHY

1. Banfield G, Tandon P, Solomons N: Hoarse voice: An early symptom of many conditions. Practitioner 244:267–271, 2000.
2. Berke GS, Kevorkian KF: The diagnosis and management of hoarseness. Compr Ther 22:251–255, 1996.
3. Garrett CG, Ossoff RH: Hoarseness. Med Clin North Am 83:115–23,1999.
4. Green G, Bayman N, Smith R: Pathogenesis and treatment of juvenile onset recurrent respiratory papillomatosis. Otolaryngol Clin North Am 33:187–207, 2000.
5. Gumpert L, Kalach N, Dupont C, Contencin P: Hoarseness and gastroesophageal reflux in children. J Laryngol Otol 112:49–54,1998.
6. Hanson DG, Jiang JJ: Diagnosis and management of chronic laryngitis associated with reflux. Am J Med 108 (Suppl 4a):112S–119S, 2000.
7. McMurray JS: Medical and surgical treatment of pediatric dysphonia. Otolaryngol Clin North Am 33:1111–1126, 2000.
8. Mishra S, Rosen CA, Murry T: Acute management of the performing voice. Otolaryngol Clin North Am 33:957–966, 2000.
9. Nostrant TT: Gastroesophageal reflux and laryngitis: A skeptic's view. Am J Med 108 (Suppl 4a):149S–152S, 2000.
10. Ormseth EJ, Wong RK: Reflux laryngitis: Pathophysiology, diagnosis, and management. Am J Gastroenterol 94:2812–2817, 1999.
11. Rosen CA, Anderson D, Murry T: Evaluating hoarseness: Keeping your patient's voice healthy. Am Fam Physician 57:2775–2782, 1998.
12. Rosen CA: Phonosurgical vocal fold injection: Procedures and materials. Otolaryngol Clin North Am 33:1087–1096, 2000.
13. Rosen CA, Murry T: Nomenclature of voice disorders and vocal pathology. Otolaryngol Clin North Am 33:1035–1046, 2000.
14. Rubin J, Sataloff R, Korovin G, Gould W: Diagnosis and Treatment of Voice Disorders. Tokyo, Igaku-Shoin, 1995.
15. Sataloff RT: Evaluation of professional singers. Otolaryngol Clin North Am 33:923–956, 2000.
16. Zeitels SM: Phonomicrosurgery I: Principles and equipment. Otolaryngol Clin North Am 33:1047–1062, 2000.

33. OTOLARYNGOLOGIC MANIFESTATIONS OF HIV

Scottie B. Roofe, M.D., and Daniel W. Watson, M.D.

1. What is the risk of acquiring HIV infection from a blood transfusion?
The risk of receiving HIV-positive blood in the U.S. is estimated to be 1 in 225,000.

2. What is the duration of developments of clinical AIDS following infection with HIV?
The median incubation period between infection with HIV and development of clinical AIDS is approximately 10 years.

3. What is the survival rate after a patient is diagnosed with AIDS?
As of 1995, more than 60% of patients developing AIDS died within 3 years, and 90% within 8 years.

AIDS Indicator Diseases

Infectious diseases	Neoplastic diseases
Pneumocystis carinii pneumonia	Kaposi's sarcoma
Cytomegalovirus retinitis	Primary lymphoma of the brain
Esophageal candidiasis	Non-Hodgkin's lymphoma of B-cell or
Cryptococcosis, extrapulmonary	unknown immunologic phenotype if small
Cryptosporidiosis with diarrhea persisting > 1 mo	noncleaved or immunoblastic sarcoma
Coccidioidomycosis, disseminated	
Toxoplasmosis of the brain	**Others**
Disseminated histoplasmosis	HIV encephalopathy (AIDS dementia)
Disseminated mycobacterial disease (other than	HIV wasting syndrome
by *M. tuberculosis*)	CD4 count <200
Extrapulmonary disease caused by *M. tuberculosis*	
Recurrent nontyphoid *Salmonella*	
Isosporiasis with diarrhea persisting > 1 mo	

From Tami T, Lee K: AIDS and the otolaryngologist. SIPAC from AAOHNS, 1993, p 23, with permission.

4. Name the most common viral opportunistic pathogen seen with HIV infection.
Cytomegalovirus (CMV). Infection can lead to chorioretinitis, pneumonia, esophagitis, colitis, encephalitis, and hepatitis.

5. An AIDS patient with the complaint of dysphagia is noted to have a white lesion involving the supraglottis and piriform sinus. A biopsy reveals gram-positive organisms, foamy macrophages, and sulfur granules. What is the diagnosis?
Actinomycosis. Although unusual in the larynx, actinomycosis should be included in the differential diagnosis of laryngeal lesions in patients with AIDS because they are at risk for opportunistic infections. The tissue in actinomycosis is necrotic and contains colonies of micro-organisms called "sulfur granules." The treatment course is prolonged, with 4–6 weeks of intravenous penicillin, followed by oral therapy for at least 6 months.
Tetracycline may be used in those patients allergic to penicillin.

6. A known HIV-positive patient presents with severe mucosal ulceration of his oral cavity. A mucosal smear (Tzanck prep) reveals altered epithelial cells. What is the most likely etiology?
The most likely etiology is **herpes simplex virus** (HSV). The herpetic infection in immunocompromised patients differs from typical HSV in that the former occurs anywhere in the oral cavity, is more extensive, and does not resolve without treatment with antiviral therapy, such as acyclovir.

7. Name the most common oral neoplasm in patients with AIDS.

Kaposi's sarcoma is by far the most common oral lesion affecting patients with AIDS. It is more common in homosexual and bisexual patients than in those patients who contract HIV from other sources. The palate is the site of involvement in greater than 95% of oral cavity Kaposi's. Kaposi's lesions have been treated surgically, with low-dose radiation therapy, laser, photodynamic therapy, intralesional vinca alkyloids, and alpha interferon.

8. An intravenous drug user presents with multiple translucent papules on his face and neck. What is the most likely diagnosis?

The most likely diagnosis is **molluscum contagiosum,** a disease related to poxvirus infection that occurs in up to 13% of the AIDS population. In non-immunosuppressed patients, the disease is usually confined to the groin. However, it may occur anywhere in the HIV-immunosuppressed patient and may present as translucent, centrally umbilicated papules over the face, neck, scalp, and eyelids. The lesions usually measure 2 to 5 mm, but may grow to 1–2 cm in diameter in some cases. Microscopically, numerous intracytoplasmic inclusion bodies are seen involving the lower epidermis.

Unlike in the immunocompetent individual in whom the disease usually resolves spontaneously, the disease in AIDS patients follows a chronic relapsing course. Treatment includes surgical excision, curettage, or cryotherapy.

These lesions must be distinguished from **bacilliary epitheliod angiomatosis,** a papular eruption similar in appearance to molluscum, but thought to be infected with Gram-negative coccobacilli. Treatment of bacilliary epitheliod angiomatosis is with erythromycin.

9. Otoscopic examination of a young female patient with AIDS with the complaint of decreased hearing reveals a polypoid mass in the external auditory canal. Biopsy of the mass reveals multiple cystic organisms in granulomatous background. This polyp is most likely related to infection with what opportunistic organism?

Pneumocystis carinii is the causative organism. Polyps in the external auditory canal in AIDS patients may be manifestations of both *P. carinii* and tuberculous infections. *Pneumocystis* may also present as a cyst under the skin of the external auditory canal and gradually enlarge until the canal is occluded. Patients may present with hearing loss, otalgia, otorrhea, tinnitus, and a polypoid mass visible in the external auditory canal. Microscopically, clear, oval cysts of *P. carinii* are present within confluent necrotic granulomas and can be identified by Gomori methanamine silver stain. Patients with extrapulmonary manifestations of pneumocystis infection usually have no evidence of active pulmonary disease.

10. What are the most common organisms causing acute otitis media in the pediatric HIV-infected patient?

Acute otitis media is much more common in the pediatric HIV-infected patient than those not infected with HIV. The most common organisms encountered in acute otitis media in these patients, however, do not differ from the general population. *Streptococcus pneumoniae, Haemophilus influenzae,* and *Moraxella catarrhalis* are most common.

Treatment is usually different from that of immunocompetent individuals and usually involves antibiotics to cover these organisms. Tympanocentesis may help in identifying pathogens in those patients refractory to broad-spectrum antibiotics.

11. Why is allergic rhinitis more common in HIV-infected patients?

Allergic rhinitis is two times more common in HIV-positive patients. Although there is a decline in the number of T helper cells and total number of lymphocytes, there is a polyclonal B cell activation and an increased production of all classes of antibodies, including IgE. The increase in IgE production has been associated with an increase in atopic symptoms, including allergic rhinitis. Symptoms are usually controlled with topical nasal steroids and antihistamines.

12. A 40-year-old male recently diagnosed with HIV infection presents for evaluation of an essentially asymptomatic lesion, which is white, irregular, and corrugated, on the lateral border of his tongue. What is the most likely diagnosis?

Hairy leukoplakia is a lesion of the HIV-positive patient that is located almost exclusively on the lateral tongue and has a fairly typical appearance as a white, raised, irregular lesion with vertical corrugations. Its diagnosis is made almost exclusively on appearance. Histologically, marked parakeratosis and epithelial hyperplasia are present, with little inflammation of the underlying connective tissue. Epstein-Barr virus has been associated.

The lesions tend to wax and wane and generally require no treatment; however, some studies have shown that their presence heralds the progression to full-blown AIDS. In studies, the probability of AIDS developing with the onset of hairy leukoplakia is 48% in 16 months and 83% in 31 months. Lesions may respond to therapy with acyclovir, zidovudine, or podophyllum resin.

13. A 25-year-old female patient with AIDS presents with a slowly enlarging, soft, and rubbery mass on the left side of her neck. A fine needle aspiration biopsy reveals evidence of intracellular acid-fast bacilli in macrophages. What is your diagnosis?

The most likely diagnosis is **tuberculous lymphadenitis** (scrofula). The lymph nodes are typically rubbery and soft. A draining sinus may occur in 5% of tuberculous lymph nodes. A purified protein derivative (PPD) skin test with controls may assist in the diagnosis. Histologically, caseating granulomas are seen, with intracellular acid-fast bacilli identified on Ziehl-Nielsen stain. Because it is difficult to histologically differentiate nontuberculous mycobacteria, such as *Mycobacterium scrofulaceum, M. avium-intracellulare,* and *M. kansasii,* from tuberculous strains, definitive diagnosis relies on culture of the specimen.

Empiric therapy with multi-drug coverage should be initiated while awaiting the results of the culture. Multi-drug resistance is becoming more and more common; therefore many investigators recommend that therapy be initiated with a four-drug regimen to include isoniazid, rifampin, pyrazinamide, and ethambutol or streptomycin. Therapy for atypical mycobacterial includes clarithromycin or azithromycin with ethambutol and/or rifabutin.

Note that atypical mycobacterial sites of infection include the larynx and the ear.

14. An HIV-positive male with recent onset of oral Candidiasis presents with retrosternal pain and dysphagia. Barium swallow reveals a "cobblestone" appearance. What is the most likely etiology?

Esophageal candidiasis is the most likely etiology. It presents with retrosternal pain and dysphagia, or occasionally is asymptomatic. Barium swallow or esophagoscopy makes the diagnosis. A classic **cobblestone appearance** is seen on the barium swallow, and white plaques with ulcerations are seen on endoscopy. Symptoms should resolve with aggressive antifungal therapy, but if they persist, biopsy should be performed to rule out other etiologies such as Kaposi's sarcoma or cytomegalovirus esophagitis.

15. Describe the recommended treatment for Kaposi's sarcoma (KS).

The treatment for KS is often multimodal and is recommended for symptomatic relief. Primary treatment may include radiation therapy, usually at low levels. Surgical excision, photodynamic therapy, laser excision, topical tretinoin gel, intralesional injection of vinblastine, and cryotherapy may be considered. In addition, single-agent or combination systemic chemotherapy or immunomodulation with interferon alpha may be beneficial.

16. A 14-year-old female patient with AIDS complains of nasal obstruction, worsening headache, and black nasal discharge. A coronal CT scan of her sinuses reveals bony erosion in the lateral nasal wall and inferior orbit. What should be the most concerning infectious etiology in your differential diagnosis?

Fungal sinusitis should be at the top of your list. Immunocompromised patients have increased potential for development of invasive fungal sinusitis. Clinically, the patient may appear toxic and complain of severe pain. Headache may indicate intracranial or skull base involvement. Diagnostic nasal endoscopy demonstrates friable erythematous mucosa, or the mucosa may appear dark and necrotic from intravascular invasion of the organism, essentially depriving the tissue of its vascular supply. Several pathogens such as *Aspergillus fumigatus* and *Rhizopus* may cause invasive infections.

Management includes urgent and aggressive surgical debridement as well as intravenous anti-fungal agents such as amphotericin-B. A high mortality and morbidity rate is characteristic of invasive fungal sinusitis.

17. A 10-year-old male with AIDS has a complaint of left-sided facial pain and nasal discharge. This unilateral nasal obstruction is treated for maxillary sinusitis with broad-spectrum antibiotics. A subsequent CT scan of the sinuses reveals a large, left intranasal mass occluding the left ostiomeatal complex. After biopsy, the pathologist tells you that the tissue has a characteristic "starry-sky" appearance. What is your diagnosis?

The patient has a **Burkitt's lymphoma.** The non-Hodgkin's lymphomas are the most frequent malignancy in children with immunosuppression from HIV. Most children with lymphomas with AIDS present with fever and weight loss and typically demonstrate extranodal manifestations. They may present with disease in a variety of sites, including the nasal cavity, paranasal sinuses, and nasopharynx. These lesions frequently cause nasal obstruction or symptoms of sinusitis such as unilateral nasal drainage, headaches, or facial pain. The majority of these lymphomas are high-grade malignancies of B-cell origin andmay be of Burkitt's (small noncleaved) or immunoblastic origin.

The Burkitt's lymphoma **starry-sky appearance** is so-named because of its diffuse growth pattern characterized by the presence of many macrophages containing phagocytized and cellular debris interspersed in a small cell infiltrate.

Treatment is per standard chemotherapy protocols.

18. A 24 year-old male with a history of progressive nasal obstruction despite treatment with topical nasal steroids and antihistamines presents to you for evaluation. A fiberoptic exam reveals a markedly enlarged adenoid pad. Should you be concerned?

Considering the title of this chapter, the answer is yes. Nasal obstruction and congestion are caused by a wide variety of disorders and often occur in HIV-positive patients. Adenoid hypertrophy is a common cause. The presence of an enlarged adenoid pad in an otherwise asymptomatic patient is suspicious for HIV. It is thought that Epstein-Barr virus or cytomegalovirus causes proliferation of B cells in lymphoid tissue in HIV-positive patients; thus, hypertrophy of Waldeyer's ring. The usual presenting symptoms are nasal obstruction and recurrent serous otitis media secondary to eustachian tube obstruction.

19. What is Ramsay Hunt Syndrome?

Ramsay Hunt sydrome, or **herpes zoster oticus,** is a vesicular eruption of the ear and face with ipsilateral facial paralysis. It is thought to be caused by reactivation of a latent varicella-zoster virus. Patients may have intense otalgia, vesicular eruptions, sensorineural hearing loss, tinnitus, and vertigo. Herpes zoster infections have been reported in up to 16% of AIDS patients.

20. HIV-infected patients often present with acute and chronic sinus problems. What are the indications to perform sinus lavage in an HIV patient with sinusistis?
- Failure to respond to initial medical therapy
- Complication of sinusitis
- Severe systemic toxicity from sinusitis

These are not absolute indications, but merely guidelines. As AIDS patients become more immunocompromised, unusual pathogens are seen in sinusitis, including *Legionella, Alternaria, Cryptococcus, Candida,* and *Acanthamoeba.*

21. An AIDS patient presents with tender, bleeding gums and erythema at the gumline. Explain the concerns you might have with this presentation.

HIV-associated periodontitis and gingivitis are much more severe in the immunocompromised patient. The process of HIV gingivitis, HIV periodontitis, acute necrotizing ulcerative gingivitis (ANUG), and necrotizing stomatitis represent a continuum of disease from moderate to severe. In ANUG the gingiva appear red and swollen, then subsequently undergo necrosis, turning yellow-gray. There is often significant destruction of periodontal soft tissue.

22. An HIV-infected patient presents with asymptomatic, bilateral parotid swelling of 3- to 4-month duration. A CT scan shows bilateral cystic lesions within the parotid. What is your diagnosis?

Salivary gland disease is not uncommon in HIV patients. In particular, lymphoepithelial cysts are fairly common, usually involving the tail of the parotid. The cysts are often bilateral, multiloculated, and contained within the parotid fascia. The etiology is unknown, although these lesions exhibit reactive lymphocytes which infiltrate parotid tissue. Salivary flow is usually preserved, and amylase is normal.

Other diagnoses to consider include **parotid neoplasms** such as Kaposi's sarcoma and non-Hodgkin's lymphoma.

23. How should benign lymphoepithelial cysts be managed?

Some advocate parotidectomy with facial nerve dissection, while others advocate needle aspiration. Recurrence is common. Therapeutic attempts have included intralesional tetracycline or doxycycline sclerosis, or low-dose radiation therapy.

24. You are performing a procedure on an HIV patient and experience a needle stick with a 21-gauge hollow-bore needle. What do you do?

It is important that you have a protocol for dealing with needle sticks. Most institutions have their own guidelines, but in general these are the steps recommended:
   1. Wash the wound (data is lacking regarding the efficacy of antiseptics while washing).
   2. Assess the type of exposure (1 in 200–300 needle sticks from an infected source will transmit HIV).
   3. Consider starting post-exposure prophylaxis (PEP).
   4. If PEP is warranted, start within 1–2 hours of exposure.
   5. If the patient's ELISA is negative, then it is reasonable to stop PEP.
   6. Get retested at 3–4 weeks post-exposure, then at 3 months, and 6 months.
   7. PEP is usually given for 4 weeks with monitoring of side effects.
   8. Basic regimen: zidovudine 300 mg with lamivudine 150 mg po BID
NOTE: All drugs and drug doses should be verified prior to administering for PEP.

BIBLIOGRAPHY

 1. Cock KM, Weiss HA: The global epidemiology of HIV/AIDS. Trop Med Int Health 5:A3–9, 2000.
 2. Colebunders R, Verdonck K, Nachega J: Impact of new developments in antiretroviral treatment on AIDS prevention and care in resource-poor countries. AIDS Pt Care STDS 14:251–257, 2000.
 3. Dezube BJ: Acquired immunodeficiency syndrome-related Kaposi's sarcoma: Clinical features, staging, and treatment. Semin Oncol 27:424–430, 2000.
 4. Donovan B, Ross MW: Preventing HIV: Determinants of sexual behavior. Lancet 355:1897–1901, 2000.
 5. Goedert JJ: The epidemiology of acquired immunodeficiency syndrome malignancies. Semin Oncol 27:390–401, 2000.
 6. Gotch F, Rutebemberwa A, Jones G, et al: Vaccines for the control of HIV/AIDS. Trop Med Int Health 5:A16–21, 2000.
 7. Gourevitch MN: The epidemiology of HIV and AIDS. Current trends. Med Clin North Am 80(6):1223–1238, 1996.
 8. Hunt SM, Miyamoto RC, Cornelius RS, et al: Invasive fungal sinusitis in the acquired immunodeficiency syndrome. Otolaryngol Clin North Am 33:335–347, 2000.

9. Keithley JK, Swanson B, Murphy M, et al: HIV/AIDS and nutrition: Implications for disease management. Nurs Case Mgt 5:52–59; quiz 60–62, 2000.
10. Miller RF: Prophylaxis of *Pneumocystis carinii* pneumonia: Too much of a good thing? Thorax 55(Suppl 1):S15–22, 2000.
11. Moazzez AH: Head and neck/AIDS. Am Fam Physician 57:1814–1822, 1998.
12. Nicoll A, Killewo J: Science, sense, and nonsense about HIV in Africa. Commum Dis Pub Health 3:78–79, 2000.
13. Ozsoy M, Ernst E: How effective are complementary therapies for HIV and AIDS? A systematic review. Int J STD AIDS 10:629–635, 1999.
14. Orgain JC: HIV/AIDS: A global epidemic. J Natl Med Assn 92:313–314, 2000.
15. Phelan JA: Oral manifestations of human immunodeficiency virus infection. Med Clin North Am 81(2):511–531, 1997.
16. Reisacher WR: Manifestations of AIDS in the head and neck. South Med J 92:684–697, 1999.
17. Rose MA, Clark-Alexander B: Coping styles of caregivers of children with HIV/AIDS: Implications for health professionals. AIDS Pt Care STDS 13:335–342, 1999.
18. Ruprecht RM, Hofmann-Lehmann R, Rasmussen RA, et al: 1999: a time to re-evaluate AIDS vaccine strategies. J Human Virol 3:88–93, 2000.
19. Schiff NF: Kaposi's sarcoma of the larynx. Ann Otol Rhinol Laryngol 106(7 Pt 1):563–567, 1999.
20. Tami TA: Laryngeal pathology in the acquired immunodeficiency syndrome: Diagnostic and therapeutic dilemmas. Ann Otol Rhinol Laryngol 108(2):214–220, 1999.
21. Truitt TO, Tami TA: Otolaryngologic manifestations of human immunodeficiency virus infection. Med Clin North Am 83(1):303–315, 1999.
22. Wistuba II, Behrens C, Gazdar AF: Pathogenesis of non-AIDS-defining cancers: A review. AIDS Pat Care STDS 13:415–426, 1999.

34. ANTIMICROBIAL THERAPY IN OTOLARYNGOLOGY

Jay H. Lee, M.D. and Bruce W. Jafek, M.D., FACS, FRSM

1. What factors need to be considered when choosing an antibiotic?

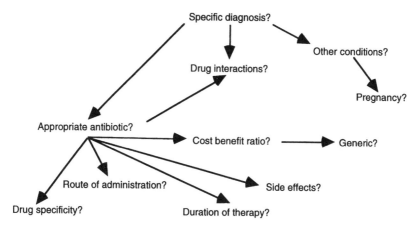

- Specific diagnosis—antibiotics may be administered for a proven infection, suspected infection, or prophylaxis against a possible infection. Clinical presentation and Gram stain may help guide the clinician with specific antibiotic therapy.
- Antibiotic specificity—may be determined with laboratory testing. Always consider local bacterial resistance patterns and ask whether penetration into specific anatomical compartments (e.g., central nervous system) is necessary.
- Route of administration—depends on type and severity of infection
- Duration of therapy—depends on type and severity of infection
- Concurrent medical conditions—including physical ailments, renal/hepatic function, immune status, and pregnancy
- Other medications—possible drug interactions
- Previously identified drug allergy
- Potential side effects—must be discussed with the patient
- Cost—consider generic formulation. But a less expensive medication that is *ineffective* should not be substituted for the more expensive but *effective* treatment.

2. In which situations would you consider the use of more than one antibiotic?

Multiple antibiotic use would provide wider coverage in the setting of a polymicrobial infection. Secondly, some antibiotics cooperate synergistically to increase net bactericidal activity (e.g., penicillin and aminoglycosides), the whole being greater than the sum of its parts. Lastly, multiple-drug therapy would prevent the emergence of resistant strains during a long course of treatment in cases such as tuberculosis.

3. What needs to be considered when treatment appears to have failed?

The physician must consider multiple scenarios in this situation: an incorrect presumptive diagnosis may be made, the targeted organism may not be the true pathogen, an abscess may require surgical drainage, a foreign body may be a nidus for infection, a bacterial superinfection with a resistant organism may emerge, noncompliance by the patient may occur, and, finally, an adverse drug reaction by the antibiotic may cause persistent fever.

4. What is the clinical spectrum of the penicillins? What are their side effects?

Penicillins are β-lactams that inhibit bacterial cell wall synthesis; they are bactericidal and penetrate well into the cerebrospinal fluid (CSF) in the presence of inflammation.

Activities of the Penicillins

ANTIBIOTIC	ACTIVE AGAINST	SIDE EFFECTS
Penicillin V or K	*Streptococcus pyogenes* Most *Streptococcus pneumoniae* Many oral anaerobes	Hypersensitivity: rash (5%), anaphylaxis (1/10,000)

Antistaphylococcals
  Methicillin
  Oxacillin
  Dicloxacillin
	Staphylococcus aureus
	Pneumococcus species
	Streptococcus species
	Many anaerobes
		Hypersensitivity

Aminopenicillins
  Ampicillin
  Amoxicillin
	Many *Haemophilus influenzae*
	Escherichia coli
	Proteus species
	Streptococcus pyogenes
	Most *Streptococcus pneumoniae*
	Most anaerobes
		Hypersensitivity

Augmented penicillins (with
  β-lactamase inhibitor)
  Amoxicillin/clavulanate
  Ampicillin/sulbactam
	Haemophilus influenzae
	Moraxella catarrhalis
	Staphylococcus aureus
	Most *Streptococcus pneumoniae*
	Most anaerobes
		Hypersensitivity

Antipseudomonals
  Ticarcillin
  Carbenicillin
  Piperacillin
	Pseudomonas aeruginosa
	Most gram-negatives
		Hypersensitivity

Adapted from Fairbanks DNF: Antimicrobial therapy in otolaryngology–head and neck surgery. In Lee KJ (ed): Essential Otolaryngology–Head and Neck Surgery. Norwalk, CT, Appleton & Lange, 1995, pp 427–436.

5. How are cephalosporins categorized? What is their clinical spectrum?

The cephalosporins belong to the same family of β-lactams as penicillins and thus their mechanism of action is similar to that of the penicillins. They are categorized into first-, second-, and third-generation agents. The first-generation agents are most active against gram-positive cocci: *Staphylococcus aureus,* streptococci, and most pneumococci. They are also active against a few gram-negative organisms. The second-generation agents are active against the gram-positive cocci but also against *Haemophilus influenzae* and *Moraxella catarrhalis.* The third-generation agents are more active against gram-negative bacteria, including *H. influenzae, M. catarrhalis,* and *Neisseria gonorrhoeae.* In addition, the third-generation cephalosporin, ceftazidine, is highly active against *Pseudomonas aeruginosa.* More recently, a fourth-generation cephalosporin, cefepime, provides one of the broadest antibiotic coverages and is typically used for nosocomially acquired mixed infections.

6. Should cephalosporins be avoided in the penicillin-hypersensitive patient?

Since cephalosporins have a similar structure to the penicillins, a patient with a history of penicillin anaphylaxis should avoid cephalosporins. However, cephalosporins can be used safely in patients with a history of penicillin rashes.

7. What other β-lactam antibiotics may be used for head and neck infections?

Imipenem and aztreonam; these antibiotics are administered parenterally and are widely bactericidal. **Imipenem** exerts the broadest spectrum of activity of any antimicrobial agent which includes *S. aureus, Streptococcus pyogenes, Streptococcus pneumoniae, N. gonorrhoeae*, and most gram-negative bacteria and anaerobes. Penicillin-allergic patients may also be hypersensitive to imipenem. **Aztreonam** is effective in penicillin-hypersensitive patients against aerobic gram-negative pathogens.

8. What are the macrolides? What is their clinical spectrum?

The macrolides inhibit the 50S subunit of bacterial ribosomes. They are bacteriostatic agents that are used for respiratory tract infections. They include erythromycin, azithromycin, and clarithromycin. Erythromycin is active against most streptococci, *S. aureus, H. influenzae* (with a sulfonamide), *Mycoplasma, Legionella, Chlamydia, Corynebacterium diphtheriae, Bordetella pertussis*, and *Clostridium tetani* (tetanus). Side effects include nausea, cramps, vomiting, and reversible jaundice. Azithromycin and clarithromycin have similar activity except that they are active against *Haemophilus* species as a single agent. In addition, they cause less nausea, and clarithromycin can be taken with meals. One should be cautious when prescribing erythromycin or clarithromycin to patients taking theophylline; both are hepatically metabolized and could cause higher (toxic) serum concentrations of theopylline.

9. What is the clinical spectrum of clindamycin? What are its side effects?

Clindamycin also inhibits the 50S subunit; it is a bacteriostatic agent that concentrates in bone. It is highly effective against anaerobic infections of the aerodigestive tract, including *Bacteroides fragilis*. It is also effective against *S. aureus* (including methicillin-resistant strains), *S. pyogenes*, and penicillin-resistant strains of *S. pneumoniae*. Its side effects include nausea, cramps, and diarrhea. In addition, it can cause pseudomembranous colitis due to overgrowth of *Clostridium difficile*.

10. What are the limitations of the tetracyclines? When should they be used?

The tetracyclines are inexpensive bacteriostastic agents to which most streptococcal, staphylococcal, and *H. influenzae* infections have become resistant. They are effective against *Mycoplasma, Chlamydia*, and *Legionella* infections. They should only be used in respiratory infections when they are proven sensitive by culture. Side effects include the staining of enamel, and they should thus be avoided in children under age 10 and in pregnant women. As a teratogen, it may also cause fetal growth inhibition and congenital limb abnormalities.

11. When should chloramphenicol be used for head and neck infections?

Chloramphenicol binds irreversibly to the 50S subunit to prevent protein synthesis. It has broad-spectrum activity against all gram-positive cocci and most gram-negative bacteria. However, *Pseudomonas* is resistant. Chloramphenicol penetrates the CSF more effectively than any other antibiotic. Because of potentially fatal bone marrow suppression (1 of 24,000 patients), it should be used only in life-threatening infections when other effective agents are unavailable.

12. Which oral agents are available for treatment of pseudomonal infections of the head and neck?

The only agents available for the treatment of head and neck infections by *Pseudomonas* are the fluoroquinolones including ciprofloxacin, ofloxacin, and levofloxacin. The quinolones bind the bacterial DNA gyrase to prevent replication. These antibiotics are bactericidal and also active against *H. influenzae, M. catarrhalis*, and *N. gonorrhoeae* and many gram-positive organisms. However, the quinolones should be reserved primarily for pseudomonal infections, and they should not be used as a first-line antibiotic in common respiratory and pharyngeal infections. There are already resistant strains of pneumococci, streptococci, and staphylococci because of its abundant use. Interestingly, structural alterations of DNA gyrase and changes in the membrane porins responsible for drug transport to the quinolones have contributed to recent resistance.

13. How should the aminoglycosides be administered? What is their clinical spectrum?

The aminoglycosides are not effective orally and are thus available only for parenteral use. They are effective against hospital-acquired infections including *Escherichia coli, Serratia, Kleb-*

siella, Proteus, and *Enterobacter.* When combined with β-lactam agents, they are particularly effective against *Pseudomonas.* Anaerobic infections are almost universally resistant to the aminoglycosides. Side effects include oto- and nephrotoxicity.

14. In addition to β-lactams and clindamycin, which agent has activity against anaerobes?
Metronidazole is highly active against protozoa and anaerobic infections including *B. fragilis* and *C. difficile.* It penetrates the CSF well. However, metronidazole is inactive against all aerobic infections. When this drug is administered, alcohol must be avoided because of metronidazole's antabuse-like effect. It is the antibiotic of choice for the treatment of *C. difficile*–associated pseudomembranous enterocolitis.

15. What agent is most commonly used for methicillin-resistant strains of *Staphylococcus aureus (MRSA)*?
Vancomycin is unrelated to other antimicrobial groups, but, similar to the penicillins, it inhibits cell wall synthesis. It is often used for treatment of infections caused by MRSA. It is also active against the streptococci. Vancomycin is only available in parenteral form, but when it is given orally, it is active against pseudomembranous colitis from *C. difficile.* Vancomycin should be reserved only for serious infections, since it is still effective against strains that already have acquired resistance to other antibiotics. Side effects include oto- and nephrotoxicity.

16. How should a carrier of a nasopharyngeal infection be treated?
Rifampin is useful for prophylaxis and treatment of patients who carry *H. influenzae* and meningococcus. When combined with other antistaphylococcal agents, it is useful against resistant *S. aureus.* It is also active against streptococci, *Legionella,* and anaerobes. Side effects include hepatic and renal dysfunction.

17. When are sulfonamides effective for the treatment of bacterial infections?
Sulfonamides inhibit bacterial growth (bacteriostatic) by disrupting the metabolism of folinic acid. When sulfonamides are used in combination with trimethoprim, it can be a powerful agent in the treatment of infections caused by *H. influenzae, M. catarrhalis,* and some streptococci. It is unaffected by β-lactamase and is appropriate for chronic bronchitis, sinusitis, and otitis media. It has not been effective against anaerobes. Side effects include rash/photosensitivity, erythema multiforme (Stevens-Johnson syndrome), and aplastic anemia.

18. Which agents should be used to treat acute and chronic otitis media?
The first-line antibiotic for treating acute otitis media is often amoxicillin. Of the most common pathogens implicated in this infection, amoxicillin effectively treats *S. pneumoniae,* but 20% of *H. influenzae* strains and 80% of *M. catarrhalis* strains are resistant. These pathogens are covered by the inexpensive trimethoprim-sulfamethoxazole preparations, but pneumococcal coverage is less effective. Although more expensive, erythromycin plus sulfonamide, amoxicillin plus clavulanic acid, cefixime, and cefuroxime combat all of these organisms. These should be considered second-line antibiotics.
Chronic otitis media with effusion usually harbors the same pathogens as the acute form and is treated with the same agents.

19. How does the treatment of sinusitis differ from that of otitis media?
Acute sinusitis is caused by the same organisms that cause otitis media, and drug choices are similar. Intracranial and orbital complications of acute sinusitis require agents that penetrate the blood-brain barrier, which include ceftriaxone, cefuroxime, ampicillin plus chloramphenicol, and vancomycin plus aztreonam. Chronic sinusitis is caused by anaerobic organisms and often *S. aureus.* Effective agents include amoxicillin plus clavulanic acid, clindamycin, cephalexin, and dicloxacillin. Fungal infections should be treated with ketoconazole. Pseudomonal infections are often associated with extensive nasal polyposis and are treated with ciprofloxacin.

20. Which agents are useful for treating tonsillitis?

Bacterial tonsillitis is most often caused by *S. pyogenes*. However, a number of anaerobic organisms may also be present in a mixed infection. Penicillin is often ineffective because of the production of β-lactamase by these organisms. Second-line alternatives include clindamycin, amoxicillin plus clavulanic acid, dicloxacillin, and cephalexin. If the infection is mononucleosis, the amoxicillin will cause a severe rash in 50% of cases. Culture may be indicated, either to rule out *Streptococcus* or to determine the causative organism in difficult cases.

21. When should pharyngitis be treated with antibiotics? Which antibiotic should be used?

Antibiotics should be given to the sore throat patient when bacterial infection is suspected, such as with *S. pyogenes* (group A β-hemolytic), *Mycoplasma, Chlamydia,* and gonococcus. Bacterial infection is favored when there is a history of contact with a bacterially infected individual, prolonged or severe sore throat, severe erythema or exudate, and lymphadenopathy. Penicillin's effectiveness is limited by β-lactamase-producing bacterial strains but may be administered. Effective alternatives include a macrolide or cephalexin.

22. When should antibiotic therapy be administered to the patient with epiglottitis? Which antibiotic?

Airway management takes priority in these patients. Antibiotics should be administered once the airway is secured. *H. influenzae* (type B) is often implicated in this infection. Antibiotics should be administered parenterally and may include ampicillin plus sulbactam, ampicillin plus chloramphenicol, or a second- or third-generation cephalosporin such as ceftriaxone.

23. When should croup be treated with antibiotics?

Croup is usually caused by a virus but may become secondarily infected with *S. aureus* or *H. influenzae*. Antibiotics should be administered when thick yellow secretions are encountered. The same antibiotics that are used to treat epiglottitis may be used for secondary infections initiated by croup.

24. Should laryngitis be treated with antibiotics?

Laryngitis is usually a viral infection that resolves with a few days of voice rest. Antibiotics may be necessary if the viral infection becomes secondarily infected with bacteria such as *Mycoplasma, Chlamydia,* and *H. influenzae*. Prolonged hoarseness suggests such a secondary infection and is effectively covered with erythromycin plus sulfonamide or amoxicillin plus clavulanic acid.

25. Which organisms predominate in deep neck abscesses? How should they be covered?

Deep neck abscesses and chronic intracranial infections spreading from the ears or sinuses are usually caused by mixed bacteria with a predominance of anaerobes. Clindamycin is a good antibiotic choice, covering anaerobic organisms and all cocci. If a pseudomonal infection is suspected, a quinolone should be added. If central nervous system (CNS) penetration is required, nafcillin plus metronidazole should be utilized.

26. What agents should be used when treating mastoiditis?

Acute mastoiditis with a subperiosteal abscess is usually caused by the same organisms that cause acute otitis media, and therefore antibiotic choices are similar. Ceftriaxone is a good initial choice, because the pneumococci and *H. influenzae* may extend intracranially. Chronic suppurative otomastoiditis requires additional coverage for *S. aureus, Proteus* species, anaerobes, and possibly *Pseudomonas*.

27. What therapy is necessary for acute otitis externa?

Combination topical antibiotic therapy is necessary for the draining ear of acute otitis externa. Pseudomonal infections are covered by polymyxin, and *S. aureus, Proteus* species, and others are covered by neomycin. Cortisporin includes both of these preparations. Lastly, boric and acetic acid suspensions have been found to be helpful in these infections.

28. What are the polyenes? When are they used by otolaryngologists?

The polyenes are antifungal agents and include nystatin and amphotericin B. Nystatin is available only in topical and oral preparations and is useful only for oral candidiasis. It is not absorbed systemically. An oral suspension is swished around in the mouth and swallowed. Amphotericin B binds to fungal cell walls, causing leakage and cell death. It is also poorly absorbed from the gastrointestinal tract and is thus limited to intravenous use. Lower doses that are administered for 1 to 2 weeks are used to treat esophageal candidiasis. High doses are required for treating documented infections due to *Aspergillus* species or zygomycosis. Therapy duration is determined by total cumulative dose, which should be 2–3 g. Side effects of amphotericin B include fever, rigors, hypotension, and a dose-related reversible nephrotoxicity. A liposomal formulation can be used to provided targeted delivery for renal patients or for those who cannot tolerated the standard formulation.

29. Can any additional agents be used for treating candidiasis?

The azoles, including cotrimazole, ketoconazole, fluconazole, and itraconazole, may be used in candidiasis. In addition, fluconazole may be used when treating histoplasmosis, coccidioidomycosis, cryptococcosis, and paracoccidioidomycosis. Itraconazole is approved for the treatment of pulmonary and extrapulmonary blastomycosis and histoplasmosis.

30. Which antiviral agents are used by the otolaryngologist?

The number of effective antiviral agents is sharply limited. Acyclovir may be used for prophylaxis or treatment of herpes infections. Amantadine is effective against influenza type A and is used primarily for severe infections, especially in the immunocompromised patient. Zidovudine and didanosine are used in patients infected with HIV.

31. What major mechanisms allow antibiotic resistance?

The emergence of antibiotic-resistant bacteria challenges the current concepts of antimicrobial therapy. Two important pathogens to otolaryngologists are MRSA and vancomycin-resistant *Enterococcus faecalis*. The former slowly developed in communities with the rampant use of penicillins, and the latter was borne quickly in hospitals with the indiscriminate use of vancomycin. Four major mechanisms include inactivation of the antibiotic (e.g., β-lactamase), prevention of access of the antibiotic to its target, change in the structure of the antibiotic's target, and active efflux of the antibiotic from the cell.

32. How can we control antibiotic resistance?

Through long experience with resistant strains, many lessons have been learned. These constants reveal that resistance evolves from a low-grade resistance to a high-grade. Secondly, resistant strains tend to be resistant to multiple antibiotics, and, most importantly, resistance is due, ironically, to antibiotic use. Recommended measures to contain the antibiotic resistance are threefold. First, surveillance is crucial; systematic collection of data helps monitor new emerging strains and sensitivity patterns. Secondly, the restraint of antibiotic use is the key. Lastly, simple concepts such as barrier methods and hand washing provide the basis for the prevention of transmission.

CONTROVERSIES

33. When should prophylactic antibiotics be administered to patients undergoing surgery of the head and neck?

This question has received much attention, and an abundance of clinical research has revolved around it. Overall, a decreased wound infection rate has been shown for patients undergoing surgery when appropriate short-term antibiotic prophylaxis has been implemented. Although these findings have not been found to be statistically significant, prophylactic antibiotics should not be withheld for the purpose of minimizing hospital costs. Prophylactic antibiotic therapy has been shown clearly to be of benefit in patients undergoing **clean** (infection rate <5%) operations with a foreign-body implant. This is not as evident for **clean-contaminated** (infection rate <10%) operations, in which the field is sterile initially but a mucosal barrier is crossed or a hollow viscus entered during the operation (e.g., sinonasal surgery or mastoidectomy). The **contaminated** (infection rate >80%) wound results from a major lapse in sterile technique or exposure to acute nonpurulent inflammation. These wounds clearly benefit from the administration of prophylactic antibiotics. The **dirty** wound is the infected traumatic wound that is contaminated with bacteria or environmental debris. "Prophylaxis" in this situation would be a misnomer.

34. What is the appropriate timing for administration of surgical prophylactic antibiotics?

The effective use of prophylactic antibiotics depends on the appropriate timing of their administration. Although most head and neck surgeons agree that prophylactic antibiotics are necessary, many disagree as to the dosing schedule. The current recommendation is that parenteral antibiotics be administered within 30 minutes of the initial incision. If they are given more than 2 hours prior to surgery, levels of the antibiotic in serum and tissues may be low or absent during the procedure. Although some surgeons have advocated continuation of antibiotics for 2 to 5 days after a procedure, a single day of administration is adequate.

35. What determines which antibiotics should be given to the patient who is undergoing head and neck surgery?

The chosen agent should efficacious against the microorganisms likely to cause infectious complications in that particular anatomical site. In addition, safety profile and cost should be considered. For example, parenteral administration of a first-generation cephalosporin is appropriate for clean procedures (e.g., thyroidectomy) in which common infecting organisms include *S. aureus* and *S. epidermidis*. Procedures that frequently involve contamination with anaerobic organisms require appropriate coverage with an antibiotic such as clindamycin.

BIBLIOGRAPHY

1. Blair EA, Johnson JT, Wagner RL, et al: Cost analysis of antibiotic prophylaxis in clean head and neck surgery. Arch Otolaryngol Head Neck Surg 121:269–271, 1995.
2. Erbeedling EJ, Rompalo AM: Current concepts in antibiotic therapy. In Cummings CW (ed): Otolaryngology Head and Neck Surgery, 3rd ed. St. Louis, Mosby, 1998, pp 102–107.
3. Fairbanks DNF: Microbiology, infections, and antibiotic therapy. In Bailey BJ (ed): Head and Neck Surgery—Otolaryngology, 2nd ed. Philadelphia, Lippincott, 1998, pp 72–79.
4. Hessen MT, Kaye D: Principles of selection and use of antibacterial agents. In vitro activity and pharmacology. Infect Dis Clin North Am 14:265–279, 2000.
5. Johnson JT: Principles of antibiotic prophylaxis. In Johnson JT (ed): Infectious Diseases and Antimicrobial Therapy of the Ear, Nose, and Throat. Tokyo, WB Saunders, 1997, pp. 589–592.
6. Kaye KS, Fraimow HS, Abrutyn E: Pathogens resistant to antimicrobial agents: Epidemiology, molecular mechanisms, and clinical management. Infect Dis Clin North Am 14:293–319, 2000.
7. Klein JO: Nonimmune strategies for prevention of otitis media. Pediatr Infect Dis J 19(5 Suppl):S89–92, 2000.
8. Kotra LP, Vakulenko S, Mobashery S: From genes to sequences to antibiotics: prospects for future developments from microbial genomics. Microbes Infect 2:651–658, 2000.
9. Rubinstein E: Antimicrobial resistance—pharmacological solutions. Infection 27 (Suppl 2):S32–34, 1999.
10. Shah S, Rosenfeld R: Antimicrobial therapy in otolaryngology. In Lucente FE (ed): Essentials of Otolaryngology. Buenos Aires, Lippincott, 1999, pp 404–416.
11. Stalam M, Kaye D: Antibiotic agents in the elderly. Infect Dis Clin North Am 14:357–369, 2000.
12. Walsh C: Molecular mechanisms that confer antibacterial drug resistance. Nature 406:775–781, 2000.
13. Witte W, Klare I, Werner G: Selective pressure by antibiotics as feed additives. Infection 27 (Suppl 2):S35–38, 1999.

35. PHARMACOLOGY IN OTOLARYNGOLOGY

Scottie B. Roofe, M.D., Daniel Watson, M.D., and Stephen G. Batuello, M.D.

1. What is the pathophysiology of aminoglycoside-induced ototoxicity?

Aminoglycosides, such as gentamicin, destroy the sensory and supporting cells of the organ of Corti in a systematic manner, beginning with the outer hair cells of the lower turns and progressing toward the apex; thus the audiologic findings of early high-frequency hearing loss. The incidence of ototoxicity varies among the different aminoglycosides, with neomycin among the strongest and netilmicin among the weakest ototoxins. The incidence for gentamicin ototoxicity ranges from 6% to 16% for cochlear and 9% to 15% for vestibular toxicity.

2. Is vancomycin ototoxic?

The predominant ototoxic response of vancomycin appears mainly to affect the cochlea. Tinnitus and high-frequency hearing loss are recognized complications of vancomycin therapy and may be antecedents to complete deafness. The incidence of otoxicity is variable but appears to be related to a cumulative dose rather than the daily dosage. This must be considered when treating patients of advancing age and weight as well as those with renal impairment. The ototoxicity associated with vancomycin is characterized by damage to the auditory receptor cells, initially affecting high-frequency hair cells in the basal turn, then middle- and low-frequency hair cells. As with aminoglycosides, the hair cell degeneration is irreversible. Ototoxicity may be additive with concomitant use of vancomycin with an aminoglycoside. The toxic potential of vancomycin may be less than previously thought, because initial published reports of ototoxicity may represent impurities in the early preparations or use in cases complicated by renal failure.

3. What is the role for omeprazole in reflux laryngitis?

Laryngeal manifestations of gastroesophageal reflux disease (GERD) include hoarseness, dry cough, cervical dysphagia, or globus sensation, as well as structural abnormalities such as vocal cord ulcers, granulomas, laryngitis, and subglottic stenosis. There is some evidence that GERD may play a role in the pathophysiology of laryngeal carcinoma. The pathogenesis is likely related to microaspiration of acid and pepsin. Therefore, antisecretory agents are believed to be effective therapy. Omeprazole acts as a proton-pump inhibitor to markedly reduce the amount of acid produced by the stomach and has been shown to improve symptoms and laryngoscopic findings in patients with laryngeal manifestations of GERD. There are, of course, other antireflux and H_2 blockers that treat GERD, but omeprazole is a model for management.

4. What are the indications for botulinum toxin (Botox) in the otolaryngologist's practice?

Botox has been described for treatment of dystonic and spasmodic disorders of the head and neck such as cervical torticollis, hemifacial spasm, and oromandibular dystonia. Its use has been described extensively for spasmodic dysphonia. In addition, it has been used as an effective treatment for pharyngoesophageal segment hypertonicity or spasm in laryngectomees with poor tracheoesophageal speech. Botox is also used in facial plastic surgery for treatment of cervicofacial rhytids in hyperfunctional areas such as around the eyes and on the forehead.

5. Describe the mechanism of action of botulinum toxin.

Botulinum toxin is produced by the bacterium *Clostridium botulinum*. When injected, it acts to irreversibly block the presynaptic release of acetylcholine, resulting in a localized muscle paralysis.

6. Describe the pharmacologic management of xerostomia.

Xerostomia is defined as a dry mouth related to decrease or lack of saliva. It is often present in patients as a side-effect of medications and in patients with autoimmune diseases such as

Sjögren's syndrome, and it is a very frequent complaint in patients following head and neck irradiation. In addition to nonpharmacologic means of managing xerostomia such as changes in diet plans and food preparations, sialogogues may be used to stimulate residual gland activity. Pilocarpine has been used to stimulate additional secretions by its muscarinic-cholinergic properties. There may be increased efficacy by administering the drug during head and neck irradiation, prior to manifestations of symptoms. The drug is contraindicated in patients with bowel obstruction, asthma, and chronic obstructive pulmonary disease (COPD). Dosages above 20 mg per day are generally avoided because of toxic side effects. Besides sialogogues, various commercial saliva substitutes have been used by some patients, especially during the night or prior to eating. Recently, the selective cytoprotective agent amifostine has shown some promise in the treatment of radiation-induced xerostomia by decreasing free-radical formation in salivary glands.

7. What are some of the advantages of second-generation antihistamines over first-generation drugs?

In contrast to first-generation antihistamines, second-generation agents are lipophobic molecules that do not readily cross the blood-brain barrier. Examples of second-generation agents include fexofenadine, loratidine, cetirizine, and terfenadine (no longer available). These drugs have the advantage of a much lower incidence of patient sedation. Studies have shown that patients who are taking second-generation drugs perform better on tests of reaction time, cognition, attention, and manual dexterity than those taking first-generation agents. Unlike first-generation agents, the second-generation drugs do not appear to potentiate alcohol-induced impairment.

8. When should one consider pharmacologic therapy for the treatment of tinnitus?

Multiple medications have been proposed for use in the treatment of tinnitus, including tocainide, carbamazepine, benzodiazepines, tricyclic antidepressants, gingko, and lidocaine. Tinnitus patients with sleep disturbance and/or major depression probably should be considered for medical therapy. Of the drugs mentioned, only tricyclic antidepressants have currently been found to have a significant advantage over placebo, especially with respect to sleep interference. There are a number of new drugs in various investigational stages.

9. Which drugs are associated with increased serum theophylline levels?

Erythromycin, ciprofloxacin, cimetidine, propranolol, and high-dose allopurinol may significantly raise serum theophylline levels. This relationship is important to remember because of the many asthmatic patients who receive long-term theophylline therapy. Signs and symptoms of theophylline toxicity include nausea, restlessness, ventricular arrythmias, convulsions, and even death. The more serious presentations are not necessarily preceded by the milder symptoms.

10. What is octylcyanoacrylate? What is it used for?

You might wonder why an otolaryngologist would use such a compound, but in fact the cyanoacrylates are fast becoming an area of keen interest. The most popular brand, Ethicon's Dermabond, is currently used for skin closure in lieu of subcuticular monofilament skin closure. Studies have shown that it has roughly the breaking strength of a 5-0 monofilament suture.

Cosmetically, the results have been excellent. There is also interest in and ongoing research on the utility of these substances in the middle ear to stabilize ossicular prostheses.

11. What is rhinitis medicamentosa?

Rhinitis medicamentosa is the medical name for "hooked-on-Afrin-nose." It is a cycle of dependence on over-the-counter nasal decongestant sprays such as Afrin (oxymetazoline). It begins innocently enough; the patient uses the spray to help with breathing, the nose opens up due to vasoconstriction of engorged turbinate erectile tissue, then when the spray wears off, the engorgement returns. With time, the engorgement is less responsive to vasoconstriction and usually worsens, resulting in a boggy and edematous nasal mucosa ("rebound"). The patient uses the spray more often than recommended, until he or she seeks help to end the cycle. Often a short course of oral steroids with a topical nasal steroid will be required to provide relief of symptoms, but the patient must discontinue the Afrin.

12. What drugs are commonly associated with ototoxicity?

Streptomycin	Minocycline
Neomycin	Quinine
Kanamycin	Quinidine
Tobramycin	Salicylates
Amikacin	Cisplatin
Netilmicin	Ethacrynic acid
Vancomycin	Furosemide
Erythromycin	

13. What pharmacologic agents are used to treat Ménière's disease?

Currently a variety of pharmacologic treatment regimens are available for Ménière's disease. Initially, it might respond to antivertiginous drugs such as meclizine or Valium, diuretics, and caffeine restriction. If this is unsuccessful, direct treatment of the labyrinth has been helpful. In general, this therapy centers around some form of treatment with either steroid or gentamicin. Both drugs can be administered intratympanically, through a myringotomy or special tube, to the vicinity of the round window membrane. Various transport mediums have been used to prolong the duration of exposure to the round window membrane, such as impregnating Gelfoam with the drug or mixing the drug with hyaluronic acid.

14. What is the mechanism of action of cromolyn sodium?

Cromolyn sodium indirectly blocks the uptake of calcium by the mast cell, thus preventing degranulation and release of vasomotor substances such as histamine, when the cell is exposed to an allergen. Cromolyn stabilizes the mast cell membrane.

15. Why is it that some sinus and ear infections do not respond to amoxicillin?

The bacteria that cause acute otitis media and sinusitis are nearly identical. The most common organisms in children are *Streptoccus pneumoniae, Haemophilus influenzae, and Moraxella catarrhalis*. Most cases of *H. influenzae* are nontypable rather than *H. influenzae* type B. Of importance, both *H. influenzae* and *M. catarrhalis* may be β-lactamase producers and thus amoxicillin resistant. Resistance varies across the country but in some cases may be greater than 50%. Drugs such as amoxicillin-clavulanate (Augmentin) or drugs that do not rely on the β-lactam ring for efficacy may be useful in these resistant cases. Other reasons for therapeutic failure include penicillin resistance other than β-lactamase and disease of viral origin.

16. Is there any medical therapy available for recalcitrant nasal polyps?

Steroid therapy has long been a standard treatment for difficult-to-treat nasal polyps. Many otolaryngologists will treat with a "burst" of oral steroid followed by a taper. The duration varies. In addition, a nasal steroid will likely provide some relief as well. More recently, the antileukotrienes have been studied to determine their effect on sinonasal polyposis. One study of 26 patients showed 72% subjective improvement with antileukotriene therapy and 50% objective alleviation of sinonasal polyposis. More investigation is underway into this treatment regimen.

17. Should ampicillin be prescribed for otitis media in a patient who regularly takes birth control pills?

Some antibiotics, when given for >10–14 days, interact with oral contraceptives and reduce their effectiveness. Ampicillin, penicillin V, sulfonamides, and tetracyclines have all been shown to have such as effect. Patients should be advised of this increased risk, and other methods of contraception should be employed for at least one cycle after the drug has been discontinued.

18. What is in Cortisporin Otic Suspension?

Cortisporin Otic Suspension or the generic equivalent is a commonly used otologic preparation. You should be familiar with its contents before randomly dispensing it. Cortisporin is made up of neomycin, polymyxin B, and 1% hydrocortisone. The polymyxin has some antifungal property, whereas the neomycin has antibacterial coverage. Neomycin is well known to cause skin irritation when used topically. In patients who complain of redness and itching around the ear canal after use, suspect a neomycin reaction. The hydrocortisone component should help with itching and inflammation; however, in some warmer climates it may enhance fungal growth. Cortisporin comes in a suspension or a solution. The suspension has particulate matter and does not readily penetrate a wick placed in the ear canal. The solution, however, is less likely to cause pain on application.

19. What are the maximum recommended doses of lidocaine, lidocaine with epinephrine, and cocaine?

Lidocaine is an amide that inhibits action potentials by interrupting the flow of sodium ions across cell membranes. *Plain lidocaine* should not be given in excess of 4.5 mg/kg, not to exceed 300 mg.

Lidocaine with epinephrine is more slowly absorbed because of the vasoconstrictive effects of the epinephrine; the maximum dose is 7.0 mg/kg, to a maximum of 500 mg.

Cocaine is an ester used in the head and neck as an anesthetic and a potent vasoconstrictor. It blocks the reuptake of norepinephrine and dobutamine at adrenergic nerve endings. Cocaine is metabolized by plasma and liver cholinesterases. The maximum dose of cocaine is 3 mg/kg or around 200 mg. A standard "bottle" contains 4 mL of 4% cocaine, which is a total of 160 mg per bottle.

20. True or false: Medicinal leeches are still used in otolaryngology.

True! *Hirudo medicinalis* is a medicinal leech approximately 25–40 mm in length. It is sold commercially and used for a variety of plastic and reconstructive procedures, generally when venous outflow needs to be re-established. Medicinal leeches have been around for 2500 years. In addition to drawing off blood (approximately 50 mL of blood "ooze" in 48 hours for one leech), there are vasodilator and anticoagulant properties to leech saliva, which provide the real therapeutic benefits. Information on leeches can be found at www.leechesusa.com.

21. Pharmacology not only applies to drugs, but also to products that affect wound healing, tissue strength, and tissue replacement. Name two biologic substances that are used in the head and neck for these reasons.

AlloDerm, manufactured by LifeCell Corporation, is human donor skin stripped of the epidermis and all of the cells in the dermis. The remaining material is a collagen framework that provides strength. There are no components left to cause rejection or inflammation. AlloDerm has been used since 1992 for burn patients and recently expanded use includes augmentation for facial defects, septal perforation repair, and even tympanic membrane grafting.

Another substance is **hydroxyapatite (HA) cement.** There are various forms of this on the market. Essentially it is interlinked calcium phosphate molecules. HA is the primary mineral component of teeth and bone. HA cement is not osteogenic, but osteoconductive; it can serve as a scaffold on which bone can grow into macropores (220–300 μm). It has been used for various facial bony contour irregularities with good success.

CONTROVERSIES

22. Can Ketorolac be safely used for post-tonsillectomy pain?

Ketorolac is a nonsteroidal, anti-inflammatory potent analgesic. Its postoperative analgesic efficacy approaches that of morphine in nonotolaryngologic surgery. Unlike narcotics, it does not cause respiratory depression or decreased gastric motility. However, Ketorolac does have antiplatelet activity via inhibition of prostaglandin synthesis. Therefore, there is concern about increased risk of postoperative hemorrhage. In one randomized study, post-tonsillectomy bleeding rates were noted to be 18.9% in the Ketorolac group compared with 7% in the group treated with meperidine for postoperative pain. The study did not gain statistical significance, but noted a trend toward increased hemorrhage with Ketorolac. The manufacturer of Ketorolac warns that its use is contraindicated in major surgery because of the increased risk of bleeding.

23. Who is best able to coordinate the otolaryngology patient's drug regimen?

Usually the otolaryngologist. However, with changing patterns of medical care provision (e.g., the emergence of HMO and "primary care physician") acute otolaryngologic care is often provided by the patient's primary care provider, and the patient has often received one or two rounds of medications before he or she is referred to the otolaryngologist. In this case, the otolaryngologist must be familiar with the primary- and secondary-line drugs, along with their cost-benefit ratios, but will usually coordinate the patient's care until the acute condition is stabilized. On other occasions, however, (e.g., chemotherapy) the otolaryngologist often recommends referral to another specialist and no longer participates directly in the patient's care, although he or she may provide follow-up (e.g., re-examine the patient for recurrence). The balance between disciplines is usually individualized, although some referral patterns may also be dictated by the patient's insurance plan.

24. How do placebos work?

Many studies suggest that problems such as pain and depression respond particularly well to placebos. Blood pressure, cholesterol levels, and heart rate are also affected by placebos, as are, surprisingly, warts. On average, about a third of people taking placebos in controlled studies report a benefit.

Since 1960, this effect has been accepted, although investigators don't yet understand its origin. Some factors are obvious: Some of the improvement in drug trials may be spontaneous and reflect random fluctuations in disease symptoms. Also, people participating in trials may report improvement because that's what they expect researchers want to hear, and they wish to cooperate. But other factors are at work also. For example, patients receiving "morphine" placebos report more pain relief than those receiving "aspirin" placebos. Also, "brand name aspirin" placebos are more effective than "generic" aspirin placebos. So patients' perception of the treatment plays a role in the result.

The effects of placebo are also found to vary from country to country. Placebos were more effective in treating ulcers in Germany than in Brazil. Any treatment, active or not, is more effective if the doctor tells the patient, "This is a powerful medicine." So the placebo response is thought to be both a conscious response to the intent of therapy and an unconscious response to treatment from a respected professional (or even a witch doctor).

Patients are "conditioned" to expect relief if a drug is given. Even the taste and appearance of a drug appears to be important, although it is not clear whether "bad tasting" or "good tasting" drugs "work better." Those with observable side effects, such as pain at the injection site, appear to be more effective than those without.

25. Why is there debate about the use of placebos?

The placebo effect has raised concerns by both advocates and opponents. Ethicists warn that new drugs must be tested against "the best current treatment" and that using placebos is unethical, even when the risk is low. In October 2000, the World Medical Association, meeting in Edinburgh, amended the Declaration of Helsinki, suggesting that "the rights of the individual patient [to the best available treatment] take precedence over the rights of science and society in general." They pointed out that even briefly taking a patient off blood pressure medications and substituting a placebo may cause irreversible side effects. In such cases, informed consent from a volunteer, even one who says he or she understands the risks involved, may be ethically untenable. Poor studies may result in the future, however, if placebo controls are omitted.

On the other hand, an article in the *New York Times* of January 9, 2000, suggested that if placebos work, "why not *use* [emphasis added] them as medicines?" The economic advantages are obvious. The author concluded, "There are real questions about the need for deception in achieving benefits. If you're not a bit troubled by the placebo effect, as well as intrigued by it, you haven't been paying attention."

These questions have earned their place in the controversy section. It's controversial how placebos work, and if or how you should use them, but the placebo effect really does exist and must be part of any consideration of drug or therapeutic approach efficacy.

HERBAL MEDICINE

A growing number of patients are using herbal products for preventive and therapeutic purposes. Because the manufacturers are not required to submit proof of the efficacy and safety of these drugs, adverse effects and drug interactions associated with herbal remedies are largely unknown. There are a number of over-the-counter "herbs" and vitamins that need to be taken into consideration in managing the otolaryngology patient. For example, vitamin E, St. John's Wort, aspirin, and ibuprofen prolong bleeding. Gingko biloba, proposed to improve cognition, has been reported to cause spontaneous bleeding and may interact with anticoagulants and antiplatelet agents. Ephedrine-containing products have been associated with adverse cardiovascular events, seizures, and death. Ginseng has been implicated as a cause of decreased response to warfarin. Inquiry about these and other herbal (often included in multidrug formulations) and over-the-counter preparations, which many patients don't really think of as "drugs," is therefore an important part of the medical history, especially in the preoperative patient.

BIBLIOGRAPHY

1. Bailey R, Sinha C, Burgess LP: Ketorolac tromethamine and hemorrhage in tonsillectomy: A prospective, randomized, double-blind study. Laryngoscope 107:166–169, 1997.
2. Buntzel J: Selective cytoprotection with amifostine in concurrent radiochemotherapy for head and neck cancer. Ann Oncol 9(5):505–509, 1998.
3. Christensen D: Medicinal mimicry. Sometimes placebos work—but how? Science News 152:74–75, 2001.
4. Crawford WW: Comparative efficacy of terfenadine, loratidine, and astemizole in perennial allergic rhinitis. Otolaryngol Head Neck Surg 118:668–673, 1999.
5. Cupp MJ: Herbal remedies: Adverse effects and drug interactions. Am Fam Physician 59:1239–1244, 1999.
6. Dobie RA: A review of randomized clinical trials in tinnitus. Laryngoscope, 109:1202–1211, 1999.
7. Gendeh BS: Vancomycin administration in continuing ambulatory peritoneal dialysis: The risk of ototoxicity. Otolaryngol Head Neck Surg 118:551–558, 1998.
8. Metz DC, Childs ML, Ruiz C, et al: Pilot study of the oral omeprazole test for reflux laryngitis. Otolaryngol Head Neck Surg 116:41–46, 1997.
9. Schacht J: Aminoglycoside ototoxicity: Prevention in sight? Otolaryngol Head Neck Surg 118:674–677, 1998.
10. Xerostomia. In Gluckman JL (ed): Renewal of Certification Study Guide, Dubuque, IA, Kendall/Hunt, 1998, pp 282–285.
11. Zormeier MM: Botulinum toxin injection to improve tracheoesophageal speech after total laryngectomy. Otolaryngol Head Neck Surg 120:314–319, 1999.

V. Endoscopy

36. LARYNGOSCOPY

Arvin K. Rao, M.S. IV, and Bruce W. Jafek, M.D., FACS, FRSM

1. What is laryngoscopy?

Visual examination of the interior of the larynx, or "voicebox."

2. What are the indications for laryngoscopy?

Visualization of the larynx with mirror laryngoscopy is part of the complete examination of the head and neck. Moreover, examination of the nasopharynx and larynx with indirect laryngoscopy is indicated in evaluation of hoarseness, suspected nasopharyngeal or laryngeal cancer, suspected laryngeal foreign body, chronic sinusitis, chronic cough, recurrent otitis media, and halitosis.

3. What is indirect laryngoscopy?

Examination of the larynx indirectly with a mirror, angulated telescope, or flexible, fiberoptic laryngoscope. Alternatively, direct laryngoscopy is the direct visual examination of the larynx with a rigid laryngoscope, performed under topical, regional block, or general anesthesia. The mirror examination is termed "indirect" because you do not visualize the larynx itself but only see it in the mirror, while during the direct examination you look at the larynx itself (sometimes through a microscope or other scope, to provide a magnified image). The direct method is best when closer inspection of the larynx is indicated, whereas the indirect method is more useful for rapid screening of laryngeal function.

4. How is mirror laryngoscopy performed?

Mirror laryngoscopy is performed with a laryngeal mirror, head mirror, and light source, with the patient in the "sniffing position" (the head extended on the neck and the neck flexed on the torso). The examiner gently grasps the patient's tongue with a gauge pad and elevates the upper lip with his or her index finger. The warmed mirror is placed into the patient's oropharynx and into contact with the soft palate and uvula, with care taken to avoid touching the posterior pharyngeal wall or the posterior tonsillar pillars. With proper placement of the mirror, the epiglottis and vocal folds come to view, and the examiner proceeds to visualize the larynx at rest, during respiration, and during vocalization.

5. How is fiberoptic laryngoscopy performed?

This procedure is performed through the patient's nose, which avoids the problems associated with touching the deep pressor receptors of the tongue base and prevents the uncooperative patient from biting your expensive fiberoptic laryngoscope! The more patent of the two nasal passages is first sprayed with a vasoconstrictor (e.g., 0.5% ephedrine) and then with a local anesthetic (e.g., lidocaine). Alternatively, 1% cocaine may be used, accomplishing both anesthesia and vasoconstriction. To keep the scope from fogging, it may be first dipped into warm water. The flexible scope is guided into the nasopharynx, then turned inferiorly past the palate and the uvula to visualize the larynx.

6. Fiberoptic laryngoscopy seems much simpler. What are its advantages and disadvantages over direct laryngoscopy?

The primary advantage is simplicity and patient comfort. The procedure is easily accomplished in the office and provides a good view of the larynx. Moreover, fiberoptic laryngoscopy can permit visualization of the larynx in patients with a vigorous gag reflex or arthritic changes in the neck who are unable to extend their head. This procedure is disadvantageous because the picture is obtained using a fiberoptic bundle, and the view of the larynx is not as good as with a Hopkins rod telescope or direct visualization with or without the microscope. Although not impossible, biopsy or vocal cord injection is more complex via fiberoptic laryngoscopy, and other surgical manipulation (e.g., dilatation) is nearly impossible.

7. What are the structures examined with indirect laryngoscopy?

The otolaryngologist systematically examines the symmetry, motion, color, and surface architecture of the base of the tongue, hypopharygeal wall, vallecula, epiglottis, aryepiglottic folds, arytenoids, piriform sinus, false and true vocal folds, first tracheal rings, and introitus of the esophagus. The scope may be passed down into the trachea only if a superior laryngeal nerve block has first been performed and the trachea topically anesthetized (e.g., by spraying with lidocaine). Minor differences in color can alert the examiner that the vocal folds may not be at the same level. Of course, the examiner also observes for more obvious inflammation, polyps, papillomas, and tumors.

8. Can vocal cord biopsies and injections be performed without direct laryngoscopy?

Yes. Biopsy samples can be obtained using a curved biopsy forceps and a mirror or a fiberoptic laryngoscope. However, this procedure requires an extremely skilled otolaryngologist and cooperative patient. Similarly, injections can be made directly into the vocal cord (e.g., Teflon or fat injection for vocal cord medialization) with this technique. Botulinum injections into the vocal cords can be performed either with this technique or via the cricothyroid membrane.

9. Name the intrinsic muscles of the larynx. What is their innervation?

Cricothyroid, posterior cricoarytenoid, lateral cricoarytenoid, transverse and oblique arytenoid, thyroarytenoid, and vocalis muscles. The recurrent laryngeal is a motor, parasympathetic, and visceral afferent nerve that originates from the vagus nerve, passes inferior to the aortic arch on the left and subclavian artery on the right, and innervates all the intrinsic muscles of the larynx with the exception of the cricothyroids. The cricothyroid muscles are supplied by motor fibers of the superior laryngeal nerve.

10. How is anesthesia obtained for manipulation of the larynx?

Cocaine or lidocaine/ephedrine can be used in the nose if the fiberoptic laryngoscope is employed. These agents are not necessary if the mirror rests on the soft palate, as in mirror laryngoscopy. Anesthesia of the larynx can then be achieved by dripping 1% cocaine through a curved cannula; by percutaneously delivering 1 to 2% lidocaine through the cricothyroid membrane; or by anesthetizing the superior laryngeal nerve.

11. What is superior laryngeal nerve anesthesia?

The superior laryngeal nerve (SLN) provides sensory innervation to the epiglottis, aryepiglottic folds, and upper larynx. Passing downward, the SLN parallels the carotid artery, until a branch (internal branch) swings anteriorly to cross and then pierce the superior aspect of the thyrohyoid membrane. It is here that the nerve is accessible to infiltration of anesthesia.

The otolaryngologist's left (nondominant) index finger is placed in the trough between the hyoid superiorly and thyroid cartilage inferiorly (over the thyrohyoid membrane). This finger is advanced posteriorly and laterally until the pulsations of the carotid artery are palpable. The common carotid artery lies posteriorly and is avoided and protected with the index finger. Through a 25-gauge needle, 2% lidocaine without epinephrine is injected approximately 1 cm deep into the tissues, just off the tip of the palpating index finger. This injection is just anterior to the posterior edge of the hyoid bone or superior cornua of the thyroid cartilage. Usually an injection of 2 mL/side provides excellent anesthesia. Alternatively, the needle is inserted until the patient complains of pain in the ear (via Arnold's nerve), but this is usually unnecessary. The area of injection is then massaged briefly to promote spread through the tissues. A similar injection is then carried out on the other side.

12. Why is lidocaine *without* epinephrine preferred?
Lidocaine spreads through the tissues easily, obviating the need to inject the SLN directly. This spread is inhibited by epinephrine because of the associated vasoconstriction.

13. What other endoscopic procedures are used to evaluate the larynx?
Two of the most important recent methods of evaluating the larynx prior to manipulation are **videolaryngoscopy** and **videolaryngostroboscopy.** These examinations are best done with the transoral rigid telescope with a rigid-rod quartz lens system (e.g., Ward-Berci scope) but can be done with the flexible laryngoscope. They are the best ways to assess the dynamic function of the larynx, as observation during both quiet breathing and during a variety of tasks is possible. The addition of a video camera (videolaryngoscopy) produces an enlarged image that may be recorded for detailed evaluation or saved for comparison with future examinations. Videolaryngoscopy also allows accurate evaluation of the closing and opening pattern of the larynx.

The addition of the stroboscope provides a flashing light to simulate a slowed vocal cord vibration and further facilitates evaluation of dynamic laryngeal function, particularly the mucosal wave of the vocal folds. The stroboscope has a microphone to sense the fundamental frequency of the vibrations and coordinates the flashing light to the same frequency. If the light flashes at the fundamental frequency, the stroboscope will freeze one image in the vibratory cycle. The slowed motion allows the most accurate assessment of the mucosal wave. This wave may be impaired by scarring, edema, or subtle defects in the mucosa. With stroboscopy, lesions such as very early carcinoma may be best seen as an adynamic segment of the vocal cord.

The **videoendoscopic swallowing study** (also called flexible endoscopic swallowing examination, or FESE) is a relatively simple and widely available method to evaluate dysphagia. A fiberoptic nasolaryngoscope is used to assess the anatomy and function of the palate, pharynx, and larynx, salivary pooling, and sensation. Then, swallowing is assessed with various consistencies of boluses. The examination cannot adequately evaluate the phases of swallowing or aspiration that occurs with swallowing, but can assess the anatomy and sensation of the patient and the ability to swallow.

14. Name the other ancillary tests used for the evaluation of laryngeal function.
Acoustic analysis measures fundamental frequency, spectral analysis, and perturbation (shimmer=loudness, and jitter=pitch).
Aerodynamic ability is an aerodynamic assessment of flow and pressure.
Photoglottography and **electroglottography**
Electromyography provides information about the nerves and muscles of the larynx.
Cineradiography is used to evaluate laryngeal closure and other functions.
Aspiration tests

15. What are the indications for direct laryngoscopy?
• When evaluation with indirect laryngoscopy is inadequate to assess suspected or actual pathology within the larynx (e.g., hoarseness, laryngeal tumor) or when indirect laryngoscopy is impossible.
• Palpation is required to distinguish vocal folds paralysis from fixation.
• Therapy or biopsy within the larynx (e.g., removal of vocal cord polyp, subglottic dilatation). Some experienced laryngologists are able to achieve biopsy and some therapeutic approaches indirectly.

- As a preliminary step to intubation (the anesthesiologist typically uses a scope with a curved blade and visualizes only the posterior larynx).
- As a preliminary step to the insertion of a rigid bronchoscope (rarely required).

16. How is direct laryngoscopy performed?

If general anesthesia is employed, the patient is placed supine and intubated. The neck is then extended and the scope inserted. With insertion, it is important to avoid injury to the lips, tongue, or teeth. The initial landmark is the uvula, followed by the epiglottis. The epiglottis is lifted superiorly into the patient's anterior neck, allowing visualization of the larynx. At this point, the operator can stabilize the patient's head by holding the scope with the palm of the nondominant hand on the patient's forehead. Alternatively, the patient can be "suspended" with various devices (e.g., Benjamin). This arrangement allows the microscope to be positioned so that the surgeon may proceed with both hands.

17. Are there any other tricks to direct laryngoscopy?

The larynx is usually cocainized prior to manipulation (4% cocaine-soaked neurosurgical patties are placed on the laryngeal mucosa).

18. Why use cocaine, if the patient is already under general anesthesia?

The cocaine serves three purposes:
- It is a vasoconstrictor and therefore minimizes bleeding if biopsy samples are to be obtained.
- It is an anesthetic and minimizes the potential for laryngospasm upon extubation, a problem due to irritation from bleeding.
- Cocaine decreases the laryngocardiac reflex.

19. Why does laryngospasm occur?

During recovery, especially during stage II anesthesia, the glottis occasionally "clamps" closed. This action is probably a primitive defense mechanism in response to an irritant and acts to protect the lower respiratory tree. It usually "breaks up" as the patient starts breathing spontaneously. However, reanesthetizing the patient, especially with paralytic agents, is occasionally required.

20. What is the laryngocardiac reflex?

Observers have noted that pressure on the larynx occasionally produces bradycardia or cardiac arrest. This response is believed to be due to reflexive laryngocardiac innervation, although the neural pathways are not precisely defined. Anesthetizing the larynx prior to manipulation avoids this problem.

21. How do the various types of laryngoscopes differ?

Each type of laryngoscope is designed to deal with a certain type of problem encountered during laryngoscopy. One has an "anterior flare" (anterior commissure scope) and allows for improved visualization of the anterior commissure of the larynx. Another is "wasp-waisted" (constricted in the middle) and minimizes pressure on the teeth. Another has a broad viewing point and facilitates the use of the microscope. Another has a "double bill," which allows the larynx to be spread somewhat, facilitating the use of a laser for a transoral supraglottic laryngectomy.

22. What are the special postoperative considerations with direct laryngoscopy?

This procedure is usually performed on an outpatient basis. Voice rest is indicated for 7–10 days if a biopsy sample has been obtained, especially if the lesion involved most of a vocal cord. One or two doses of 8–10 mg dexamethasone IV (4 hours apart) minimizes postoperative edema. Cool mist is also soothing if the cord has been biopsied.

23. What are the potential complications associated with direct laryngoscopy?

The most common is inadvertent injury to the lips, tongue, or teeth. You should be able to avoid this by watching these areas carefully during the procedure. A tooth guard minimizes pressure on the teeth. Laryngospasm and the laryngocardiac reflex are discussed earlier (see Questions 19 and 20). If one cord has had its mucosa violated, great care should be taken to protect the anterior commissure mucosa on the opposite side to avoid anterior laryngeal webbing.

CONTROVERSIES

24. Is laryngoscopy best done under local or general anesthesia?
Direct laryngoscopy is usually done under general anesthesia, but in the cooperative, preferably sedated patient, direct laryngoscopy can be done under local or regional block anesthesia. However, the real decision to use local, regional block, or general anesthesia relates to the purpose. A detailed examination of the larynx can easily be accomplished under local anesthesia in the office. Laryngeal manipulation, on the other hand, may require general anesthesia, depending on the skill of the operator, the specific procedure to be performed, and patient preference.

25. What is the optimal position for direct laryngoscopy?
The "sniffing position," with the head extended on the neck and the neck flexed, is considered the optimal position for direct laryngoscopic examination of the vocal folds. Nonetheless, the optimal position relates to the purpose of the direct laryngoscopy. Flexion of the head on the neck and flexion of the neck can provide optimal glottal exposure for endotracheal intubation in patients predisposed to difficulty in direct examination of the glottis. Alternatively, the sniffing position is the optimal position for microlaryngoscopy because it allows the use of the largest laryngoscope.

SUSPENSION OR HAND-HELD LARYNGOSCOPY?

The choice of laryngoscopy technique depends on procedure and desired result of examination. For simple examination of the larynx or minimal biopsying, under general anesthesia, holding the laryngoscope in the nondominant hand shortens the procedure and minimizes tooth injury. For prolonged procedures (e.g., use of the laser or microscope), suspension is probably indicated. Outpatient laryngoscopy with local or no anesthesia is always, of course, "hand-held," although it may be fiberoptic, mirror, or rod-amplified.

BIBLIOGRAPHY

1. Armstrong M, Mark LJ, Synder DS, et al: Safety of direct laryngoscopy as an outpatient procedure. Laryngoscope 107:1060–1065, 1997.
2. Bastian RW: Contemporary diagnosis of the dysphagic patient. Otolaryngol Clin North Am 31:489–506, 1998.
3. Bucx MJ: Right- or left-handed laryngoscopy? Anaesthesia 55:395–396, 2000.
4. Fried MP, Moharir VM, Shinmoto H, et al: Virtual laryngoscopy. Ann Otol Rhinol Laryngol 108:221–226, 1999.
5. Hochmann II, Zeitels SM, Heaton JT: Analysis of the forces and position required for direct laryngoscopic exposure of the anterior vocal folds. Ann Otol Rhinol Laryngol 108:715–723, 1999.
6. Kempen PM: Arytenoid subluxation caused by laryngoscopy and intubation. Anesthesiology 92:1505–1507, 2000.

7. Kleinsasser O: Microlaryngoscopy and Endolaryngeal Microsurgery: Technique and Typical Findings, 3rd ed. (translated by PM Stell) Philadelphia, Hanley & Belfus, 1992.
8. Kurien KM: Maintaining optimal head positioning for laryngoscopy [letter]. Anaesth Intensive Care 26:331, 1998.
9. Langmore SE: Role of flexible laryngoscopy for evaluating aspiration. Ann Otol Rhinol Laryngol 107(5 Pt 1):446, 1998.
10. Levitan RM, Higgins MS, Ochrock EA: Contrary to popular belief and traditional instruction, the larynx is sighed one eye at a time during direct laryngoscopy [letter]. Acad Emerg Med 5:844–846, 1998.
11. Muehlberger T, Kunar D, Munster A, et al: Efficacy of fiberoptic laryngoscopy in the diagnosis of inhalation injuries. Arch Otolaryngol Head Neck Surg 124:1003–1007, 1998.
12. Vanner RG, Clarke P, Moore WJ, et al: The effect of cricoid pressure and neck support on the view at laryngoscopy. Anaesthesia 52:896–900, 1997.

37. ESOPHAGOSCOPY

Bruce W. Jafek, M.D., FACS, FRSM, and Stephen G. Batuello, M.D.

1. What are the indications for esophagoscopy?

Diagnostic indications: dysphagia, odynophagia, atypical chest pain, hematemesis, suspected gastroesophageal reflux, webs, strictures, and neoplasia

Therapeutic indications: removal of foreign bodies, sclerotherapy, myotomy, dilation, and coagulation of bleeding

2. When is esophagoscopy contraindicated?

Aneurysm of the thoracic aorta

Severe deformities of the cervical or thoracic spine (flexible esophagoscopy may be possible)

Uncooperative or combative patient

Severe erosive burns to the esophagus

Chronic administration of high-dose steroids

Laryngeal edema

3. What are the potential complications of esophagoscopy?

Esophageal perforation	Hypotension
Trauma to the lips, tongue, or oral mucosa	Arrhythmias
Fracturing or dislocation of the teeth	Pneumothorax
Aspiration pneumonia	Bleeding
Respiratory depression	

The most common complication of esophagoscopy, esophageal perforation, occurs in 1–2% of cases.

4. What are the symptoms of esophageal perforations?

Pain and tachycardia (early signs), followed by fever, hematemesis, hypotension, and shock.

5. How is an esophageal perforation diagnosed?

The patient with fever after esophagoscopy should be presumed to have a perforation until proven otherwise. Chest radiography and Gastrografin contrast studies should be performed immediately to determine the extent of extravasation. The white blood cell count is usually elevated. An electrocardiogram is obtained to rule out possible myocardial ischemia, either as the coexisting result of the perforation or as the etiology of the symptoms rather than perforation.

6. Why does the esophagus have a greater propensity to rupture than other sites of the alimentary tract?

The esophagus has no serosal layer. This anatomic fact, combined with the presence of negative intrathoracic pressure, makes the esophagus more susceptible to perforation.

7. Describe the technique of rigid esophagoscopy.

In general, esophagoscopy should not be performed without a preoperative esophagogram viewable during the procedure. Rigid esophagoscopy is best tolerated by the patient under general anesthesia. The patient is positioned with the shoulders at the free end of the operating table, the head in the neutral position on the occiput with the chin "jutted," and the neck flexed initially; a tooth guard is usually used. The lubricated esophagoscope is introduced and the uvula first visualized (assuring midline placement). The scope is then advanced in the midline, and the next landmark is the epiglottis. The esophagoscope then is carefully advanced posteriorly to the level of the cricopharyngeus muscle, the most dangerous location of the procedure. The lumen is always maintained in the center of the visual field as the instrument is advanced slowly toward the stomach, and the esophagus is carefully examined to and through the gastroesophageal junction. The esophagoscope is never advanced unless it moves easily and the lumen is visible at all times. The esophagus may be re-inspected during careful removal of the instrument by "corkscrewing" out to visualize the full circumference of the lumen.

8. **At what distances from the incisor teeth are major esophageal landmarks encountered in the adult? In the 3-year-old? In the 1-year-old?**

	ADULT	3-YEAR-OLD	1-YEAR-OLD
Cricopharyngeus	12–16	9–11	8–10
Aorta	20–24	13–15	12–14
Esophageal hiatus	35–38	20–23	18–20
Cardia	38–42	25–27	21–22

Distances are in cm.

9. **Where are the three areas of anatomic narrowing of the esophagus?**

The upper esophageal sphincter, or **cricopharyngeus,** is at the level of the cricoid cartilage. The anterior compression by the **aortic arch and left mainstem bronchus** is approximately 20–25 cm from the upper incisors in the adult. The **gastroesophageal junction** is 40–45 cm away. These locations are significant because they are common sites for foreign bodies to lodge, and swallowed corrosive liquids may produce more damage in these areas.

10. **Where are most esophageal foreign bodies found?**

Foreign bodies of the upper aerodigestive tract in the pediatric population are a common occurrence. Despite significant advances in prevention, first aid, and endoscopic technology, they remain a diagnostic and therapeutic challenge. Early diagnosis is the key to successful and uncomplicated management of these accidents.

Ninety-five percent of esophageal foreign bodies are located just inferior to the cricopharyngeus muscle. The force of this powerful sphincter muscle and the pharyngeal constrictors can transmit objects into the esophagus but they cannot be transported further by the esophageal musculature. The remaining 5% of foreign bodies are normally found in regions of anatomic narrowing of the esophagus: the gastroesophageal junction and the indentations of the esophagus caused by the arch of the aorta and left mainstem bronchus.

11. **Where is Killian's triangle?**

Killian's triangle is an area of weakness in the posterior esophagus. Specifically, it is located in the midline pharyngoesophageal segment, above the cricopharyngeus muscle and below the midline raphe of the inferior constrictor. This is the location of Zenker's diverticulum, a mucosal sac that protrudes between the oblique and transverse fibers of the cricopharyngeus muscle. This sac is thought to be formed by the repeated pulsion forces created by the contracting pharyngeal constrictors.

12. **How is a Zenker's diverticulum diagnosed and treated?**

A Zenker's diverticulum is diagnosed primarily by history. About 70% of patients with a Zenker's diverticulum are over 60 years old. They typically report gradual-onset dysphagia of long duration, with food "sticking" at the level of the suprasternal notch. Another typical feature is regurgitation of the undigested food from the pouch with a foul odor and taste. Physical examination may show a palpable mass in the left neck, posteroinferior to the sternocleidomastoid muscle. Barium swallow is diagnostic and shows a pouch with multiple radiographic lucencies from retained food.

The treatment of Zenker's diverticula has paralleled its presumed pathophysiology. With the development of technical facilities to better evaluate the pharyngoesophageal region, incomplete relaxation of the upper esophageal sphincter seems to represent the key element in the development of high pharyngeal pressures with a subsequent outpouching responsible for the diverticulum formation. Many studies have justified **cricopharyngeal myotomy** as an essential component in the treatment of pharyngoesophageal diverticula because it represents an efficient therapy with little morbidity. A **diverticulopexy** (identifying the pouch and suturing it superiorly to reverse its dependent positioning in the erect patient) should be added for pouches between 1 and 4 cm, and a diverticulectomy should be performed for sacs greater than 5 cm for best relief of symptoms. Other treatment modalities have recently been used, such as the endoscopic division of the common wall between the cervical esophagus and the diverticulum with electrocautery (Dohlman's procedure), a laser, or a stapling device. This method is gaining popularity because it achieves a good clinical outcome, especially in high-risk patients. However, more studies are needed to confirm its long-term effectiveness.

13. How are midthoracic and lower esophageal diverticula managed?

Periesophageal inflammation, most commonly secondary to tuberculosis, used to be a frequent cause of *midthoracic diverticula*. Today, the majority of these diverticula are the result of esophageal motility disorders. Although many patients are asymptomatic, it is the underlying motility disturbances that produce most symptoms. A barium esophagogram is the best study to show midthoracic diverticula. Esophageal manometry may be difficult to perform because of obstruction of passage of the motility catheter by the diverticulum, but it is useful in defining the cause of the diverticulum and directing therapy. Esophagoscopy is helpful in the assessment of complications or associated esophageal abnormalities; it adds little to the evaluation of the diverticulum. In patients requiring surgery, a diverticulectomy with a myotomy performed on the esophageal wall opposite the diverticulum is the preferred treatment. Lesser procedures have been reported to be successful in select patients.

Minimally invasive approaches are ideally suited to treat *diverticula of the lower esophagus*. The most commonly reported procedure is a laparoscopic diverticulectomy and myotomy, particularly when the diverticulum is located within 10 cm of the lower esophageal sphincter. Treatment is the same as for the open approach: Symptomatic patients are offered surgical treatment, the diverticulum is excised without compromise of the esophageal lumen, the proximal extent of the myotomy is dictated by preoperative manometry, and postoperative evaluation is performed to exclude recurrence and gastroesophageal reflux. The results of laparoscopic treatment of esophageal diverticula are similar to the results reported in the open procedure.

14. A child has ingested a caustic substance, but physical examination reveals no oral or pharyngeal burns. Is there cause for concern?

Yes. After caustic ingestion, there is little correlation between the presence of burns on the lips, oral cavity, and pharynx and the presence of burns in the esophagus. If the substance is crystalline (e.g., detergent), there is greater chance of proximal burning, because these substances are harder to swallow and the immediate pain prevents further ingestion. Liquid substances, on the other hand, are more likely to produce distal burns. Nevertheless, observation is indicated based on history alone.

15. What intervention is required after a caustic ingestion?

If the airway is compromised on presentation, it should be controlled with intubation or tracheotomy if the supraglottic structures are severely burned. All patients should be kept NPO (nothing by mouth), supported with intravenous fluids, and observed for acute complications. These include laryngeal edema with airway obstruction, esophageal perforation with mediastinitis, gastric perforation with peritonitis, and tracheoesophageal fistula with pneumonia. Esophagoscopy under general anesthesia is performed as soon as possible after the ingestion; after 12 hours it should probably *not* be performed, owing to increased risk of perforation due to damage to and resultant necrosis of the esophagus. It is used to determine whether a burn is present and the extent of the burn. A feeding tube may be placed carefully if severe or circumferential burns are encountered, although this is controversial. If burns are encountered, antibiotics and steroids are initiated. Antibiotics are shown to prevent intramural spread of infection and mediastinitis, and steroids have been found to help prevent formation of strictures if given in the first 24–48 hours. A contrast esophagogram is performed at 6 weeks to evaluate for stricture.

16. Which type of caustic ingestion causes more severe esophageal injury: acid or alkaline?

Acid causes coagulation necrosis, which creates a barrier to deeper penetration. *Alkaline* agents, however, cause a liquefaction necrosis and therefore tend to penetrate more quickly and deeply through tissue layers. Nevertheless, strong acids may produce severe burns and strictures.

17. What is Barrett's esophagus?

Barrett's esophagus occurs more frequently than previously anticipated. The diagnosis of Barrett's esophagus is made by endoscopic biopsy. The normal squamous epithelium of the esophagus is found to be replaced by a specialized columnar epithelium of any length. Patients with more than 5 years of gastroesophageal reflux symptoms (GERD), particularly those 50 years of age or older, should undergo (usually) flexible esophagoscopy to detect Barrett's esophagus. With the recognition of Barrett's esophagus as a premalignant lesion (subsequent development of adenocarcinoma), the crucial issue is surveillance for detection of dysplasia. Although the natural history of dysplasia is incompletely defined, it is clear that patients with dysplasia have a higher risk for adenocarcinoma than those without dysplasia. Recent studies have shown that p53 protein accumulation appears to be an earlier and more specific/sensitive marker than dysplasia of malignant potential in Barrett's esophagus.

18. How is Barrett's esophagus managed?

The management of Barrett's esophagus often involves a multidisciplinary evaluation. Photodynamic therapy seems to be able to control high-grade dysplasia within Barrett's esophagus about 80% of the time. Long-term results are not available, but the treatment is promising. Given the success with surgical intervention, however, use of photodynamic therapy should be reserved for nonsurgical candidates at the current time. The complications that occur with photodynamic therapy (stricture and even perforation) are not trivial and must be weighed against the potential benefits. Other forms of management include argon plasma coagulation or endoscopic mucosal resection. Both proton pump inhibitor therapy and laparoscopic fundoplication represent major advances in the prevention of GERD, and therefore Barrett's esophagus. The possibility of reversing Barrett's esophagus in selected high-risk patients offers major hope for the future prevention of adenocarcinoma of the esophagus.

19. Describe the technique of flexible esophagoscopy.

Flexible endoscopes are more easily passed from the oropharynx into the esophagus and may be used with local or topical anesthesia. With the patient in the sitting or decubitus position (to minimize aspiration), the endoscope is introduced past the cricopharyngeus muscle as the patient swallows. The esophagus and stomach are then inspected during cautious advancement of the instrument. The major problem with this technique is that positive pressure (insufflation) is required to distend the esophagus to permit inspection and the superior 10–15 cm of the esophagus is not well seen.

CONTROVERSIES

20. How do you treat an esophageal perforation?

The patient should receive nothing by mouth. Additional treatment depends on whether there is a *known* or a *suspected* perforation. Either way, most clinicians would start broad-spectrum antibiotics, but a few would hold these, fearing that they would "mask" an infection. The patient's vital signs and white blood cell count are followed closely. Oral suctioning of saliva, rather than swallowing, is helpful.

If the perforation is suspected, a Gastrografin swallow is obtained. If there is no perforation, the patient is started on oral liquids and monitored, depending on the suspicion of unrecognized perforation in spite of the swallow. If the patient remains afebrile, without pain, the diet is advanced as the possibility of perforation is ruled out.

If the perforation is confirmed on Gastrografin swallow, the treatment depends on the location. If it is in the cervical esophagus, above the thoracic inlet, observation for 4–5 days may be indicated. Some otolaryngologists would do an immediate drainage procedure and leave a drain in place 4–5 days before advancing it slowly. Assuming that the perforation is in the thoracic esophagus, early exploration is indicated, unless contraindicated by the patient's general condition.

If symptoms resolve and there is no evidence of infection in 7–10 days, the Gastrografin contrast may be repeated to reassess the perforation. If there is no evidence of leakage, the diet may be advanced slowly and the patient closely observed. Antibiotics are discontinued if there is no evidence of recurrent infection. Should symptoms persist or recur, surgical exploration with drainage is usually indicated.

21. Which is better, rigid or flexible esophagoscopy?

Because each procedure has advantages and disadvantages, many endoscopists consider them as adjunctive rather than mutually exclusive techniques. In general, rigid esophagoscopy provides better visualization of the pharynx and upper esophageal sphincter, more controlled foreign-body removal, direct visualization during dilation, easier debulking of tumor, and easier securing of biopsies. Flexible esophagoscopy obviates the need for general anesthesia, allows inspection of the stomach and duodenum, and can be used to maneuver through tortuous anatomy.

22. Should esophagoscopy always be performed in cases of caustic ingestion?

Some authors have identified caustic ingestion as an absolute contraindication to endoscopy, but others report the necessity of evaluating the esophagus so that appropriate treatment can be instituted. However, it is generally agreed that esophagoscopy is contraindicated in cases of severe burns or evidence of laryngeal edema. Most also agree that it is contraindicated for patients on high-dose steroids. The generally accepted dictum is that if esophagoscopy is performed, it should be terminated as the site of the "first significant burn" is visualized to avoid stretching (and rupturing) impaired tissue.

23. Can bleeding esophageal varices be managed endoscopically?

Bleeding esophageal varices are a frequent and sometimes fatal complication of portal hypertension. Prompt resuscitation and arrest of hemorrhage are the immediate goals. Vasoactive therapy to reduce portal pressure is administered on presentation. Early endoscopy is indicated to make a definitive diagnosis and initiate appropriate therapy. Both the control of acute variceal bleeding and elective variceal eradication to prevent recurrent bleeding can be achieved endoscopically. After the acute bleeding episode, follow-up therapy is instituted either to obliterate the varices or to chronically lower portal hypertension pharmacologically to reduce the risk of rebleeding; a combination of both therapies may be used.

In contrast to acute and elective treatment, the role of endoscopy in asymptomatic patients who have never had bleeding remains controversial because of the rather disappointing results obtained from prophylactic sclerotherapy. Most published controlled trials showed that prophylactic sclerotherapy had no effect on survival. In some studies, neither survival rate nor bleeding risk was improved. Active surveillance of those at risk of developing varices is, however, advocated. Long-term beta-blocker therapy has been demonstrated to be effective in both the primary prevention of variceal hemorrhage and the prevention of rebleeding in those who have already bled.

Despite a multitude of therapeutic regimens and ongoing clinical trials, the rate of mortality from this condition remains disappointingly high.

BIBLIOGRAPHY

1. Baker ME, Zuccaro G Jr, Achkar E, et al: Esophageal diverticula: Patient assessment. Semin Thorac Cardiovasc Surg 11:326–336, 1999.
2. Lambert R: Endoscopic treatment of esophagogastric tumors. Endoscopy 30:80–93, 1998.
3. Mayoral W, Fleischer DE: The esophacoil stent for malignant esophageal obstruction. Gastrointest Endosc Clin North Am 9:423–430, 1999.
4. McCormack G, McCormick PA: A practical guide to the management of oesophageal varices. Drugs 57:327–335, 1999.
5. Mokhashi MS, Hawes RH: The ultraflex stents for malignant esophageal obstruction. Gastrointest Endosc Clin North Am 9:413–433, 1999.
6. Morgan R, Adam A: The radiologist's view of expandable metallic stents for malignant esophageal obstruction. Gastrointest Endosc Clin North Am 9:431–435, 1999.
7. Nelson D: The wallstent I and II for malignant esophageal obstruction. Gastrointest Endosc Clin North Am 9:403–412, 1999.
8. Radu A, Wagnieres G, van den Bergh H, et al: Photodynamic therapy of early squamous cell cancers of the esophagus. Gastrointest Endosc Clin North Am 10:439–460, 2000.
9. Rahmani EY, Rex DK, Lehman GA: Z-stent for malignant esophageal obstruction. Gastrointest Endosc Clin North Am 9:395–402, 1999.
10. Rice TW, Baker ME: Midthoracic esophageal diverticula. Semin Thorac Cardiovasc Surg 11:352–357, 1999.

38. BRONCHOSCOPY

Bruce W. Jafek, M.D., FACS, FRSM

1. Describe the embryologic development of the trachea and bronchi.

A median **tracheobronchial groove** appears in the ventral wall of the embryonic pharynx during the third week of development. As this groove deepens, the **lateral septae** grow together and fuse to divide the esophagus from the trachea. Superiorly, the fusion is incomplete, forming the laryngeal inlet. The **caudal end** of the embryonic trachea elongates and divides into two lateral outgrowths, the **right and left lung buds.** These buds grow out into the **coelom,** which forms the primitive **pleural cavity.** The buds are enveloped in splanchnic mesoderm from which the connective tissues of the lungs and bronchi develop. Subsequent divisions of the lung buds form the lobes of the lungs and progressively smaller divisions of the tracheobronchial tree (e.g., bronchopulmonary segments down to alveolar sacs).

2. What are the functions of the trachea and bronchi?

The trachea and bronchi conduct air from the upper aerodigestive cavity. The larynx serves to protect these airways. While the air is being conducted to the periphery of the lung, it is being conditioned by the ciliated tracheobronchial epithelium. This specialized epithelium traps and expels small foreign bodies (e.g., 1- to 5-μm particles), propelling them back up to the pharynx where they are swallowed. Larger foreign bodies may trigger the cough reflex. The air also is warmed and humidified by exposure to the tracheobronchial epithelium and mucus, although most of this activity occurs in the nose. In addition to these respiratory functions, the trachea and bronchi have a lesser role in vocal resonation, providing the column of air from the lung to the vocal cords (generator function).

3. Describe the structure of the trachea and bronchi.

The trachea extends from the larynx to the carina. It is supported by horseshoe-shaped cartilages with membranous connections. At approximately the level of the 5th thoracic vertebra, the trachea divides into the right and left main bronchi. Posteriorly, the trachea is closed by fibrous tissue. Interspersed in the fibrous membranes are smooth and voluntary (trachealis) muscle fibers. As the bronchi divide and become progressively smaller, the cartilages become less complete, until the alveoli are formed. At this point, there is no cartilage present. The tracheobronchial tree is lined by a ciliated respiratory epithelium.

4. What biomechanical characteristics of the trachea must be considered for reconstructive surgery?

The trachea is a dynamic organ that expands and contracts longitudinally in response to the demands of deglutition, respiration, and gravity. Following tracheal resection, reconstruction must allow the trachea to resume its dynamic functions. The upper tracheal segments assume a larger stress load than the lower tracheal segments following trachea resection. By severing the suprahyoid musculature from the hyoid, you can loosen the trachea superiorly, and by severing intrathoracic connective tissue, you can loosen the trachea inferiorly. This allows maximal tracheal resection of five or more rings and subsequent reconstruction without tension.

5. What is "open" bronchoscopy? When is it indicated?

Open, or rigid, bronchoscopy was the first type of bronchoscopy developed. During this procedure, a rigid hollow tube measuring 6–8 mm in its inside diameter is inserted through the larynx into the tracheobronchial tree. Specialized telescopes, such as the Hopkins rod telescope, and other specialized magnification devices may be inserted into the bronchoscope to facilitate observation of the tracheobronchial tree.

This procedure is indicated for the evaluation of actual or suspected tracheobronchial pathologic lesions (e.g., hemoptysis, neoplasm) and tracheobronchial therapy (e.g., foreign-body removal, dilatation). It is especially useful for the establishment of an emergency airway via the oral route. Open bronchoscopy is limited by two major disadvantages: (1) it is technically difficult to visualize tissue beyond the second order of bronchi, even with mirrors; and (2) this procedure is associated with significant discomfort, and the patient almost always requires general anesthesia.

6. What is the Hopkins rod?
Optical telescopes, used to magnify the tracheobronchial tree, initially used a lens or series of lenses separated by air. Hopkins, an ingenious British inventor, reversed the traditional design, replacing the former air spaces with a series of glass rods and then replacing the former lens with small air spaces. As a result, this system allows a much larger viewing angle with greatly increased illumination and resolution. The use of this viewing telescope through the rigid endoscope has revolutionized the field of endoscopy.

7. What is "closed" bronchoscopy? When is it indicated?
Closed, or flexible, bronchoscopy was popularized by Ikeda in 1971. In this technique, a flexible bronchoscope is inserted through the larynx and into the lungs. This instrument is approximately 5 mm in diameter and carries a viewing channel via light-bearing, flexible, coherently arranged glass fibers. One or two noncoherent glass fiber bundles carry the light. Another open channel permits suctioning or biopsy. Closed bronchoscopy is indicated to inspect the second- to fifth-order bronchi for peripheral or upper lobe lesions, to evaluate radiographically negative hemoptysis, and to evaluate patients whose lung spaces are inaccessible with rigid bronchoscopes (e.g., kyphosis). It is also used to retrieve small foreign bodies and to evaluate occult carcinoma (radiographically negative, sputum-positive). Unfortunately, closed bronchoscopic images are not as sharp as the images that are obtained with a rigid bronchoscope and telescope.

8. Which type of anesthesia is used for bronchoscopy?
For flexible bronchoscopy, topical local anesthesia usually suffices. Rigid bronchoscopy can also be performed under local anesthesia with sedation. This includes glossopharyngeal and superior laryngeal nerve blocks, supplemented by spraying local anesthesia through the scope as it is advanced. However, general anesthesia is more commonly used for rigid bronchoscopy.

9. Describe the landmarks seen as the bronchoscope is introduced and advanced.
The flexible scope is commonly inserted through the nose. This provides a path to the larynx, via the pharynx, and avoids the contamination of the tongue. (More importantly, this route prevents the patient from biting your several-thousand-dollar instrument in half!) As the scope is advanced, landmarks seen include the posterior choana, pharynx, larynx, vocal cords, and tracheal rings.

Insertion of the rigid bronchoscope is facilitated by remaining close to the midline. The landmarks, in sequence, are the uvula, epiglottis, larynx, and tracheal rings. The patient's head is retroflexed on the occiput to recreate the "sniffing position." To expose the larynx, the tongue is displaced anteriorly.

10. What is the first endobronchial landmark?
Once the scope traverses the larynx, you should see the cartilaginous rings of the trachea and the carina. If you are too far posteriorly, you enter the esophagus, which lacks the rings and carina of the trachea, identifying your error.

11. How many divisions does the lung have?
The bronchoscopist should regard the lungs as being divided according to bronchial distribution, rather than by fissures. Starting at the carina, there is a left and right lung. The right lung has three major divisions existing from the right main, or mainstem, bronchus. These divisions are the upper, middle, and lower lobes. The left lung has two divisions, the upper and the lower

lobe. A third division on the left, corresponding to the middle lobe on the right, is called the lingula. The lingula shares its initial bronchus with the upper lobe.

12. How many bronchopulmonary segments are there in the right lung? In the left?
   In the American nomenclature, there are 10 segments on the right and 8 on the left. Variations in anatomy include an occasional subapical division. Each bronchopulmonary segment has its own bronchus and blood supply.

Right Lung (10 segments)	Left Lung (8 segments)
Upper lobe	Upper lobe
Apical	Apical-posterior
Posterior	Anterior
Anterior	Lingula
Middle lobe	Lateral
Superior	Inferior
Medial	Lower lobe
Lower lobe	Superior
Superior	Anteromedial basal
Lateral basal	Lateral basal
Medial basal	Posterior basal
Posterior basal	
Anterior basal	

13. Beyond the bronchopulmonary segments, how do you indicate location of findings?
   Examination of this area requires an extended anatomic nomenclature to describe the site of the findings. One system correlates closely with the endobronchial system. An "a" represents the more anterior and a "b" the more posterior segments as the endoscopist views the patient internally and progresses to the more peripheral bronchopulmonary tree. Using this system, a lesion in a sub-sub-subsegmental (fifth-order) bronchus in the right lung could be designated RB1b1β, and the location is described reliably to another endoscopist.

14. What is the eparterial bronchus? Why is it vitally important?
   The right upper lobe bronchus is the eparterial (above the artery) bronchus. This bronchus passes over the right pulmonary artery. The left upper lobe bronchus passes *under* the left pulmonary artery. This difference is important to remember when obtaining biopsies. If a deep biopsy (e.g., with a 5-mm cup forceps) is taken from the right upper lobe divider ("spur"), or secondary carina, the pulmonary artery may be violated, with obviously disastrous results.

15. If you encounter major bleeding when performing a bronchoscopy, how is it managed?
   The *only* treatment for major bleeding, such as with a pulmonary artery biopsy, is the immediate placement of the rigid bronchoscope down the opposite main bronchus. This allows ventilation of the "good" lung until the thoracic surgeon can open the chest and control the bleeding. Any attempt at suctioning or local endobronchial control is disastrous, as both lungs fill rapidly with blood. Once this blood clots, it is impossible to extract. Because ventilation is impossible, the patient suffocates. Immediate action is the only life-saving measure.

16. What non-neoplastic lung conditions are commonly evaluated with bronchoscopy?
   Bronchoscopy is indicated for nearly all patients with prolonged respiratory disease. Specific non-neoplastic indications include unexplained chronic cough, stridor, wheezing, hemoptysis, noncardiac shortness of breath, suspected foreign body, stenosis, vocal cord paralysis, neck mass, obstructive emphysema, atelectasis, and radiographic abnormalities. Of course, each of these indications may result in the finding of a neoplasm. The differential diagnosis is dependent on specimens gathered for microbiology, cytology, or pathology at the time of bronchoscopy. Therapeutic aspiration of secretions or foreign-body retrieval may also be performed.

17. How are endobronchial foreign bodies removed?

Smaller foreign bodies may be removed with a cup forceps via the fiberoptic bronchoscope. Removal of larger foreign bodies may require the use of intricate foreign-body forceps and complex maneuvers. Organic foreign bodies may be especially tricky, because they tend to swell (e.g., bean), cause inflammatory responses (e.g., peanut), and break up. This prevents their complete removal, and the fragment may be lodged further down the tracheobronchial tree. If all else fails, open removal with a thoracotomy or partial lobectomy may be required.

18. How does tuberculosis appear on bronchoscopy in the lung?

The incidence of tuberculosis is again increasing, unfortunately, and resistance is also increasing. Characteristically, tuberculosis appears as a "cottage cheese" exudate. It is associated with surprisingly little inflammatory response in the epithelium. When this diagnosis is suspected, special stains for acid-fast bacilli may help with early confirmation. This facilitates early therapy, as the organisms are often fastidious and difficult to culture. It is important to protect the endoscopist, anesthesiologist, and other staff from accidental inoculation. Protection can be facilitated by interposing a glass or Plexiglas shield over the viewing channel. This step is, of course, an important routine precaution in the age of human immunodeficiency virus and antibiotic-resistant organisms. Special precautions are also indicated when cleaning the operating room and instruments after the case.

19. What kinds of samples should you obtain by bronchoscopy?

Depending on the evaluated condition, biopsies, brushings, washings, or specimens for culture are obtained. Translobar lung biopsies may also be indicated, especially when the suspected diagnosis is pneumocystis.

20. How are these samples obtained?

Biopsies are generally obtained with the cup forceps through the open bronchoscope or with the flexible-cup forceps through the closed scope. Often, the flexible forceps are not withdrawn through the small biopsy channel; instead, they are withdrawn to the opening, and the scope and biopsy are withdrawn together, which avoids dislodging the biopsy in the channel.

Brushings are obtained with a tiny stiff-bristled brush. The brush can be withdrawn through the biopsy channel, but it should be irrigated into a trap at the conclusion of the procedure to retrieve all cells for cytologic examination. Alternatively, a sheathed brush can be used to retain all possible cells.

Washings are obtained by flushing the suspicious segment with physiologic saline and retrieving the washings into a sterile trap.

Specimens for culture can be obtained in the same fashion.

Translobar lung biopsy (see question 23).

21. How does cancer appear in the lung?

The most common cancer of the lung is squamous cell carcinoma. Since this is an epithelial lesion, it presents as an irregularity of epithelial lining. Some adjacent blood vessels may be somewhat tortuous, and the lesion is usually raised. In more advanced cases, the lumen may be completely occluded.

22. How is a "sputum cytology" obtained?

Because neoplastic cells commonly exfoliate, they may be found in the sputum. Because early-morning specimens are the most concentrated with these cells, the patient is asked to cough deeply and produce samples when he or she awakens. The samples are examined by the trained pathologist, usually using Papanicolaou or other stains. They are examined for the usual malignancy criteria (pleomorphism, increased nuclear/cytoplasmic ratios, etc). Newer technology uses lasers to identify suspicious cells, which are then visually evaluated by the pathologist.

23. Why are translobar lung biopsies performed? How are they performed?

If the lung is diffusely involved (e.g., *Pneumocystis carinii* pneumonia or metastatic disease), the fiberoptic bronchoscope is advanced to the periphery, and the biopsy forceps are advanced blindly until gentle resistance is encountered. The patient is advised to "take a deep breath," and the biopsy cups are advanced further. The patient is then asked to exhale. This maneuver brings lung tissue into the biopsy cups. The biopsy sample is removed along with the scope. This procedure carries the associated danger of creating a pneumothorax if the biopsy is performed too peripherally.

CONTROVERSIES

24. Is a bronchial adenoma benign?

Bronchial adenomas were formerly classified as benign neoplasms, but this is now known to be incorrect. Histologically, two types of adenoma are recognized, a *carcinoid* type with uniform, benign-appearing, cuboidal cells, and a *cylindromatous* type, with equally benign-appearing cells. Both tend to present with hemoptysis and appear at endoscopy as a reddish mass. Both tend to bleed vigorously on biopsy. Both also tend to cause problems of distal obstruction. Here the similarities cease. Metastases are occasionally seen with the carcinoid variant, and endobronchial resection is often helpful. In contrast, the cylindroma is clearly malignant, and resection is indicated.

26. Which is better, rigid or flexible bronchoscopy?

Although some may advocate one method over the other, each has specific limitations and indications (see Questions 5 and 7). Depending on the problem, the bronchoscopist should be able to perform either technique.

BIBLIOGRAPHY

1. Ahmad M, Dweik RA: Future of flexible bronchoscopy. Clin Chest Med 20:1–17, 1999.
2. Baughman RP, Pina EM: Role of bronchoscopy in lung cancer research. Clin Chest Med 20:191–199, 1999.
3. Dweik RA, Stoller JK: Role of bronchoscopy in massive hemoptysis. Clin Chest Med 20:89–105, 1999.
4. George PJ: Fluorescence bronchoscopy for the early detection of lung cancer. Thorax 54:180–183, 1999.
5. Hopper KD: CT bronchoscopy. Semin Ultrasound CT MR 20:10–15, 1999.
6. Ikeda S: Flexible bronchofiberscope. Ann Otol Rhinol Laryngol 79:916–925, 1970. (A classic)
7. Jackson C, Jackson CL: Bronchoesophagology. Philadelphia, W.B. Saunders, 1950. (Another classic)
8. Kennedy TC, Miller Y, Prindiville S: Screening for lung cancer revisited and the role of sputum cytology and fluorescence bronchoscopy in a high-risk group. Chest 117(4 Suppl 1):72S–79S, 2000.
9. Liebler JM, Markin CJ: Fiberoptic bronchoscopy for diagnosis and treatment. Crit Care Clin 16:83–100, 2000.
10. Mares DC, Wilkes DS: Bronchoscopy in the diagnosis of respiratory infections. Curr Opin Pulm Med 4:123–129, 1998.
11. Miller JI Jr: Rigid bronchoscopy. Chest Surg Clin North Am 6:161–167, 1996.
12. Niederman MS: Bronchoscopy in nonresolving nosocomial pneumonia. Chest 117(4 Suppl 2):212S–218S, 2000.
13. Nusair S, Kramer MR: The role of fibre-optic bronchoscopy in solid organ, transplant patients with pulmonary infections. Respir Med 93:621–629, 1999.
14. Raoof S, Rosen MJ, Kahn FA: Role of bronchoscopy in AIDS. Clin Chest Med 20:63–76, 1999.
15. Stradling P: Diagnostic Bronchoscopy: A Teaching Manual, 6th ed. New York, Churchill Livingstone, 1991.

39. MEDIASTINOSCOPY

Bruce W. Jafek, M.D., FACS, FRSM, and Marvin Pomerantz, M.D.

1. What is mediastinoscopy?

Mediastinoscopy is a method for exploring and biopsying lesions in the superior mediastinum. It can be used to define the resectability of bronchogenic cancer, determine cancer spread prior to thoracotomy, and provide pathologic confirmation of mediastinal masses. Mediastinoscopy assists in the accurate staging of lung cancer. It helps to identify patients who will gain little benefit from a thoracotomy, therefore sparing them the risks of a major surgical procedure. It is, however, used less frequently in the classic manner as time goes on, as newer video-assisted procedures become more widely available.

2. Who is the "father of mediastinoscopy"?

Eric Carlens, who described the endoscopic technique in 1959.

3. What are the indications for mediastinoscopy?

Absolute and Relative Indications for Mediastinoscopy

Absolute indications
    Presence of enlarged mediastinal lymph nodes (> 1.5 cm) on CT scan
Relative indications
    Presence of T2 or T3 primary lesion
    Presence of lesions located within the inner third of the lung field
    Presence of adenocarcinoma or large-cell undifferentiated tumors on preoperative biopsy
    Presence of small-cell cytology on preoperative biopsy with apparently resectable stage 1 lesions
    Suspected presence of multiple primary lesions or synchronous lung tumors
    Presence of vocal cord paralysis in the setting of left upper lobe primary lesion
    Intent to use neoadjuvant therapy

From Sugarbaker DS, Strauss GM: Advances in surgical staging and therapy of non-small-cell lung cancer. Semin Oncol 20:163–172, 1993, with permission.

4. How is the dissection made in preparation for mediastinoscopy?

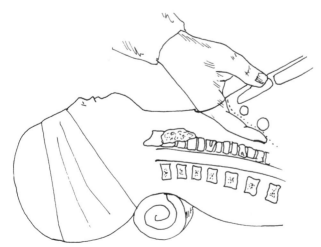

Dissection into the mediastinum. (From Jepsen O: Mediastinoscopy. Copenhagen, Munksgaard, 1966, with permission.)

The patient is placed on the back with a roll under the shoulders. A 2- to 3-cm curvilinear incision is made just above the suprasternal notch and is carried deeper until the pretracheal fascia is reached. The fascia is then incised to confirm the presence of tracheal rings. Blunt finger dissection is carried down into the superior mediastinum, with careful palpation anteriorly for the innominate artery. The dissection must be performed beneath the innominate artery to avoid injury to this vessel. Usually, the tip of the surgeon's finger can reach the carina and may feel the pulsation of the aortic arch deep in the superior mediastinum. The mediastinoscope is then inserted, and the necessary diagnostic or therapeutic measures are performed.

5. What are the divisions of the mediastinum? Why are these important?

The mediastinum is systematically divided into **superior** and **inferior** halves. The inferior portion is further divided into **anterior, middle,** and **posterior** portions. Ordinarily, only lesions that occupy the superior mediastinum are accessible to mediastinoscopy. Intrathoracic metastases are commonly found in the superior mediastinum, as are primary mediastinal tumors such as lymphoma and germ cell tumors. The heart occupies the middle mediastinum. Neurogenic neoplasms commonly are found in the posterior mediastinum.

6. Where is the innominate artery in the mediastinum?

The innominate artery is usually in the anterior mediastinum. Mediastinoscopy occurs deep to and inferior to this vessel. In approximately 25% of cases, the innominate may rise above the suprasternal notch, where it may be subject to injury.

7. How far down in the thorax can you reach with mediastinoscopy?

Mast and Jafek reported a fairly consistent distance of 11 cm from the cricoid cartilage to the carina in adults. The mediastinoscopist should find this well within the range of the 14.5-cm mediastinoscope. This gives access to an average of 31 mediastinal lymph nodes.

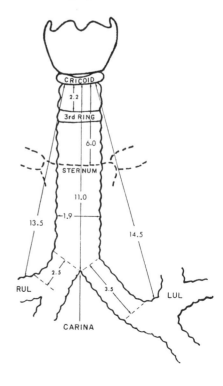

Distances between major cervical and mediastinal landmarks (in cm). RUL = right upper lobe, LUL = left upper lobe. (From Mast WR, Jafek BW: Mediastinal anatomy for the mediastinoscopist. Arch Otol 101:596–599, 1975, with permission.)

8. Where are you unable to reach (and shouldn't try to)?

Lymph nodes that are extremely anterior and those in the aortopulmonary window are difficult to reach by standard mediastinoscopy. Lymph nodes in the posterior mediastinum (posterior subcarinal and paraesophageal nodes) are inaccessible.

9. How does the lymphatic drainage of the lungs relate to tumor spread?

A number of lymph node groups are identified within the chest, and there are many anatomic variations in normal lymphatic drainage of the lungs and adjacent esophagus. Under pathologic conditions, blockage of lymph nodes may lead to collateral and retrograde lymph flow, resulting in deviations from predicted lymphatic spread patterns in bronchogenic carcinoma. Generally, sidedness (e.g., right lung to right nodes) and position (e.g., superior lung field to superior lymph nodes) are maintained. However, a major part of the left lung lymphatics may drain into the inferior tracheobronchial nodes and subsequently into the right paratracheal nodes. Therefore, the site of the primary tumor helps to guide the mediastinoscopist to the proper node chain.

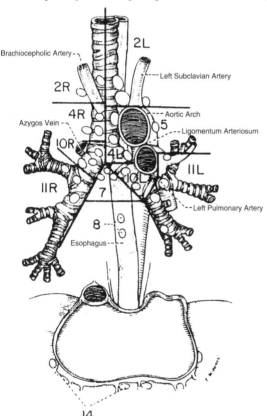

X   **Supraclavicular nodes.**

2R **Right upper paratracheal nodes.** Nodes to the right of the midline of the trachea, between the intersection of the caudal margin of the brachiocephalic artery with the trachea and the apex of the lung or above the level of the aortic arch.

2L **Left upper paratracheal nodes.** Nodes to the left of the midline of the trachea, between the top of the aortic arch and the apex of the lung.

4R **Right lower paratracheal nodes.** Nodes to the right of the midline of the trachea, between the cephalic border of the azygos vein and the intersection of the caudal margin of the brachiocephalic artery with the right side of the trachea or the top of the aortic arch.

4L **Left lower paratracheal nodes.** Nodes to the left of the midline of the trachea, between the top of the aortic arch and the level of the carina, medial to the ligamentum arteriosum.

5   **Aortopulmonary nodes.** Subaortic and paraaortic nodes, lateral to the ligamentum arteriosum or the aorta or left pulmonary artery, proximal to the first branch of the left pulmonary artery.

6   **Anterior mediastinal nodes.** Nodes anterior to the ascending aorta or the innominate artery.

7   **Subcarinal nodes.** Nodes arising caudal to the carina of the trachea but not associated with the lower lobe bronchi or arteries within the lung.

8   **Paraesophageal nodes.** Nodes dorsal to the posterior wall of the trachea and to the right or the left of the midline of the esophagus below the level of the subcarinal region. (Nodes around the descending aorta should also be included.)

9   **Right or left pulmonary ligament nodes.** Nodes within the right or left pulmonary ligament.

10R **Right tracheobronchial nodes.** Nodes to the right of the midline of the trachea, from the level of the cephalic border of the azygos vein to the origin of the right upper lobe bronchus.

10L **Left peribronchial nodes.** Nodes to the left of the midline of the trachea, between the carina and the left upper lobe bronchus, medial to ligamentum arteriosum.

11 **Intrapulmonary nodes.** Nodes removed in the right or left lung specimen, plus those distal to the mainstem bronchi or secondary carina (includes interlobar, lobar, and segmental nodes)

14 **Superior diaphragmatic nodes.** Nodes adjacent to the pericardium within 2 cm of the diaphragm.

10. Why do you aspirate lesions or lymph nodes prior to biopsy?

When a mass is encountered, you may not be able to palpate it directly to evaluate for pulsation. Therefore, before biopsying any mass, you should aspirate it to ensure that it is not a vascular structure. As carefully as possible, lesions should be bluntly dissected to inspect the lesion for consistency. This may be difficult and time-consuming if a lymph node exhibits extracapsular spread and adherence to adjacent tissue. Blind biopsies should never be performed during mediastinoscopy.

11. What happens if you enter the aortic arch, pulmonary artery, or innominate artery?

Major vascular injury is the most dangerous complication of this procedure. Direct pressure should be placed on the area, optimally by a finger, and an immediate sternotomy should be performed to control the bleeding. However, this may not be possible, and the patient may exsanguinate. The superior vena cava, azygos vein, and other vessels are also at risk, but injury to these structures is less likely to lead to patient death.

12. What are some common complications that occur with mediastinoscopy?

In addition to major vascular injury, which is the most hazardous complication, other vital structures in the immediate vicinity of the operative field also pose potential hazards. If the surgeon has a thorough knowledge of the relevant anatomy and follows a gentle, meticulous approach, the risk of complications should be very low. Described complications include pleural damage leading to pneumothorax or hemothorax, left recurrent laryngeal nerve damage, tracheal or esophageal trauma, mediastinitis, wound infection, and tumor seeding. In patients with superior vena caval syndrome, special care is necessary due to venous engorgement.

13. What tests should be performed prior to mediastinoscopy to evaluate resectability of lung cancer?

A number of preoperative studies may be helpful in determining resectability, including radiographs, full-chest computed tomographic (CT) scan, bronchoscopy, and cardiac and pulmonary function tests. By means of these examinations, as many as 50% of all diagnosed patients may be found to have unresectable tumors; in this case, biopsy may still be indicated in the mediastinum, to obtain diagnostic tissue, but thoracotomy may be avoided. The role of positron emission tomography (PET) scan is yet to be defined.

14. What are the absolute contraindications to thoracotomy?

Absolute contraindications to thoracotomy, and therefore unresectability, are **invasive growth** into the mediastinum and **advanced small-cell carcinoma.** Although most thoracic surgeons feel that a single distal lymph node does not exclude the possibility of resection, **contralateral spread** or **fixation** is also an absolute contraindication to thoracotomy.

15. How is lung cancer staged?

Staging of Lung Cancer: TNM Classification

Primary Tumor (T)

Tx   Tumor proven by the presence of malignant cells in bronchopulmonary secretions but not visualized roentgenographically or bronchoscopically, or any tumor that cannot be assessed (as in retreatment staging).

T0   No evidence of primary tumor.

Tis Carcinoma *in situ*

T1   A tumor that is ≤ 3.0 cm in greatest dimension, surrounded by lung of visceral pleura, and without evidence of invasion proximal to a lobar bronchus at bronchoscopy.

T2   A tumor > 3.0 cm in greatest diameter or a tumor of any size that either invades the visceral pleura or has associated atelectasis or obstructive pneumonitis extending to the hilar region. At bronchoscopy, the proximal extent of demonstrable tumor must be within a lobar bronchus or at least 2.0 cm distal to the carina. Any associated atelectasis or obstructive pneumonitis must involve less than an entire lung.

Continued on next page.

T3   A tumor of any size with direct extension into the chest wall (including superior sulcus tumors), diaphragm, or mediastinal pleura or pericardium without involving the heart, great vessels, trachea, esophagus, or vertebral body, or a tumor in the main bronchus within 2 cm of the carina without involving the carina.

T4   A tumor of any size with invasion of the mediastinum or involving heart, great vessels, trachea, esophagus, vertebral body, or carina, or presence of malignant pleural effusion.

Nodal Involvement (N)

N0   No demonstrable metastasis to regional lymph nodes.

N1   Metastasis to lymph nodes in the peribronchial or ipsilateral hilar region, or both, including direct expansion

N2   Metastasis to ipsilateral mediastinal lymph nodes and subcarinal lymph nodes

N3   Metastasis to contralateral mediastinal lymph nodes, contralateral hilar lymph nodes, and ipsilateral or contralateral scalene or supraclavicular lymph nodes.

Distant Metastasis (M)

M0   No (known) distant metastasis

M1   Distant metastasis present—Specify site(s)

From Miller JD, Gorenstein LA, Patterson GA: Staging: The key to rational management of lung cancer. Ann Thorac Surg 53:170–178, 1992, with permission.

Stage Groupings for Lung Cancer

Occult carcinoma	Tx	N0		M0
Stage 0	Tis		Carcinoma in situ	
Stage I	T1	N0		M0
	T2	N0		M0
Stage II	T1	N1		M0
	T2	N1		M0
Stage IIIa	T3	N0		M0
	T3	N1		M0
	T1–3	N2		M0
Stage IIIB	Any T	N3		M0
	T4	Any N		M0
Stage IV	Any T	Any N		M1

From Shields TW: General Thoracic Surgery, 5th ed. Philadelphia, Lea & Febiger, 2000, with permission.

16. How does sarcoid appear by mediastinoscopy?

Classically, mediastinal lymph nodes that have been affected by sarcoid are described as symmetrically enlarged, nonadherent, and somewhat purplish in color. A biopsy of a clinically involved lymph node should yield a positive diagnosis 80–90% of the time. In cross-section, affected nodes appear to possess microscopic noncaseous granulomas, leading to a "pebbly, salt crystal" gross description.

17. What is a "pawn broker" sign?

Historically, pawn brokers suspended three brass balls in front of their shop to identify it. On a radiograph, the marked, symmetrical, and enlarged mediastinal lymph nodes characteristic of sarcoid resemble this symbol. At mediastinoscopy, biopsies of these lymph nodes provide a very reliable method of diagnosis.

18. Does a positive tuberculosis isolate from the mediastinum indicate active tuberculosis?

Bronchogenic carcinoma and tuberculosis may be difficult to distinguish because they generate similar clinical pictures. Mediastinal lymph nodes may harbor healed childhood tuberculosis and may yield positive histology. However, this does not necessarily indicate that the identified intrathoracic disease process is caused by tuberculosis. In addition, attempts to make a diagnosis of tuberculosis by means of mediastinal biopsies are generally not rewarding.

19. How is the diagnosis of silicosis made?

The diagnosis of pulmonary silicosis may be difficult, especially when minimal changes are present on radiograph. Also, silicosis may coexist with tuberculosis, bronchogenic carcinoma, or other intrathoracic pathologic lesion. When mediastinal nodes are biopsied in a patient with silicosis, they are often densely fibrotic and adherent to surrounding structures. Polarized light microscopy showing birefringent crystals is diagnostic for silicosis.

20. What other lesions do you encounter during mediastinoscopy?

Although mediastinoscopy is most commonly used to evaluate the resectability of primary lung tumors, other lesions may be evaluated. Sarcoidosis, metastatic tumors, tuberculosis, mediastinal cysts, lymphoma, Hodgkin's disease, malignant liposarcoma, silicosis, histoplasmosis, thymoma, germ cell tumors, neurogenic tumors, substernal thyroids, and parathyroid adenomas are not rare. Ward even described the removal of a foreign body, a bullet, from the mediastinum. Therefore, the mediastinoscopist must be prepared to evaluate a number of possibilities at surgery.

21. What vascular anomalies can occur in the superior mediastinum?

Knowledge of vascular anomalies of the mediastinum is essential to the mediastinoscopist. The embryologic development of the aortic system is complex, and a number of anomalies may be present. These anomalies include a double aortic arch, anomalous innominate artery, anomalous left common carotid artery, and aberrant right subclavian artery. A right aortic arch with an anomalous right recurrent laryngeal nerve and left ligamentum arteriosum may also be present. Aneurysms may be found in any vessel, most frequently the aorta, and should be diagnosed prior to biopsy.

22. Do other uses exist for mediastinoscopy?

Surgeons have described using the mediastinoscope to assist in the application of heart electrodes for atrial-triggered pacemakers. The mediastinoscope has also been considered for evaluating the resectability of esophageal neoplasms. Approaches to any intrathoracic region are theoretically possible, depending on the length of scope employed. The mediastinoscope has even been used to assist in removing thrombus from pulmonary arteries.

23. How accurate is the standard chest radiograph in evaluating mediastinal metastases?

Mediastinal nodes are apparent on standard chest radiographs when they are large enough to distort the normal mediastinal silhouette or cause widening of the cairn. The standard chest radiograph is hardly sensitive, however; in one study, 72% of patients with positive mediastinoscopy had a normal chest radiograph.

24. What is the diagnostic sensitivity and specificity of mediastinoscopy?

> 90%.

CONTROVERSIES

25. Instead of a diagnostic mediastinoscopy, wouldn't it be simpler and safer to do a supraclavicular fat pad biopsy?

Simpler and safer, yes, but a supraclavicular fat pad biopsy has a much smaller positive yield for intrathoracic disease. Therefore, this technique is now largely of historical interest, except where there is clinical adenopathy in the supraclavicular region or when it is used as a preliminary step in the diagnosis of tuberculosis.

26. A patient with lung cancer has radiologic lymph nodes < 1 cm in the mediastinum. Is mediastinoscopy indicated?

Although some would say that mediastinoscopy is indicated, most would argue that it is probably not beneficial, as the positive yield in this situation is only 10–15%.

27. What contrast studies are helpful in the preoperative evaluation of a patient with lung cancer?

Although some advocate preoperative contrast studies, Miller et al. pointed out that routine radionuclide scans of brain, liver, and bone have no useful role in patients who do not have clinical or laboratory evidence of metastases to these sites. CT studies of the head and abdomen and nuclear bone scans are therefore reserved for patients with (1) signs of symptoms of metastatic disease at any site, (2) a histologic diagnosis of small cell cancer, (3) a previous history of malignancy, and (4) a high risk of resection.

28. Are patients with positive mediastinal lymph nodes candidates for resection?
Attitudes vary from one extreme to the other. Some surgeons consider the presence of malignant mediastinal nodes as a contraindication to thoracotomy and lung resection because the survival rates in these situations are extremely low. At the other extreme, some surgeons recommend lung resection and mediastinal node dissection even when contralateral nodes are involved. This group hopes to improve the salvage rate in a class of patients who have an otherwise dismal prognosis. The most reasonable approach utilizes neoadjuvant therapy for positive N2 nodes. The appropriate therapy for tumors with positive N3 nodes is still unclear.

BIBLIOGRAPHY

1. Aabakken L, Silvestri GA, Hawes R, et al: Cost-efficacy of endoscopic ultrasonography with fine-needle aspiration vs. mediastinotomy in patients with lung cancer and suspected mediastinal adenopathy. Endoscopy 31:707–711, 1999.
2. Barendregt WB, Deleu HW, Joosten HJ: The value of parasternal mediastinoscopy in staging bronchial carcinoma. Eur J Cardiothorac Surg 9:655–658, 1995.
3. Carlens E. Mediastinoscopy: A method for inspection and tissue biopsy in the superiormediastinum. Dis Chest 36:343–352, 1959. (*A classic*)
4. Ginsberg RJ: Extended cervical mediastinoscopy. Chest Surg Clin North Am 6:21–30, 1996.
5. Jepsen O: Mediastinoscopy. Copenhagen, Munksgaard, 1996. (*A classic*)
6. Kirschner PA: Cervical mediastinoscopy. Chest Surg Clin North Am 6:1–20, 1996.
7. Mast WR, Jafek BW: Mediastinal anatomy for the mediastinoscopist. Arch Otol 101:596–599, 1975.
8. Mentzer SJ, Swanson SJ, DeCamp MM, Bueno R, Sugarbaker DJ: Mediastinoscopy, thoracoscopy, and video-assisted thoracic surgery in the diagnosis and staging of lung cancer. Chest 112 (Suppl):239S–241S, 1997.
9. Serna DL, Aryan HE, Chang KJ, et al: An early comparison between endoscopic ultrasound-guided fine-needle aspiration and mediastinoscopy for diagnosis of mediastinal malignancy. Am Surg 64:1014–1018, 1998.
10. Urschel JD: Conservative management (packing) of hemorrhage complicating mediastinoscopy. Ann Thorac Cardiovasc Surg 6:9–12, 2000.
11. Ward PH, Jafek BW, Harris P: Interesting and unusual lesions encountered during mediastinoscopy. Ann Otol Rhinol Laryngol 80:487–491, 1971.

VI. Tumors

---

40. SALIVARY GLAND TUMORS

Bruce W. Jafek, M.D., FACS, FRSM

---

1. Name the most common benign tumors of the salivary glands.

Pleomorphic adenoma   Benign cyst
Warthin's tumor   Lymphoepithelial lesions
Monomorphic adenoma   Oncocytoma

2. What are the most common malignant tumors of the salivary gland?

Mucoepidermoid carcinoma   Adenocarcinoma
Malignant mixed   Adenoid cystic carcinoma
Acinic cell carcinoma   Epidermoid carcinoma

Some of these malignancies are low-grade, some are intermediate-grade, and some are high-grade. Mucoepidermoid is the most common malignant tumor of the parotid.

3. What are the types of adenoid cystic carcinoma? Why is typing important?

Adenoid cystic carcinomas are typed **tubular, cribriform,** and **solid.** The solid has the worst prognosis and the tubular the best

4. Where do adenoid cystic carcinomas metastasize?

Ninety percent of metastases occur to the lung. These can be resected, with prolongation of patient survival.

5. How does a tumor of the salivary gland typically present?

Patients usually have a clinical history of a slowly enlarging, painless mass in the area of an involved salivary gland (e.g., below the ear for the parotid). Any mass of this type should be considered a tumor until proved otherwise. "Malignant" tumors present in exactly the same way that benign ones do, leading to occasional delay in diagnosis. Pain or neural involvement (e.g., paresis of a branch of the facial nerve) is more common with malignancy and is therefore a more ominous sign.

6. How is salivary gland disease evaluated?

Salivary gland disease is strongly suspected on the basis of the **history** and **physical examination.** Bimanual **palpation** of the involved gland is helpful in evaluating enlargement of the gland or presence of a mass. Palpation of the gland may also express pus or dislodge a stone, assisting in diagnosis. **Sialography,** cannulation of the duct with instillation of contrast material to facilitate radiographic studies, is uncommon except when it is used to confirm benign lymphoepithelial disease. **Computed tomography, magnetic resonance imaging,** and other techniques (e.g., technetium-99 scanning) help to visualize actual or suspected neoplasms, but may not be indicated unless deep extension is suspected. Most of these studies only confirm the presence of a mass.

7. What are the important aspects of the history and physical examination in a patient with a suspected salivary gland tumor?

Historical information should include the rate of growth and presence or absence of pain. Other related history (e.g., keratoconjunctivitis, arthritis) might direct you toward a non-neoplastic cause of salivary gland enlargement, for example Sjögren's syndrome. Other conditions that might produce salivary gland enlargement include bulimia, actinomycosis, tuberculosis, parotitis, mumps, Sjögren's syndrome, and parotid lymphadenitis.

Physical examination should be directed toward determining the size of the mass, skin fixation, cervical adenopathy, and function of all branches of the facial nerve. A complete otolaryngologic examination is obviously in order, focusing on the exclusion of surface neoplasms of the upper aerodigestive tract that might have metastasized to the preparotid lymph nodes.

8. Do any conditions predispose to salivary gland malignancy?

The only apparent influence in the pathogenesis of salivary gland malignancy seems to be a history of radiation exposure to the gland.

9. Why is a facial nerve palsy in association with a parotid mass significant?

A facial nerve palsy suggests that the underlying mass is malignant and has invaded the nerve, producing the dysfunction. Coexisting palsy or paresis is uncommon with benign neoplasms, but may occur secondary to pressure.

10. Why shouldn't the parotid mass be biopsied directly?

- Risk of injury to the facial nerve. The tumor may have displaced the facial nerve to an abnormal location, and the surgeon may inadvertently injure the nerve because of its unexpected position.
- Risk of tumor spillage. Tumor spillage increases the incidence of recurrence, even for benign lesions.

A fine-needle aspiration is 95% sensitive, and therefore, many surgeons regard it as a very appropriate diagnostic tool. Other surgeons may prefer to do a superficial parotidectomy primarily, as this procedure is therapeutic as well as diagnostic.

11. How do low-grade and high-grade salivary gland malignancies differ in clinical behavior?

Among the malignant salivary gland tumors, some behave in a relatively benign fashion, whereas others are relatively aggressive. The relatively benign or low-grade tumors include acinic cell carcinoma, low-grade mucoepidermoid carcinoma, and "malignant" oncocytoma. The relatively aggressive or high-grade tumors include adenoid cystic carcinoma, squamous cell carcinoma, adenocarcinoma, carcinoma ex pleomorphic adenoma, and high-grade mucoepidermoid carcinoma. In general, as a rule of thumb, benign tumors of the salivary glands behave in a less "benign" fashion than benign tumors do usually and malignant tumors are less "malignant" than most malignant tumors.

12. Describe the staging system for salivary gland tumors.

1997 American Joint Commission Staging System

TUMOR	
Tx	Tumor extent unknown or can't be assessed
T0	No evidence of primary tumor
T1	Tumor < 2 cm in greatest diameter, without parenchymal extension
T2	Tumor > 2 cm but < 4 cm in greatest diameter, without parenchymal extension
T3	Tumor > 4 cm but < 6 cm in greatest diameter, or extraparenchymal extension without facial nerve involvement
T4	Tumor > 6 cm in greatest diameter, or invades skull base, or with facial nerve involvement

All categories are subdivided:
  a. No local extension
  b. Local extension, defined as clinical evidence of skin, soft tissue, bone, or nerve invasion

Continues on next page.

LYMPH NODES

N0	No regional lymph node metastasis
N1	Metastasis in a single ipsilateral lymph node, < 3 cm in greatest diameter
N2a	Metastasis in a single ipsilateral lymph node > 3 cm but < 6 cm in greatest diameter
N2b	Metastases in multiple ipsilateral lymph nodes, none > 6 cm in greatest diameter
N2c	Metastases in bilateral or contralateral lymph nodes, none > 6 cm in greatest diameter
N3	Metastasis in a lymph node > 6 cm in greatest diameter
Distant metastasis	
M0	No distant metastasis
M1	Distant metastasis

13. How are parotid malignancies of the various grades managed?

Group 1: This group includes T1 and T2N0 low-grade malignancies (mucoepidermoid low-grade and acinous). Excision of the tumor with a cuff of normal tissue is recommended. Regional lymph nodes should be evaluated at the time of surgery. The facial nerve is preserved.

Group 2: This group includes T1 and T2N0 high-grade malignancies (adenocarcinoma, malignant mixed, undifferentiated, and squamous). Total parotidectomy with excision of digastric nodes and preservation of the facial nerve is recommended. If the nerve is involved, it is resected back to clear margins on frozen section and immediately grafted. All patients receive wide-field radiation to include the upper-echelon nodes.

Group 3: This group includes T3N0 or any N+ high-grade cancers and recurrent cancers. Radical parotidectomy with sacrifice of the facial nerve and modified neck dissection is recommended for N0 tumors. Radical neck dissection is recommended for N+ tumors. If there is evidence of facial nerve involvement into the mastoid, the nerve must be followed until negative margins are obtained. Primary nerve grafting is recommended. Postoperative radiation therapy is given to a wide field, from skull base to clavicle.

Group 4: This group includes all T4 tumors. In addition to radical parotidectomy and neck dissection, surgery may sometimes include resection of the masseter muscle, buccal fat pad, skin, mandible, ear canal, mastoid, or other involved structures as necessary. Postoperative radiotherapy is routine, and the facial nerve is grafted.

14. How is a parotid tumor removed?

Previously, tumors were "shelled out," which resulted in frequent recurrence. Current technique dictates excision of the tumor with a surrounding cuff of normal parotid tissue. This procedure is usually accomplished with a superficial lobectomy. The facial nerve must be carefully identified and spared.

15. During an operation on the parotid, where do you find the facial nerve?

This is a classic secret! The facial nerve is most often located just inferior to the external auditory canal, where it exits the stylomastoid foramen, approximately 6 cm medial to the tympanomastoid suture. The "tragal pointer" points at the stylomastoid foramen, and hence the trunk of the nerve, here. The surgeon must know other ways to find the nerve in difficult cases. The facial nerve is just superficial to the retrofacial (hence the name) vein at the inferior portion of the gland. The nerve trunk is found just superior to the cephalic portion of the posterior belly of the digastric muscle. The nerve lies just superficial to the styloid process on its posterolateral aspect. Occasionally (especially in the case of larger tumors, overlying the area of the stylomastoid foramen), the facial nerve must be found by retrograde dissection. The marginal mandibular branch of the facial nerve passes over the facial artery and vein at the anterior border of the masseter. The zygomatic branch crosses the zygomatic arch two-thirds of the way from the tragus to the lateral canthus of the eye. If all else fails, the otolaryngologist can drill out the mastoid process to identify the nerve (cortical mastoidectomy) and follow the nerve peripherally.

16. What if the tumor is in the deep "lobe" of the parotid?

Fortunately, deep lobe tumors are uncommon, as they necessitate a complex surgery. The facial nerve is identified, and a superficial lobectomy is performed. The nerve is then carefully freed from the underlying tumor, if the nerve is not invaded, and the tumor is removed with a cuff of normal gland.

17. What constitutes an "adequate operation" for a benign mixed tumor?

The pressure of an expanding benign mixed tumor compresses the surrounding salivary parenchyma, resulting in fibrosis and creating what is referred to as **false capsule.** The false capsule is frequently incomplete, and tumor may project through the dehiscences and contact surrounding gland tissue. The lack of a complete capsule is a compelling reason for removing these tumors with wide margins. Once, these tumors were treated with enucleation, but this surgery resulted in an unacceptably high rate of recurrence, often as high as 40% over a 30-year period. Enucleation has now been largely abandoned in favor of superficial parotidectomies.

18. If a benign mixed tumors recurs, what action should be taken?

A recurrent mixed tumor is to be feared. It often represents not a discrete mass but a multiplicity of nodules. A recurrence may appear in the previous scar, subcutaneous tissue, superficial or deep parotid parenchyma, facial nerve sheath, or perichondrium of the external meatus. Further attempts at surgery may be fruitless given the widespread nature of this condition, and further surgery is highly likely to cause damage to the facial nerve. Therefore, radiation may be the best treatment. An eventual malignancy is seen in 2–5% of cases.

19. Is radiotherapy indicated in the treatment of a parotid tumor?

Indications for postoperative radiation therapy include:

High-grade tumors   Documented lymph node metastasis
Gross or microscopic residual disease   Extraparotid extension
Tumors involving or close to the facial nerve Deep lobe cancers
Recurrent disease   All T3 and T4 cancers

20. Discuss the potential complications following parotid surgery.

Common complications include skin slap necrosis, hematoma, infection, and salivary fistula. **Hematoma** is generally related to inadequate hemostasis at the time of surgery. Treatment involves evacuation of the hematoma and hemostasis. **Salivary fistula** is a rare complication and usually responds to treatment with pressure dressings. It usually presents as an opening in the suture line below the lobule of the ear. A **temporary facial paresis** may occur in 10% of patients. It is seen more commonly in older patients, those with circulatory compromise (diabetes), and patients with deep lobe tumors. Permanent facial nerve dysfunction is uncommon (< 2% of patients). **Frey's syndrome** may occur in as many as 40% of parotid surgeries.

21. What is Frey's syndrome?

Frey's syndrome, also called **gustatory sweating,** is flushing and sweating of the skin overlying the surgical site. It occurs because of the postoperative growth of the interrupted preganglionic parasympathetic nerve branches to the parotid into the more superficial sweat glands. It may also occur following submandibular gland excision. The diagnosis is usually made from the history but can be confirmed by the starch-iodine test.

22. How is the starch-iodine test done?

Paint the affected skin with iodine, allow it to dry, dust the skin with starch, and feed the patient. The appearance of a bluish discoloration on the overlying skin is diagnostic. It is due to a reaction of the starch and iodine in the presence of moisture (sweat).

23. How do you treat Frey's syndrome?

Although Frey's syndrome is usually a very minor problem, it may require treatment.

Jacobsen's neurectomy involves surgically interrupting the preganglionic parasympathetic nerves in the ear, which run to the parotid. Frey's syndrome may also be treated by re-elevating the skin flap and placing tissue, such as fascia, under the flap to prevent re-innervation. Parasympatholytic creams such as 1% glycopyrrolate lotion may also be applied to the skin.

24. Which parotid masses occur in children?

Parotid masses in children are very unusual, with only 3% of all parotid neoplasms occurring in the first 16 years of life.

Mixed tumors are by far the most common benign epithelial neoplasm in children. The peak incidence occurs at 10 years of age. The tumor behavior and treatment do not differ from those of similar tumors in adults.

Hemangiomas are the next most common, accounting for nearly 10% of all childhood parotid swellings. These tumors are usually present at birth and are located at the angle of the mandible. They are most common in white females. Whether these are true neoplasms or vascular malformations is an unresolved controversy.

Well-differentiated mucoepidermoid carcinoma is the most common malignant tumor in children.

CONTROVERSIES

25. Do benign parotid tumors ever undergo malignant degeneration?

Yes, but rarely. **Carcinoma ex pleomorphic adenoma** has been described. On the other hand, some pathologists argue that the tumor was malignant from the beginning. These masses have been known to grow at an extremely slow rate over many years and then suddenly grow very rapidly. Because the rate changes so rapidly, it appears that some sort of malignant transformation has occurred.

26. Are fine needle aspirates (FNAs) of salivary masses reliable?

FNAs of the salivary glands are notoriously hard to read, with both false negatives and false positives. Their accuracy is directly related to the experience of the pathologist, as well as the preservation technique of the aspirate. "Excisional" biopsy as the initial approach may be best in the younger patient without HIV risk factors (see also Chapter 29, Question 19, for explanation). Excisional biopsy is probably indicated, also, in "nondiagnostic" aspirates in patients without contraindication.

27. Are diagnoses based on frozen sections of salivary tumors reliable?

This remains an area of controversy. It is often difficult for the pathologist to make a definitive diagnosis of a salivary gland neoplasm with frozen sections. The pathologist may require a second opinion and may need to send the specimen to an outside center before a definitive diagnosis can be reached. Many otolaryngologists are reluctant to proceed with a major, destructive operation, risking permanent facial nerve damage, based on a frozen section diagnosis that may or may not be correct. Therefore, these otolaryngologists may perform a superficial parotidectomy and close, with the intention of performing a definitive operation later, should the final pathology require this. The accuracy of the frozen section reading is often related to the experience of the pathologist.

28. Is a neck dissection indicated in the treatment of salivary malignancies?

This is only an issue in the case of selected high-grade salivary malignancies. Most otolaryngologists feel that it is indicated only when there is palpable, preoperative adenopathy or when a positive fine-needle aspirate of the involved mass has been obtained. The risk of occult metastasis to the cervical nodes is < 25%.

SALIVARY GLAND MALIGNANCY METASTASES

Cervical lymph node metastases are not common in patients with cancer of the major salivary glands. The reported incidence of clinical nymph node metastases is 16% carcinomas of the parotid and 8% for submandibular and sublingual gland carcinomas. These regional metastases, when they occur, have a profound effect on prognosis. The 5-year survival rate for patients with previously untreated parotid cancer is 74% when the regional lymph nodes are not involved and only 9% when they are clinically histologically positive. The corresponding figures for patients with submandibular gland cancers are 41% and 9%.

~Medina JE: Neck dissection in the treatment of cancer of major salivary glands.
Otolaryngol Clin North Am 31:815, 1998.

BIBLIOGRAPHY

1. Carlson GW: The salivary glands: Embryology, anatomy, and surgical applications. Surg Clin North Am 80:261–273, 2000.
2. Dawson AK, Orr JA: Long-term results of local extension and radiotherapy in pleomorphic adenoma of the parotid. Int J Radiat Oncol Biol Phys 11:451–455, 1985.
3. English GM (ed): Otolaryngology, vol 5 [ch 30–31]. Philadelphia, J.B. Lippincott, 2000.
4. Gallo O: New insights into the pathogenesis of Warthin's tumor. Euro J Cancer Part B Oral Oncol 31B:211–215, 1995.
5. Medina JE: Neck dissection in the treatment of cancer of major salivary glands. Otolaryngol Clin North Am 31:815–822, 1998.
6. Sinha UK, Ng M: Surgery of the salivary glands. Otolaryngol North Am 32:887–906, 1999.
7. Spiro RH: Changing trends in the management of salivary tumors. Semin Surg Oncol 11:240–245, 1995.
8. Spiro RH: Management of malignant tumors of the salivary glands. Oncology (Huntington), 12:671–680; discussion 683, 1998.
9. Stewart CJ, MacKenzie K, McGarry GW, et al: Fine-needle aspiration cytology of salivary gland: A review of 341 cases. Diagn Cytopathol 22:139–146, 2000.
10. Sur RK, Donde B, Levin V, et al: Adenoid cystic carcinoma of the salivary glands: A review of 10 years. Laryngoscope 107:1276–1280, 1997.
11. Westra WH: The surgical pathology of salivary gland neoplasms. Otolaryngol Clin North Am 32:919–943, 1999.

41. TUMORS OF THE ORAL CAVITY AND PHARYNX

Vincent D. Eusterman, M.D., D.D.S.

1. Name the anatomic structures making up the oral cavity.

The oral cavity, extending from the vermilion border of the lips to the circumvallate papillae and the junction of the hard and soft palate, is composed of eight areas.

Lips	Retromolar gingiva
Buccal mucosa	Floor of the mouth
Lower alveolar ridge	Hard palate
Upper alveolar ridge	Oral tongue (anterior two-thirds of tongue)

2. What are the anatomic subdivisions of the pharynx?

The human pharynx is divided into three anatomic areas: the **nasopharynx** between the skull base and hard palate, the **oral pharynx** between the hard palate and hyoid bone, and the **hypopharynx** between the hyoid bone and lower portion of the cricoid cartilage. Each of these three areas is divided into subunits, which is beneficial for cancer staging. The larynx is not considered part of the pharynx but is significant for tumor staging when involved in the spread of pharyngeal cancer.

- Nasopharynx:
  Posterior superior wall (skull base to the hard palate)
  Lateral wall (including the fossa of Rosenmüller and eustachian tube torus and orifice)
  Inferior wall (superior surface of the soft palate)
- Oropharynx:
  Tongue base (posterior one-third of tongue)
  Vallecula
  Tonsils
  Tonsillar fossa
  Faucial pillars
  Inferior surface of the soft palate
  Pharyngeal wall
- Hypopharynx:
  Pharyngoesophageal junction (postcricoid area)
  Pyriform fossa
  Posterior pharyngeal wall

3. What is the most common benign tumor of the oral cavity and pharynx?

Squamous papilloma. Unlike its nasal and laryngeal counterparts, oral papillomas are not locally invasive, and malignant degeneration is rare. Human papillomavirus (HPV) has been implicated as the cause; however, polymerase chain reaction (PCR) studies of oral papilloma DNA show no evidence of HPV types 6a or 11a, suggesting that HPV may influence oral tumor development differently.

4. Which are the most common odontogenic neoplasms?

Odontogenic neoplasms arise from dental lamina (early ectoderm invagination into the jaw) or any of its derivatives. The **dentigerous cyst** is the most common follicular odontogenic neoplasm, constituting 95% of follicular cysts and 34% of odontogenic cysts. Multiple cysts can be seen in basal cell nevus syndrome and cleidocranial dysostosis. Aggressive neoplasms such as **odontogenic keratocysts** and **ameloblastoma** develop from the epithelial wall of a dentigerous cyst.

5. Which genetic disease is related to multiple osteomas of the jaw?

Osteomas are benign tumors in the oral cavity that may be related to **Gardner's syndrome.**

This autosomal dominant hereditary defect of connective tissue consists of polyposis of the large bowel, epidermoid cysts of the skin, and multiple osteomas of the facial bones. The large bowel polyps appear late to a 40% incidence of malignant degeneration.

6. **What hard palate lesion appears as a painless ulcer and is often confused with malignancy?**
   Uninformed physicians often mistake **necrotizing sialometaplasia** for carcinoma and may treat it as such without an appropriate biopsy to confirm its benign nature. Histologic features include coagulative necrosis of minor salivary glands along with prominent squamous metaplasia of acini and ducts and pseudoepitheliomatous hyperplasia.

7. **List some etiologic factors associated with cancer of the oral cavity and pharynx.**
   Tobacco smoking (cigarettes, cigars, pipes)   Sunlight exposure (carcinoma of the lower lip)
   Smokeless tobacco use   Epstein-Barr virus (nasopharyngeal
   Use of betel nut   carcinoma)
   Heavy alcohol consumption   Plummer-Vinson syndrome (cancer of the
                                                   tongue and hypopharynx)
   Those who use tobacco and alcohol have a 15-fold increase for oral cancer when compared to those who abstain from both.

8. **Describe the premalignant lesions of the oral cavity and pharynx.**
   All white or red patches should be viewed with suspicion:
   Leukoplakia, or white lesions, demonstrate invasive squamous cell carcinoma in 8% of cases, while the remainder represent a spectrum of epithelial hyperplasia (80%), dysplasia (30%), and carcinoma in situ (2%).
   Lichen planus appears as a white lace pattern on the buccal mucosa and has a squamous cell transformation rate of about 4%.
   Erythroplakia, or red velvety plaques on the floor of mouth or gingiva, carry a much higher risk of malignancy than leukoplakia.

9. **What is the most common malignancy of the oral cavity?**
   About 90% of all carcinomas of the oral cavity and pharynx are **squamous cell carcinomas.** Other tumor types include minor salivary gland tumors, sarcomas, lymphomas, and melanoma.

10. **Why do oral and pharyngeal neoplasms cause ear pain?**

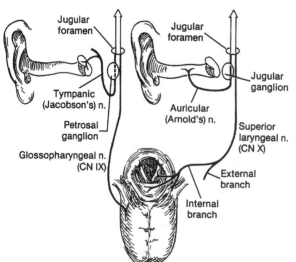

Pathways for referred pain from the oropharynx to the ear. (From Thawley SE, O'Leary MO: Malignant neoplasms of the oropharynx. In Cummings CW, et al (eds): Otolaryngology–Head and Neck Surgery, 3rd ed. St. Louis, Mosby, 1998, with permission.)

Cancers in the oropharyngeal region, which is supplied by cranial nerves IX and X, may cause **referred otalgia,** as the ear also receives sensory innervation along branches of the same nerves and sensory nuclei. A patient complaining of otalgia may be erroneously diagnosed with otitis or temporomandibular joint disease and may be treated with bite splints, antibiotics, or analgesics, while a throat cancer goes undiagnosed.

11. What is the most common oral minor salivary gland cancer? Where is it likely to occur?

Adenoid cystic carcinoma is the most common, accounting for 40% of all minor salivary gland malignancies. Adenocarcinoma (30%) and mucoepidermoid carcinoma (20%) are second and third, respectively. In the oral cavity, most salivary gland cancers occur in the posterior aspect of the hard palate near the greater palatine foramen.

12. The triad of nasal obstruction, nasopharyngeal mass, and recurrent epistaxis in a young male usually represents what nasopharyngeal neoplasm?

Angiofibromas (juvenile nasopharyngeal angiofibromas) are the most common benign tumors of the nasopharynx. Accounting for < 0.05% of head and neck tumors, they are vascular neoplasms that occur only in males, usually during pubescence. This triad of symptoms indicates the presence of an aggressive and destructive neoplasm. If the patient is from China, **nasopharyngeal carcinoma** should also be in the differential diagnosis.

13. What is the etiology of nasopharyngeal carcinoma?

Nasopharyngeal carcinoma (NPC) accounts for 0.25% of all cancers among North American whites, but it accounts for approximately 18% of all malignant tumors among North American Chinese. In southern China, this rate is even higher, where it is the most common cancer in males and the third most common in females. There is a significant increase in HLA-A2 and HLA-B-SIN-2 in Chinese patients with NPC, but this association is not absolute. Other potential etiologic factors include the Epstein-Barr virus, polycyclic hydrocarbons, nitrosamine ingestion, and chronic rhinosinusitis, although the etiology is probably multifactorial.

14. What is the differential for a neck mass?

Remember the mnemonic **KITTENS:**

K Congenital-development (sebaceous cysts, branchial cleft cysts, thyroglossal duct cysts, lymphangioma/hemangioma, dermoid cysts, ectopic thyroid tissue, laryngocele, pharyngeal diverticulum, thymic cysts)

I Infectious-inflammatory (lymphadenitis: bacterial, viral, granulomatous, tuberculous, cat-scratch, actinomycosis, fungal)

T Toxin (unlikely)

T Traumatic (hematoma)

E Endocrine (thyroid, parathyroid, carotid body, tumor, multiple endocrine neoplasia)

N Neoplastic (metastatic: unknown primary, epidermoid carcinoma, melanoma, adenocarcinoma, breast, lung, kidney, gastrointestinal tract; primary: thyroid, lymphoma, salivary, lipoma, angioma, carotid body tumor, rhabdomyosarcoma)

S Systemic, psychiatric

15. How do you evaluate a solitary neck mass?

The first step is a thorough **history** and **head** and **neck examination,** including flexible nasopharyngoscopy. A negative finding on examination and low suspicion for malignancy may indicate an inflammatory node, which can be observed over 2–4 weeks with or without antibiotics. If the lesion persists or enlarges or if the clinical examination finding is suspicious for neoplasm, **fine-needle aspiration** for cytology and culture should be performed. A negative aspirate should not be accepted if the clinical suspicion for malignancy is high and repeat FNA or open biopsy may be required. **Imaging studies** of the neck (magnetic resonance imaging, computed tomography), chest radiography, and **gastrointestinal work-up** (if indicated by fine-needle aspiration) should be done before the lesion is biopsied. An open biopsy should be preceded by **panen-doscopy** (pharyngoscopy, laryngoscopy, esophagoscopy, and bronchoscopy) for an occult primary tumor. Multiple random **biopsies** of the most common occult sites (nasopharynx, tonsil, tongue base and valleculae, and pyriform sinus) should follow a negative panendoscopy; unilateral tonsillectomy, if the tonsils are present, is preferable to tonsil biopsy). If an open biopsy of the neck mass is to be performed during the panendoscopy, the patient and surgeon should be prepared for a neck dissection if metastatic squamous cell carcinoma is found.

16. Why is lymphatic drainage of the oral cavity and pharynx a consideration in treating malignancy?

Carcinoma of the oral cavity and pharynx metastasize at different rates and in different directions. Pharyngeal tissues have abundant lymphatics, and tumors often metastasize earlier and to a greater extent. Also, "silent areas" exist in the pharynx, where lesions of the valleculae or pyriform sinus will remain asymptomatic for a longer time, resulting in great metastatic potential. Tongue-based lesions have extensive bilateral drainage and produce regional metastasis in as many as 70% of cases. Soft palate and other midline tumors spread to bilateral nodes approximately 30–40% of the time. Oral cancers, especially gingival cancers, rarely metastasize. Therefore, the location of the primary tumor and its lymphatic drainage must be taken into consideration when planning treatment of metastatic spread to the neck and other distant sites.

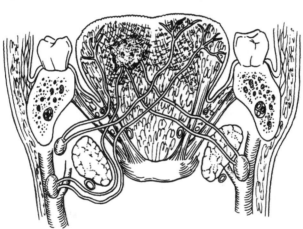

Bilateral lymphatic drainage of the base of the tongue. (From Thawley SE, O'Leary MO: Malignant neoplasms of the oropharynx. In Cummings CW, et al (eds): Otolaryngology– Head and Neck Surgery, 3rd ed. St. Louis, Mosby, 1998, with permission.)

17. How do the rates of occult neck metastasis differ with respect to anatomic site in oral cavity and pharyngeal cancers?

The incidence of occult metastasis increases with the size of the primary tumor and the site. Oral cavity sites such as the tongue (34%) and floor of the mouth (30%) tend to have a high incidence of occult metastasis. In contrast, the lower alveolar ridge (19%) and buccal mucosa (9%) fare much better. Pharyngeal sites such as the pyriform sinus (38%) and tongue base (22%) also have a high incidence of occult metastasis, while the posterior pharynx (0%) is associated with virtually none. With this information, the management of an N0 neck should include surgical or radiation therapy to the nodes that drain the primary tumor.

18. How is cancer of the oral cavity and pharynx staged?

Primary tumors of the oral cavity and oropharynx are predominantly staged according to tumor size. Tumors of the nasopharynx and hypopharynx are staged by the involvement of subsites.

Staging of Oral Cavity and Pharynx Cancer

Oral Cavity and Oropharynx
T1   Tumor < 2 cm
T2   Tumor > 2 but < 4 cm
T3   Tumor > 4 cm
T4   Tumor invades adjacent structures, such as cortical bone, tongue, skin, maxillary sinus, or soft
      tissues of neck.
Nasopharynx
T1   Tumor limited to 1 nasopharyngeal subsite
T2   Involvement of < 1 nasopharyngeal subsite
T3   Invasion of nasal cavity and/or oropharynx
T4   Invasion of skull and/or cranial nerves
Hypopharynx
T1   Tumor limited to 1 hypopharyngeal subsite
T2   Involvement of > 1 hypopharyngeal subsite or adjacent area *without* fixation of the hemilarynx
T3   Involvement of > 1 hypopharyngeal subsite or adjacent area *with* fixation of the hemilarynx
T4   Tumor of adjacent structures (neck soft tissue, etc.)

Neck node staging. (From Lee KJ: the vestibular system and its disorders. In Lee KJ (ed): Essential Otolaryngology–Head and Neck Surgery. Norwalk, CT, Appleton & Lange, 1995, p 539, with permission.)

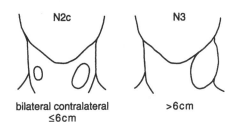

TNM staging of cancers of the oral cavity and pharynx. (From Lee KJ: The vestibular system and its disorders. In Lee KJ (ed): Essential Otolaryngology–Head and Neck Surgery. Norwalk, CT, Appleton & Lange, 1995, p 539, with permission.)

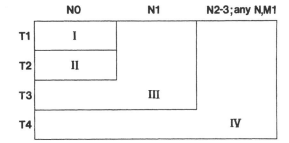

19. A 3.5-cm cancerous-appearing lesion is observed in the tonsillar fossa. It spreads down onto the tongue base, into the vallecula, and to the midline. The patient's neck has a large 3-cm matted node at the angle of the jaw. The remaining examination is incomplete. How is this tumor staged?

T2N2bMx. This lesion is contained entirely within the oral pharynx and is therefore staged similarly to oral cancers, with the T stage being determined by size, not by subunit involvement.

Because the tumor is between 2–4 cm, it is considered a T2 lesion. The jugulodigastric node is matted, representing multiple nodes. Therefore, instead of a single node of 3 cm or less (N1), the nodal status increases to N2b. The presence of the matted nodes also moves the patient from stage III disease to stage IV disease. The "x" means that the staging category cannot be assessed; therefore, Mx designates that distant metastases are unaddressed.

20. What is the treatment of carcinoma of the oral cavity?

Radiation therapy and surgery have proved to be equally efficacious when used to treat stage I and Ii tumors of the oral cavity. Stage III and IV tumors are treated with combination therapy, which consists of surgery with either preoperative or postoperative radiation. As the location of the tumor proceeds anatomically from the front of the lips to the hypopharynx, prognosis becomes poorer.

21. Is chemotherapy effective for the treatment of regionally advanced carcinoma of the oral cavity and pharynx?

Three methods of chemotherapy in local and regional sites in the head and neck have been utilized. **Neoadjuvant chemotherapy,** or induction chemotherapy, is given prior to surgery or irradiation. **Conventional adjuvant chemotherapy** is given after surgery and irradiation. Neither of these methods has improved disease control and survival when compared with regional treatment alone. In contrast, randomized studies looking at **combined modality therapy** (chemotherapy concomitantly with radiation therapy), using 5-fluorouracil or cisplatin in addition to radiation therapy, have found improved disease control and survival over irradiation alone.

22. How do you reconstruct the pharynx following pharyngectomy for cancer?

Oral and pharyngeal tissue following ablative therapy were initially reconstructed with **free skin grafting, local skin flaps,** and **skin muscle flaps.** Owing to the hypovascular effect following radiation therapy, reconstructions often failed because of wound breakdown, fistula formation, and stenosis. **Regional muscle-skin flaps** (pectoralis, trapezius, and latissimus dorsi) had improved outcomes due to the fact that the transferred tissue was vascularized and nonirradiated. These flaps are the current workhorses in head and neck reconstruction. Although time-consuming and expensive, **free vascularized flaps** have been highly successful. Free vascularized flaps are useful in replacing missing tissue with similar tissue and, in most cases, restore sensation, contour, and function.

CONTROVERSIES

23. What is an N0 neck? Why is it controversial?

If there is no clinical or radiographic evidence of nodal spread from a primary oral or pharyngeal cancer, the neck is considered to have an N0 cervical node status. Treatment of the N0 neck is controversial because it can range from close observation with clinical and radiographic examination to surgery or radiation. Because of the high risk of occult metastases, pathologically N0 necks (necks that are clinically negative—no palpable disease—but are found at surgery to harbor histologic metastases) are uncommon with tongue–base lesions, tonsillar fossa lesions, T3 or T4 oral tumors, and T3 or T4 pharyngeal tumors. Observation of the clinically negative neck under these circumstances is not recommended. Surgical treatment of suspected unilateral neck disease should be done with a **functional neck dissection.** For primary tumors with a higher incidence of occult bilateral cervical metastases, bilateral neck irradiation or neck dissections are performed. Patients with advanced cancer and clinically negative necks have no significant differences in neck cancer recurrence rates when the different treatment modalities—elective neck irradiation, neck dissection, and combined treatment—are compared.

—»•«—

THE "COMMANDO" PROCEDURE

The term *commando,* or composite resection, in head and neck surgery refers to the resection of the pharyngeal primary lesion (usually tonsil and lateral pharyngeal wall) in continuity with a partial mandibulectomy and a radical neck dissection with primary closure. This procedure was described by Hayes Martin in the 1930s and is still considered radical therapy today. When originally described, legend has it that it was named for the brave Commandos of wartime fame. The patient had to be similarly brave to undergo the operation. Alternatively, it may have been named for the surgeon, who was characterized by his or her bravery in *performing* the operation! The author feels that the former is probably more likely, given the absence of antibiotics and relatively primitive anesthetic and surgical techniques of the times. Commando procedures with primary closure may leave significant cosmetic and functional handicaps, including facial deformity, malocclusion, nasal regurgitation, aspiration, and speech and deglutition difficulties.

—»•«—

BIBLIOGRAPHY

1. Akervall J, Wennerberg J, Mertens F: Chromosomal abnormalities in squamous cell carcinoma of the head and neck. Adv Otorhinolaryngol 56:261–267, 2000.
2. Batsakis JG, Suarez P: Mucosal melanomas: A review. Adv Anat Pathol 7:167–180, 2000.
3. Ganly I, Soutar DS, Kaye SB: Current role of gene therapy in head and neck cancer. Eur J Surg Oncol 26:338–343, 2000.
4. Hicks MJ, Flaitz CM: Oral mucosal melanoma: Epidemiology and pathobiology. Oral Oncol 36:152–169, 2000.
5. Hyde N, Hopper C: Oral cancer: The importance of early referral. Practitioner 243:753, 756–758, 760–761 passim, 1999.
6. Jones A: A general review of he p53 gene and oral squamous cell carcinoma. Ann R Australasian Coll Dent Surg 14:66–69, 1998.
7. Kamer AR, Krebs L, Hoghooghi SA, et al: Proliferative and apoptotic responses in cancers with special reference to oral cancer. Crit Rev Oral Biol Med 10:58–78, 1999.
8. Khuri FR, Shin DM, Glisson BS, et al: Treatment of patients with recurrent or metastatic squamous cell carcinoma of the head and neck: Current status and future directions. Semin Oncol 27(4 Supp 8):25–33, 2000.
9. List MA, Stracks J: Evaluation of quality of life in patients definitively treated for squamous carcinoma of the head and neck. Curr Opin Oncol 12:215–220, 2000.
10. Nemeth Z, Somogyi A, Takacsi-Nagy Z, et al: Possibilities of preventing osteoradionecrosis during complex therapy of tumors of the oral cavity. Pathol Oncol Res 6:53–58, 2000.
11. Polverini PJ, Nor JE: Apoptosis and predisposition to oral cancer. Crit Rev Oral Biol Med 10:139–152, 1999.
12. Posner MR, Colevas AD, Tishler RB: The role of induction chemotherapy in the curative treatment of squamous cell cancer of the head and neck. Semin Oncol 27(4 Suppl 8):13–24, 2000.
13. Rose BR, Thompson CH, Tattersall MH, et al: Squamous carcinoma of the head and neck: Molecular mechanisms and potential biomarkers. Austral N Z J Surg 70:601–606, 2000.
14. Scully C, Porter S: ABC of oral health: Oral cancer. Br Med J 321(7253):97–100, 2000.
15. Wertheimer-Hatch L, Hatch GF 3rd, HatchB S KF, et al: Tumors of the oral cavity and pharynx. Wrld J Surg 24:395–400, 2000.

42. ODONTOGENIC CYSTS, TUMORS, AND RELATED JAW LESIONS

Bruce W. Jafek, M.D., FACS, FRSM

1. What is the differential diagnosis for a mass in the jaw (mandible or maxilla)?

Masses of the jaw generally can be classified into three categories: neoplastic, infectious/inflammatory, and congenital. In addition, the jaws are unique in that they contain teeth, and, therefore, each category can be broken down further into masses related to the teeth (odontogenic) and masses not related to the teeth (nonodontogenic).

2. Name the two most common cystic lesions of the jaw.

Periapical cysts are the most common, representing approximately 55% of jaw cysts. These are inflammatory and odontogenic in origin. They are secondary to inflammation at the apex of a nonvital tooth. They are therefore related to overall poor dental hygiene, and additional dental disease is usually noted in other teeth. Although often asymptomatic, patients may report pain either with biting or percussion. Radiographically, these cysts present as an area of radiolucency attached to a root apex.

Follicular (or dentigerous) cysts are developmental and odontogenic in origin, accounting for about 10% of jaw cysts. These cysts form around the crown of an unerupted but fully formed tooth. Radiographically, they present as a radiolucency at the crown of an unerupted tooth, usually a third molar or canine. Follicular cysts may be quite large (up to 5 cm in diameter).

3. Why is an odontogenic keratocyst (OKC) often difficult to diagnose? Why is its differentiation from other types of cysts important?

OKCs can be difficult to diagnose because they often have a radiologic and/or histologic appearance consistent with other less aggressive cysts. These may occur in association with the crown of an unerupted tooth, thus resembling a follicular cyst, or in association with a tooth root, thus resembling a periapical cyst. Histologically, OKCs can easily be mistaken for follicular cysts, as both have a thin connective tissue wall lined by a thin layer of stratified squamous epithelium. There are, however, specific criteria for the diagnosis of OKC, and these must be evaluated by an experienced pathologist.

The importance of differentiating an OKC from other cysts lies in the fact that OKCs have a very high recurrence rate. Treatment consists of enucleation and curettage, but recurrence rates of 10–60% can be expected. Therefore, the postoperative follow-up for these cases must be much more vigilant and long-term.

4. A patient presents with multiple odontogenic keratocysts and basal cell carcinomas. What genetic syndrome do you suspect?

Basal cell nevus syndrome is associated with the development of multiple odontogenic keratocysts and basal cell carcinomas. This autosomal dominant syndrome affects patients at a young age. The syndrome may be associated with bifid ribs, a wide nasal bridge, and mandibular prognathism, and 85% of patients have calcification of the falx cerebri and 65% have palmar pitting.

5. A patient presents with a swelling in the upper buccal-gingival sulcus. The patient's history is significant for a Caldwell-Luc procedure 1 year ago. What lesion should you consider?

This patient has probably developed a **retention cyst.** This is an inflammatory *non*odontogenic cyst with an iatrogenic cause. A Caldwell-Luc procedure may result in the entrapment of sinus epithelium within the incision tract, forming a retention cyst. Typically, retention cysts are lined with ciliated, columnar (i.e., respiratory) epithelium. Simple excision is usually curative.

6. What is the oral cavity counterpart to basal cell carcinoma of the skin?

Ameloblastoma. The ameloblastic cell resembles the basal cell of basal cell carcinoma. The clinical behavior of an ameloblastoma also resembles that of basal cell carcinoma, as both show local growth and invasion but limited metastatic potential.

7. Describe the characteristics of an ameloblastoma.

Ameloblastomas are benign neoplasms of odontogenic origin. They are rare tumors, accounting for only 1% of all tumors and cysts of the jaws. They arise from odontogenic epithelium or the enamel organ and thus are classified as benign epithelial odontogenic tumors. About 20% of ameloblastomas are associated with impacted teeth or dentigerous cysts. There are several types of ameloblastomas. These lesions may occur at any age, although those associated with a dentigerous cyst or impacted tooth typically occur before the age of 40. The average age at presentation is 34–38 years. The usual symptom is a painless swelling. Radiologically, a multiloculated, radiolucent area resembling "soap bubbles" or "honeycomb" is pathognomonic. These tumors are benign but locally invasive, and the treatment of choice is wide local excision. Histologically, they show a characteristic pattern of follicles lined by tall columnar cells with reversed nuclear polarity. The epithelium is supported by a mature collagenous stroma.

8. How does a malignant ameloblastoma differ from an ameloblastic carcinoma?

In a **malignant ameloblastoma,** the cells retain their benign histologic pattern, but these cells are found to metastasize to lung and lymph nodes. In an **ameloblastic carcinoma,** the cells appear cytologically malignant and metastasize to lung and lymph nodes. Both have a very poor prognosis.

9. What is an ossifying fibroma?

An ossifying fibroma is a slow-growing, nonodontogenic, benign tumor of the mandible and, less frequently, maxilla. This lesion is most common in women in their third to fourth decades. It presents as a well-circumscribed, marble-like mass in the bone. The tumor follows an expansile course and can attain a substantial size. It usually grows slowly, destroying the normal bone and producing facial asymmetry. Radiologically, it can be radiopaque or radiolucent. Normal radiologic landmarks are distorted. With large masses, there can be evidence of both bone destruction and bone formation. The histologic picture demonstrates collagenous stroma and cementoid deposits. Treatment involves excision and curettage.

10. How does fibrous dysplasia affect the jaw?

This benign, hamartomatous lesion affects the maxilla more frequently than the mandible. It most commonly presents in the first or second decade of life. Patients are generally asymptomatic, but this painless swelling may lead to a unilateral facial deformity. Normal bone is replaced by fibrous tissue that calcifies in an abnormal pattern. Radiographically, this lesion has diffuse margins and a "ground-glass" appearance. Fibrous dysplasia is generally associated with a good prognosis. However, a **juvenile aggressive** type of fibrous dysplasia is associated with a rapidly destructive lesion that obliterates tooth buds and is refractory to treatment. Polyostotic fibrous dysplasia may be associated café-au-lait spots and precocious puberty as **Albright's syndrome.**

11. What is cherubism?

Cherubism is a benign, self-limited disease of the jaw bones. This rare congenital disorder displays an autosomal dominant inheritance pattern. It is more common in males and usually presents prior to age 5 with premature tooth displacement and loss. Symmetric mandibular enlargement may lead to a mild cosmetic deformity, giving these children a round, cherub-like face. Radiographically, the lesions are bilateral, multiple, multilocular, well-defined radiolucencies with a thin or absent cortex. The prognosis is generally favorable. Some patients may require facial contouring, but these features generally regress spontaneously by puberty.

12. What history and physical findings are useful in evaluating a patient with jaw swelling?

A complete history and physical examination is the first step in the work-up of a patient with swelling in the jaw. A slow-growing, painless, nonspecific swelling is the usual scenario. Pain or paresthesia may be an indication of neural invasion or compression and must raise the suspicion of a malignant process. Alternatively, pain may be an indication of recent infection of a benign process. Other indicators that raise the suspicion for malignancy include pathologic fractures, malocclusion, and trismus. A bruit over the mass or in the common carotid raises the suspicion of a vascular malformation or tumor.

13. Which tests are basic in the work-up for a swelling in the jaw?

The **panoramic (Panorex) radiograph** is indispensable in the work-up of a swelling in the jaw. The location of the lesion, density of the lesion, presence or absence of septa or loculations, and reaction of surrounding bone and teeth all give specific clues as to the etiology. Well-demarcated lesions surrounded by sclerotic bone are most likely slow-growing and benign. Proximity to teeth, especially diseased teeth, suggests an odontogenic origin. Ill-defined lytic lesions with resorption of bone and neighboring teeth are more likely malignant or at least locally aggressive. A **CT scan** will more accurately identify cortical thinning and local invasion.

A **fine-needle aspiration** (FNA) may be helpful prior to open biopsy. Although the FNA likely will not identify the tumor, it may aid in the identification of a vascular malformation or tumor, preventing the disastrous result of an open biopsy of such a lesion. The final diagnosis usually requires an **open biopsy,** which can be combined with curative procedures, such as curettage or enucleation.

14. Name the three basic treatment modalities for these cysts and tumors of the jaw.

Odontogenic cysts and tumors can be treated by one of three different modalities:

Simple enucleation, with or without curettage, can be used to treat the more benign lesions.

Marginal or segmental resection of the lesion and surrounding bone is usually used for benign but more locally invasive tumors and cysts.

Composite resection of bone and surrounding soft tissues is used for malignant tumors.

15. Which lesions can be treated with enucleation and curettage?

Enucleation and curettage is adequate treatment for virtually all odontogenic cysts and many odontogenic tumors. Odontogenic tumors in this category include odontoma, ameloblastic fibroma and fibro-odontoma, adenomatoid odontogenic tumor, calcifying odontogenic cyst, cementoblastoma, and central cementifying fibroma. The odontogenic keratocyst is a notable exception in this category.

16. What lesions can be treated with marginal or segmental resection of the mandible?

Marginal resection of the mandible involves the resection of only a margin of the mandible, usually the alveolar margin. Segmental resection, on the other hand, involves the resection of a complete segment; that is, the full height of the mandible is resected along a certain portion. Either of these modalities may require reconstruction using some type of bone graft or plate. This modality is appropriate for persistent or locally invasive lesions, including odontogenic keratocyst (especially if recurrent), ameloblastoma, Pindborg tumor, odontogenic myxoma, ameloblastic odontoma, and squamous odontogenic tumor.

17. Which lesions require a composite resection?

Composite resection of bone and surrounding soft tissues may be required for *malignant* tumors of the jaws, especially if there is obvious involvement of the adjacent tissues. A CT scan is helpful in delineating the extent of involvement and in the preoperative planning. These tumors include malignant ameloblastoma, ameloblastic carcinoma, ameloblastic fibrosarcoma or odontosarcoma, or primary intraosseous carcinoma.

18. A patient with an adenomatoid odontogenic tumor undergoes surgery, but portions of the tumor are difficult to access and are left in the maxilla. Should a "second-look" operation be performed to assess recurrence?

Surprisingly, the answer is no. Adenomatoid odontogenic tumors occur in females under the age of 20. Two-thirds occur in the mandible, and most are anterior to the permanent molars. These tumors have a rapid life cycle, which culminates in amyloid and calcific material replacing the cells. Therefore, recurrence is rare, even if the entire tumor is not removed at the time of surgery.

19. What complications may be associated with adenomatoid odontogenic tumors?

Recurrence
Infection
Rapid increase in size
Pathologic fracture of the mandible

CONTROVERSIES

20. How is fibrous dysplasia of the jaw managed?

Treatment of fibrous dysplasia generally consists of conservative surgery, involving shaving and recontouring of the bone. The treatment is cosmetic in nature. No attempt should be made to remove all of the diseased bone, as there is no distinct border. Controversy arises as to the timing of this surgery, and even its necessity. Fibrous dysplasia nearly always "burns itself out" around the age of puberty. Malignant transformation, although rare, can occur.

21. Can a patient wear false teeth if the mandible is reconstructed?

In general, yes. However, the patient may or may not be able to chew food, depending on the size and location of the defect in the mandible and on the type of reconstruction. Controversy exists as to how and when mandibular reconstruction is performed. If the resected segment of the mandible is relatively short and is located at the angle, then some surgeons argue that no reconstruction is necessary. The patient may wear a denture but will not be able to chew with any significant force. Other surgeons favor reconstructing this defect with one sort of bone graft or another, with the goal of giving the patient a strong enough mandible to chew. Similar controversy exists for defects in other segments of the mandible.

22. Which cysts are known to be "fissural"?

In the past, several types of nonodontogenic, developmental cysts were thought to arise from epithelium trapped between fusing embryonic processes. Today, it is known that the **median palatal cyst** is the only true fissural jaw cyst. It is formed by the growth of epithelium that is trapped between the fusing embryonic palatal shelves. Median palatal cysts are rare and present as a prominent midline palatal mass. In the past, it was argued that nasopalatine duct cysts, globulomaxillary cysts, and nasoalveolar cysts were also fissural. However, these arguments have been disproved.

BIBLIOGRAPHY

1. Bataineh AB, al Qudah M: Treatment of mandibular odontogenic keratocysts. Oral Surg Oral Med Oral Pathol Oral Radiol Endod 86:42–47, 1998.
2. Ching AS, Pak MW, Kew J, et al: CT and MR imaging appearances of an extraosseous calcifying epithelial odontogenic tumor (Pindborg tumor). Am J Neuroradiol 21:343–345, 2000.
3. Eversole LR: Malignant epithelial odontogenic tumors. Semin Diagn Pathol 16:317–324, 1999.
4. Han MH, et al: Cystic expansile masses of the maxilla: Differential diagnosis with CT and MR. Am J Neuroradiol 16:333–338, 1995.
5. Henderson JM, Sonnet JR, Schlesinger C, et al: Pulmonary metastasis of ameloblastoma: Case report and review of the literature. Oral Surg Oral Med Oral Pathol Oral Radiol Endod 88:170–176, 1999.
6. Iordanidis S, Makos C, Dimitrakopoulos J, et al: Ameloblastoma of the maxilla. Aust Dent J 44:51–55, 1999.

7. Manor Y, Merdinger O, Katz J, et al: Unusual peripheral odontogenic tumors in the differential diagnosis of gingival swellings. J Clin Periodont 26:806–809, 1999.
8. Melrose RJ: Benign epithelial odontogenic tumors. Semin Diagn Pathol 16:271–287, 1999.
9. Philipsen HP, Reichart PA: Adenomatoid odontogenic tumour: facts and figures. Oral Oncol 35:125–131, 1999.
10. Philipsen HP, Reichart PA: Calcifying epithelial odontogenic tumour: Biological profile based on 181 cases from the
11. Literature. Oral Oncol 36:17–26, 2000.
12. Takata T, Miyauchi M, Ogawa I, et al: So-called 'hybrid' lesion of desmoplastic and conventional ameloblastoma: Report of a case and review of the literature. Pathol Int 49:1014–1018, 1999.
13. Toida M: So-called calcifying odontogenic cyst: Review and discussion on the terminology and classification. J Oral Pathol Med 27:49–52, 1998
14. Tomich CE: Benign mixed odontogenic tumors. Semin Diagn Pathol 16:308–316, 1999.
15. Yoshiura K, Tabata O, Miwa K, et al: Computed tomographic features of calcifying odontogenic cysts. Dento maxillo fac Radiol 27:12–16, 1998.

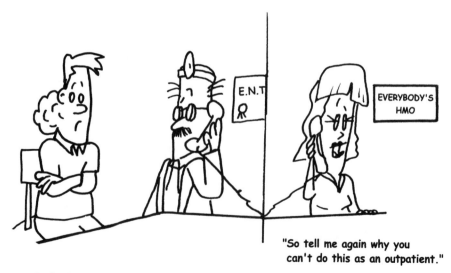

"So tell me again why you can't do this as an outpatient."

Jim Gough

43. TUMORS OF THE NOSE AND PARANASAL SINUSES

Mark R. Mount, M.D.

1. What are the most common benign tumors of the nose and sinuses?
Osteomas are the most common benign tumors, followed by **hemangiomas** and **papillomas.**

2. An inverted papilloma is a benign tumor often misdiagnosed as a nasal polyp. Why is it important to make the correct diagnosis?
Ten to 15% of inverting papillomas will transform into squamous cell carcinoma. If the polyp is simply excised, it may recur aggressively with bony destruction and intracranial extension. Overall, recurrence rates vary from 27–73%.

3. When should one suspect that a nasal polyp might be an inverted papilloma?
These tumors are less translucent than polyps. They are usually unilateral and more commonly present with epistaxis. As a rule, you should biopsy all unilateral nasal polyps in the clinic before surgery unless they are obviously vascular.

4. Which viruses are associated with sinonasal papillomas?
As with genital condylomas, skin warts, and laryngeal papillomas, sinonasal papillomas often contain human papilloma virus (HPV). Epstein-Barr virus recently has been found in 65% of inverted papillomas.

5. What is the clinical significance of HPV when it is present in inverted papilloma?
When HPV is present, there is a higher likelihood of both malignancy and recurrence. HPV types 6 and 11 are associated with benign papillary tumors, whereas types 16 and 18 are weakly associated with malignant degeneration. However, the presence of any HPV strongly predicts recurrence. In one study, 13 of 15 patients with recurrent papilloma were HPV positive, and 10 of 10 patients without recurrence were HPV negative.

6. Does location of a papilloma in the nose affect prognosis?
Yes. A septal papilloma is virtually always a squamous papilloma, with almost no malignant potential. Most lateral nasal wall papillomas, however, are inverted papillomas, which are more aggressive and may become malignant.

7. Unilateral epistaxis in a teenage boy should alert the physician to rule out what tumor?
A **juvenile angiofibroma** is a benign vascular tumor that occurs almost exclusively in adolescent males; various hormonal influences have been suspected, but none have been consistently shown to be abnormal. The presenting symptoms are usually unilateral epistaxis and obstruction. The tumor appears as a smooth lobulated mass. Because it is highly vascular, biopsies should be avoided. Diagnosis is made by inspection and CT scan. Treatment is primarily surgical, as the tumor may be quite aggressive.

8. Why is juvenile angiofibroma rarely seen in men over 30 years of age?
It's unknown. However, this type of tumor is thought to regress spontaneously in many or all patients. There are several reports of residual tumor completely regressing after surgery. Despite the good prognosis, resection of the mass is prudent. This expansive tumor may invade the cranial vault or orbit with devastating consequences before it regresses.

9. What is a pyogenic granuloma?

A pyogenic granuloma, or lobular capillary hemangioma, is a common benign polypoid lesion of the mucosa, usually seen on the septum. It is vascular and may bleed spontaneously. Although it may involute spontaneously, treatment is excision.

10. What is epiphora?

Epiphora is the symptom of **excessive tearing** caused by blockage of the nasolacrimal duct. It is most often a surgical complication. If this symptom presents in a patient who has had no facial surgery, nasal or maxillary sinus tumors obstructing the duct should be considered.

11. Which is the most common malignancy of the nose and paranasal sinuses?

Squamous cell carcinoma accounts for 70% of these cancers, followed by adenocarcinoma (5–10%) and adenoid cystic carcinoma (5–10%). Less common tumors include undifferentiated transitional cell carcinoma, olfactory esthesioneuroblastoma, lymphoma, and malignant melanoma.

12. Where do nose and sinus cancers typically originate?

The maxillary sinus is the most common site (55%), followed by the nasal cavity (35%), ethmoid sinus (9%), and, rarely, sphenoid sinus. Septal cancers are exceedingly rare.

13. Are there any risk factors associated with developing nasal or sinus malignancies?

Certain industrial workers have a predisposition for sinonasal malignancies. Nickel workers have an increase of 100–870 times the normal rate of sinus squamous cell carcinoma. These cancers may develop after 10 or more years of exposure and after 20 years of latency. Wood dust and, to a lesser extent, leatherworking and furniture-making chemicals are exclusively associated with adenocarcinoma. Other inhalants associated with these malignancies include chrome pigment, radium dial paint, mustard gas, and hydrocarbons. Tobacco has shown no association with nasal and sinus cancers. The incidence of nasal and sinus malignancies in males is twice that of females.

14. How do patients with paranasal sinus tumors present?

Usually, patients experience prolonged sinusitis, especially unilateral. Patients may develop epistaxis, numbness, swelling, or nasal congestion. Patients with maxillary sinus tumors may have loose upper teeth or suddenly poor-fitting dentures. Rarely, a patient may experience trismus, palatal numbness, or diplopia. Pain is often a late and therefore ominous symptom. Ethmoid sinus tumors usually spread into vital structures before causing symptoms. They may invade the anterior cranial fossa, orbits, maxillary sinuses, or sphenoid sinuses. Usual symptoms include unilateral nasal obstruction, severe headache, and/or diplopia. The sphenoid sinus lies just inferior and anterior to the optic chiasm and pituitary gland. It lies between the carotid arteries. Tumors in this area present as headache, diplopia, or vision loss. Invasion of the skull base exists in 50% of cases.

15. Does computed tomography (CT) or magnetic resonance imaging (MRI) better evaluate nasal and maxillary tumors?

CT is much better at evaluating bony invasion and destruction. Therefore, it is essential for proper evaluation and preoperative planning. MRI is also useful if there is possible central nervous system or orbital involvement, as MRI is better at distinguishing dura from tumor.

16. What is Ohngren's line?

Ohngren's line is an imaginary line extending from the medial canthus of the eye to the angle of the mandible. Tumors *above* the line have a poorer prognosis because of their tendency to metastasize superiorly and posteriorly. Tumors *below* the line are more easily resected and carry a better prognosis.

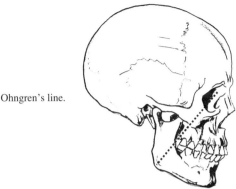

Ohngren's line.

17. Where do nose and sinus tumors metastasize?

To cervical or retropharyngeal nodes. The incidence of cervical metastases on presentation is about 10%, although up to 44% of cases will eventually metastasize to the cervical area. Only 10% of patients ever develop distant metastases.

18. What are the most accepted therapies for cancer of the nose and paranasal sinuses?

Surgery is the mainstay therapy and can be curative if resection is complete. Obviously, surgery is more easily performed on small tumors. Options for resection include inferior maxillectomy, medial maxillectomy, and total maxillectomy. Most centers use postoperative **radiation therapy** for large tumors, positive margins, perineural or perivascular invasion, or lymph node metastases. However, considering the morbidity of radiation in this area, its use is controversial—100% of eyes receiving 58 cGy will develop severe panophthalmopathy with severe corneal ulceration, and 86% of eyes receiving 28–54 cGy will develop cataracts and visual disturbances. Owing to the low overall incidence of nose and paranasal cancer, few studies have adequately compared various therapies. The eventual mortality for all nose and sinus tumors is > 50%.

19. What approaches are available to perform a medial maxillectomy?

Lateral rhinotomy is an incision that traverses the lateral base of the nose, curves around the alar sidewall to the midline, and splits the lip. It affords excellent exposure but leaves a scar. Sometimes the incision is extended under the eye near the lid margin. **Midface degloving procedure** is primarily an intraoral incision in the gingivobuccal sulcus. Intranasally, a transfixion incision is connected to bilateral intercartilaginous incisions. These allow the nose and upper lip to be peeled away from the maxilla. This maneuver spares the patient an external scar but substantially reduces exposure. Also, this technique may cause nasal stenosis.

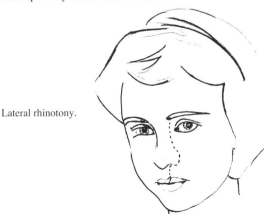

Lateral rhinotony.

20. Is there any role for chemotherapy?

As in many head and neck cancers, chemotherapy's use is expanding. Because it alone does not improve survival, it has been traditionally reserved for end-stage palliation. New protocols show promise for combination chemotherapy with surgery or radiation.

CONTROVERSIES

21. How should an inverting papilloma be removed at its initial presentation?

Aggressively: The traditional and proven approach for treating an inverting papilloma or early carcinoma has been a lateral rhinotomy incision with a **medial maxillectomy.** Because the incidence of malignant change is > 10%, complete removal of the tumor is imperative. Even benign tumors have recurrence rates of up to 70% after conservative resection. Intranasal endoscopic techniques are simply inadequate for total excision and have limited data to support their use.

Conservatively: The **endoscopic approach** to resecting inverted papilloma is gaining popularity. If the tumor does not extend into the maxillary sinus, it may be easily and completely removed with this procedure. A medial maxillectomy is a major procedure with definite morbidity and leaves the patient with a visible deformity. If the tumor can be removed without this operation, it is to the patient's advantage. Several recent authors support the use of this technique with data showing good local control. Treatment should be individualized, but the endoscopic approach is a safe and effective method in appropriate patients.

22. Should orbital exenteration be performed routinely for advanced sinus cancers?

Yes: Despite the obviously unpleasant effect of removing the entire orbit, there is evidence, presented by Ketcham and Van Buren, that this procedure may double the survival rate of patients with ethmoid tumors (50% vs. 30%). Even if exenteration is avoided, the patient will surely go blind in the same eye after radiation therapy. Although unilateral blindness is a functional problem, new techniques in reconstruction and prosthetics have minimized the cosmetic issues caused by exenteration.

No: Although it may be difficult to cure a cancer that invades the orbit, the decision to remove the eye should be heavily weighed. The Ketcham study is contradicted by at least two other studies. One must seriously consider the cosmetic and psychological devastation to the patient before proceeding with exenteration. Use of an aggressive eye-sparing protocol, including preoperative radiation with or without chemotherapy has been shown to effectively treat these cancers and save sight.

BIBLIOGRAPHY

1. Beck JC, McClatchey KD, Lesperance MM, et al: Presence of human papillomavirus predicts recurrence of inverted papilloma. Otolaryngol Head Neck Surg 113:49–55, 1995.
2. Bielamowicz S, Calcaterra TC, Watson D: Inverting papilloma of the head and neck: The UCLA update. Otolaryngol Head Neck Surg 109:71–76, 1993.
3. Buchwald C, Franzmann MB, Jacobsen GK, Lindeberg H: Human papillomavirus in sinonasal papillomas: A study of 78 cases using in situ hybridization and polymerase chain reaction. Laryngoscope 105:66–71, 1995.
4. Catalano PJ, Sen C: Management of anterior ethmoid and frontal sinus tumors. Otolaryngol Clin North Am 28:1157–74, 1995.
5. Choi KN, Rotman M, Aziz H, et al: Concomitant infusion cisplatin and hyperfractionated radiotherapy for locally advanced nasopharyngeal and paranasal sinus tumors. Int J Radiol Oncol Biol Phys 39:823–829, 1997.
6. Lund VJ: Optimum management of inverted papilloma. J Laryngol Otol 114:194–197, 2000.
7. Lyons BM, Donald PJ: Radical surgery for nasal cavity and paranasal sinus tumors. Otolaryngol Clin North Am 24:1499–1521, 1991.
8. Macdonald MR, Le KT, Freeman J, Hui MF, Cheung RK, Dosch HM: A majority of inverted sinonasal papillomas carries Epstein Barr virus genomes. Cancer 75:2307–2312, 1995.

9. Martel MK, Sandler HM, Cornblath WT, et al: Dose-volume complication analysis for visual pathway structures of patients with advanced paranasal sinus tumors. Int J Radiol Oncol Biol Phys 38:273–284, 1997.
10. McCary WS, Levine PA, Cantrell RW: Preservation of the eye in the treatment of sinonasal malignant neoplasms with orbital involvement. Arch Otolaryngol Head Neck Surg 122: 657–659, 1996.11. Meyers EN, Carrau RL: Neoplasms of the nose and paranasal sinuses. In Bailey BJ, Calhoun KH (eds): Head and Neck Surgery—Otolaryngology, Philadelphia, J.B. Lippincott, 1998.
12. Sham CL, Woo JK, van Hasselt CA: Endoscopic resection of inverted papilloma of the nose and paranasal sinuses. J Laryngol Otol 112:758–764, 1998.
13. Spiessl B, et al (ed): UICC TNM Atlas, 3rd ed. Berlin, Springer-Verlag, 1989.

44. LARYNGEAL CANCER

Vincent D. Eusterman, M.D., D.D.S., and Timothy J. Downey, M.D.

1. How frequent is laryngeal cancer? Where does it occur in the larynx?

Laryngeal cancer accounts for 1–5% of all malignancies diagnosed annually, or about 3–8 per 100,000 population. In the United States, this represents about 11,000 new cases annually, with 3700 deaths annually, for a mortality rate of 1.6/10,000. Laryngeal cancer is more common in men (8:1), having a peak incidence in the sixth to seventh decades with an average age of onset at 60–62 years.

Laryngeal cancer generally occures in the glottis (67%), followed by supraglottic (31%) and supraglottic (2%) areas. Ninety-five percent of glottic cancers arise from the true vocal cords. When diagnosed, laryngeal cancer is confined to the larynx in 60% of the cases, 25% will develop regional metastasis, and 15% will have distant metastasis. The incidence of multiple synchronous primary tumors (occurring at the same time) is 0.5–1%, and the incidence of metachronous tumors (occurring at different times) is 5–10%, with lung the most common site.

2. What risk factors predispose to laryngeal carcinoma?

The most important risk factors are **smoking** and **alcohol abuse**. When these two factors are both present, the risk is 50% greater than the additive risk of each. Smokers are 6–39 times more likely to get laryngeal carcinoma than nonsmokers. Less than 5% of laryngeal cancer patients have *no* smoking history. Less important risk factors include esophageal reflux, radiation, presence of laryngocele, and history of juvenile papillomatosis.

3. What types of cancers are found in the larynx?

- Squamous-cell carcinoma (carcinoma in situ; well,   94%
  moderately, and poorly differentiated; spindle-cell variant)
- Verrucous carcinoma   2–4%
- Adenocarcinoma (nonspecific adenocarcinomas, adenoid   1%
  cystic carcinomas, mucoepidermoid carcinomas)
- Sarcomas (fibrosarcoma, chondrosarcoma, malignant   1%
  fibrous histiocytoma, rhabdomyosarcomas)
- Metastatic tumors (melanoma, renal-cell, prostate,   Rare
  breast, lung, stomach)

4. How does laryngeal cancer present?

Glottic carcinoma presents with **hoarseness** as the cardinal symptom. Sore throat, dysphagia, otalgia, and odynophagia may exist alone or with other symptoms. Airway obstruction and hemoptysis are late findings, less common in glottic cancer, and often require emergency treatment.

Supraglottic carcinoma presents with hoarseness (laryngeal fixation, mass effect), odynophagia, dysphagia, otalgia (tongue base, pharyngeal extension), and neck mass.

5. Are laryngeal cancer and lung cancer related?

Yes. In all probability, the inciting factor for laryngeal cancer has a similar effect on lung mucosa. A laryngeal cancer patient has about a 5–10% chance of developing a second primary cancer in the lung after laryngeal therapy and should be followed closely with laryngeal examinations and chest radiographs.

6. Do squamous cell carcinomas of the larynx express oncoproteins?

Cytogenetic evidence has revealed a probable multistep process of carcinogenesis in laryngeal squamous cell carcinomas. Deletions in chromosome 3p and 18q, as well as amplification and over-expression of c-*erb*-B, *int*-2, *bcl*-1, $p21^{N-ras}$, and other oncogenes have been found in some laryngeal carcinomas. Approximately 60% of laryngeal squamous cell carcinomas show mutations of the *p53* tumor suppressor gene. It has been postulated that *p53* may be one of the genetic elements by which tobacco-associated mutagens produce an oncogenic effect on the larynx. However, clinical studies of the overexpression of p53 protein in laryngeal tumors have yielded inconsistent results with regard to survival, metastasis, and response to therapy. Further research in the molecular biology of head and neck carcinomas is necessary to provide ideal cytogenetic markers for detecting premalignant lesions, primary tumors, and metastases as well as determining response to chemotherapy and radiation and prognosis.

7. Have viruses been implicated as causative factors for laryngeal carcinoma?

The herpes simplex virus has been associated with early reports of squamous cell carcinoma of the larynx. Human papilloma virus (HPV), most commonly associated with upper respiratory papillomas and verrucous carcinomas, has also been detected in 5% to 50% of laryngeal squamous carcinomas. HPV probably alters the normal regulation of mucosal squamous cell proliferation by binding the transforming proteins it encodes to the tumor suppressor gene products of *p53* and other oncogenes. Malignant transformation probably requires additional contributing factors such as smoking and alcohol.

8. Describe the anatomic divisions of the larynx. Discuss the way cancer affects these subdivisions.

The larynx is subdivided into three areas: supraglottis, glottis, and subglottis. The **supraglottis** extends from the tip of the epiglottis to the ventricular fold. It has extensive lymphatics that feed the pre-epiglottic space and the neck bilaterally. The incidence of nodal metastasis varies from 25–50% depending on the tumor stage of the primary; 20–35% are bilateral. The **glottis** begins at the ventricular fold and extends 1 cm inferior to the vocal cord. It is the most common laryngeal site for cancer that invades the pre-epiglottic space through cartilage perforations access the "paraglottic space," which communicates with the entire larynx. Fortunately, this region has limited lymphatic drainage and spread to the neck nodes occurs in < 10% of cases. Tumors are detected early because of hoarseness. They are often slow-growing, well-differentiated tumors that extend in predictable ways. The **subglottis** begins 1 cm inferior to the vocal cord and proceeds to the inferior border of the cricoid cartilage. Subglottic carcinoma is often silent and poorly differentiated

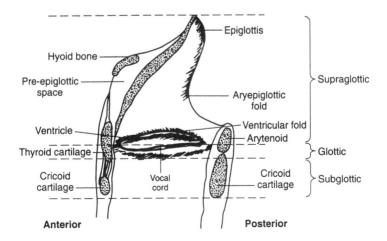

Anatomic subdivisions of the larynx. (From Eisele DW, Clifford AR, Johns ME: Cancer of the larynx, paranasal sinuses, and temporal bone. In Lee KJ (ed): Essential Otolaryngology, 6th ed. Norwalk, Connecticut, Appleton & Lange, 1995, p 556, with permission.)

and extends to and through the cricoid cartilage to involve the paratracheal and cervical lymphatics in a large number of the cases. Prognosis is poor because of the advanced stage at the time of diagnosis. Each division is affected differently, each requires different management, and each has its own prognosis. An accurate diagnosis of cancer in each of these regions is important.

9. What is the significance of the paraglottic space?
This space surrounds the glottis and acts as a conduit for cancer to spread between all divisions of the larynx. Cancers that extend between regions are considered transglottic tumors and have a high incidence of cartilage invasion and a poorer prognosis.

10. What is pyriform sinus cancer? What is its significance to the larynx?
The pyriform sinus is the inferior extent of the hypopharynx just before it turns into the cervical esophagus. It is a funnel-shaped mucosa-lined sinus that invaginates between and around the thyroid and cricoid cartilages. It opens during swallowing to direct food into the esophagus. It is also the site of hypopharyngeal cancer, which is often silent. Medial-wall pyriform sinus cancers invade the larynx through the paraglottic space. Laterally, they invade the thyroid cartilage or pharyngeal wall. They often present late as a neck mass, often with a history of referred ear pain, and require aggressive combined therapy. Three-year survival is about 40% with treatment.

11. What barriers exist in the larynx to check the spread of cancer?
The **quadrangular membrane** above the false cords and the **conus elasticus** between the true cords and cricoid cartilage act as barriers to the spread of cancer. The thyroid and cricoid cartilage is lateral to these structures, and when they become invaded, it suggests a poor prognosis (T4).

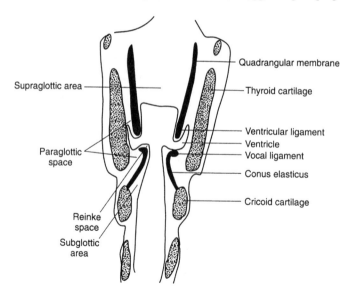

Coronal section of the larynx illustrating the barriers to the spread of cancer. (From Eisele DW, Clifford AR, Johns ME: Cancer of the larynx, paranasal sinuses, and temporal bone. In Lee, KJ (ed): Essential Otolaryngology, 6th ed. Norwalk, Connecticut, Appleton & Lange, 1995, p 557, with permission.)

12. What are the patterns of endolaryngeal lymphatic drainage?
There is a rich superficial lymphatic system throughout the mucosa that is not compartmentalized. The deep system, however, arises from midline structures in the supraglottis and subglottis that form lateral cell masses in the glottis. The deep system drains ipsilaterally, except at the subglottis and pre-epiglottic space, where bilateral drainage occurs.

13. How is laryngeal carcinoma staged?

The American Joint Committee on Cancer (AJCC) uses the TNM classification for laryngeal cancer by anatomic region. Nodal and metastatic staging is identical to that for other forms of head and neck cancers. A hoarse patient with a left fixed cord and a single left 2-cm neck mass would have at least a T3N1Mx classification.

Staging System for Laryngeal Carcinoma

Glottis	
T1	Tumor to vocal cords (involving anterior or posterior commissure) with normal mobility
T1a	Tumor limited to one vocal cord
T1b	Tumor involving both cords
T2	Tumor extending to supra- or subglottis with impaired vocal cord mobility
T3	Tumor confined to larynx with vocal cord fixation
T4	Tumor invading through thyroid cartilage and/or with direct extralaryngeal spread
Supraglottis	
T1	Tumor limited to 1 subsite of supraglottis with normal vocal cord mobility
T2	Tumor involving > 1 subsite of supraglottis or glottis, with impaired vocal cord mobility
T3	Tumor limited to larynx with vocal cord fixation; tumor may invade postcricoid area, medial pyriform sinus, or pre-epiglottic space
T4	Tumor invades beyond thyroid cartilage and/or with extralaryngeal spread
Subglottis	
T1	Tumor limited to subglottis
T2	Tumor extending to glottis with or without impaired vocal cord mobility
T3	Tumor limited to larynx with vocal cord fixation
T4	Tumor invading beyond cricoid or thyroid cartilages, with extralaryngeal tissue spread

14. What is a "fixed cord"?

Vocal cords that have motor neural injury or tumor invasion into the thyroarytenoid muscle or arytenoid cartilage can be "fixed in place," or immobile. A nonworking cord is considered "fixed," and the alert clinician should evaluate the patient for cancer, either in or around the larynx or over the pathway of the vagus and recurrent laryngeal nerve. There are many other causes of vocal cord paralysis (traumatic, infective, congenital, idiopathic, iatrogenic), but neoplastic sources should be ruled out first. Laryngeal cancers with mobile cords are usually staged T1 or T2; however, when cord fixation is present, the stage increases to T3, which drops 5-year survival from 80–95% to 30–57%.

15. How do the survival rates for laryngeal cancer vary by T stage?

Survival is measured as the percent 5-year cure rate. Increased nodal disease reduces these figures significantly, depending on nodal stage.

Supraglottic

T1–T2	75% with either surgery or radiation alone
T3–T4	23% with radiation alone, 52–83% with surgical salvage or surgery alone

Glottic

T1–T2	70–95% with either modality alone
T3	30–40% with radiation with surgical salvage, 50–80% with surgery alone
T4	20% with radiation, 40% with surgery and neck dissection, 50% for combined surgery and radiation

Subglottic

T1–T2	70% with combined therapy
T1–T4	36% with radiation and surgical salvage, 42% with surgery alone

16. How is laryngeal cancer treated?

Current thought concerning treatment for laryngeal cancer supports "organ-sparing" therapy for voice preservation. **Radiation therapy** is ideal for organ-sparing and works well for cases of disease in the lower stages. **Surgical therapy** has evolved to organ-sparing techniques, including partial laryngectomy (horizontal supraglottic, vertical hemilaryngectomy), laryngofissure and cordectomy, and laser cordectomy. Controversy arises with higher stages of disease; patients who do not want to lose their voices can undergo an organ-sparing protocol with **combination therapy** (chemotherapy and radiation). However, these and lower-staged radiation failures generally result in total laryngectomy. Near-total laryngectomy is a surgical procedure to treat advanced-stage disease by constructing a physiologic mucosal shunt with the remaining arytenoid to produce speech. This procedure requires a tracheostomy.

17. Discuss the patient criteria for performing a horizontal supraglottic laryngectomy.

Important to any conservative surgery for laryngeal cancer is that control of the tumor takes precedence over voice preservation. Physiologic parameters are an important consideration with supraglottic laryngectomy. The patient should have near-normal pulmonary function testing and be younger than 65 years of age. Som and Sisson have described criteria that include a 5-mm anterior commissure clearance, normal vocal cord mobility, no cartilage invasion, no tongue extension within 5 mm of the circumvallate papillae, and no extension to postcricoid, arytenoid, interarytenoid, prevertebral fascia, or pyriform sinus apex. Lesions > 3 cm or with fixed cervical nodes are also a contraindication to surgery.

18. Following total laryngectomy, what options are available for alaryngeal speech?

The **electrolarynx** is the most simple and most common method of alaryngeal speaking. The device is a battery-powered, vibratory, buzzing instrument that when held against the neck or cheek produces speech. The upper aerodigestive tract articulates the sound. The electrolarynx can be mastered very quickly. **Esophageal speech** is the most difficult form of alaryngeal speech to master. Esophageal speakers ingest air into the esophagus by oropharyngeal trapping and, as the air is released, the mucosa of the upper esophagus and lower pharynx vibrates, producing sound. Esophageal speech produces a more natural sound than the electrolarynx. Therapy begins 3 to 6 weeks after surgery and takes longer to master. **Tracheoesophageal puncture** (TEP) is the third form. It reqires the placement of a small plastic tube at the time of the laryngectomy or as a secondary procedure. On exhalation, the patient digitally occludes the tracheostoma, and tracheal air is passed through the prosthesis into the upper esophagus, which vibrates. Intelligible speech can be attained as quickly as 1 to 2 days. Early rates of success have been reported at around 90%.

19. Describe some of the glottic reconstructive options after conservation laryngeal surgery for early glottic carcinoma.

Options range from advancing local tissue to free tissue grafts for larger tumors. The most frequently reported procedures are the **strap muscle flaps** and **epiglottic or hemiepiglottic laryngoplasty.** Ogura and Biller first developed the **unipedicled** sternohyoid muscle flap in 1969. Following a hemilaryngectomy, the inferiorly based pedicle from the ipsilateral sternohyoid muscle is inserted into the larynx and sutured into the defect left from the excision of the vocal cord and arytenoid. Bailey, in 1975, described the use of a **bipedicled** strap muscle flap for the hemilaryngectomy defect. A vertical incision is made through the ipsilateral sternohyoid muscle from the hyoid bone to the cricoid cartilage, creating two vertical strips of muscle. The anterior flap is then rotated into the larynx and sutured in the defect. Epiglottic and hemiepiglottic laryngoplasty following hemilaryngectomy is accomplished by a split-thickness total or partial epiglottic flap pulled down and secured to the cricoid cartilage. Rotating it posteriorly to reconstruct an arytenoid creates a closure that can protect the airway and produce vocal sounds.

CONTROVERSIES

20. What is the treatment for T1 glottic carcinoma of the larynx?

Surgery and radiation are effective treatments for early glottic carcinoma. However, surgical proponents feel that radiation should be held in reserve, as failure of radiation often results in laryngectomy. Radiation therapy is longer in duration, requiring 6 weeks of therapy, and the expense is considerable. Surgery may only require one treatment as an outpatient. Voice quality is also an area of controversy. Many surgeons feel that the results are better with radiation, although some surgeons feel that postoperative voice is comparable. The radiated larynx can have vocal dysfunction from post-treatment swelling and may proceed to complete dysfunction from radiation-induced chondronecrosis.

21. Should the N0 neck in laryngeal cancer be treated when using primary radiation therapy?
Controversy exists for the treatment or nontreatment of the N0 neck in laryngeal cancer. Recommendations vary depending on the site, location, and extent of tumor. In glottic cancer, occult metastasis occurs in 14–16% of patients, whereas a higher incidence of 20–38% occurs in those with supraglottic tumors. The highest rate of occult metastasis is seen in patients with pyriform sinus neoplasms. When the risk of occult cervical metastasis is high ($> 15\%$), consideration should be given to include regional nodes in the planned radiation fields for the primary tumor. Patients with positive clinical adenopathy should have a neck dissection.

22. Can conservation surgery be utilized after failure of radiation therapy for laryngeal cancer?
Radiation failures can be treated with conservation surgery to include cordectomy, hemilaryngectomy, and subtotal laryngectomy. These patients must not have clinically palpable cervical lymphadenopathy and should have been candidates for conservation surgery prior to radiotherapy. Controversies exist concerning the application of these procedures after post-irradiation recurrences. Some investigators apply the same accepted criteria for hemilaryngectomy, whereas others place more stringent limitations on conservation surgery for these recurrent tumors. Although conservation surgery is possible for some previously irradiated tumors, the majority will require total laryngectomy for salvage. Hemilaryngectomy for salvage of irradiation failures has had reported local control rates as high as 80%.

23. Can transoral carbon dioxide laser resection of supraglottic carcinoma be as effective as conventional open resection?
Newer techniques to remove cancer without opening the neck are being described. Rudert has shown that survival for all T stages treated by transoral carbon dioxide laser resection were comparable to the outcome after conventional open partial resection. This technique has lower morbidity with less need for tracheostomy and has no age limit. Patients with advanced inoperable tumors treated with this technique may not require palliative radiotherapy or tracheostomy. Adequate resection techniques are essiential for success.

24. What is the treatment for anterior commissure glottic cancer?
No natural barrier exists to the spread of cancer from the anterior vocal commissure into the thyroid cartilage, where it attaches. Often, these tumors are understaged, and deep invasion diminishes the effectiveness of radiation therapy. Zohar et al. found local control rates of 90% with conservation surgery versus 72% with radiation. There are no well-controlled prospective studies that compare radiation therapy for this site. Woodhouse and others feel that anterior commissure involvement does not affect the outcome for radiation therapy and believe that it remains the preferred method of initial treatment.

LARYNGEAL CANCER COMORBIDITY

Previous studies have evaluated the effects of comorbidity on survival in patients with cancer. A group of 152 patients with laryngeal cancer were assigned CCI scores and were categorized into low- and high-grade comorbidity groups for comparison. Age adjustments were performed. Low- versus high-grade comorbidity was a valid predictor of survival independent of TNM (tumor, nodes, and metastases) stage. Low-grade comorbidity was present in 126 patients; their median survival was 41 months. High-grade comorbidity was present in 26 patients; their median survival was 8 months ($P = 0.0002$). The addition of the age factor to the CCI score did not improve the prognostic ability. There was no difference in CCI groups with respect to tobacco and alcohol use, gender, treatment modality, or mean time to recurrence. The incidence and severity of complications were also similar in the two groups. The CCI is a strong predictor of survival in patients with laryngeal cancer.

~Sabin, Ear Nose Throat J 78:578, 1999

BIBLIOGRAPHY

1. Becker M: Neoplastic invasion of laryngeal cartilage: Radiologic diagnosis and therapeutic implications. Eur J Radiol 33:216–229, 2000.
2. Devaney SL, Ferlito A, Rinaldo A, et al: The pathology of neck dissection in cancer of the larynx. Orl J Otorhinolaryngol Relat Spec 62:204–211, 2000.
3. Ferlito A, Rinaldo A: The pathology and management of subglottic cancer. Eur Arch Otorhinolaryngol 257:168–173, 2000.
4. Ferlito A, Rinaldo A: Paraneoplastic syndromes in patients with laryngeal and hypopharyngeal cancers. Ann Otol Rhinol Laryngol 109:109–117, 2000.
5. Ferlito A, Rinaldo A, Marioni G: Laryngeal malignant neoplasms in children and adolescents. Int J Pediatr Otorhinolaryngol 49:1–14, 1999.
6. Gillison ML, Forastiere AA: Larynx preservation in head and neck cancers. A discussion of the National Comprehensive Cancer Network Practice Guidelines. Hematol-Oncol Clin North Am 13:699–718, vi, 1999.
7. Gluckman JL, Farrell ML, Kelly DH: Vocal rehabilitation following total laryngectomy. In Cummings CW, et al (ed): Otolaryngology—Head and Neck Surgery. St. Louis, Mosby, 1998.
8. Greenman J, Homer JJ, Stafford ND: Markers in cancer of the larynx and pharynx. Clin Otol Allied Sci 25:9–18, 2000.
9. Hoffman HT, McCulloch TM: Management of early glottic cancer. In Cummings CW, et al (ed): Otolaryngology—Head and Neck Surgery. St. Louis, Mosby, 1998.
10. Hogikyan ND, Bastian RW: Surgical therapy of glottic and subglottic tumors. In Thawley SE, et al (ed): Comprehensive Management of Head and Neck Tumors, 2nd ed. Philadelphia, W.B. Saunders, 1999.
11. Kau RJ, Alexiou C, Stimmer H, et al: Diagnostic procedures for detection of lymph node metastases in cancer of the larynx. Orl J Otorhinolaryngol Relat Spec 62:199–203, 2000.
12. MacKenzie RG, Franssen E, Balogh JM, et al: Comparing treatment outcomes of radiotherapy and surgery in locally advanced carcinoma of the larynx: a comparison limited to patients eligible for surgery. Int J Radiol Oncol Biol Phys 47:65–71, 2000.
13. Mendenhall WM, Tannehill SP, Hotz MA, et al: Should chemotherapy alone be the initial treatment for glottic squamous cell carcinoma? Eur J Cancer 35:1309–1313, 1999.
14. Myers EN, Fagan JF: Management of the neck in cancer of the larynx. Ann Otol Rhinol Laryngol 108:828–832, 1999.
15. Rudert HH, Werner JA, Hoft S: Transoral carbon dioxide laser resection of supraglottic carcinoma. Ann Otol Rhinol Laryngol 108(9):819–827, 1999.
16. Schaefer SD, Leach JL: Diagnosis and treatment of cancer of the glottis and subglottis [self-instructional package]. Rochester, MN, American Academy of Otolaryngology-Head and Neck Surgery Foundation, 1999.
17. Schwartz MR: Pathology of laryngeal tumors. In Thawley SE, et al (ed): Comprehensive Management of Head and Neck Tumors, 2nd ed. Philadelphia, W.B. Saunders, 1999.
18. Spafford MF, Koeppe J, Pan Z, et al: Correlation of tumor markers p53, bcl-2, CD34, CD44H, CD44v6, and Ki-67 with survival and metastasis in laryngeal squamous cell carcinoma. Arch Otolaryngol Head Neck Surg 122(6):627–632, 1996.
19. Stewart MG, Chen AY, Stach CB: Outcomes analysis of voice and quality of life in patients with laryngeal cancer. Arch Otolaryngol Head Neck Surg 124:143–148, 1998.
20. Szyfter K, Szmeja Z, Szyfter W, et al: Molecular and cellular alterations in tobacco smoke-associated larynx cancer. Mutat Res 445:259–274, 1999.

45. TUMORS OF THE TRACHEA AND TRACHEOBRONCHIAL TREE

Phillip L. Massengill, M.D., and Douglas M. Sorensen, M.D., FACS

1. Describe the anatomy of the trachea.

The adult trachea averages 11 cm in length and is composed of 18–22 incomplete cartilaginous rings. Each incomplete ring has a posterior membranous segment. Posteriorly, the trachea lies against the esophagus, and anteriorly, the thyroid isthmus crosses the level of the second or third tracheal ring. The innominate artery crosses the trachea inferiorly. The tracheal extension begins 2 cm below the vocal cords and extends inferiorly to the carina.

2. What is the arterial supply to the trachea?

The inferior thyroid, subclavian, internal thoracic, supreme intercostal, innominate, and superior and middle bronchial arteries.

3. What are common signs and symptoms of tracheal tumors?

Most patients present with a troublesome cough, dypsnea on exertion, and, eventually, wheezing and stridor. The most common signs and symptoms are cough (37% of patients), hemoptysis (41%), and signs of progressive airway compromise to include shortness of breath on exertion (54%), wheezing and stridor (35%), and dysphasia or hoarseness (7%). Dypsnea is the most prominent symptom, although wheezing and stridor are more prominent in adenoid cystic carcinoma. Wheezing often may lead to diagnostic error and can delay the diagnosis. Patients may demonstrate recurrent attacks of pneumonitis. Hemoptysis is more prominent in squamous cell carcinoma.

4. What is the differential diagnosis of a tracheal neoplasm in an adult?

Tracheal tumors are rare, representing only 2% of all upper airway tumors. Ninety percent of adult tracheal neoplasms are malignant, and 10% are benign.

Differential diagnosis:
Squamous cell carcinoma
Adenoid cystic carcinoma
Heterogeneous group:
    Malignant: adenocarcinoma, adenosquamous carcinoma, small-cell carcinoma, mucoepidermoid carcinoma, sarcoma, melanoma
    Benign: squamous papillomata, pleomorphic adenoma, granular cell tumor, fibrous histiocytoma, leiomyoma, chondroma, chondroblastoma

5. How does the differential diagnosis of a primary tracheal neoplasm differ in the pediatric age group?

Although 90% of tracheal tumors in the adult are malignant, the opposite is true in children: 90% of tracheal tumors in children are benign. Of the benign neoplasms, squamous papilloma and hemangioma are the most common. Chondroma, osteochondroma, osteoma, and fibroma are much less common. Although rare, malignant pediatric tracheal neoplasms include squamous cell carcinoma, adenoid cystic carcinoma, sarcoma, and adenocarcinoma.

6. Name the two most common malignant primary tracheal tumors. What are their distinguishing characteristics?

Squamous cell carcinoma	**Adenoid cystic carcinoma**
Strongly associated with smoking	Not associated with smoking

Lymph node metastasis common	Lymph nodes rarely involved
Grows rapidly and aggressively	Slow growing and indolent
Invades mediastinal structures	Displaces mediastinal structures
Occurs predominantly in men	Even sex distribution
Exophytic or ulcerative	May extend submucosally
May have contiguous lung lesion	Recurs after many years

7. What are the most common secondary tracheal tumors?

A secondary tracheal tumor is a malignant tumor that involves or invades the trachea from an adjacent site. These tumors are often incurable. They are (in order of frequency)

Laryngeal carcinoma
Bronchogenic carcinoma, from a main bronchus
Esophageal carcinoma, commonly associated with a fistula
Metastatic breast carcinoma, lymphoma, or other head and neck cancer
Thyroid carcinoma of any variety, usually anaplastic

8. What are the primary diagnostic techniques used for tracheal neoplasms?

Initially, **radiographic plain films** should be obtained, including a chest radiograph (anteroposterior and lateral views) and plain films of the neck. **Fluoroscopy** can further demonstrate functional asymmetry of the vocal cords and provides information concerning the extent of the lesion. A neck **computed tomographic (CT) scan** may further delineate the tumor's extratracheal extension. **Barium swallow** is helpful to establish or rule out esophageal involvement by extension. **Rigid bronchoscopy** with biopsies should be performed to confirm diagnosis in the operating room. **Pulmonary function tests** give information about the status of the underlying lung parenchyma distal to the obstruction.

9. How is the airway managed in a patient with a tracheal neoplasm?

Airway control is best accomplished in the operating room. The initial evaluation should be performed with rigid bronchoscopy using rigid telescopes to assess the level and degree of tracheal obstruction. Tracheal tumors may present with varying degrees of airway obstruction, and endotracheal intubation may be difficult or impossible. Intubation is best accomplished in the operating room with inhalational anesthesia without paralytics. This requires a team effort between the anesthesiologist and the otolaryngologist. Patients presenting with near total obstruction (90%) may benefit from CO_2 laser partial resection of the lesion, as a temporizing measure, prior to surgical therapy. Patients presenting with total obstruction may require tracheotomy.

10. How are benign tracheal tumors treated?

Respiratory papillomas are the most common benign tumors of the trachea. About 1500 patients are treated annually for this disorder, with most cases being in children. The disease is caused by infection with human papillomavirus (HPV), with HPV-6C being the most common and virulent subtype. Fifty-four percent of children with this disease are born to women with vulvar papilloma. HPV subtypes (6 and 11), which can be venereal warts, also cause papillomatosis. In the pediatric patient, multiple sites are involved throughout the laryngotracheobroncheal tree. In contrast, the adult patient usually has a single lesion or discrete site of involvement. Treatment of symptomatic, benign tracheal lesions primarily involves endoscopic ablation. Currently, the CO_2 laser may be used to vaporize benign neoplasms from the tracheal wall. If the tumor appears to be friable and bleeding occurs, the Nd:YAG laser may be used for its ability to deeply coagulate.

11. How does the surgeon prevent tracheal wall perforation while using laser therapy in the airway?

Perforation of the tracheal wall can be avoided by delivering the laser energy parallel to the tracheal wall. In addition, the laser settings of time and wattage should be appropriate to avoid deep tissue destruction.

12. What is the role of surgery in treating malignant tracheal tumors?

Most malignant tracheal tumors carry a poor prognosis, and treatment is directed toward palliation. Tracheal resection is the mainstay of therapy, with primary anastomosis performed on the free ends of the trachea.

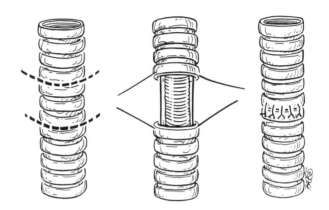

End-to-end reanastomosis of the trachea. (From Cardoso et al. In Cummings CW, et al: Otolaryngology–Head and Neck Surgery, 3rd ed. St. Louis, Mosby Publishers, 1998, with permission.)

13. What are the various surgical approaches for tracheal resection?

Most tumors of the upper trachea can be approached through a low collar incision in the neck with the option to extend exposure through the upper sternum. Midtracheal tumors can be approached with an extended low collar incision or through a full median sternotomy. Lower tracheal tumors located at or near the carina require a combination approach, which involves a neck incision and a right posterolateral thoracotomy incision.

14. How much of the trachea can be resected?

Up to one-half of the trachea can be resected and still be reconstructed with a primary anastomosis. The trachea is 10–11 cm long in the adult. Therefore, roughly 5–6 cm can be resected.

15. What are some options for reconstructive techniques for tumors that involve the carina?

There are at least 12 possible resections. (See figure next page.)

16. What maneuver gives the most distance for tracheal reconstruction?

Neck flexed (15–30 degrees) gives approximately 4.5 cm of length. The surgeon can gain 2.5 cm with a supralaryngeal release, 1.3 cm with increased neck flexion, 1.4 cm with mobilization of the right hilus and inferior pulmonary ligament, 3.0 cm with full mobilization of the right hilus, 0.9 cm with dissection of the pulmonary artery and vein intrapericardially, and, finally, 2.7 cm with reimplantation of the left mainstem bronchus.

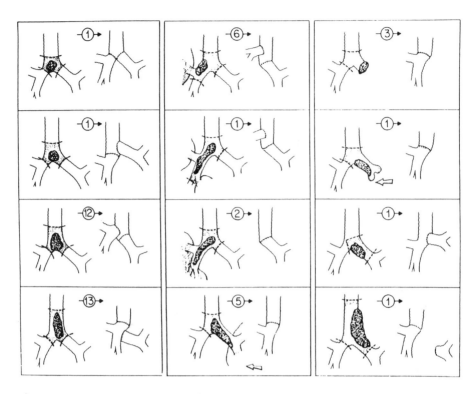

Twelve possible carina resections. (From Mathisen DJ. In Bailey BJ, et al (eds): Head and Neck Surgery—Otolaryngology, 2nd ed. Philadelphia, Lippincott, 1998, p 1796, with permission.)

17. What are the complications of a tracheal resection and reconstruction?
- Wound infection is a potential complication, as with any surgery. Drainage should be implemented and appropriate antibiotics should be administered.
- Anastomotic dehiscence may be caused by ischemia or undue tension on the anastomotic suture line.
- Aspiration may be due to transection of one or both recurrent laryngeal nerves.
- A tracheal-innominate artery fistula is a rare but serious complication.
- A suture line granuloma can usually be treated successfully by endoscopy.
- Restenosis is caused by ischemia or undue tension on the anastomosis.

18. Name two maneuvers to prevent dehiscence of the tracheal anastomosis.
1. To prevent ischemia, the surgeon should avoid circumferentially dissecting around two or more consecutive tracheal rings.
2. To avoid excessive tension, the surgeon should perform a suprahyoid release. In this procedure, the suprahyoid muscle is severed to allow the neck to easily flex. The patient's neck should remain in this flexed position to avoid excessive tension.

19. What is the role of radiation and chemotherapy in treating malignant tracheal tumors?
Both squamous cell carcinoma and adenoid cystic carcinoma are radiosensitive. Therefore, most patients are treated with postoperative irradiation. Radiation therapy alone will not provide a cure, but when radiation is combined with surgery, a three-fold increase in survival rates has been reported as compared to treatment with surgery alone. Chemotherapy has not been shown to be effective in treating tracheal tumors.

CONTROVERSY

20. What is the long-term survival for patients with tracheal tumors?
Patients with adenoid cystic carcinoma who are treated with tracheal resection and postoperative radiation have a 5-year survival rate of 75%. Patients with squamous cell carcinoma who receive the same therapeutic management have a 5-year survival rate of 49%. Meaningful long-term follow-up is lacking because of the rarity of this disorder.

BIBLIOGRAPHY

1. Azar T, Abdul-Karim FW, Tucker HM: Adenoid cystic carcinoma of the trachea. Laryngoscope 108:1297–1300, 1998.
2. Desai DP, Holinger LD, Gonzalez-Crussi F: Tracheal neoplasms in children. Ann Otol Rhinol Laryngol 107(9 Pt 1):790–796, 1998.
3. Glazer HS, Siegel MJ: Imaging of tracheal tumors. In Cummings CW, et al (eds.): Otolaryngology—Head and Neck Surgery. St. Louis, Mosby, 1998, pp 2299–2313.
4. Green GE, Bauman NM, Smith RJ: Pathogenesis and treatment of juvenile onset recurrent respiratory papillomatosis. Otolaryngol Clin North Am 33:187–207, 2000.
5. Grillo HC: Management of tracheal tumors. Am J Surg 143:697, 1982. (A *classic*)
6. Harcourt JP, Worley G, Leighton SE: Cimetidine treatment for recurrent respiratory papillomatosis. Int J Pediatr Otorhinolaryngol 51:109–113, 1999.
7. Katsimbri PP, Bamias AT, Froudarakis ME, et al: Endobronchial metastases secondary to solid tumors: Report of eight cases and review of the literature, Lung Cancer 28:163–170, 2000.
8. Lange TH, Magee MJ, Boley TM, et al: Tracheobronchial glomus tumor. Ann Thorac Surg 70:292–295, 2000.
9. Mathisen DJ: Primary tracheal tumor management. Surg Oncol Clin North Am 8:307, 1999.
10. Menaissy YM, Gal AA, Mansour KA: Glomus tumor of the trachea. Ann Thorac Surg 70:295–297, 2000.
11. Regnard JF, Fourquier P, Levasseur P: Results and prognostic factors in resections of primary tracheal tumors: A multicenter retrospective study. The French Society of Cardiovascular Surgery. J Thorac Cardiovasc Surg 111:808–813; discussion 813–814, 1996.
12. Sie KC, Tampakopoulou DA: Hemangiomas and vascular malformations of the airway. Otolaryngol Clin North Am 33:209–220, 2000.
13. Soga J, Yakuwa Y: Bronchopulmonary carcinoids: An analysis of 1,875 reported cases with special reference to a comparison between typical carcinoids and atypical varieties. Ann Thorac Cardiovasc Surg 5:211–219, 1999.
14. Tasker AD, Flower CD: Imaging the airways. Hemoptysis, bronchiectasis, and small airways disease. Clin Chest Med 20:761–773, viii, 1999.
15. Vinod SK, Macleod CA, Barnes DJ, et al: Malignant fibrous histiocytoma of the trachea. Respirology 4:271–274, 1999.

46. TUMORS OF THE ESOPHAGUS

John P. Campana, M.D.

1. What are the major categories of esophageal tumors? Which types are most common?

Less than 1% of esophageal tumors are benign. The most common benign tumor is leiomyoma. The most common malignant tumor used to be squamous cell carcinoma (SCCA). However, in the last several decades, the incidence of adenocarcinoma (AC) has increased to the point where about half the cancers are SCCA and half are AC. The increased incidence of AC probably relates to the increased incidence of Barrett's esophagus and gastroesophageal reflux (GER). AC is usually found in the lower esophagus because of this. Most cancers are in the middle and lower third of the esophagus. Rarely are primary cancers found in the cervical esophagus that are not extensions of laryngeal or hypopharyngeal cancer. SCCA and AC account for 95% of esophageal tumors.

Major Categories of Esophageal Tumor

BENIGN	MALIGNANT
Nonepithelial	**Carcinoma**
Myomas	Squamous cell carcinoma
Leiomyoma	Adenocarcinoma
Fibromyoma	Adenoid cystic carcinoma
Lipomyoma	Mucoepidermoid carcinoma
Fibroma	Small-cell carcinoma
Vascular tumors	Undifferentiated
Hemangioma	
Lymphangioma	**Sarcoma**
Mesenchymal tumors	Leiomyosarcoma
Reticuloendothelial	Fibrosarcoma
Lipoma	Osteosarcoma
Myxofibroma	Synovial sarcoma
Giant cell tumor	Hemangiopericytoma
Neurofibroma	Kaposi's sarcoma
Osteochondroma	Rhabdomyosarcoma
	Liposarcoma
	Malignant mesenchymoma
Epithelial	
Papilloma	
Polyp	**Lymphoproliferative**
Adenoma	Malignant lymphoma
Mucous cyst	Hodgkin's disease
	Plasmacytoma
Heterotopic tumors	
Gastric mucosal tumor	**Mucosal melanoma**
Melanoblastic tumor	
Sebaceous gland tumor	**Metastatic or direct invasion from**
Granular cell myoblastoma	Lungs/bronchi
Pancreatic gland tumor	Larynx
Thyroid nodule	Thyroid

Adapted from Wurster CF, Sisson GA: Neoplasms of the trachea/esophagus. In Cummings CW, et al (eds): Otolaryngology–Head and Neck Surgery, 3rd ed. St. Louis, Mosby, 1998; and Begin LR: The pathobiology of esophageal cancer. In Roth JA (ed): Thoracic Oncology. Philadelphia, W.B. Saunders, 1989.

2. What are the epidemiologic characteristics of esophageal tumors?

Esophageal SCCA represent 1.5% to 2% of all human malignancy and 5% to 7% of gastrointestinal malignancies. In the United States, esophageal cancer is mostly a disease of men between the ages 50–70 who use alcohol and tobacco. Men are affected three to five times more often than women and have mortality rates four to six times higher than women. African-Americans are four to five times more likely than whites to get esophageal cancer. The overall annual incidence of esophageal SCCA in the United States is less than 10/100,000, with approximately 12,000 new cases of esophageal SCCA per year and almost an equal number of deaths. In certain parts of China, Iran, and the former Soviet Union, the incidence is over 100/100,000 males.

3. Name the risk factors for esophageal tumors.

Nutritional, vitamin, and mineral deficiencies; radiation exposure; chemical exposures (nitrates, nitrites, petroleum oils); repeated ingestion of extremely hot liquids; and partial gastrectomy have all been associated with an increased incidence of esophageal malignancy. A history of achalasia, chronic esophagitis, strictures, Plummer-Vinson syndrome, tylosis, and caustic ingestion increase the risk of these cancers. Human papillomavirus and genetic predisposition may also play a role in their development.

4. What are Barrett's esophagus, Plummer-Vinson syndrome, and tylosis? How do they relate to esophageal cancer?

Barrett's esophagus is metaplasia of the distal esophagus from stratified squamous mucosa to glandular stomach-like epithelium. This usually occurs in response to GER. This disorder is usually associated with AC.

Plummer-Vinson syndrome is characterized by dysphagia due to degeneration of the esophageal musculature, microcytic hypochromic anemia, and splenomegaly. It is also associated with achlorhydria with atrophy and inflammation of the mouth, pharynx, and upper end of the esophagus. Fissures at the corners of the lips (angular stomatitis) may be present. Patients may have spoon-shaped, concave nails. Pharyngoesophageal webs can occur that sometimes require dilation. This disorder is more prevalent in women than men. Patients have an increased risk of developing a pharyngeal or upper esophageal SCCA.

Tylosis is a rare autosomal dominant disease. The patients have hyperkeratosis of the palms of the hands and feet. They have a 95% chance of having SCCA by the age of 65.

5. How do esophageal tumors present?

Small benign lesions may be asymptomatic or present with mild dysphagia. Patients sometimes feel the sensation of pressure in the chest or neck. These neoplasms can occasionally bleed, resulting in hemoptysis or anemia. Rare pedunculated lesions can be regurgitated into the mouth and occasionally into the region of the vocal cords, causing airway obstruction. Cancers of the esophagus tend to grow rapidly. They usually present with progressive dysphagia, pain, weight loss, and malaise. Hemoptysis may be a recurrent problem. Fatal hemorrhage can occur from invasion into major mediastinal vessels. Tumor invasion can also cause hoarseness from the involvement of the recurrent laryngeal nerve or aspiration from a tracheoesophageal fistula. Unrelenting cough and regurgitation plague some patients. Back pain can occur in patients with mediastinal involvement.

6. Which diagnostic methods are most often used to evaluate esophageal tumors?

Some routine laboratory tests are recommended. Hematocrit is a useful check for anemia. A low albumin level is common from dysphagia and malnutrition. Alkaline phosphatase and bilirubin can be elevated from liver metastases. Elevated calcium levels can occur from bone metastases. There is a serum marker, CA19-9, that is occasionally used to follow responses to treatment. It is not sensitive enough to use as a screening or diagnostic tool.

Chest radiographs, barium swallows, esophagoscopy, brush cytology, biopsy, endoscopic ultrasonography (EUS), computed tomography (CT), magnetic resonance imaging (MRI), and positron emission tomography (PET) all have utility.

7. What information can a chest radiograph reveal to the clinician regarding esophageal tumors?

A chest radiograph for a benign lesion is usually unremarkable, but it can show a mediastinal density if the mass is large. In malignancies, chest radiographs can reveal tumor and lymph node densities in the mediastinum, displacement of normal mediastinal structures, aspiration pneumonitis and pneumonia, air/fluid levels in the esophagus, pulmonary metastasis, and pleural effusions.

8. Describe the characteristic findings for esophageal tumors on barium swallow.

A barium swallow can usually delineate *extraluminal* from *intraluminal* tumors. Leiomyomas are intramural neoplasms that narrow the lumen extrinsically. Although the mucosa can ulcerate with leiomyomas, it is usually intact with a smooth outline, and the tumor does not affect peristalsis. Dilation proximal to a benign lesion is rare. Malignancies of the esophagus usually have an irregular, ulcerated mucosa with luminal narrowing in a "shelf-like" or concentric, annular fashion and dilation proximal to the mass. This finding is sometimes described as an "apple-core" lesion. Stenosis and overt obstruction are sometimes seen. Metastatic lymph nodes often displace or leave an impression on the esophagus. A barium swallow may also reveal tracheoesophageal fistulas.

9. What nontumor findings can be confused with tumors on esophageal barium studies?

Normal extrinsic impressions from the aortic arch, left mainstem bronchus, and left atrium can occasionally mimic tumors, especially if these structures are dilated or tortuous. Reflux stenosis (Schatzki's ring), scleroderma strictures, Barrett's esophagus with ulceration and stricture, cricopharyngeal spasm with and without associated diverticula (Zenker's), foreign bodies, diffuse esophageal spasm, lower esophageal spasm due to achalasia and reflux, congenital bands, webs, cysts, duplications, and vascular rings can all occasionally be confused with esophageal tumors.

10. What can endoscopy add to the work-up?

Esophagoscopy can provide tissue for histopathologic evaluation, help dilate stenoses, and aid in the placement of endoprosthetic stents for palliation in advanced cases. Ulcerated, fungating, polypoid, pedunculated, and verrucous lesions should be biopsied. Small cancers confined to the mucosa without lymph node metastasis can be resected endoscopically. However, conventional wisdom dictates that intramural lesions with intact mucosa should not be biopsied. These are usually benign leiomyomas, and biopsies make subsequent thoracotomy excision more difficult. This issue has recently been questioned, and some centers are finding endoscopic aspiration lumpectomy to be safe and effective for small esophageal leiomyomas.

11. Can other diagnostic modalities supplement the endoscopic evaluation?

Absolutely. Endoscopic ultrasonography (EUS) is probably the most valuable diagnostic tool for local tumor and nodal staging. Usually, EUS can correctly determine the tumor depth and nodal stage (mediastinal, perigastric, and celiac nodes) of an esophageal malignancy. Occasionally, laryngoscopy and bronchoscopy are added to the endoscopic work-up to check for second primary malignancies, which can occur in up to 5% of patients, and to evaluate the trachea and bronchi for invasion or fistulization. Some centers add thoracoscopy and a mini-laparotomy or laparoscopy to the staging work-up. With improved CT, MRI, and PET scanning, surgical staging of this sort is falling out of favor. These open procedures are still sometimes done to biopsy suspicious tissue if needed as part of the work-up.

12. When evaluating an esophageal malignancy, is any additional information obtained from a CT scan that can justify the cost? Is MRI better?

Esophageal cancer spreads directly to surrounding structures, through the bloodstream, and via lymphatic channels. Most of these malignancies directly involve a major mediastinal structure (trachea, left mainstem bronchus, or aorta) and have already spread to regional lymphatics (cervical, mediastinal, or celiac nodes) at the time of diagnosis. CT scans of the chest and abdomen reveal invasion of mediastinal structures, nodal metastasis, and distant metastasis to the liver, lungs, pleura, adrenals, and other sites. MRI is not usually considered superior to CT, but it is occasionally used in the work-up of these malignancies.

13. What role does PET scanning play?

Considering the overall grim prognosis of esophageal cancer, many clinicians advocate PET scanning to screen for metastasis to the liver, lungs, and skeleton. It appears to be superior to anatomic imaging with CT and MRI when it comes to finding distant metastasis.

14. How do you stage esophageal cancer?

SCCA and AC have similar survival rates despite the epidemiologic differences. Eighty-five to 95% of patients have lymph node involvement at the time of surgical treatment. Twenty-five to 30% have metastases to the liver, lung, and bone at presentation. Esophageal cancers are staged with the American Joint Committee on Cancer (AJCC) protocols:

Primary tumor (T):
   Tx: Cannot assess
   T0: No evidence of primary tumor
   Tis: Carcinoma-in-situ (high-grade dysplasia)
   T1: Invades lamina propria or submucosa
   T2: Invades muscularis propria
   T3: Invades adventitia
   T4: Invades adjacent structures

Regional lymph nodes (N):
   Nx: Cannot assess
   N0: No evidence
   N1: Present

Distant metastasis (M):
   Mx: Cannot assess
   M0: No evidence
   M1: Present

Stage 0	T0N0, TisN0
Stage I	T1N0
Stage IIA	T2N0, T1N1
Stage IIB	T3N0, T2N1
Stage III	T3N1; T4, any N
Stage IV	Any T, any N, M1

15. What are the survival rates for patients with esophageal cancer?

The overall 5-year survival rate for patients with squamous cell cancer of the esophagus is usually < 15%, regardless of treatment modality. Lymph node involvement cuts survival in half for each T stage. Survival rates decrease with increasing stage.

Stage I	18–55%
Stage IIA	14–38%
Stage IIB	6–27%
Stage III	4–17%
Stage IV	0–2%

16. What are the goals of palliation?

Appropriate goals are maximizing function with regard to eating and speaking while minimizing pain for as long as possible. Chemotherapy, radiation therapy, and surgery are used, often in combination. Some tumors can be palliated by dilation and placement of an esophageal stent, including the newer self-expanding metal stents. A stent can also be employed in the presence of a tracheoesophageal fistula to help prevent continued pulmonary contamination. Iatrogenic perforation is not uncommon with these devices. An occasional tumor can be debulked using endoscopic laser techniques (Nd:YAG), bipolar cautery, injection with absolute alcohol or chemotherapeutics, intraluminal brachytherapy, or photodynamic therapy. External beam radiation therapy can be used as palliation in selected patients, with many getting relief of their dysphagia for the remainder of their lives.

There is evidence indicating that the use of concurrent chemotherapy and radiation is superior to radiation therapy alone for palliation of locally advanced esophageal carcinoma. Selected patients may benefit from transhiatal esophagectomy or surgical bypass of an obstructed esophagus without actual tumor removal, usually using a substernal gastric pull-up. Tracheotomy, gastrostomy, and jejunostomy do not give good palliation in most patients but must be considered in selected cases.

Pain control and emotional support are helpful. Most pain can be relieved with appropriate doses of narcotics. Addiction is obviously not an issue in these very sick, terminal patients. Adequate patient and family counseling regarding terminal issues, such as resuscitation status, should be provided. Hospice programs may be of great benefit to both the patient and family. To ensure that analgesia is adequate and to provide emotional support, frequent follow-up is indicated.

17. What role does chemotherapy play in the curative therapy for esophageal malignancies?

Used alone, chemotherapy cannot cure and is considered palliation only. Although there are sporadic reports of reasonable palliation using chemotherapy, no randomized studies are available that reveal statistically significant improvements in survival. The response is usually poor. Most regimens are combinations, including cisplatin and 5-fluorouracil, but multiple other combinations have been tried. Chemotherapy-related morbidity and mortality are problems in themselves. As part of multimodality therapy, chemotherapy is often used. But, there is no significant increase in survival using preoperative chemotherapy compared with surgery alone. Several biologic agents, such as anti-growth factor antibodies, are being investigated in combination with chemotherapy.

18. Is radiation therapy helpful in treating esophageal malignancies?

Yes. Squamous cell cancers of the esophagus are moderately radioresponsive. When radiotherapy is used alone as a definitive treatment, the best reported results yielded a 5-year survival of 20% (20/99 patients). Most reported results are not as good and have rates below 10%. This disparity may be due to the fact that radiation therapy has been historically considered palliation, and more advanced tumors may have been selected for this treatment. Radiation is usually used in a multimodality protocol also involving surgery, chemotherapy, or both. Preoperative and postoperative radiation therapy have been studied extensively and do not definitively improve 5-year survival. In spite of this, it is widely used and thought by most people to increase local control.

19. What are the complications of radiation therapy used for esophageal carcinoma?

Radiation therapy has its own complications. It can cause bleeding, tracheoesophageal fistula, perforation into the mediastinum, radiation pneumonitis and fibrosis, myelitis of the spinal cord, and strictures. If radiation is followed by surgery, increased operative complications, such as anastomotic leakage, and increased perioperative mortality from high doses to the lungs are observed. These negative effects are counterbalanced by the observation that occasionally there is no viable tumor left in the esophagus in surgical resection specimens after preoperative radiation therapy.

20. Does surgery alone, as a single-modality therapy, have much to offer these patients?

Many people believe that surgery is the single best treatment for this disease. If the malignancies are detected early and confined to the mucosa or submucosa, aggressive surgery involving esophagectomy and cervical, mediastinal, and abdominal lymph node dissection can lead to 5-year survival rates of up to 73.2%, with a 2.3% operative mortality rate. Other surgical series report a 34% 5-year survival rate, but most cancers were stage I and II lesions. Photodynamic therapy alone can provide cure in some early-stage cancers. Unfortunately, most lesions are more advanced at presentation, and the outcome with surgery alone is similar to radiation alone, with overall 5-year survivals < 15% in most series. Perioperative mortality is usually about 5% but can be significant, with some series reporting rates of up to 20%. These results may be skewed because they often include procedures done for palliation as well as for cure—only 30–50% of patients are considered "resectable" at presentation, but many more are considered "operable" for palliation. Most patients have been losing weight and have coexistent chronic lung disease. It is important to try to optimize both their nutritional and pulmonary status for a week or two prior to surgery.

21. What types of surgery are employed in esophageal carcinoma?

Cervical esophageal carcinomas often require bilateral neck dissections and complete laryngopharyngectomy with gastric pull-up, colon interposition, jejunal free flap, or other free flap for reconstruction. Resections for "cure" of all other esophageal cancers usually require a "three-hole" technique, combining a cervical approach, laparotomy, and right thoracotomy to remove all tumor and regional nodes. Left thoracotomies are anatomically more difficult because of the physical interference offered by the heart and aortic arch. A transhiatal esophagectomy via cervical and abdominal incisions is usually considered a palliative procedure because midesophageal segments are dissected without direct vision, and complete mediastinal lymph node dissection is difficult, if not impossible. Reconstruction after esophagectomy is usually accomplished using a gastric pull-up or colon interposition. If the patient has had previous gastric surgery or if there is tumor involvement of the stomach, colon interposition is the procedure of choice.

22. What is anatomically unique about the esophagus that leads to increased postoperative complications?

The esophagus is the only part of the alimentary canal that does not have a fibrous serosal layer. Anastomosis with esophageal remnants tends to heal poorly, resulting in more anastomotic leaks and postoperative morbidity and mortality.

23. Is chemoradiation alone a viable curative alternative?

Some studies report 5-year survival rates of up to 25% for chemoradiation with less morbidity and mortality than esophagectomy alone. Some centers consider chemoradiation the treatment of choice. Esophagectomy can still be used later for palliation and occasional cure, although the operative morbidity goes up after chemoradiation.

24. Does combining all three treatment modalities do anything to improve survival in patients with this disease?

Trimodality therapy involving preoperative radiation and chemotherapy followed by curative surgery holds promise. The average median survival is about 18 months in most studies. However, there are studies that report 3-year and 5-year survival rates of 54% and 36%, respectively. There is probably some selection bias in these studies, with only lesions considered "resectable" being entered into this aggressive protocol.

CONTROVERSY

25. Is there consensus regarding the best treatment for esophageal cancer?

NO! After appropriate staging, the decision is usually made between the physician team, patient, and family to treat for cure versus palliation. Surgery has been the historical mainstay for both palliation and cure. However, the paradigm has been shifting in the treatment of esophageal cancer. Since most patients have advanced disease at diagnosis, survival is poor even with the most aggressive operative protocols. Aggressive surgery is often plagued by major complications, and several "organ preservation" protocols have been explored. The only definitive thing that can be said about the treatment of esophageal cancer is that there is no single definitive treatment plan for every patient. Multimodality therapy is usual. The entire area of treatment is controversial.

BIBLIOGRAPHY

1. Ajani JA: Current status of new drugs and multidisciplinary approaches in patients with carcinoma of the esophagus. Chest 113:112S–119S, 1998.
2. Axelrod AM, Fleischer DE: Esophageal Tumors. In Sleisenger MH, Fordtran JS, Feldman M, Scharschmidt BF (eds): Gastrointestinal and Liver Disease, 6th ed. Philadelphia, WB Saunders, 1997.
3. Begin LR: The pathobiology of esophageal cancer. In Roth JA (ed): Thoracic Oncology. Philadelphia, W.B. Saunders, 1989.
4. Coia LR: Chemoradiation: A superior alternative for the primary management of esophageal carcinoma. Semin Radiat Oncol 4(3):157–164, 1994.
5. Corti L, Skarlatos J, et al: Outcome of patients receiving photodynamic therapy for early esophageal cancer. Int J Radiat Oncol Biol Phys 47(2):419–424, 2000.
6. Haddad NG, Fleischer DE: Neoplasms of the esophagus. In Castell DO (ed): The Esophagus, 2nd ed. Boston, Little, Brown, 1995.
7. Heitmiller RF, Forastiere AA, et al: Neoadjuvant chemoradiation followed by surgery for resectable esophageal cancer. Recent Results Cancer Res 155:97–104, 2000.
8. Kato H, Tachimori Y, et al: Cervical, mediastinal, and abdominal lymph node dissection (three-field dissection) for superficial carcinoma of the thoracic esophagus. Cancer 72:2879–2882, 1993.
9. Wurster CF, Sisson GA: Neoplasms of the trachea/esophagus. In Cummings CW, et al (eds): Otolaryngology—Head and Neck Surgery. St. Louis, Mosby, 1993.
10. Zhang DW, Cheng GY, et al: Operable squamous esophageal cancer: Current results for the east. World J Surg 18:347–354, 1994.

47. THYROID AND PARATHYROID TUMORS

Catherine Winslow, M.D., Margaret K.T. Squier, M.D.,
and James I. Cohen, M.D., Ph.D.

1. What is a thyroid nodule?

A thyroid nodule is a discrete mass in the thyroid gland. The prevalence of thyroid nodules on physical examination has been estimated at approximately 6% in women and 1–2% in men. These statistics increase up to 10-fold when ultrasonographic or necropsy data are considered. The conditions that produce nodules may be benign, such as a solitary cyst, or life-threatening, such as an undifferentiated carcinoma. Because thyroid nodules are common and also potentially serious, the clinician must be prepared to evaluate and treat them methodically.

2. A patient presents with a lump on one side of her thyroid gland. What is the chance that it is malignant?

The likelihood of a nodule being malignant varies between 5 and 20% depending on whether the method of nodule detection is clincal examination or ultrasonography.

3. What factors increase the likelihood of a nodule being malignant?

Pregnant patients, children with nodules, patients with a history of radiation to the head and neck, and older patients who are male have a higher chance of having a malignant nodule.

4. What benign diseases cause local thyroid enlargement?

About half of clinical thyroid nodules are seen in the setting of a dominant nodule in a nodular goiter. A benign goiter is a common response of the thyroid gland to inadequate thyroid hormone levels. It can occur for physiologic reasons (during puberty, menses, and pregnancy), because of low iodine intake, from congenital defects in thyroid hormone production, or secondary to "goitrogenic" foods and drugs. Other benign causes of focal enlargement include cysts, teratomas, and, on occasion, abscesses, as in acute suppurative (pyogenic) thyroiditis, an uncommon complication of upper respiratory infection or of pyogenic infection elsewhere in the body. Unilateral lobe agenesis can also produce an asymmetric thyroid gland. The autoimmune diseases Hashimoto's thyroiditis and Graves' disease, in contrast, are relatively common causes of diffuse thyroid enlargement. Other forms of thyroiditis include subacute, painless, and Riedel's thyroiditis.

5. Which is the most common benign tumor of the thyroid?

Most benign tumors of the thyroid are follicular adenomas. Histologically and functionally, they are similar to normal thyroid tissue, but they take up radioactive iodine and can be distinguished as "warm" or "hot" spots on a radioiodine scan owing to the relative increase in tissue density compared to the surrounding gland. Eventually, they may overwhelm the normal function of the thyroid and produce chemical thyrotoxicosis. They can also undergo hemorrhagic necrosis and produce localized pain. A necrosed adenoma may appear as a cold nodule on a radioiodine scan and therefore be mistaken for a carcinoma.

6. What is the most common type of thyroid malignancy?

Papillary adenocarinoma. Eighty-five percent of thyroid cancers fall into this subtype. Other possible malignancies include follicular adenocarcinoma, medullary carcinoma, and undifferentiated (anaplastic) adenocarcinoma as well as lymphomas and metastases from kidney, lung, esophagus, and breast.

7. How is the prognosis for well-differentiated thyroid malignancy determined?

Age, sex, and extent of tumor are the main prognostic indicators. Females under 40 years of age with minimal invasion and nuclear euploidy tend to have a more favorable prognosis.

8. Do papillary and follicular carcinoma differ in their pathways of spread?

With papillary carcinoma, metastasis is generally occurs by lymphatic spread. Eighty percent of children and 20% of adults will have palpable lymph nodes at diagnosis. Distant metastatic spread (most commonly to lungs and bone) is relatively rare. Papillary adenocarcinoma carries a good prognosis for survival, even if disease is metastatic. Follicular carcinomas differ in that only 7% of follicular carcinomas spread to the lymph nodes, but this cancer more often spreads through the blood to the lungs, bone, and liver. Follicular adenocarcinoma carries a poorer prognosis than papillary adenocarcinoma.

9. Are any laboratory criteria of value in detecting or following thyroid carcinoma?

Medullary carcinoma may arise from the calcitonin-secreting parafollicular cells of the thyroid, or C-cells. These cells are neuroectodermal in origin and join the thyroid gland as it descends from the base of the tongue. Because they secrete calcitonin, calcitonin immunoreactivity can be used as an identifier of this type of cancer. Serum calcitonin and CEA levels can also prove useful.

10. How do the various multiple endocrine neoplasia (MEN) syndromes differ?

MEN I (Wermer's syndrome)—hyperparathyroidism, pancreatic islet cell tumors, pituitary tumors, gastric carcinoid

MEN IIA (Sipple's syndrome)—thyroid medullary carcinoma, pheochromocytoma, hyperparathyroidism

MEN IIB—thyroid medullary carcinoma, pheochromocytoma, mucosal neuromas, ganglioneuromas, marfanoid habitus

11. How is a well-differentiated thyroid carcinoma treated?

Surgical excision is the only effective treatment for well-differentiated thyroid cancer. Great controversy exists as to the extent of thyroidectomy and nodal dissection that constitutes adequate resection.

12. How is a poorly differentiated thyroid carcinoma treated?

Widespread local, regional, and distant metastasis at the time of presentation precludes surgical excision in the vast majority of these patients at the time of presentation. Radiation and chemotherapy are often used to try to control the disease locally but are rarely successful.

13. A diagnosis of papillary-follicuar carcinoma was returned on a thyroid specimen. Does this just indicate an indecisive pathologist?

A papillary-follicular carcinoma is a tumor with microscopic evidence of both types. It behaves clinically as a papillary carcinoma, with lymphatic metastasis and a favorable prognosis.

14. Which type of thyroid cancer cannot be found in a lingual thyroid? Why?

Lingual thyroid carcinomas are exceedingly rare but do occur. Medullary carcinoma is not found in a lingual thyroid, as the parafollicular cells only join the gland on its descent.

15. How is a patient with a thyroid nodule evaluated to determine malignancy?

The history should assess for the awareness of a neck mass, pain, dyspnea, voice changes, or dysphagia. Patients may identify symptoms of infection, hyper- or hypothyroidism, or impingement on neck structures. The clinician should ask about the duration of symptoms, recent growth of the mass, and the patient's age, place of birth, history of radiation exposure, and the personal and family history of thyroid ailments and cancer. High-risk factors for malignant disease include a family history of medullary carcinoma and rapid growth of the nodule; moderate risk factors include age < 20 or > 60, history of irradiation to the neck, and male gender.

The physical examination is a key aspect of the thyroid nodule evaluation. It should emphasize whether the thyroid is enlarged symmetrically or asymmetrically; the number, size, smoothness, fixation, and hardness of any nodules palpated; and whether local structures, such as the trachea, have been displaced. Regional lymphadenopathy should be noted. High-risk factors include firm consistency of the nodule, dysphonia (suggesting vocal cord paralysis), fixation of the nodule to adjacent structures, and regional lymphadenopathy. A nodule > 4 cm in diameter is a moderate risk factor.

16. What is a delphian node?

Also known as the **cricothyroid node,** the delphian node is a common site of thyroid carcinoma metastases and sits anteriorly over the cricothyroid membrane.

17. Is there a role for fine needle aspiration in determining diagnosis?

The most used test for thyroid nodules is **fine-needle aspiration cytology** (FNAC). Given a qualified cytologist and an adequate specimen, this is the test of choice. Early fears that this technique would lead to seeding of the needle track with malignant cells and contribute to spread of the disease have not been borne out clinically. FNAC is also relatively simple to perform and less expensive than either ultrasonography or radioiodine scanning.

18. If a thyroid cyst can be easily aspirated, is there a need for further intervention?

Aspirates should always be sent for pathologic examination, as papillary carcinoma can be cystic. If the aspirate is negative for malignancy, careful observation with or without thyroid suppression will suffice. A positive or suspicious result warrants further treatment.

19. What should you tell a patient undergoing thyroid surgery?

Because surgery poses a risk to the recurrent laryngeal nerve, a baseline preoperative evaluation of vocal cord function should be obtained. Voice changes may occur from damage either to the recurrent laryngeal nerve or to the superior laryngeal nerve. The superior laryngeal nerve supplies the cricothyroid muscle, a tensor of the vocal cord.

The potential need for life-long thyroid hormone replacement should be discussed with patients. Also, inadvertent parathyroidectomy may occur and, if complete, may require life-long calcium and vitamin D replacement therapy.

20. What is a nonrecurrent laryngeal nerve?

The recurrent laryngeal nerve, a branch of the vagus nerve, embryologically loops around the fifth arch. On the left side, the fifth arch is represented by the aortic arch and ductus arteriosus. On the right, the fifth and sixth arches disappear, and the nerve loops around the subclavian artery. In patients with anomalous subclavian arteries, the nerve arises directly from the vagus, hence, a nonrecurrent nerve. A nonrecurrent laryngeal nerve is more likely to be injured during surgery because of its location.

21. How can potential traction injury to the nerve be decreased?

Steroids given preoperatively or postoperatively decrease the incidence of recurrent laryngeal nerve injury from 10% to 3%.

22. Would a patient with *unilateral* vocal cord paralysis have more difficulty with voice or breathing?

Unilateral vocal cord paralysis causes problems with hoarseness (breathiness, loss of volume), not breathing.

23. Would a patient with *bilateral* vocal cord paralysis have more difficulty with voice or breathing?

Over time, because the vocal cords tend to migrate medially, patients with bilateral vocal cord paralysis may have problems with breathing.

24. A patient has undergone a near-total thyroidectomy and has difficulty breathing in the recovery room. Describe the evaluation and management of this patient.

An immediate evaluation of the wound should be made. If evidence of a hematoma exists, the wound should be opened. Immediate intubation or urgent tracheotomy may be necessary;

however, if possible, fiberoptic laryngoscopy to assess vocal cord position and function should be done first.

25. What options are available to improve the voice of a patient with unilateral vocal cord paralysis?

Medialization procedures to close the glottic gap, either by transoral injection of the paralyzed vocal cord or externally by thyroplasty or arytenoid adduction, are available.

26. What options are available to assist a patient with bilateral vocal cord paralysis?

Tracheotomy will restore the airway but is usually unacceptable on a long-term basis to patients. Endoscopic partial cordectomy or arytenoidectomy (endoscopic or external) as well as reinnervation procedures can be tried to restore an adequate glottic gap that allows breathing without complete compromise of voice.

27. You take a patient with papillary carcinoma to the operating suite and discover tracheal invasion. What do you do now?

Complete macroscopic removal of all tumor should be achieved even if it necessitates removal and reconstruction of parts of the laryngotracheal complex. Residual microscopic disease can be treated by postoperative radioactive iodine. If the patient is unprepared for this possibility, then the case should be terminated and the operation completed at a later time.

28. When is a thyroid scan performed?

Preoperatively, thyroid scans are used in the management of thyroid nodules only if there is a suspicion that the nodule is hyperfucntioning. Postoperatively, thyroid scans are done 6 to 8 weeks after the surgery, when the patient has recovered from surgery, to determine the presence or absence of residual disease.

29. Should thyroid hormone replacement therapy be started after surgery if a patient is scheduled to have a scan?

Although thyroid hormone replacement will lower the level of thyroid-stimulating hormone (TSH) and therefore cause less iodine uptake, thyroid hormone replacement with a short-acting preparation can be started postoperatively to facilitate recovery and then withheld 1–2 weeks prior to the planned thyroid scan.

30. What is the usual dose of radioiodine for a thyroid scan?

Less than 50 millicuries is generally given for residual uptake in the thyroid bed. 100–200 millicuries is generally given in cases in which a significant risk of residual thyroid cancer is believed to exist.

31. Do patients who have undergone lobectomy for thyroid malignancy need thyroid hormone replacement?

Postoperative replacement is advocated by many surgeons, regardless of thyroid hormone levels, to decrease TSH stimulation of any remaining thyroid tissue.

32. How are the parathyroid glands identified?

The glands are tan and oval, and they weigh approximately 35 mg. Parathyroid tissue will sink in normal saline, as opposed to fat, which will float. Ultimate identification should be histologic.

33. Can anything be done if a parathyroid gland is accidentally removed?

If the surgeon suspects that a parathyroid gland has been removed with the thyroid tissue, a small sample can be sent for pathologic verification. If parathyroid tissue is identified, the gland can be reimplanted in the sternocleidomastoid muscle or forearm. Calcium levels should be followed closely postoperatively.

34. What clinical signs are seen with parathyroid malignancy?

Parathyroid carcinoma is often associated with hypercalcemia (usually >15 mg/dL), pathologic fractures, nephrocalcinosis, or a palpable neck mass.

CONTROVERSIES

35. What is the best management for a small (< 2 cm) unilateral papillary carcinoma?

Surgery is indicated. Beyond that, opinions differ significantly. One school of thought is that a lobectomy is sufficient for eradication of disease. This is supported by the low rate of mortality associated with small well-differentiated thyroid carcinomas. However, some surgeons prefer a total thyroidectomy, citing the high incidence of multifocal disease. Studies are equivocal as to whether a second surgery for a contralateral lobectomy imparts a higher morbidity. A total thyroidectomy is indicated if a patient will receive radioiodine ablation.

36. Should all patients with well-differentiated thyroid carcinomas receive radioiodine?

Many surgeons work in close association with endocrinologists, and they decide this issue together. Again, owing to the high survival rate and low recurrence of small, well-differentiated thyroid carcinomas, many surgeons do not believe that radioiodine treatment following successful surgery is necessary. However, some believe that the relatively low rate of morbidity associated with the treatment and the potential for eradication of any small but unseen pockets of tumor speaks for providing this therapy to all patients. Distant metastases, local invasion of muscle or tracheal wall, and numerous multifocal lesions are all indications for therapy.

HÜRTHLE CELL TUMOR OF THE THYROID

This subtype of follicular adenocarcinoma tends to occur in older patients. It generally is more invasive and carries a worse prognosis. The Hürthle cell has eosinophilic cytoplasm, the function of which is unknown. It may or may not take up radioactive iodine on a scan.

BIBLIOGRAPHY

1. Belfiore A, Rosa GL, Giuffrida D, et al: The management of thyroid nodules. J Endocrinol Invest 18:155–158, 1995.
2. Boigon M, Moyer D: Solitary thyroid nodules: Separating benign from malignant conditions. Postgrad Med 98:73–80. 1995.
3. Goretzki PE, Simon D, Dotzenrath C, et al: Growth regulation of thyroid and thyroid tumors in humans. World J Surg 24:913–922, 2000.
4. Hamburger JI: Diagnosis of thyroid nodules by fine-needle biopsy: Use and abuse. J Clin Endocrinol Metab 79:335–339, 1994.
5. Learoyd D, Messina M, Zedenius J, et al: Molecular genetics of thyroid tumors and surgical decision-making. World J Surg 24:923–933, 2000.
6. Lumachi F, Zucchetta P, Angelini F, et al: Tumors of the parathyroid glands. Changes in clinical features and in noninvasive localization studies sensitivity. J Exp Clin Cancer Res 19:7–11, 2000.
7. Mazzaferri EL: Management of a solitary thyroid nodule. N Engl J Med 328:553–559, 1993.
8. Noyek A, Friedberg J: Thyroglossal duct and ectopic thyroid disorders. Otolaryngol Clin North Am 14:187, 1981.

 9. Rifat SF, Ruffin MT: Management of thyroid nodules. Am Fam Physician 50:785–790, 1994.
10. Segal K, Fridental R, Lubin E, et al: Papillary carcinoma of the thyroid. Otolaryngol Head Neck Surg 113:356, 1996.
11. Wiersinga WM: Is repeated fine-needle aspiration cytology indicated in (benign) thyroid nodules? Eur J Endocrinol 132:661–662, 1995.
12. Woeber KA: Cost-effective evaluation of the patient with a thyroid nodule. Surg Clin North Am 75:357–336, 1995.

48. VASCULAR TUMORS OF THE HEAD AND NECK

Catherine Winslow, M.D., and Mark K. Wax, M.D.

1. What are paragangliomas? From what tissues are they derived?

Paragangliomas derive from paraganglionic cells. These cells derive from sympathogonia, which in turn are derived from neural crest cells. The greatest concentration of paraganglionic cells is located adjacent to the aorta in the adrena medulla, but there is also a large collection of more diffusely distributed cells in the head and neck region. These cells have the ability to produce catecholamines and are chromaffin positive. This has led to the confusing terminology applied to these tumors. Chemodectoma and chromaffin or non-chromaffin positive are other terms used to describe these tumors.

2. Where are paragangliomas commonly found?

Paragangliomas of the head and neck can be found in any area where paraganglionic tissue is located. The carotid body bifurcation (carotid body tumor) is the most common location. Glomus jugulare (arising at the jugular bulb in the temporal bone) is the next most common. Paragangliomas on the promontory of the cochlea in the middle ear (glomus tympanicum) and on the vagal nerve (glomus vagale) are seen in decreasing frequency. Paragangliomas have also been reported in the larynx and low neck.

3. How do paragangliomas present?

A carotid body tumor, the most common paraganglioma of the head and neck, presents as a painless, slow-growing mass in the upper neck. The growth rate is approximately 0.5 cm/year. It is not until carotid body tumors become quite large that they begin to affect cranial nerves at the base of the skull. Glomus jugulare tumors present as a bluish mass behind the eardrum found on physical examination. Because of their location in the temporal bone, their primary presenting symptom is cranial nerve involvement (IX, X, and XI).

4. What is the diagnostic work-up of a carotid body tumor?

Physical examination will reveal a pulsatile mass in the region of the carotid bifurcation. The mass will move laterally or anteroposteriorly but does not move up and down because of its fixation to the bifurcation of the carotid. A computed tomographic (CT) scan with contrast or magnetic resonace imaging (MRI) with gadolinium will often provide the diagnosis and superior anatomic extent. Angiography reveals splaying of the internal and external carotid artery at the bifurcation (Lyre's sign). Magnetic resonance angiography (MRA) is also diagnostic. *Under no circumstances should an open neck biopsy be performed*, as this may lead to torrential and uncontrollable bleeding. Routine screening for urinary metanephrines and VMA and serum catecholamines is probably only indicated for multiple or familial paragangliomas or in the presence of catecholamine-related symptoms. However, considering the hazards associated with operating on a previously unsuspected, metabolically active tumor, an argument can be made for performing these studies in all cases.

5. What is the inheritance pattern of familial paragangliomas?

Although most paragangliomas are sporadic in nature, up to 10% are familial in nature. This is important, since a higher incidence of multicentric tumors exists in the patient with the familial pattern. Thus, all patients require investigation to rule out multicentric tumors. In the familial pattern, the gene is expressed in an autosomal dominant pattern with maternal imprinting.

6. Discuss the treatment options for carotid body tumors.

Surgical excision of carotid body tumors is curative. One-third of cases will require carotid artery resection with reconstruction. Up to one-third of cases will have a cranial nerve palsy postoperatively, most commonly the superior laryngeal nerve; the marginal mandibular and hypoglossal nerves are also at risk in the surgical approach. Radiation therapy has been used extensively in glomus jugulare tumors, but *not* for carotid body tumors. It has been shown to stop growth and cause fibrosis of the vascularity and even some involution of the tumor. It should be considered when surgical resection is contraindicated.

7. What is the difference between a glomus tympanicum and a glomus jugulare?

Glomus tympanicum tumors arise in the middle ear on the promontory of the cochlea. The morbidity associated with resecting them is minimal. They present with conductive hearing loss or a blue mass behind the tympanic membrane on examination. Glomus jugulare tumors arise from paraganglionic tissue in the jugular bulb. Their site of origin is in the temporal bone. Their growth involves a great deal of bone destruction. Tumors of the jugular foramen put the IX, X, and XI nerves at risk, and resection in this region involves a combined skull base procedure.

8. How do you tell the difference between a malignant paraganglioma and a benign paraganglioma?

Paragangliomas have a low potential for malignancy. They are typically composed of two cell types: epithelioid cells (Zellballen) in nests separated in a trabeculated fashion by vascularized connective tissue. Neural elements are peripherally located. Histologic diagnosis of malignancy is not possible in this tumor. Reported figures range from 2–50% based on pathology alone. Thus, most authors agree that histologic appearance does not correlate well with growth behavior. The only admissible criteria for malignancy is the presence of distant metastasis. This runs approximately 10%.

9. Discuss the management of a glomus jugulare tumor.

Glomus jugulare tumors typically arise in the temporal bone. They are intimately involved with the structures exiting through the jugular foramen (cranial nerves IX, X, and XI). Surgical resection involves radical skull base surgery with some compromise of these cranial nerves. The resulting aspiration, dysphagia, and possible facial nerve injury make radiotherapy an attractive alternative. With modern skull base techniques, total resection with excellent rehabilitation of the patient is possible. Radiation therapy has been shown to stabilize tumors, or possibly cause the tumors to involute.

10. A 13-year-old male presents with a history of unilateral nasal congestion, epistaxis, and anosmia. Physical examination reveals a large purplish mass in the symptomatic nasopharynx. What diagnosis should you consider?

Juvenile nasopharyngeal angiofibromas occur exclusively in males, often presenting with nasal congestion, epistaxis, or anosmia. These tumors are hormonally responsive and usually occur during adolescence. Although they are histologically benign, they may be locally invasive and have the potential to spread intracranially. A suspected nasopharyngeal angiofibroma can be evaluated with carotid arteriography, CT, and biopsy. Treatment involves surgery, often with preoperative embolization. Radiation therapy is reserved for unresectable cases. These vascular tumors are associated with a high recurrence rate.

11. An adolescent female is diagnosed with juvenile nasopharyngeal angiofibroma. How should you proceed?

This diagnosis is unlikely. Although nasopharyngeal angiofibroma is the most common vascular lesion in the nasal cavity, it occurs only in males. If there is doubt, chromosomal analysis may be pursued.

12. A child develops a rapidly enlarging hemangioma on her face. Her parents beg you to remove the lesion surgically. What is the appropriate treatment?

Hemangiomas are the most common head and neck tumors in children. They are more frequently found in females than males (3:1). The typical history is a period of rapid enlargement followed by gradual involution. Fifty percent have involuted by age 5, and 70% by age 7. Despite the cosmetic deformity in the period of enlargement, it is wise to wait for the natural progression of the lesion.

13. A child with a large hemangioma develops a coagulopathy. What is this entity? How is it managed?

Kasabach-Merritt syndrome is an unusual but feared entity related to large hemangiomas. A disseminated intravascular coagulation–like syndrome with platelet trapping is characteristic. It is treated by transfusion of clotting factors and platelets as necessary, in addition to addressing the lesion responsible.

14. Describe the Sturge-Weber syndrome.

This congenital syndrome, of unknown etiology, is characterized by venous angioma of the cerebral leptomeninges and port-wine nevi in a distribution of the first and second trigeminal branches. The mouth and nasal mucosa are frequently involved with angiomas. The occipital and posterior lobes may have calcifications, and patients may exhibit ophthalmologic problems. Seizure disorders are also associated.

15. A child presents to you with a history of stridor. Physical examination is remarkable for a facial hemangioma. What is the likely cause of the child's stridor?

Hemangiomas may occur in the larynx as well as on the skin. In adults, most laryngeal hemangiomas are supraglottic, whereas in children most are subglottic. About 50% of children with subglottic hemangiomas also have cutaneous lesions. Therefore, a child with a cutaneous hemangioma and stridor should be evaluated for a laryngeal tumor. These children frequently need tracheostomies to protect their airways.

16. How is the management of a port-wine stain different than that of a hemangioma?

A port-wine stain, also known as **nevus flammeus**, is a dark-purple, irregularly shaped patch that usually occurs on the face or neck. It grows with the skin and is not elevated. These patches are usually large and located in conspicuous regions, and surgical excision is challenging. However, laser surgery has had promising results. In general, most uncomplicated hemangiomas involute over several years with no treatment. Treatment of any lesion involves risks such as scarring and poor cosmetic result. Thus, only hemangiomas that do not spontaneously resolve are candidates for treatment.

17. What types of lasers are used to treat cutaneous vascular lesions?

The CO_2 laser is rapidly becoming outdated in the treatment of vascular lesions. It remains highly effective for small lesions such as telangiectasias. Argon and KTP lasers have wavelengths specific for hemoglobin, which enhances their ability to treat such lesions. YAG lasers (and also argon) have been associated with involution and arrest of growth of hemangiomas. The laser best suited for cutaneous vascular lesions is currently the pulsed dye laser. It is excellent for port-wine stains.

18. What other treatment options are available for vascular lesions of the head and neck?

Small cutaneous lesions may be treated with laser therapy, local injection of steroids, systemic steroid therapy, or local injection of sclerosing agents. Large lesions not amenable to local treatment may require more extensive therapy. An example of this would be a JNA or glomus tumor. Preoperative embolization and surgical extirpation are usually required. In lesions extending beyond the skull base, radiation may be of benefit by compromising the blood supply to the lesion.

19. What is a cystic hygroma?

A cystic hygroma, also known as a cystic lymphangioma, is a benign neck mass caused by lymphatic dilation. Most often presenting by the second year of life, cystic hygromas are commonly painless, soft, and compressible. Although these lesions may be small and unrecognized for long periods of time, patients often present after the lesions have undergone rapid enlargement.

CONTROVERSY

20. An infant with a large facial and submental lymphangioma has stridor. What is the best management of this child?

The child may suffer airway compromise if a cystic hygroma is associated with pharyngeal compression or laryngeal involvement. Therefore, a tracheotomy may be necessary. Complete surgical excision is the only successful treatment. Surgery may require a multistaged procedure, and recurrence is uncommon if all visible disease is excised. A 50% recurrence is cited with partial excision alone. Extensive involvement of the tongue may actually require a subtotal glossectomy.

BIBLIOGRAPHY

1. Adams GL, Latchaw RE: Carotid body tumor. In Gates GA (ed): Current Therapy in Otolaryngology—Head and Neck Surgery, 5th ed. St. Louis, Mosby, 1994.
2. Browne JD, Jacob SL: Temporal approach for resection of juvenile nasopharyngeal angiofibromas. Laryngoscope 110:1287–1293, 2000.
3. Charles NC, Palu RN, Jagirdar JS: Hemangiopericytoma of the lacrimal sac. Arch Ophthalmol 116:1677–1680, 1998.
4. Clarke SR, Hebert AF: Tumors of the parapharyngeal space. J La St Med Soc 151:597–600, 1999.
5. Danesi G, Panizza B, Mazzoni A, et al: Anterior approaches in juvenile nasopharyngeal angiofibromas with
6. intracranial extension. Arch Otolaryngol Head Neck Surg 122:277–283, 2000.
7. Dillard DG, Cohen C, Muller S, et al: Immunolocalization of activated transforming growth factor beta-1 in juvenile nasopharyngeal angiofibroma. Arch Otolaryngol Head Neck Surg 126:723–725, 2000.
8. Enjolras O: Vascular tumors and vascular malformations: Are we at the dawn of a better knowledge? Pediatr Dermatol 16:238–241, 1999.
9. Howard DJ, Lund VJ: The role of midfacial degloving in modern rhinological practice. J Laryngol Otol 113:885–887, 1999.
10. Kuppersmith RB, Teh BS, Donovan DT, et al: The use of intensity modulated radiotherapy for the treatment of extensive and recurrent juvenile angiofibroma. Int J Pediatr Otorhinolaryngol 52:261–268, 2000.
11. Lewark TM, Allen GC, Chowdhury K, et al: Le fort I osteotomy and skull base tumors: A pediatric experience. Arch Otolaryngol Head Neck Surg 126:1004–1008, 2000.
12. Marianowski R, Wassef M, Herman P, et al: Nasal haemangiopericytoma: Report of two cases with literature review. J Laryngol Otol 113:199–206, 1999.
13. Murray A, Falconer M, Mcgarry GW: Excision of nasopharyngeal angiofibroma facilitated by intra-operative 3d-image guidance. J Laryngol Otol 114:311–313, 2000.
14. Powell J: Update on hemangiomas and vascular malformations. Curr Opin Pediatr 11:457–463, 1999.
15. Sabini P, Josephson GD, Yung RT, et al: Hemangiopericytoma presenting as a congenital midline nasal mass. Arch Otolaryngol Head Neck Surg 124:202–204, 1998.
16. Wylie JP, Slevin NJ, Johnson RJ: Intracranial juvenile nasopharyngeal angiofibroma. Clin Oncol R Coll Radiol 10:330–333, 1998.

49. CUTANEOUS NEOPLASMS OF THE HEAD AND NECK

Vincent D. Franco, Jr., M.S. III, Ryan L. Van De Graff, M.D., and Tyler Lewark, M.D.

1. Can sun damage lead to precancers?

Sun damage to the skin can be seen in photo-aging, which results in mottled hyperpigmentation and wrinkling. The sun damage can lead to precancers such as actinic keratosis and lentigo maligna.

2. What do seborrheic keratoses look like? Are these lesions worrisome?

Seborrheic keratoses are very common skin lesions. They usually present as well-defined, elevated plaques that have a "stuck-on" appearance. A waxy, soft scale may be present. Seborrheic keratoses have no malignant potential and are unrelated to sun exposure. Treatment is not necessary, but may be requested for cosmetic reasons. Bothersome lesions can be effectively removed with cryosurgery.

3. What are actinic keratoses?

Actinic keratoses are scaly or warty growths that appear on sun-exposed regions of skin. They are well-circumscribed patches or papules that are usually skin-colored or brown. When inflamed, they are often pink or red The most distinctive feature on clinical examination is their sandpaper-like scale. The amount of scale varies considerably and may be detectable only with palpation. Lesions may also appear markedly hyperkeratotic with a very thick scale.

The definitive diagnosis requires biopsy with histopathologic examination. Actinic keratoses are premalignant and have a 12% risk of becoming squamous cell carcinama (SCC) if untreated. Recognizing and treating them is a method of skin cancer prevention (secondary prevention). Because there is a spectrum from actinic keratosis to Bowen's disease (SCC in situ) to SCC, it is sometimes necessary to biopsy a lesion that has features that appear more suspicious than a typical actinic keratosis. It is difficult to predict which lesions will develop into malignancies; therefore, many clinicians perform a biopsy or treat prophylactically.

Effective treatments include superficial shave excision, cryotherapy, trichloroacetic acid peel, and topical 5-fluorouracil.

4. Who is most at risk for actinic keratoses?

Actinic keratoses occur most commonly on fair or light-skinned individuals who tan poorly and sunburn easily. People of Northern European descent, who have blonde or red hair, blue eyes, and scant pigmentation, are especially at risk. Deeply tanning people and those with black or brown skin usually develop these lesions only with extreme, long-standing sun exposure. Actinic keratoses are caused by exposure to ultraviolet (UV) light, and it is clear that the intensity and duration of sun exposure are important to their development. However, the mechanism that leads to this disordered regulation of growth is unknown.

5. What is ultraviolet light?

All energies that move at the speed of light are collectively referred to as electromagnetic radiation or "light." Various types of light differ in their wavelength, frequency, and energy. Ultraviolet light is light with wavelengths between 150 and 300 nm. Ultraviolet-B (UV-B) is a section of the UV spectrum, with wavelengths between 270 and 320 nm.

6. Why is the amount of UV-B received dependent on location?

Cloud cover: The radiation in UV-B exposure depends on the cloud cover's thickness.

Latitude and elevation: At the high-latitude polar regions, the sun is always low in the sky. Because sunlight passes through more atmosphere, more of the UV-B is absorbed. For this reason, average UV-B exposure at the poles is over a thousand times lower than at the equator.

Proximity to an industrial area: Mainly because of the protection offered by photochemical smog. Industrial processes produce ozone, one of the more irritating components of smog, which absorbs UV-B. This is thought to be one of the main reasons that significant ozone losses in the Southern Hemisphere have not been mirrored in the Northern Hemisphere.

7. What are the health effects of UV-B light?

Genetic damage: DNA absorbs UV-B light and the absorbed energy can break bonds in the DNA. Proteins present in the cell nucleus repair most of the DNA breakages, but unrepaired genetic damage of the DNA can lead to skin cancers.

The cancer link: The principle danger of skin cancer is to light-skinned peoples. A 1% decrease in the ozone layer will cause an estimated 2% increase in UV-B irradiation; it is estimated that this will lead to a 4% increase in basal cell carcinomas (BCC) and 6% increase in squamous cell carcinomas (SCC).

8. What is the most common skin malignancy?

Basal cell carcinoma (BCC) is the most common, accounting for 80% of non-melanoma skin cancers. BCCs occur largely (85%) on the head and neck. In addition, they are by far the most common malignant tumor of any organ. More than 25% of diagnosed cancers in the United States each year is BCC.

9. What are the risk factors for BCC?

Light skin, fifth decade, and sun exposure. Light skin and the duration of UV radiation exposure are the major risk factors for BCC. However, because the distribution of BCC does not correlate directly with degree of sun exposure, the relationship between BCC and UV radiation is unclear. Additional risk factors include ionizing radiation, scars, and arsenic exposure. Immunosuppressed patients have a modestly increased risk for developing BCC, which may be more aggressive in this population.

10. What are some of the pathologic features of BCC?
- Locally invasive but almost never metastasizes
- Gross pathology—pearly papules
- Basal cell tumors have "palisading" nuclei

11. What is another name for the basal cell nevus syndrome?

Also called Gorlin's syndrome, basal cell nevus syndrome is an autosomal dominant genetic condition (mapped to 9q chromosome).

12. What is basal cell nevus syndrome?

A rare (600 cases) autosomal dominant syndrome that predisposes the affected individual to multiple nevoid BCCs, ondontogenic keratocysts, ocular abnormalities, rib abnormalities, medulloblastomas and other neoplasms, and a wide range of other anomalies. Affected patients usually present with multiple BCCs between puberty and their mid-30s, with seizures and characteristic cutaneous lesions. The number of lesions varies from patient to patient and ranges from a few to thousands. They can become locally invasive and cause significant destruction. Complete cutaneous examinations every 3–6 months are required for early diagnosis and treatment.

13. What are the diagnostic criteria for basal cell nevus syndrome?

Diagnosis requires two major criteria, or one major and one minor criteria. Major criteria: > two basal cell carcinomas, < 30 years old, odontogenic keratocysts, palmar pits, flax calcification, and family history. Minor criteria: rib or vertebral anomalies, macrocrania, fribroma, medulloblastoma, lymphomesenteric cysts.

14. What is the most common type of BCC?
Nodulo-ulcerative BCC.

15. Describe the clinical types of BCC.

Clinical Types of Basal Cell Carcinomas

Nodulo-ulcerative	Most common type. Begins as small, pearly telangiectatic papule and slowly enlarges. Forms central ulcer surrounded by rolled pearly border.
Pigmented	Similar to nodulo-ulcerative, but instead with brown pigmentation.
Superficial	Occurs predominantly on trunk. Appears as slightly indurated, scaling, erythematous patches. May resemble patches of eczema, psoriasis, tinea, or excoriation.
Morpheaform	Occurs almost exclusively on face and often mistaken for a scar. Flat or slightly depressed, indurated, yellowish plaques without defined border.
Fibroepitheliomas	Raised, moderately firm, slightly pedunculated or sessile lesions. Mildly erythematous with a smooth skin surface.

16. Are BCCs aggressive? What factors suggest that a BCC will be aggressive?
In general, BCCs are locally invasive, slowly spreading, and have very low metastatic potential. **Morpheaform tumors** are undoubtedly the most aggressive type and also have the highest recurrence rate. **Local nerve involvement** by neurophilic spread has been associated with increased aggressiveness. This occurs in approximately 1% of BCCs, most of which are of the infiltrating type. **Tumor location** also seems to influence BCC behavior, with central face tumors tending to be more aggressive and having an increased recurrence rate. Greater recurrence risk has also been seen with **large tumors.**

17. What is Mohs' micrographic surgery?
Originally devised by Frederick Mohs in the 1930s, this technique significantly decreases the recurrence rate of certain skin cancers. Completeness of excision is assessed with *intraoperative* histopathologic tumor examination. A precise mapping technique allows the surgeon to identify the exact location of remaining cancer tissue. The usual approach today involves freezing a surgical specimen, cutting horizontal sections from its base, and examining these sections for residual tumor. A later attempt was made to use Mohs' name as an acronym, by characterizing this as *M*icro-*O*ncologic *H*istologically controlled *S*urgery.

18. Why is Mohs' micrographic surgery performed for BCC?
Mohs' surgery is most effective for tumors that invade by direct extension from the primary site. Accordingly, BCCs are excellent candidates. The overall 5-year recurrence rate for primary BCCs is estimated at 1%. Mohs' technique should be considered when a BCC is recurrent or possesses a diameter > 2 cm, aggressive histology, or ill-defined border. It should also be considered when a BCC of the head and neck region occurs in a high-risk location, such as the nose, periorbital area, ears, or lips. The advantage of Mohs' procedure is that it allows complete, histologically verified tumor excision without the loss of wide margins of normal skin and without the risk of inadequate margins that may leave tumor behind. Mohs' surgery offers survival and metastatic (spread of cancer) rates equal to those of wide surgical excision, yet with significantly narrower margins and without the risk of local recurrence due to incomplete excision.

19. Are additional treatments available for BCC?
Effective management of primary BCC usually involves early diagnosis and surgery. Surgical excision, curettage with electrodesiccation, and cryosurgery has 5-year recurrence rates of

10.1%, 7.7%, and 7.5%, respectively. Radiation therapy also is effective in treating BCC, with a 5-year recurrence rate of approximately 9%. Less aggressive treatment with topical 5-fluorouracil has received recent support. In addition to primary tumor treatment, adequate follow-up is important for early diagnosis of recurrence. Because they are at risk for developing a second lesion, patients should be taught to recognize the early features of skin cancer.

20. How prevalent are cutaneous squamous cell carcinomas of the head and neck?

Cutaneous squamous cell carcinoma (CSCC) is the second most common skin cancer. It accounts for 20% of all cutaneous malignancies, over 95% of which arise on the head and neck. The diagnosis is typically made during the seventh decade of life, and males are more likely to develop these lesions. Development of CSCC has been associated with arsenic exposure.

21. Where is arsenic found?

The major source of occupational exposure to arsenic in the United States is in the manufacture of pesticides, herbicides, and other agricultural products. High exposure to arsenic fumes and dust may occur in the smelting industries; the highest concentrations most likely occur among roaster workers.

Arsenic has a predilection for skin and is excreted by desquamation of skin and in sweat, particularly during periods of profuse sweating. It also concentrates in nails and hair. Arsenic in nails produces Mee's lines (transverse white bands across fingernails) appearing about 6 weeks after onset of symptoms of toxicity.

22. What factors predispose to CSCC development?

The etiology of CSCC seems to involve interplay between extrinsic and intrinsic factors. The most commonly implicated extrinsic factor is long-term unprotected exposure to **ultraviolet light.** The wavelengths of light responsible for skin erythema and sunburn are associated with carcinogenesis. **Chemical exposure** is another extrinsic factor implicated in CSCC development. Inciting chemicals include arsenic, soot, coal tar, paraffin oil, petroleum oil, and asphalt. A high incidence of **human papillomavirus** presence has been detected in certain cases and may be another extrinsic factor in CSCC carcinogenesis. This finding also may be related to immune system dysfunction and may not be an independent etiologic factor. **Immunosuppression** appears to be an important intrinsic factor for CSCC development, with the patient's impaired ability to respond immunologically to UV radiation perhaps being one of the most important carcinogenic mechanisms. **Age** is clearly a risk factor for CSCC development. However, some argue that aging may be a manifestation of altered immunologic function and therefore not an independent etiologic factor.

23. How often is CSCC cured?

The 5-year cure rate for CSCC ranges from 75–90%. Of the approximately 5000 deaths that occur yearly from non-melanoma skin cancer, 75% are due to head and neck CSCCs. The incidence of metastasis varies between 0.3–3.7%, and the 5-year survival rate for these patients is only 25%.

24. What factors affect recurrence and prognosis of CSCCs?

Factors include anatomic site, etiology, histologic features, tumor size, depth of invasion, and the patient's immune status. Lesions arising from the external ear, lip, and temple are more likely to recur. Increased recurrence is also seen when lesions arise from areas previously exposed to gamma radiation or from chronic lesions including wounds, burn scars, and ulcers. Survival and cure rate decrease as lesion size increases, especially when lesions are > 2–3 cm in diameter. Invasion below the coiled region of the sweat glands or penetration into muscle, cartilage, bone, parotid gland, or perineurium increases the recurrence risk. Patients with lesions containing a larger percentage of well-differentiated cells have increased survival. Immune factors also affect prognosis. The amount of immune dysfunction varies directly with metastasis incidence. In addition, this population has a higher incidence of multiple primary tumors and a poorer prognosis.

25. What is Bowen's disease?

Bowen's disease is an intraepidermal squamous cell carcinoma that usually spreads along the epidermal plane. It may invade the dermis and metastasize in 20–25% of cases. On examination, it is a slowly growing, reddened, scaly patch that may become nodular with invasion. These lesions usually occur on sun-exposed areas, although they may occur on non-exposed areas in black people. When involving the oral mucosa, the lesion appears as a velvety, reddened macule that becomes elevated and may ulcerate. Approximately 30% of patients with this disease develop invasive squamous cell carcinoma.

26. A patient in the clinic has a 3-cm lesion over his right temple, which he states has tripled in size over the last month. You suspect CSCC. Are you likely to be correct?

Although this lesion may be CSCC, it is most likely a **keratoacanthoma.** This lesion is often difficult to distinguish from CSCC, both clinically and histopathologically. Unlike CSCCs, keratoacanthomas rapidly enlarge, reaching their full size in about 2 months. They are usually smooth, firm, dome-shaped, verrucous nodules filled centrally with keratin craters. Involution usually occurs within 2–6 months and may leave a depressed scar. Large central face or lip lesions may be aggressive. Deep tissue invasion has been reported, and metastases may be seen in cases with multiple lesions refractory to treatment.

27. How are BCC and CSCC staged? How are they graded?

The American Joint Committee on Cancer has developed a classification system for skin carcinoma that applies to both clinical and pathologic staging. Bowen's disease is included and should be classified as Tis.

The 1992 American Joint Committee on Cancer
Staging System for Cutaneous Melanoma

DEFINITIONS	
Primary tumor (pT)*	
• pTX	Primary tumor cannot be assessed
• pTO	No evidence of primary tumor
• pTis	Melanoma in situ (atypical melanocytic hyperplasia, severe melanocytic dysplasia), not an invasive lesion (Clark level I)
• pT1	Tumor 0.75 mm or less in thickness and invades the papillary dermis (Clark level II)
• pT2	Tumor more than 0.75 mm but not more than 1.5 mm in thickness and/or invades the papillary reticular-dermal interface (Clark level III)
• pT3	Tumor more than 1.5 mm but not more than 4 mm in thickness and/or invades the reticular dermis (Clark level IV)
pT3a	Tumor more than 1.5 mm but not more than 3 mm in thickness
pT3b	Tumor more than 3 mm but not more than 4 mm in thickness
• pT4	Tumor more than 4 mm in thickness and/or invades the subcutaneous tissue (Clark level V) and/or satellite(s) within 2 cm of the primary tumor
pT4a	Tumor more than 4 mm in thickness and/or invades the subcutaneous tissue
pT4b	Satellite(s) within 2 cm of primary tumor
Lymph node (N)	
• NX	Regional lymph nodes cannot be assessed
• N0	No regional lymph node metastasis
• N1	Metastases ≤3 cm in greatest dimension in any regional lymph node(s)
• N2	Metastases >3 cm in greatest dimension in any regional lymph node(s) and/or in transit metastases
N2a	Metastases >3 cm in greatest dimension in any regional lymph node(s)
N2b	In transit metastases
N2c	Both (N2a and N2b)
Distant metastases (M)	
• MX	Presence of distant metastases cannot be assessed
• M0	No distant metastases
• M1	Distant metastases

Table continues on next page.

| M1a | Metastases in skin or subcutaneous tissue or lymph node(s) beyond the regional lymph nodes |
| M1b | Visceral metastases |

STAGE GROUPING			
I	pT1	N0	M0
	pT2	N0	M0
II	pT3	N0	M0
	pT4	N0	M0
III	Any pT	N1	M0
	Any pT	N2	M0
IV	Any pT	Any N	M1

*If there is a discrepancy between tumor thickness and level, the pT category is based on the less favorable finding.
Adapted from Balch MC, Houghton AN, Sober AJ, Soon S-J: Cutaneous Melanoma, 3rd ed. St. Louis, Quality Medical Publishing, 1998.

28. Describe the clinical features of xeroderma pigmentosum.

Xeroderma pigmentosum is an autosomal recessive disorder in which patients have a defect in the DNA-repair system responsible for detecting and excising damaged DNA segments. The most common cause of DNA damage is UVB radiation. The initial clinical manifestation is an abnormal response to sunlight, with patients having a delayed-onset erythema and prolonged response after sun exposure. Early freckling and pigment abnormalities also occur. The incidence of skin malignancies in this population is very high. The median age that patients present with a skin cancer is 8 years. Malignancies include BCC and CSCC, and the overwhelming majority occur on the face, head, or neck. Melanomas have been estimated to occur 2000 times more often than expected in the general population.

29. What is melanoma?

Melanoma is a highly malignant tumor of the skin that is usually darkly pigmented. It is sometimes called malignant melanoma. Melanoma had been on the rise in the United States in the last few decades and is becoming more common every year. This is a very serious kind of skin cancer that can cause death. If this cancer is caught early, when it is very small, it can be cured. Early detection and treatment can prevent deaths and morbidity. A melanoma can grow in a mole that you have had for years. Or it can grow in a spot that never had a mole before. Many benign growths can resemble melanoma, so a suspicious growth should receive a full-depth biopsy to make a definitive diagnosis.

30. How is melanoma diagnosed?

Melanoma is diagnosed by the "ABCDE" Guidelines:

Asymmetry	Benign lesions are symmetrical.
	Melanomas tend to have pronounced asymmetry.
Border	Benign lesions usually have smooth borders.
	Melanomas tend to have notched, irregular outlines.
Color	Benign lesions usually contain only one color.
	Melanomas frequently have variegated color.
Diameter	Benign pigmented lesions are usually < 6 mm in diameter.
Elevation	Malignant melanoma is almost always elevated, at least in part, so that it is palpable.

31. What are the risk factors for malignant melanoma of the head and neck?

- Prolonged sunlight exposure—Particularly when it occurs during early childhood and leads to sunburning
- Pre-existing pigmented lesions—About 70% of melanomas arising on the head and neck develop from a pre-existing mole
- Race and skin complexion—Fair-skinned, poorly tanning individuals with red or blonde hair are more likely to develop melanoma

- Age—Most melanomas are diagnosed in the 5th and 6th decades of life
- Family history
- Immunosuppression

32. What physical findings of a pigmented lesion suggest malignant melanoma?
The distinction between melanoma and non-melanoma pigmented lesions can be difficult. The following are characteristics of pigmented lesions suggestive of melanoma:
- Mild itch or slightly altered skin sensation
- Maximum diameter >1 cm
- Increasing size
- Irregular lateral margin
- Multiple shades of brown-black, red, and blue (color variation)
- Inflammation
- Bleeding or crusting within the lesion

33. What preventive measures should be taken for individuals who are at risk?
Patients with multiple pigmented nevi should be taught to recognize suspicious lesions and encouraged to see a physician when one is discovered. At-risk individuals should be followed by a dermatologist.

34. What are the clinical appearances of the subdivisions of malignant melanoma?

Clinical Types of Malignant Melanoma

Lentigo maligna	Predominantly occur on sun-exposed skin in older persons, with 90% on head and neck
	Appear initially as macular areas with increased pigmentation
	Neoplastic melanocytes confined to epidermis
	Lesions expand laterally across skin and may regress centrally
	Invasive phase shows densely pigmented, raised nodules with pre-existing macular area
	Melanoma cell present in dermis
Superficial spreading melanoma	40–50% of melanoma in the United States
	Usually occurs on calf or back; less common on head and neck
	Presents as irregularly shaped pigmented areas, usually >1 cm in diameter
	Border and pigmentation tend to be irregular
	Central nodules may develop over time
Nodular malignant melanoma	Occur predominantly on trunk but may occur on head and neck
	Blue-black nodule with normal surrounding skin
Acral lentiginous melanoma	Occur on hand and soles of feet, usually not found on head and neck
	Raised, densely black nodular lesions within a pigmented macular area

35. In addition to appearance, what physical features are important in assessing a possible malignant melanoma?
Thorough examination of the neck with careful palpation for **enlarged lymph nodes** is essential when assessing melanotic lymphatic metastases. In addition to the cervical lymph nodes, the preauricular, retroauricular, suboccipital, and buccinator regions should be evaluated when the location of a pigmented lesion suggests lymph node involvement.

36. How is melanoma diagnosed?
Diagnosis of melanoma is made primarily on histopathologic examination of **biopsy tissue.** Whenever possible, excisional biopsy should be performed so that the entire lesion may be examined microscopically. Shave biopsy with curettage should not be performed on any lesion suspicious for melanoma. In cases when the lesion is large or excisional biopsy is impractical, a full-thickness elliptical incision or punch biopsy provides adequate sample for diagnosis.

37. What are Breslow's Microstages?

Tumor thickness in malignant melanoma is often reported according to Breslow's Microstages. This measurement is obtained by selecting the thickest portion of a given tumor and cutting a section. After hematoxylin-eosin staining, the distance between the granular layer of the epidermis and the deepest identified tumor cell is measured. Reported in millimeters, this value is inversely proportional to survival.

BRESLOW'S MICROSTAGES	FIVE-YEAR SURVIVAL (%)
1 <0.76 mm	>98
2 0.76–1.49 mm	87–94
3 1.50–4.00 mm	66–83
4 >4.00 mm	<50

38. What are Clark's Levels?

Tumor invasion is indicated by Clark's Levels, which relate the most deeply invading tumor cells to surrounding structures. Like Breslow thickness, these levels also have prognostic significance.

CLARK'S LEVELS	FIVE-YEAR SURVIVAL (%)
1 Intraepidermal	>99
2 Invasion of papillary dermis	95
3 Fill the papillary dermis	82
4 Invasion of reticular dermis	71
5 Invasion of fat	49

39. How are malignant melanomas staged?

Staging of malignant melanoma uses maximal tumor depth to determine the tumor stage.

Staging of Melanomas

STAGE	DEFINITION
Primary tumor (T)	
Tx	Primary tumor cannot be assessed
T0	No evidence of primary tumor
Tis	Carcinoma in situ
T1	Tumor ≤ 2 cm in greatest dimension
T2	Tumor 2–5 cm in greatest dimension
T3	Tumor >5 cm in greatest dimension
T4	Tumor invades deep extradermal structures (cartilage, skeletalmuscle, and bone)
Regional lymph nodes (N)	
Nx	Regional lymph nodes cannot be assessed
N0	No regional node metastasis
N1	Regional lymph node metastasis
Distant metastasis (M)	
Mx	Presence of distant metastasis cannot be assessed
M0	No distant metastasis
M1	Distant metastasis
Histopathologic grade (G)	
Gx	Grade cannot be assessed
G1	Well differentiated
G2	Moderately well differentiated
G3	Poorly differentiated
G4	Undifferentiated

40. How is malignant melanoma treated?

The primary tumor is treated by **surgical removal.** The amount of normal skin margin resected around a malignant melanoma is determined by tumor thickness. A 1-cm margin of normal skin around the resected lesion is appropriate for tumors < 2 mm thick. Thicker melanomas require wider margins, but no more than 3 cm is necessary. Adequate margins are often difficult to obtain in the head and neck region because of the proximity of important structures, such as the eye.

Evaluation and treatment of possible regional and distant metastasis follow primary treatment. Patients with localized melanoma are at risk for regional lymphatic metastases, and elective neck dissection is advocated by many clinicians. Patients with palpable lymph nodes should undergo regional lymph node dissection. Involved nodes and those at risk for containing metastases should be removed. When multiple nodes are involved, a radical neck dissection is frequently necessary. It is not clear at present whether adjuvant radiation or systemic therapy is helpful, but initial data indicate that radiation may increase survival for patients with proven neck metastases.

41. What is the overall outcome of malignant melanoma?

The prognosis for the patient with melanoma, however, is irrespective of the subtype and depends solely on the vertical depth of invasion. Long-term survival in patients with metastic disease is only 5%. Conversely, the prognosis for patients with early disease is excellent, and this stage is often curable with simple surgical excision.

DEPTH OF INVASION	FIVE-YEAR SURVIVAL (%)
≤0.75 mm	96
0.76–1.49 mm	87
1.50–2.49 mm	75
2.50–3.99 mm	66
≥4.00 mm	47

42. What is the familial dysplastic nevus syndrome?

The familial dysplastic nevus syndrome is an autosomal dominant heritable disorder with variable penetrance and a wide range of expressivity. Affected individuals have a large number of pigmented nevi, many of which are dysplastic. Persons who have dysplastic nevi, either familial or nonfamilial, are predisposed to developing malignant melanoma. A patient with familial dysplastic nevi is approximately 400 times more likely to develop melanoma. Individuals with dysplastic nevi with no family history are six to seven times more likely to develop melanoma.

43. Where does familial dysplastic nevus syndrome occur?

Dysplastic nevi tend to appear on sun-exposed areas and are commonly found on the head and neck. When compared to benign nevi, these lesions are larger and more numerous with more variegated color, irregular borders, and papular surface. Affected individuals require careful monitoring every 3–6 months. Lesion removal with histopathologic examination should be performed when clinical features are consistent with malignant transformation.

44. How prevalent are neoplasms of the adnexa?

The adnexa are the skin appendages and include eccrine and apocrine sweat glands, hair follicles, and sebaceous glands. Malignancies of these structures are very different from those of the epidermis, and most are highly malignant. They account for approximately 0.005% of all skin lesions.

45. Which are more common, sarcomas of the skin or deeper tissue sarcomas?

Sarcomas of the dermis and subcutaneous tissue are much less common than deeper tissue sarcomas. They account for approximately 0.003% of soft tissue sarcomas. Sarcomas of the skin are usually histologically identical to deeper tumors and thus are a diagnostic challenge. Sarcomas confined to superficial structures, particularly the dermis, have a better prognosis than deeper tissue sarcomas.

46. Does Kaposi's sarcoma often occur on the head and neck?

Kaposi's sarcoma (KS), a superficial skin sarcoma, has had a dramatic increase in the number of cases in young AIDS patients, especially homosexual men. It is the initial manifestation of AIDS in 18–30% of patients. The classic KS type usually involves the lower extremities and affects elderly men of Mediterranean or Jewish descent. AIDS-associated KS differs in appearance and distribution. Lesions occur commonly on the head and neck, as well as on the arms and trunk and in all areas of the upper aerodigestive tract. Early lesions can be small and subtle, often resembling a simple bruise. These pink macules have a surrounding white halo and progress within days to indurated papules with a yellow-green halo. They usually cease growing when they attain a size of 8–15 mm and turn gray with maturation. KS lesions are highly radiosensitive, and single-agent chemotherapy regimens have been effective in treating the disease.

CONTROVERSIES

47. Should elective lymph node dissection (ELND) be performed with localized malignant melanoma?

The role of ELND is probably the most controversial aspect of malignant melanoma treatment. Proponents cite studies that demonstrate effective control of regional metastases and more accurate staging with ELND. It removes a possible source of tumor burden and allows early treatment of metastatic disease. Opponents argue that the patient undergoes unnecessary morbidity from ELND.

48. What measure is used to determine whether ELND is indicated?

Tumor thickness is the measure most often used. Most investigators argue that it should not be performed when the lesion is < 1.0 mm thick, but it has little benefit when the lesion is > 4.0 mm thick. Several studies indicate that ELND confers survival advantage for intermediate-thickness melanomas. However, other trials support the concept that positive lymph nodes are a systemic disease manifestation and show that survival is the same for patients who wait until a therapeutic lymph node dissection is necessary.

Selective lymphadenectomy following **sentinel node identification** has received recent support. The sentinel node is the first node into which the primary lesion drains. Theoretically, if this node is negative, the remaining nodes should also be negative. The procedure can be performed on an outpatient basis, using local anesthesia and small incisions. Proponents of the procedure argue that it can be used as a prognostic indicator, identifying the subgroup of melanoma patients who would be candidates for complete ELND and therefore reducing unnecessary morbidity.

49. How is distant metastatic melanoma treated?

Complete resection of a single distant metastatic melanoma can usually be achieved in two-thirds of cases. Complete resection of melanoma metastatic to multiple sites can be achieved in about one-third of cases, but 5-year survival in this group is < 10%. Soft tissue and extraregional nodal lesions are resectable in 70% of cases. Pulmonary, extrahepatic abdominal and osseous lesions can be resected in only 40% of cases.

50. Are mucosal melanomas different from cutaneous melanomas?

Mucosal melanomas behave differently than cutaneous melanomas. They are more aggressive and usually are associated with a grave prognosis. Lymph node metastases from a mucosal primary tumor are infrequent. They occur more commonly on Asians, primarily Japanese. The overall incidence of head and neck mucosal melanomas is 2%.

BIBLIOGRAPHY

1. Abel EA: Skin neoplasias including cutaneous lymphoma, melanoma, and others: Unapproved treatments or indications. Clin Dermatol 18:201–210, 2000.
2. Brown RO, Osguthorpe JD: Management of the neck in nonmelanocytic cutaneous carcinomas. Otolaryngol Clin North Am 31:841–856, 1998.
3. Edman RL, Wolfe JT: Prevention and early detection of malignant melanoma. AAFP 62:2277–2284, 2000.
4. England RJ, Stafford ND: Conservative neck surgery in squamous cell carcinoma. Surg Oncol 7:91–94, 1998.
5. Haddad FF, Costello D, Reintgen DS: Radioguided surgery for melanoma. Surg Oncol Clin North Am 8:413–426, 1999.
6. Jerant AF, Johnson JT, Sheridan CD, et al: Early detection and treatment of skin cancer. AAFP 62:357–368, 2000.
7. Kelley MC, Ollila DW, Morton DL: Lymphatic mapping and sentinel lymphadenectomy for melanoma. Semin Surg Oncol 14:283–290, 1998.
8. Kumar V, Cotran RS, Robbins SL: Basic Pathology: The Skin. W.B. Saunders, 1997, pp. 698–712.
9. Maiolino P, de Vico G: Proliferation indexes. A comparison between cutaneous basal and squamous cell carcinomas. J Clin Pathol 50:355, 1997.
10. McCord MW, Mendenhall WM, Parsons JT, et al: Skin cancer of the head and neck with clinical perineural invasion. Int J Radiat Oncol Biol Phys 47:89–93, 2000.
11. Myers JN: Value of neck dissection in the treatment of patients with intermediate-thickness cutaneous malignant melanoma of the head and neck. Arch Otolaryngol Head Neck Surg 125:110–115, 1999.
12. Neely J: The utility of sentinel node biopsy in managing melanoma. JAAPA 12:14–19, 1999.
13. Stadelmann WK, McMasters K, Digenis AG, et al: Cutaneous melanoma of the head and neck: Advances in evaluation and treatment. Plast Reconstr Surg 105:2105–2126, 2000.
14. Staffel JG, Denneny JC, Eibling DE, et al: Primary Care Otolaryngology. American Academy of Otolaryngology—Head and Neck Surgery Foundation: Skin Cancer. 2000, pp.80–82.
15. White WL, Loggie BW: Sentinel lymphadenectomy in the management of primary cutaneous malignant melanoma. Dermatol Clin 17:645–655, 1999.

50. RADIATION THERAPY FOR HEAD AND NECK CANCER

Rachel Rabinovitch, M.D.

1. What is radiation therapy (RT)?

RT is the medical use of ionizing radiation to treat malignant tumors, and less often, benign diseases. RT is most often delivered from a linear accelerator (Linac), a machine that has the ability to create a variety of radiation beams. Cobalt machines house a single radioactive cobalt source, which provides a specific low-energy radiation beam. Newer machines deliver other atomic particles, for example neutrons. Delivery of radiotherapy that originates external to a patient, as from a Linac, is called **external beam radiotherapy**. Radiation treatment can also be delivered by permanently or temporarily placing radioactive sources into a person's body; this is called **brachytherapy**. The two most commonly used types of radiation in clinical practice are photon beams (deeply penetrating) and electron beams (superficially penetrating).

2. How does radiation therapy work?

Ionizing radiation causes damage to the DNA of targeted cells (usually cancer cells) through a complicated series of atomic interactions. Most of the nuclear damage is due to the interaction of DNA with free radicals, formed by the interaction of the radiation with water molecules. Normal cells in the body are better able to repair DNA damage than tumor cells, which are less efficient at DNA repair. Following RT, damaged cells undergo mitotic cell death.

3. What are the advantages of RT in comparison with surgery?

RT, like surgery, is a local therapy, delivered to a specific body site containing a tumor and often to surrounding lymph node stations containing microscopic or gross disease. Since it is delivered on an outpatient basis, RT allows the patient to continue daily activities without interruption. A patient with numerous medical conditions, rendering him or her a poor surgical candidate, is not prevented from receiving RT, as there is no concern with the risks of anesthesia, bleeding, and so on. RT, when delivered as the primary treatment modality, is less physically deforming than surgery. Definitive RT allows for continued organ preservation and function, potentially resulting in an improved quality of life. This advantage is most evident in the treatment of tumors of the head and neck, where RT can preserve normal speech, swallowing, and breathing.

4. Are there disadvantages of RT in comparison with surgery?

In contrast to a one-time surgical procedure, RT is generally delivered on a daily basis, Monday through Friday, over 6–8 weeks. This protracted time commitment can be problematic for noncompliant or elderly patients and those living great distances from a radiation oncology facility. Another potential limitation of RT is its decreased ability to control locally advanced tumors, or those near radiosensitive critical structures (i.e., the spinal cord, optic nerves, etc). Since there is a direct correlation between tumor control and treatment dose, the radiation oncologist may be limited in delivery of the required tumoricidal dose due either to technical factors or sensitivity of surrounding normal tissues.

5. Will RT make the patient radioactive?

Patients undergoing external beam RT are never radioactive, whereas those undergoing brachytherapy procedures may be. The high-energy sources used for temporary implants necessitate that the patient remain in a shielded room for the several minutes of a high dose rate treatment, or in a single-patient hospital room for the hours of a low dose rate implant. Once the brachytherapy sources are removed, the patient is no longer a radiation risk to anyone. Permanent

brachytherapy implants, such as those used for prostate cancer, generally use low-energy iso-
topes, which are largely absorbed by the surrounding tissues.

6. What tumors can be definitively treated with radiation as the sole treatment modality?
Nearly all head and neck cancers that are T1–T2 ($<$ 4 cm) and N0–N1 (single ipsilateral
lymph nodes $<$ 3 cm) are candidates for definitive RT. These include primary tumors of the
tongue, tonsil, larynx, and hypopharynx. Exceptions include cancers of the nasopharynx, in which
external beam RT is the standard treatment regardless of T or N stage. Tumors of the salivary
glands and floor of the mouth are generally managed primarily with surgery, even if diagnosed at
an early stage. Specialized radiation techniques and RT combined with chemotherapy are appropriate nonsurgical options for larger (T3–T4, N2–N3) head and neck tumors. Adjuvant neck dissections following irradiation is often important in the management of bulky (N2–N3) neck disease.

**7. What are the standard indications for adjuvant RT following surgical resection of a
head and neck tumor?**
• Primary tumor $>$ 4 cm, invading bone or beyond the primary site (T3–T4)
• Multiple positive neck nodes
• Extracapsular nodal extension
• Positive resection margins of either the primary tumor or neck disease
• Recurrent disease

8. Who cannot be treated with RT?
Patients with collagen-vascular diseases, pregnant women, and those who have previously
received a maximal dose of RT to the head and neck region.

9. What are the common acute side effects of RT to the head and neck region?
During treatment, skin erythema, dryness, pruritus, and mild-moderate desquamation within
the treatment field are typically encountered. Hoarseness, serous otitis, mucositis, odynophagia,
and xerostomia are also common. The acute side effects of RT usually become manifest by the
second to third week of treatment and resolve within 4–6 weeks after completion. The main exception is xerostomia, which is permanent if the major salivary glands are included within the
treatment field and receive $>$2000 cGy.

10. How are these side effects managed during the course of treatment?
Moisturizers are commonly used to minimize and soothe the dermal symptoms, although
there is no single product that has proved superior to any other. Mild odynophagia is treated with
anesthetic mouth rinses, and oral analgesics (including narcotics) are indicated for more severe
pain and mucositis. On occasion, gastric tube feeding is required to maintain adequate nutrition
in a patient with severe oral/pharyngeal symptoms. Xerostomia can be minimized by prescribing
Pilocarpine (100–200 mg po TID) from the beginning of irradiation and continued for months
post-treatment.

11. Are there potential long-term complications of RT?
Serious radiation complications are unusual (with an incidence of $<$ 10%) but are difficult to
manage when they occur. The likelihood of a given patient developing long-term complications
depends on the total dose of radiation delivered, the time frame over which it was given, and the
anatomic sites included within the radiation portal. In general, the risk increases with increasing
doses delivered over shorter time periods to greater volumes of tissue. Complications include xerostomia, skin changes, hypothyroidism, osteonecrosis, bone exposure, laryngeal edema, and induction of secondary cancers. The incidence of osteonecrosis can be greatly diminished by meticulous dental care before, during, and after RT.

12. What is the most common long-term side effect of RT?

Xerostomia is the most common and bothersome long-term side effect of head and neck ir-radiation, and it results whenever major salivary glands are treated to doses > 2000 cGy. Loss of saliva negatively affects patients' quality of life because of the consequent difficulty with speech and eating, and general mouth discomfort. Dry mouth also causes an increased risk of develop-ing dental carries.

Once xerostomia has developed, intake of large amounts of liquids between and during meals and use of artificial saliva preparations are helpful interventions. Prevention of xerostomia, how-ever, is much more important. These symptoms can be minimized or even prevented through the use of pilocarpine both during and after salivary gland irradiation, and with salivary gland–sparing radiation treatment techniques.

13. What is the role of pre-RT dental evaluation?

An essential part of the radiation oncologist's care of the head and neck cancer patient is prompt referral for an evaluation by a dentist prior to starting RT. This evaluation includes de-termination of the need for any dental extractions or invasive dental procedures, which must be performed prior to initiation of RT. Two to 4 weeks of healing time are minimally required prior to starting RT. Healing of the gingiva and mandible is impaired following standard doses of RT; delay of anticipated extractions or invasive dental procedures until after RT predisposes the pa-tient to chronic and painful bone exposure and tissue necrosis.

Patients are generally provided with a prescription fluoride rinse or fitted for custom fluoride trays, to be used indefinitely following treatment. The lack of saliva and its altered pH in a dry ir-radiated mouth would otherwise predispose patients to dental caries on the exposed surfaces of teeth. Meticulous and consistent dental care completely obviates this problem.

14. What long-term skin changes are associated with RT?

Male patients may experience permanent facial alopecia in regions treated to > 6000 cGy. Other skin changes may include mild atrophy, pigmentation changes, development of skin or mu-cosal telangectasias, and submental edema.

15. What is the standard treatment for a T1N0M0 squamous cell carcinoma of the glottic larynx?

External beam RT delivered to the larynx, to a total dose of 6600 cGy in 6.5 weeks, results in a cure rate of >90%. Since the radiation is delivered to the larynx only, and not to regional lymph nodes, xerostomia does not result.

16. Is a total laryngectomy necessary in the curative management of advanced larynx cancer?

No. The Veterans Affairs Laryngeal Cancer Study Group performed a randomized trial in-volving 332 patients with stage III or IV larynx cancer in which patients received either total la-ryngectomy followed by RT or three cycles of chemotherapy (cisplatin and 5-fluorouracil) fol-lowed by RT. The results from this study demonstrated no difference in the survival rate between the two groups. Sixty-four percent of the patients in the chemo-RT arm were able to preserve la-ryngeal function. This trial established the curative role of chemoradiation as an organ-preserv-ing treatment for advanced cancers of the larynx. All patients being evaluated for advanced la-ryngeal cancer should be offered both treatment approaches. Furthermore, numerous publications have documented similar local control rates with specialized radiation techniques delivering ra-diation alone.

17. When evaluating the head and neck cancer patient, what principles guide the coordi-nation of RT and/or surgery?

It is critical to manage both the primary tumor and regional lymph nodes with one treatment modality whenever possible. This approach minimizes the toxicity and complications of com-bined modality therapy. Therefore, if the primary tumor is to be managed with surgical resection, then the regional neck lymph nodes, if at risk, should be treated with a neck dissection. Postoperative RT is added only if indicated. Likewise, when the primary tumor is to be treated with RT alone, the neck(s) should be included within the RT fields, followed by a neck dissection if necessary. When both surgery and RT are clearly necessary from the outset (i.e., large tumor and/or multiple neck nodes), the treatment modality addressing both the primary tumor and neck node(s) should be delivered first. It is unsound oncologic practice to first manage the neck with surgery, leaving the primary tumor untreated. Any wound complication would further delay initiation of definitive RT and/or potentially result in aberrant contralateral nodal drainage.

18. Explain the general dosing guidelines for treatment of the neck with RT.
A clinically negative undissected neck will be controlled with a probability of > 90% when a total dose of 5400 cGy is delivered in daily fractions of 180 cGy. Postoperative doses are higher, owing to the presence of fibrous scarring within the operative bed, resulting in decreased blood flow to the tissues at risk, which renders them less sensitive to external beam RT. A minimum dose of 5760 cGy is therefore indicated, increasing to a total dose of 6300 cGy whenever the neck dissection demonstrates extracapsular extension or other high-risk features. These dose recommendations are the result of a randomized trial from the M.D. Anderson Cancer Center that demonstrated increased failures with postoperative doses of 5400 cGy.

19. Have there been any recent technologic advances in head and neck radiotherapy?
Advances in Linac accessories and accompanying software have allowed for a new radiation technique called intensity modulated radiation therapy (IMRT). IMRT is achieved through the dynamic movement of metallic "fingers" through a radiation beam, blocking the beam from reaching the patient in a highly customized fashion. The intensity of radiation to the patient's various organs or tissues can be selectively tailored to a much greater degree with IMRT technology than through the use of standard blocking techniques. In other words, when treating a patient's tonsil cancer, for instance, a full 180 cGy can be delivered to the tumor with every treatment, while the dose to the spinal cord and ipsilateral salivary gland is just a small fraction of that dose. The full impact of IMRT technology on organ sparing and quality of life has yet to be fully explored.

20. Is RT always given once a day during the 6- to 8-week treatment course?
No. Once-daily RT treatments, generally called standard fractionation, is the traditional way of delivering radiotherapy. Investigation of altered fractionation schemes has been a major focus of head and neck radiotherapy research. The results of a recently completed radiotherapy head and neck cancer trial demonstrated that altered fractionation schemes are better than once-daily RT. When using RT alone, "accelerated hyperfractionation with concomitant boost" (delivering twice-daily treatment for the last 2 weeks of a 6-week treatment course) or "hyperfractionation" (twice daily treatment from the start of the treatment), results in improved local control and disease–free survival as compared with standard fractionation. These fractionation approaches have become the standard of care when treating patients definitively with RT alone for head and neck cancer. Future trials will compare these RT approaches with combined modality therapy (chemotherapy and RT).

21. What is the role of radiosensitizers in the use of RT to treat head and neck cancers?
Comprehensive treatment regimens for *advanced* squamous cell carcinoma of the head and neck require attention to both local tumor burden and disseminated disease. Recent protocols using cisplatin for radiosensitization of tumor cells during concomitant RT have shown progress to enhance tumor control. Cisplatin is a chemotherapeutic agent that induces DNA changes in malignant cells that may be mutagenic or lethal. Additionally, when used concurrently with radiation therapy, cisplatin acts as a radiosensitizer, increasing damage to malignant nuclear DNA to enhance the anti-neoplastic capacity of radiotherapy.
The mechanisms by which this radiosensitization occurs remain controversial, although one involves cisplatin's ability to inhibit the repair of sublethal damage in radiated tumor cells. Vari-

ations in protocols are underway, including the route of administration, dosing, scheduling, timing with surgery, and combination therapy with 5-fluorouracil and radiation. Higher response rates, prolonged mean survival, increased survival rates, longer local recurrence-free survival rates, and considerable organ preservation with the use of concurrent cisplatin and radiation have already been demonstrated. 5-fluorouracil, carboplatin, paclitaxel, and targeted monoclonal antibodies also appear to function as radiosensitizers.

CONTROVERSY

22. Which is better in the treatment of head and neck cancers: surgery or radiation?
Actually, you can't make a generalization in this area. The treatment is individualized according to the type and size of the primary tumor, presence and location of metastases, and general patient condition. And finally, the treatment options and recommendations must be discussed at length with the patient and family before the decision is reached.

BIBLIOGRAPHY

1. Colevas AD, Posner MR: Docetaxel in head and neck cancer: A review. Am J Clin Oncol 21:482–486, 1998.
2. Eisbruch A, Dawson LA, Kim HM, et al: Conformal and intensity modulated irradiation of head and neck cancer: The potential for improved target irradiation, salivary gland function, and quality of life. Acta Otorhinolaryngol Belg 53:271–275, 1999.
3. Forastiere AA: Taxoids in head and neck cancer: The American approach. Acta Otorhinolaryngol Belg 53:253–257, 1999.
4. Fu KK, Pajak TF, Trotti A, et al: A Radiation Therapy Oncology Group (RTOG) phase III randomized study to compare hyperfractionation and two variants of accelerated fractionation to standard fractionation radiotherapy for head and neck squamous cell carcinomas: First report of RTOG 9003. Int J Radiat Oncol Biol Phys 48:7–16, 2000.
5. Johnson JT, Ferretti GA, Nethery WJ, et al: Oral pilocarpine for post-irradiation xerostomia in patients with head and neck cancer. N Engl J Med 329:390–395, 1993.
6. Isaacs JH Jr, Stiles WA, Cassisi NJ, Million RR, Parsons JT: Postoperative radiation of open head and neck wounds—updated. Head Neck 19:194–199, 1997.
7. Metges JP, Eschwege F, de Crevoisier R, et al: Radiotherapy in head and neck cancer in the elderly: A challenge. Crit Rev Oncol Hematol 34:195–203, 2000.
8. Parsons JT, Mendenhall WM, Stringer SP, Cassisi NJ, Million RR: An analysis of factors influencing the outcome of postoperative irradiation for squamous cell carcinoma of the oral cavity. Int J Radiat Oncol Biol Phys 39:137–148, 1997.
9. Saunders MI: Head and neck cancer: Altered fractionation schedules. Oncologist 4:11–16, 1999.
10. Schrijvers D, Vermorken JB: Role of taxoids in head and neck cancer. Oncologist 5:199–208, 2000.
11. Senan S, Levendag PC: Brachytherapy for recurrent head and neck cancer. Hematol-Oncol Clin North Am 13:531–542, 1999.
12. Sharma VM, Wilson WR: Radiosensitization of advanced squamous cell carcinoma of the head and neck with cisplatin during concomitant radiation therapy. Eur Arch Otorhinolaryngol 256:462–465, 1999.
13. Trotti A: Toxicity in head and neck cancer: A review of trends and issues. Int J Radiat Oncol Biol Phys 47:1–12, 2000.
14. Vokes EE, Haraf DJ, Kies MS: The use of concurrent chemotherapy and radiotherapy for locoregionally advanced head and neck cancer. Semin Oncol 27(4 Suppl 8):34–38, 2000.
15. Wheeler RH, Spencer S, Buchsbaum D, et al: Monoclonal antibodies as potentiators of radiotherapy and chemotherapy in the management of head and neck cancer. Curr Opin Oncol 11:187–190, 1999.

51. CHEMOTHERAPY OF HEAD AND NECK CANCERS

Madeleine A. Kane, M.D., Ph.D.

1. What is chemotherapy?

Chemotherapy is the systemic treatment of cancer with cytotoxic drugs. These drugs are designed to have more impact on malignant cells than normal cells, but the therapeutic index is often small. Newer systemic treatments that are not, strictly speaking, chemotherapy drugs are showing some promise in chemoprevention as well as treatment.

2. What head and neck cancers may benefit from treatment with chemotherapy?

The most common histologic diagnosis for head and neck cancers is squamous cell carcinoma. This histologic type is the focus of this chapter. Response rates of over 50% have been reported with some chemotherapy regimens. Adenocarcinomas of the salivary glands have lower response rates; adenoid cystic carcinomas are indolent malignancies with little or no response to past chemotherapy. Kaposi's sarcoma of the oral cavity is sometimes treated with chemotherapy, with a response rate of 70% with paclitaxel. Lymphomas may also involve the head and neck and are usually very responsive to chemotherapy.

3. How is chemotherapy used in head and neck cancers?

Chemotherapy may be administered as (1) neoadjuvant or induction treatment; (2) adjuvant treatment; (3) concomitant treatment with radiation; (4) therapy for metastatic disease; (5) chemoprevention.

4. What is neoadjuvant or induction therapy?

In head and neck cancers, neoadjuvant or induction chemotherapy is used to induce a response (i.e., shrink the tumor significantly) prior to definitive local treatment with surgery and/or radiation therapy.

5. What is the goal of neoadjuvant chemotherapy?

The goal of this approach is to decrease the size and extent of the cancer so that definitive surgery or radiation therapy might be able to be less extensive. Chemotherapy alone in this application has not been definitely demonstrated to be of benefit, to date. Organ preservation is one potential goal of neoadjuvant chemotherapy, and chemotherapy preceding definitive radiation therapy for locally advanced laryngeal cancer permitted organ preservation in two-thirds of patients and resulted in the same 68% overall 2-year survival rate as laryngectomy followed by radiation.

6. What is adjuvant chemotherapy?

Adjuvant chemotherapy is administered after primary therapy with surgery and/or radiation has eradicated all detectable evidence of cancer, but a patient remains at high risk for recurrence owing to the size or extensiveness of the primary tumor and/or involvement of lymph nodes. Adjuvant chemotherapy alone with past treatment regimens has not been proven to benefit head and neck cancer patients, but, with the development of newer systemic treatments, studies continue.

7. Which chemotherapy agents have shown activity in head and necks cancers?

Objective response rates reported for single agents are as follows:

Docetaxel	38%	Bleomycin	21%
Paclitaxel	38%	Epirubicin	18%

Methotrexate	31%	5-fluorouracil (5Fu) (bolus)	15%
Cisplatin	28%	Vinorelbine	14%
Ifosfamide	26%	Topotecan	13%
Carboplatin	22%	Gemcitabine	6%

8. What is the role and goal of chemotherapy in patients with metastatic or recurrent head and neck cancers?

Systemic chemotherapy can play a significant role in palliating symptoms from extensive cancer, but no regimen to date has been able to induce durable complete responses. Objective response rates range from 30–90%. In addition, survival of patients may not be extended, but reduction in masses, painful infiltration of tissues, and regression of lung metastases may improve overall quality of life.

9. What is an objective response to chemotherapy?

An objective response means significant shrinkage of the tumor. Complete response is defined as disappearance of all detectable evidence of the cancer. Partial response is defined as 50% or more decrease in the sum of the products of the perpendicular diameters of all measurable disease. Stable disease is defined as a decrease in measurable tumor that is less than a 50% response, but less than 25% increase. Progressive disease is defined as a greater than 25% increase in the sum of the products of the perpendicular diameters of all measurable disease.

10. What is the rationale for using more than one chemotherapy drug at a time (combination chemotherapy)?

The use of more than one chemotherapy drug at a time reduces the chances that a population of cancer cells with resistance to a single agent will be selected for or that multidrug resistance will develop. Chemotherapy drugs selected to be used in combination are chosen for non-overlapping toxicities and non-cross resistance as far as is possible.

11. What are some commonly used active combination chemotherapy regimens in squamous cell carcinoma of the head and neck?

Cisplatin + 5FU by continuous infusion
Carboplatin + 5FU by continuous infusion
Cisplatin + paclitaxel
Cisplatin + 5FU + leucovorin + docetaxel
Methotrexate + 5FU

12. What are predictable side effects for the chemotherapy drugs commonly used to treat head and neck cancers?

Cisplatin: severe nausea; vomiting; renal failure; sodium, potassium, and magnesium wasting; peripheral neuropathy; hearing loss; anemia; anorexia; asthenia
5FU: diarrhea, mucositis, photosensitivity dermatitis, myelosuppression, fatigue
Methotrexate: mucositis, myelosuppression
Carboplatin: myelosuppression, nausea, vomiting, peripheral neuropathy, alopecia
Bleomycin: hypersensitivity reaction, fever, pulmonary toxicity (after high cumulative dose)
Paclitaxel: myelosuppression, peripheral neuropathy, nausea, vomiting, hypersensitivity reaction, alopecia
Docetaxel: myelosuppression, fluid retention, nausea, vomiting, hypersensitivity reaction, alopecia

13. What measures are taken to reduce side effects from chemotherapy drugs?

Prophylactic treatment with antiemetics is used with essentially all chemotherapy drugs. To prevent and treat severe nausea and vomiting, 5HT3 receptor blockers such as ondansetron or granisetron together with dexamethasone are used. Prochlorperazine may be adequate for drugs with low emetic potential such as 5FU, methotrexate, and bleomycin. Pretreatment and post-treatment hydration with electrolyte supplementation reduces the risk of renal failure, hearing loss, or electrolyte wasting in patients receiving cisplatin. Amifostine pretreatment also reduces the risk of renal impairment and possibly peripheral neuropathy. Dexamethasone, diphenhydramine, cimetidine, and acetaminophen are used to reduce the risk of severe hypersensitivity reaction or fever. Dexamethasone is also used to prevent fluid retention, reduce delayed emesis, and reduce myalgias and arthralgias after treatment. Severe myelosuppression may be abrogated by growth factor support with granulocyte colony stimulating factor (GCSF) or granulocyte-monocyte colony stimulating factor (GM-CSF) for neutropenia, erythropoietin for severe anemia, and/or oprelvekin for thrombocytopenia.

14. What is the role of chemotherapy combined with radiation therapy?
Several chemotherapy drugs (5FU, cisplatin, carboplatin, paclitaxel) appear to augment the efficacy of radiation therapy in low dose or in full dose. In low daily or weekly doses, little toxicity from chemotherapy is added to the side effects of radiation, and results seem to be improved. At least four randomized trials have shown statistically significant improved response rates and also overall survival when chemotherapy is added to radiation treatment for unresectable stage III or IV head and neck cancers. Local control rates are also impressively improved with the combined modality treatment compared with radiation alone.

15. What additional toxicity may be expected from chemotherapy combined with radiation therapy?
Both full-dose chemotherapy regimens including continuous-infusion 5FU and radiation therapy by itself cause mucositis as the dose-limiting toxicity. The combination may be worse, although the use of low-dose weekly chemotherapy reduces the side effects from chemotherapy without apparent loss of efficacy in local control. Myelosuppression, nausea, anorexia, and fatigue may also be worse with both modalities together. Aggressive nutritional support with enteral agents via gastrostomy tube is encouraged for patients undergoing definitive radiation treatment, especially with the addition of chemotherapy. Total parenteral nutrition is seldom needed.

16. What is chemoprevention?
Chemoprevention is treatment with systemic drug(s) to reduce the risk of development of cancer. Several clinical trials have suggested that retinoids can play a role in reduction of occurrence of squamous cell cancers of the head and neck in high-risk patients, such as those with leukoplakia. Isotretinoin (13-*cis*-retinoic acid) decreased the likelihood of development of second primary head and neck cancers in patients curatively treated for head and neck cancer, but the role of retinoids outside of a study is still controversial. Ketorolac also shows promise for the treatment of leukoplakia, a precancerous mucosal lesion.

17. What new systemic agents show promise in the treatment of head and neck cancers?
Monoclonal antibody C225, which is directed against the epidermal growth factor receptor, a growth-promoting protein that is overexpressed in the majority of squamous cell carcinomas of the head and neck, is showing promise in clinical trials when it is combined with radiation or chemotherapy. Capecitabine, an oral analogue of 5FU, is being studied as a possible substitute for continuous infusion intravenous 5FU. Gene therapy with adenoviral vectors expressing wild type p53 or HSV thymidine kinase with ganciclovir are being studied. Antisense oligodeoxynucleotides to cyclin D1 inhibited the growth of head and neck cancer cell lines in culture. Antiangiogenesis agents, farnesyltransferase inhibitors, and tyrosine kinase inhibitors are all being studied as well.

18. Why is the mucositis so severe in the treatment of head and neck cancer?
Most of the drugs currently used in the treatment of head and neck cancer cause mucositis. This side effect is made worse in patients who receive irradiation to the oral cavity, which damages the salivary glands.

19. Why is nutrition important for patients receiving chemotherapy for head and neck tumors?

Most of these patients are nutritionally depleted due to the morbidity of their aerodigestive tumor, previous surgery, or irradiation. Mucositis, nausea, vomiting, and anorexia from the chemotherapy compound the nutritional depletion, compounding the weight loss. Often, tube feedings or total parenteral nutrition are required to maintain patients' dietary needs. More recently, parenteral gastrostomy feedings have been used, especially where chemotherapy is combined with irradiation.

CONTROVERSY

20. Is it "worth it" to undergo chemotherapy for head and neck cancer?

This is another tough decision that must be individualized. Aside from the usual considerations of stage of tumor, type of tumor, and individual preference, current chemotherapy for head and neck cancer ("solid tumors") is not yet as promising as it is for some "liquid" tumors, such as some of the leukemias or lymphomas, which can be cured with chemotherapy. However, recent regimens are ever-more promising, with greater percentages of complete responders (with absence of clinical tumor for a period of time) and partial responders (decrease in size of measureable tumor of over 50% for a period of time) and less patient morbidity (e.g., loss of hair, nausea).

ECONOMICS OF CHEMOTHERAPY SUPPORTIVE MEASURES

One study comparing the cost of recombinant human erythropoietin (rHuEPO) with that of blood transfusions in the treatment of chemotherapy-induced anemia from a health care system perspective found that for a treatment period of 24 weeks, approximately 64% of rHuEPO recipients responded at an average expected cost of $12,971 per patient. *One hundred percent* of transfusion recipients responded at a cost of $481, resulting in a cost savings of $8490. From a health care system cost and outcome perspective, blood transfusion is the preferred strategy for chemotherapy-induced anemia; however, rHuEPO may be considered an effective blood-sparing alternative for patients with non–stem cell disorders. Equivalent analyses are indicated for other chemotherapeutic agents as these are often very expensive, and will become even more so as monoclonal antibodies and gene therapy leave the research laboratories and enter clinical practice.

~*Sheffield, Ann Pharmacother 31:22, 1997.*

BIBLIOGRAPHY

1. Al-Sarraf M, LeBlanc M, ShankerGiri PG, et al: Chemotherapy vs radiotherapy in patients with advanced nasopharyngeal cancer: Phase III randomized Intergroup Study 0099. J Clin Oncol 16:1310–1317, 1998.
2. Brizel DM, Albers ME, Fisher SR, et al: Hyperfractionated irradiation with or without concurrent chemotherapy for locally advanced head and neck cancer. N Engl J Med 338:1798–1804, 1998.
3. Clayman GL, Lippman SM, Laramore G, et al: Head and neck cancer. In Holland JF, Frei E III, Bast RC, et al (eds.): Cancer Medicine, 4th ed. Baltimore, William & Wilkins, 1997; pp. 1645–1710.
4. Colevas AD, Norris CM, Tishler RB, et al: Phase II trial of docetaxel, cisplatin, fluorouracil and leucovorin as induction for squamous cell carcinoma of the head and neck. J Clin Oncol 17:3505–3511, 1999.

5. Forastiere AA, Leong T, Rowinsky E, et al: A phase III comparison of high dose paclitaxel + cisplatin + GCSF versus low-dose paclitaxel + cisplatin in advanced head and neck cancers. J Clin Oncol 19:1088-1095, 2001.
6. Forastiere AA: Head and neck cancer: Overview of recent developments and future directions. Semin Oncol 27:1–4, 2000.
7. Khuri FR, Shin DM, Glisson BS, et al: Treatment of patients with recurrent or metastatic squamous cell carcinoma of the head and neck: Current status and future directions. Semin Oncol 27:25–33, 2000.
8. Khuri FR, Nemunaitis J, Ganly I, et al: A controlled trial of ONYX-015, a selectively-replicating adenovirus, in combination with cisplatin and 5-fluorouracil in patients with recurrent head and neck cancer. Nat Med 6: 879–885, 2000.
9. Shin DM, Glisson BS, Khuri FR: Phase II trial of paclitaxel, ifosfamide and cisplatin in patients with recurrent head and neck squamous cell carcinoma. J Clin Oncol 16:1325–1330, 2000.
10. Sidransky D, Schantz SP, Harrison LB, et al: Cancer of the head and neck. In: Cancer—Principles and Practice of Oncology, 6th ed. Philadelphia, Lippincott, Williams & Wilkins, 2001, pp. 789–916. (*This is a chapter with five sections; these authors have variously contributed to the five sections.*)
11. Veterans Affairs Laryngeal Cancer Study Group. Induction chemotherapy plus radiation compared with surgery plus radiation in patients with advanced laryngeal cancer. N Engl J Med 324:1685–1690, 1991.
12. Vokes EE, Haraf DJ, Kies MS: The use of concurrent chemotherapy and radiotherapy for locoregionally advanced head and neck cancer. Semin Oncol 27:34–38, 2000.
13. Vokes EE, Kies MS, Haraf DJ, et al: Concomitant chemoradiotherapy as primary therapy to locoregionally advanced head and neck cancer. J Clin Oncol 18:1652–1661, 2000.
14. Wheeler RH, Spencer S, Buchsbaum D, et al: Monoclonal antibodies as potentiators of radiotherapy and chemotherapy in the management of head and neck cancer. Curr Opin Oncol 11:187–190, 1999.

VII. Facial Plastic Surgery

52. PRINCIPLES OF GRAFTS AND FLAPS

Catherine P. Winslow, M.D., and Michael L. Lepore, M.D.

1. How do grafts and flaps differ?

A **graft** is a segment of tissue, often skin, that is transplanted *en bloc* to a recipient site where it obtains nutrients and, eventually, a blood supply from the recipient tissue. A **flap** is a segment of tissue (skin, subcutaneous tissue, muscle, bone, etc.) that is transplanted to the area of defect while maintaining attachment to its own vascular supply. A **microvascular free flap** is a segment of tissue dissected deep, with its arterial and venous blood supply, and transplanted to the area of defect. The vessels (arterial and venous) are grafted to vessels in the area of the proposed defect.

2. What are the commonly used grafts in head and neck surgery?

A **full-thickness skin graft** (FTSG) contains the epidermis and entire dermis.

A **split-thickness skin graft** (STSG) contains the epidermis and a variable amount, but not all, of the dermal layer. STSGs can be further classified as thin, intermediate, or thick.

A **dermal graft** contains dermis without any overlying epidermis. It is obtained by harvesting an STSG and then removing the overlying epidermis.

Mucosal grafts are obtained from mucosal-lined surfaces, such as the conjunctiva, oral cavity, or nasal cavity.

Bone grafts are used for mandibular and calvarium reconstruction.

Composite grafts contain more than one type of tissue, such as dermis-fat grafts and skin-cartilage-skin grafts.

3. Discuss the advantages and disadvantages of FTSGs and STSGs.

STSGs have less nutrient demand and therefore survive more readily. However, they result in more graft contracture and poorer color match, and are less resistant to trauma. FTSGs, conversely, have greater nutrient demand due to the increased thickness of the graft, and therefore do not "take" as easily. Additionally, because the entire dermis is removed, the donor bed requires an STSG unless the defect is very small and can be closed primarily. On the positive side, they suffer less contracture, are more resistant to trauma, and result in a better texture and color match than do STSGs.

4. Describe the steps involved in the survival of a skin graft.

It takes 3–4 days before blood flow to the graft is achieved. In the interim, survival of the graft depends on the arrival of nutrients and the removal of metabolic waste by diffusion. A *fibrin exudate* between graft and recipient bed is initially formed, which establishes adherence, allows for diffusion of metabolites, and establishes a framework through which vascular anastomoses will occur. After 3–4 days, *capillary buds* from both graft and recipient bed anastomose to create a neovasculature capable of supporting the graft. After 4–5 days, the infiltration of *fibroblasts* within the fibrin exudate creates a more permanent fibrin attachment.

5. What aspects of the recipient bed enhance survival of a skin graft?

The recipient bed should be level. There should not be active bleeding in the bed, as this will result in hematoma formation and limit attachment of graft to bed. However, excessive cautery of the bed will result in diminished vascular supply to the graft. Healthy granulation tissue in the bed is necessary for the creation of the fibrin exudate. In addition, the graft should be sutured in place to reduce shearing. To help reduce tenting, movement, and fluid accumulation under the graft, a bolster dressing may be used, and the graft can be incised in a number of places to allow serum egress. A skin graft will not "take" if placed on bare bone, cartilage, or tendon, and will often fail if placed on radiated tissue or infected granulation tissue. If bone, cartilage, or tendons need coverage, or if radiated tissue is involved, a flap or microvascular free flap would be a better option.

6. Name some donor sites for skin grafts used in the head and neck.

The color and thickness of skin vary for different areas of the body. The color and texture of facial skin are most closely approximated with skin from the face. The skin of the nasolabial fold and postauricular area have excellent color and texture matches to most areas of the face. The eyelids have particularly thin skin, and grafting in this area is usually best achieved by use of an upper eyelid graft from the same or contralateral eye. The donor sites for these facial grafts are almost always closed primarily, except for large postauricular grafts, which require STSGs. The supraclavicular area can provide large amounts of donor skin with texture and color matches that are reasonable but not quite as good as from nasolabial and postauricular donor sites. FTSGs from areas of the body below the clavicle are usually too thick, and the color match is poor. STSGs are usually taken from the abdomen, thigh, and back.

7. How are skin grafts harvested?

FTSGs are usually harvested with a scalpel and are cut in a plane between the dermis and subcutaneous tissue. Any subcutaneous tissue remaining should be trimmed to reduce the thickness of the graft and decrease its metabolic needs. STSGs are harvested with free-hand knives and, more commonly, dermatomes. With a dermatome, the exact thickness of the graft can be regulated. Thin (0.008–0.01 inch), intermediate (0.012–0.014 inch), or thick (0.016–0.018 inch) grafts can be harvested based on the surgeon's need. An STSG can be meshed, so that it will cover a larger area.

8. When are FTSGs and STSGs used in head and neck reconstruction?

FTSGs are most commonly used for reconstruction following cutaneous malignancies that cannot be closed primarily. STSGs are often used in head and neck surgery to reconstruct oral cavity and pharyngeal defects following ablative oncologic surgery. Defects that cannot be closed primarily and that do not require a large flap are often best treated with an STSG. In these situations, STSGs close the defect while still allowing adequate tongue mobility.

9. Describe the various types of bone grafts.

Autologous grafts (from the same person) are most popular and can be divided into three groups. **Cancellous** bone grafts consist of bone marrow and medullary bone. These grafts have the quickest revascularization and highest percentage of surviving transplanted cells. **Cortical** bone grafts consist of cortex (lamellar) bone. Revascularization is slower, and cell survival is low. **Cortico-cancellous** bone grafts contain both types. This graft has the advantages of quickly revascularized cancellous bone and strong cortical bone.

Allogeneic bone grafts do not actually provide viable cells. Instead, these grafts induce proliferation of native osteogenic cells. The most common use of allogeneic bone grafts is for mandibular reconstruction. A hollowed-out crib of mandible or iliac crest that is filled with autologous cortico-cancellous bone chips may be used.

Xenografts (grafts from other species) are no longer used.

10. When is a flap needed?

There are many instances in which a flap provides a better result than a graft. A flap can often provide an optimum result when the defect is too large for an FTSG, when the defect possesses poor vascularity (e.g., following irradiation), or when it is used to approximate color and texture match with the surrounding tissue. In addition, when bulk or composite tissue is needed, flaps are usually the best choice.

11. What are some of the basic categories of flaps?

Local skin flaps are harvested from skin in close proximity to the defect.

Regional pedicled flaps are larger flaps and can contain skin, subcutaneous tissue, muscle, and/or bone. Regional pedicled flaps are rotated into the area of the defect along their pedicle from a greater distance than local flaps.

Microvascular free flaps can originate from sites distant from the head and neck. Like regional pedicled flaps, free flaps can be composed of multiple tissue types. However, the vascular and sometimes nervous supply of the flap is isolated and then anastomosed with vessels and nerves in proximity to the defect.

12. What are random and axial pattern flaps?

The blood supply to the epidermis and dermis is derived from the dermal-subdermal plexus. The vascular supply to the flap plexus may involve an artery that directly communicates with the plexus at the proximal end of the flap (**random pattern**). In contrast, it may also involve a segmental artery that runs the length of the flap, sending multiple branches to the plexus throughout the length of the flap (**axial pattern**). The blood supply to muscle can be characterized similarly: random pattern has a random distribution of blood vessels throughout the muscle; an axial pattern has a segmental artery that courses along the fascia deep to the muscle and sends perforating branches along its distribution into the muscle.

Almost all local skin flaps have a random pattern. Regional skin flaps can have either random or axial patterns. Microvascular free flaps, by their very nature, are dependent on a particular arterial and venous supply.

13. Describe the various types of local flaps.

Advancement flap—Skin adjacent to the defect is directly advanced into the defect. Incisions are made in the lateral aspects of the flap to allow advancement of the flap. Burow's triangles are made along the proximal aspect of the flap to prevent dog-earing.

Rotation flap—As the name suggests, a flap is rotated along an arc into the defect. As with advancement flaps, Burow's triangles are often needed.

Transposition flap—The flap is passed over an incomplete bridge of skin.

Interpolated flap—The flap is passed either over or under a complete bridge of skin, which separates the flap from the defect.

14. Which anatomic structures must be considered with local flaps?

The distribution of the facial nerve should be clearly understood by the reconstructive surgeon. Of particular note is the temporal branch as it traverses the zygoma midway between the lateral canthus and the external auditory canal. The marginal mandibular branch, which can be located near the mandibular notch, is also an important consideration. The **parotid duct** also resides in a superficial location. The course of the duct is located midway between a line drawn from the tragus to the oral commissure.

15. Which tissues are commonly used in a regional flap?

There are three major types of regional pedicled flaps that are used for head and neck reconstruction: cutaneous, myocutaneous, and osteomyocutaneous flaps. **Cutaneous flaps** are composed of skin elements only and are used in the reconstruction of skin loss secondary to malignancy, radiation, or infection. **Myocutaneous flaps** are composed of skin and underlying muscle, provide more bulk than cutaneous flaps, and are used when a defect requires the additional bulk for enhanced return of form and function. **Osteomyocutaneous flaps** are used for reconstruction of the mandible and overlying soft tissue defects. Note that, in many instances, microvascular free flaps provide superior reconstructive results to regional pedicled flaps.

16. Name some commonly used regional cutaneous flaps and their vascular supply.

Regional cutaneous flaps are used for large facial defects and were commonly used for oral cavity and oropharyngeal reconstruction before the advent of more sophisticated reconstructive methods.

The **deltopectoral flap** is based on the first four perforating branches of the internal mammary artery and is an axial-pattern flap. The skin and underlying superficial fascia of the pectoralis major and deltoid muscles are contained in this medially based flap.

The **midline forehead flap** is a pedicled axial-pattern flap based on the supratrochlear artery. It could also be classified as a local flap and is used for reconstruction of dorsal nasal defects.

The **temporal flap** is an axial flap based on the superficial temporal artery.

Other regional cutaneous flaps include the thoracoacromial, nape of neck, and cervicofacial flaps, which are all random-pattern flaps based on several arteries.

17. Name some commonly used regional myocutaneous flaps and their vascular supply.

The most commonly used myocutaneous flap for head and neck reconstruction is probably the **pectoralis major flap.** This flap is an axial-pattern flap based on the thoracoacromial artery. The lateral thoracic artery also provides blood to this flap, and the flap is laterally based. A skin paddle between the nipple and sternum is harvested, and the paddle and underlying pectoralis muscle are then tunneled above the clavicle and used as needed.

The **latissimus dorsi myocutaneous flap** is an axial-pattern flap based on the thoracodorsal artery. The muscle and skin paddle are tunneled either above or below the pectoralis major muscle and into the neck.

The **trapezius myocutaneous flap** is also an axial flap based on the transverse cervical artery, which originates from the thyrocervical trunk.

The **sternocleidomastoid muscle flap** is a random-pattern flap. Its vascular supply is derived from the occipital artery superiorly, the superior thyroid artery, and the transverse cervical artery inferiorly.

18. Name some of the regional osteomyocutaneous flaps.

Osteomyocutaneous flaps are similar to previously described myocutaneous flaps (see Question 17) except that **bone** is included in these flaps. The pectoralis major flap includes an adjacent portion of rib; the sternocleidomastoid muscle flap includes an adjacent portion of clavicle; and the trapezius muscle includes an adjacent scapular spine. These have all been used for reconstructive purposes.

Because both the rib and clavicle are long bones, their blood supply is more dependent on the nutrient artery. Therefore, removal of a portion of these bones results in a more tenuous bone flap. The scapula is a flat bone; therefore, harvesting part of the scapula results in a more reliable flap because its blood supply is more dependent on periosteal vessels. Microvascular bone flaps, however, have been shown to be more reliable and are most often employed if a flap is necessary for mandibular reconstruction.

19. What are the major advantages of microvascular free flaps over regional pedicled flaps?

Microvascular free flaps hold a number of advantages over regional pedicled flaps:
- Many different postoncologic surgery defects confront the reconstructive surgeon, and the wide variety of free flaps enables the surgeon to tailor the flap to the defect much more closely than could be accomplished with regional flaps.
- Microvascular free flaps provide reliable, well-vascularized donor tissue.
- Regional flaps are limited in where they can be used by the length of the pedicle.
- The donor site defect, on the whole, is greater with regional flaps than with free flaps.
- Microvascularized free flaps can withstand subsequent radiation therapy, if necessary.

20. List some of the fasciocutaneous microvascular free flaps and their vascular pedicles.

The arterial supply of the **radial forearm fasciocutaneous flap** is the radial artery. Venous drainage is though the venae comitantes. The medial or lateral cutaneous nerves of the forearm may be used to create a sensate flap.

The **lateral thigh fasciocutaneous flap** is based on the third perforating branch of the profunda femoris artery. Venous drainage is through accompanying venae comitantes, which drain into the profunda femoris vein. The lateral femoral cutaneous nerve of the thigh may be harvested to provide sensation.

The **scapular and parascapular fasciocutaneous flaps** are based on the cutaneous scapular and cutaneous parascapular arteries, respectively, which are branches of the circumflex scapular artery. These flaps can be raised as one large flap if necessary. Venous drainage is through accompanying veins.

The **lateral arm fasciocutaneous flap** relies on the radial collateral artery, cephalic vein, and venae comitantes and the lateral cutaneous nerve of the arm.

21. Name two myocutaneous microvascular free flaps.

The **rectus abdominis myocutaneous free flap** is based on the deep inferior epigastric vessels. Multiple superficial perforating arteries radiate out from the periumbilical area, enabling generous amounts of skin to be taken with the graft. Sensation is *not* possible with this graft.

The **latissimus dorsi myocutaneous free flap** is based on the thoracodorsal artery and accompanying venae comitantes. Sensation is possible through the thoracodorsal nerve. This flap can provide a large amount of both muscle and skin.

22. What is the purpose of the gracilis myogenous microvascular free flap?

The gracilis myogenous flap is used for facial reanimation. The motor nerve to the muscle can be anastomosed with the nerve to the masseter muscle. This results in facial movement when the teeth are clenched. The motor nerve may also be anastomosed with the contralateral facial nerve to improve symmetry of movement in the midportion of the face.

23. How are flaps and grafts used in the reconstruction of the mandible?

The reconstructive method depends on the location and size of the defect, the need for additional soft-tissue reconstruction in the oral cavity, and the desire for dental implants. Bone grafts and plates are often sufficient for small lateral mandibular defects. Larger defects and anterior "Andy Gump" deformities often require microvascular free flap reconstruction. Options include iliac crest, fibula, radial forearm, and scapular-based microvascular free flaps.

24. How does a free flap survive?

Unlike a thin split-thickness graft, a large full-thickness flap does need an independent blood supply for survival. Flaps can either be *pedicled* (rotated about the native blood supply) or transferred as *free flaps*. Free flaps, because of their immediate metabolic requirements, require an immediate new blood supply. This is established by locating the vessels supplying the flap and anastomosing them (sewing them into) a blood supply at the recipient site. In head and neck reconstruction, the recipient vessels are usually the internal jugular vein and a branch of the carotid.

25. How big are the vessels that are anastomosed?

Very small! A microscope is needed to see the vessels (which range from 1–3 mm) and the suture (9–0 or 10–0). Otolaryngologists with microvascular training, as well as plastic surgeons, can perform the entire reconstruction.

26. When is a free flap necessary?

A free flap is a viable reconstructive option any time a flap is going to be required to fix a defect. This is particularly true in previously radiated patients; when a defect cannot be easily reconstructed with pedicled flaps; or when function is critical. Examples include mandibular or midface reconstruction, tongue or floor of mouth reconstruction, or reconstruction of large pharyngeal defects. Skin, soft tissue, bone, and muscle can all be replaced. Bone can be contoured to replace a specific defect. The utilities and contouring abilities of these flaps are remarkable.

27. Does the flap shrink with time?
The flap will show some decrease in size as edema subsides. Skin, fat, and fascia will not atrophy in a vascularized flap. A muscle flap will lose its innervation and show significant atrophy with time. Transposed bone should not change.

28. Does postoperative radiation injure the flap?
As the flap has a robust blood supply, it usually becomes the healthiest tissue in the head and neck. It will atrophy somewhat with radiation, but the radiation does not compromise the vascular supply.

29. How does a free flap give better function than a pedicled flap?
A free flap offers superior contouring ability and allows the surgeon to precisely fit a flap to a defect. Bone can be osteotomized, vascularized nerve grafts can be included in the flaps, and the thickness of a flap can be tailored to a specific defect.

30. What flaps have the capacity for sensory reinnervation?
The flaps that have large sensory nerves in a predictable location can have an anastomosis performed to a native sensory nerve at the recipient site. These include:
- Radial forearm flap (lateral antebrachial cutaneous nerve)
- Ulnar flap (medial antebrachial cutaneous nerve)
- Fibula (lateral sural cutaneous nerve)
- Lateral arm (posterior cutaneous nerve of the arm)
- Scapula (cutaneous branch of spinal nerve dorsal rami).

31. If the nerve is not anastomosed, will the patient ever be able to feel the flap?
Spontaneous return of sensation in a noninnervated flap has been documented. The results are unpredictable, but better for thinner fasciocutaneous flaps than for myocutaneous or osteocutaneous flaps.

32. Can motor reinnervation be achieved?
Yes. This has been described for the rectus abdominus flap and may assist in preventing atrophy of the muscle. In tongue reconstruction, innervation can be re-established by an anastomosis with the hypoglossal nerve.

33. What factors increase the risk of thrombosis?
While somewhat disputed, it is clear that vein grafting (to lengthen a pedicle) increases the risk of thrombosis. This may be due to the increased number of anastomoses. Other factors include transferring the flap into a chronic wound, postoperative fistula in the region of the pedicle, and patient factors leading to hypercoagulative states (protein c and s deficiency). Specific flaps, choice of blood thinners (such as aspirin or heparin), and patient age do not seem to be as important.

34. How can you decide if a flap is thrombosed?
There are many ways of monitoring a flap. The gold standard is direct visualization of the flap and the color of the blood with a pinprick. A normal flap is pale but warm. The blood return should be bright red. If the flap is swollen, purple, and warm, thrombosis may exist in a vein (most common). A pinprick would show fast, copious return of dark or purple blood. If there is *no* blood return in a cool, very pale flap, thrombosis may exist in the artery.

Additional methods of monitoring include Doppler checks of the pulse (usually arterial), color flow Doppler, and laser Doppler.

35. When are leeches used? How much blood can they suck out?
Leeches are effective for *short-term* maintenance of flap thrombosis, but they are not a fix for venous congestion. The flap must be salvaged in the OR. The leech attaches to the flap and sucks blood, but the efficacy of the leech is actually through an enzyme it secretes, called hirudin.

36. Why must a patient be on antibiotics if leeches are used?
Superinfection is common without prophylaxis. A bacterium, *Aeromonas hydrophilis,* is the main bug responsible for infections. Antibiotics effective for pseudomonas (such as the floxin family) are recommended.

37. How common is thrombosis?
Flap thrombosis occurs in 5–10% of free flaps. If detected immediately, the flap can be salvaged by removing the clot in the blood vessel (usually in the vein) and re-establishing the blood flow. If too long a time period elapses, a no-reflow state may exist.

38. How much time can elapse before you must take the patient back to the OR if you suspect a thrombosis?
A free flap thrombosis is an emergency, and the patient must return to the operating suite immediately. It is thought that at 4 hours of ischemic time a flap may not be salvageable, and at 6 hours little hope exists to save the flap. Jejunal flaps tolerate even less ischemia (2 hours).

39. Can you take *any* tissue and use it as a free flap?
No, but established flaps have been well documented to demonstrate the normal anatomy and blood supply. Commonly employed flaps include:

Fasciocutaneous	Osseocutaneous	Musculocutaneous
Radial forearm	Fibula	Rectus abdominus
Lateral arm	Iliac crest	Latissimus dorsi
Lateral thigh	Scapula	
Ulnar (radial forearm)		
Scapula		

40. How much of the mandible can be reconstructed?
Virtually the entirety of the mandible can be adequately reconstructed to a natural shape with a fibula free flap. The flap can even be anchored to the glenoid fossa to reconstruct the temporomandibular joint. Contouring of the fibula is done after a plate is preformed based on the native mandible. Osteotomies are made to shape the bone to the size and shape of the native jaw.

41. A patient is going to have a total laryngopharyngectomy. How can the swallow mechanism be reconstructed?
If the whole tube (pharynx) will be resected, a jejunal flap (which is harvested as a tube) or a radial forearm flap (which is tubed upon insetting) can adequately reconstruct the anatomy. A voice prosthesis can assist with postoperative language. Most patients do well, although strictures are common. If a partial pharyngectomy is performed, but the defect is too large to close primarily, a radial forearm is a nice, pliable flap for closure. A defect that extends beyond the esophageal inlet usually must be reconstructed with a gastric pull-up.

42. Are any special preoperative tests required?
The usual labs and imaging for a head and neck patient should be performed. Carefully assess the potential donor site. Only a few additional points are required:
• Radial forearm: perform an Allen's test
• Fibula: consider Doppler or angiography of the leg to assess vascular anatomy
• Rectus: ensure no previous surgery in the abdomen.

43. How is an Allen's test performed?

The nondominant hand is evaluated. The patient is asked to pump his or her fist as the examiner occludes the radial and ulnar inflow to the hand. The patient is then asked to gently release his or her fingers (not fully extend, or they will blanch). The examiner first lets go of the ulnar vessel and evaluates the refill of the thenar region. The radial artery occlusion is then released, with the examiner constantly watching the hand.

44. Why is an Allen's test necessary when doing a radial forearm?

In approximately 3–7% of patients, an abnormal Allen's test is found. This indicates noncommunication between the deep and superficial palmar arches—the radial and ulnar supply to the hand. In the worst possible case, if a radial forearm were harvested and the patient had a noncommunicating arch, necrosis of the thumb and first digit could result.

45. What artery supplies a flap?

Of course, this varies depending on the flap. A thorough review of the vascular anatomy of a region is imperative prior to performing a flap procedure.

Radial forearm—radial artery
Lateral thigh—3rd perforator of the profunda femoris
Rectus—deep inferior epigastric
Scapula—circumflex scapular
Iliac crest—deep circumflex iliac artery

Fibula—peroneal
Ulnar—ulnar artery
Lateral arm—profunda brachii
Latissimus—thoracodorsal

46. What are venae comitantes?

Venae comitantes are the veins that accompany most named arteries harvested for a flap. There are generally one or two veins of sufficient size (> 1 mm) to allow for adequate venous drainage of the flap. Since they accompany the artery, they add little to the pedicle harvest and are usually used for the venous anastomoses.

CONTROVERSIES

47. How long can a flap survive a period of ischemia before it is anastomosed?

All flaps must undergo a period of ischemia—the time between cutting the flap out of the donor site and establishing flow at the recipient site. Jejunal flaps tolerate the least ischemia, only 2 hours. Most other flaps tolerate up to 4 hours, although this is rarely necessary. If a tourniquet is used to harvest the flap (with sites such as the radial forearm or fibula), the flap tolerate a shorter period of ischemia. This is because the tourniquet induced the *primary* period of ischemia. A *secondary* ischemic insult will only add to the previous damage. The length of time a flap will tolerate secondary ischemia is roughly half that of primary ischemia. Letting the tourniquet down to allow for flap reperfusion (and washout of free radicals) lengthens the allowable ischemic period.

48 Should all patients who have undergone a flap procedure be placed on heparin?

This is a controversial question, but in general, no. An aspirin a day is usually sufficient to prevent platelet sludging. Postoperative anemia may work in favor of thrombosis prevention. Subcutaneous heparin, low-molecular-weight heparin, and dextran are preferred by some surgeons. Cost and risk of postoperative hematoma must be considered.

49. Which flaps on that list are the best to use?

It depends on the defect and the patient. For fasciocutaneous flaps, the radial forearm is the most reliable and simplest to harvest. In patients with osseocutaneous flaps, osseointegrated implants are sometimes placed. These implants are best tolerated by the iliac bone, but can also be placed into fibular flaps. The greatest bone length is provided with a fibular flap (up to 25 cm). Flaps based on the back, such as the scapula or latissimus flaps, require turning the patient midprocedure and add to the length of OR time required.

50. How long is the pedicle of a flap?

This depends on the flap. Some flaps, particularly the radial forearm, boast long pedicles (6–10 cm) that allow for anastomosis on the other side of the neck, if necessary. Most flaps allow for pedicles of up to 6 cm, depending on the patient's anatomy.

BIBLIOGRAPHY

1. Hoffmann JF, Cook TA: Reconstruction of facial defects. In Cummings CW, et al (eds): Otolaryngology–Head and Neck Surgery, 3rd ed. St. Louis, Mosby, 1998.
2. Petruzzelli GJ, Johnson JT: Skin grafts. Otolaryngol Clin North Am 27:25, 1994.
3. Shindo ML, Sullivan MJ: Muscular and myocutaneous pedicled flaps. Otolaryngol Clin North Am 27:161, 1994.
4. Urken ML, Cheney ML, Sullivan MJ, Biller HF: Atlas of regional and free flaps for head and neck reconstruction. New York, Raven Press, 1995.
5. Khori RK, Cooley BC, Kunselman AR, et al: A prospective study of microvascular free-flap surgery and outcome. Plast Recon Surg 102:711–721, 1998.
6. Wax MK, Winslow CP, Hansen J, et al: Temporomandibular joint reconstruction with free fibula microvascular flap: A retrospective analysis of results. Laryngoscope 110:977–981, 2000.
7. Close LG, Truelson JM, Milledge RA, Schweitzer C: Sensory recovery in noninnervated flaps used for oral cavity and oropharyngeal reconstruction. Arch Otol HNS 121:967–972, 1995.
8. Kimata Y, Uchiyama K, Ebihara S, et al: Comparison of innervated and noninnervated free flaps in oral reconstruction. Plast Recon Surg 104:1307–1313, 1999.
9. He W, Neligan P, Lipa J, et al: Comparison of secondary ischemic tolerance between pedicled and free island buttock skin flaps in the pig. Plast Recon Surg 100:72–81, 1997.
10. Cooley BC, Hansen FC, Dellon AL: The effect of temperature on tolerance to ischemia in experimental free flaps. J Microsurg 3:11–14, 1981.
11. Carlson GW, Schusterman MA, Guillamondegui OM: Total reconstruction of the hypopharynx and cervical esophagus: A 20-year experience. Ann Plast Surg 29:408–412, 1998.
12. Fowler JD, Li X, Cooley BC: Brief ex vivo perfusion with heparinized and/or citrated whole blood enhances tolerance of free muscle flaps to prolonged ischemia. Microsurg 19:135–140, 1999.
13. Khouri RK, Brown DM, Koudsi B, et al: Repair of calvarial defects with flap tissue: Role of bone morphogenetic proteins and competent responding tissues. Plast Recons Surg 98:103–109, 1996.

53. PRINCIPLES OF SKIN RESURFACING

Ben Lee, M.D.

1. What are the indications for skin resurfacing?

Skin resurfacing may be considered for patients with actinic keratoses, rhytids, pigmentary dyschromias, superficial scarring, radiation dermatitis, acne vulgaris, and rosacea.

2. What are the different techniques of facial skin resurfacing?

Treatment is either medical or surgical. The application of retinoic acid (Retin-A) is the most common medical treatment. Surgical treatments include chemical face peels of varying strengths, dermabrasion, laser selective photothermolysis, and injectable fillers.

3. What are the different skin types?

Fitzpatrick classified skin types according to varying degrees of reaction to ultraviolet light. The scale ranges from I–VI as listed below. There is a positive correlation between darker Fitzpatrick skin types and postinflammatory hyperpigmentation and dyschromias following peeling. Caution is therefore urged in the typical Asian, dark-skinned Hispanic, and African-American patient (Fitzpatrick IV, V, and VI).

Fitzpatrick's Skin Types

SKIN TYPE	SKIN COLOR	TANNING RESPONSE
I	White	Always burns, never tans
II	White	Usually burns, tans with difficulty
III	White	Sometimes burns, average tanning
IV	Brown	Rarely burns, tans easily
V	Dark brown	Very rarely burns, tans very easily
VI	Black	Never burns, tans very easily

4. How does the sun change the skin?

Sun exposure, or actinic radiation, primarily results in changes of the dermis. Collagen in the papillary dermis becomes disorganized as elastic fibers increase (elastosis).

5. How does aging change the skin?

The epidermis tends to remain the same thickness throughout the aging process. However, the rete ridges, which are pronounced in young healthy skin, become flattened and give the appearance of skin thinning. The papillary and reticular dermis thins with age. Likewise, elastin, ground substance, dermal cells, the microcirculation, and cutaneous nerves decrease with aging. Thicker skin will require more treatments than thinner skin to achieve the same degree of tissue removal.

6. How do you classify aged skin?

The Glogau classification groups patients as having mild, moderate, advanced, and severe photodamage on a scale of I–VI:

Type I	No wrinkles (mild)
Type II	Wrinkles in motion (moderate)
Type III	Wrinkles at rest (advanced)
Type IV	Only wrinkles (severe)

7. What is Retin-A?

Topical tretinoin (all-*trans*-retinoic acid) demonstrates diverse effects on the differentiation, metabolism, and protein synthesis activities of the keratinocyte. The commercial form, Retin-A is emulsified in a moisturizing base and applied once or twice daily. When it is used for > 6 months, it has been demonstrated to reduce elastosis and stimulate new collagen production. The overall effect is to improve rhytids, actinic keratoses, and pigmentary actinic changes.

8. What is a skin peel?

Skin peels are administered in an attempt to reverse the histologic damage created by actinic radiation, preneoplastic conditions, and the aging process. Acids or other substances are applied to the skin to destroy progressively deeper layers of epidermis and papillary dermis. New epidermis then develops from keratinocytes derived from cutaneous adnexal structures. New dermal collagen develops in the papillary dermis, arranged in compact, parallel bundles.

9. Are there different kinds of face peels?

Yes. Face-peeling solutions are usually classified according to the depth of burn that they create. Superficial peeling solutions (e.g., glycolic acids) create damage that is limited to the epidermis and papillary dermis. Medium-depth peels (e.g., trichloroacetic acid) create a burn through the upper reticular dermis. Deeper peeling solutions (e.g., phenol or "Baker's solution") create tissue damage through the mid-reticular dermis. There are different indications for the use of each of these solutions.

10. What are the indications for a deep peel?

The classic deep peel formula is the Baker-Gordon phenol formula consisting of the following:

Phenol 88%	3 mL
Croton oil	3 drops
Septisol	8 drops
Distilled water	2 mL

Besides deep rhytids, deep peels are indicated in the treatement of chronic photodamage, premalignant keratoses, and solar lentigines. Some improvement may also be seen in mild to moderate acne damage, although severe acne pitting requires more aggressive techniques such as dermabrasion or direct excision.

11. How is a peel performed?

Peels are usually performed in an outpatient setting with the patient under mild sedation. Pretreatment with Retin-A for several weeks prior to the procedure has been shown to increase the depth of the peel. The skin is degreased and prepped, and the wounding agent is applied. The application is sometimes covered with tape or ointment to increase the depth of the peel. In the postoperative period, daily cleansing with mild soap and water is performed, and either a protective dressing (e.g., vigilon) or vaseline is applied to prevent crusting. Depending on the depth of the peel, epithelialization may occur by 1 to 6 weeks. Hydroquinone is often applied in the post-peel period to minimize hyperpigmentation.

12. What are the complications of face peeling?

Generally, the deeper and more aggressive the peel is, the greater the rate of complications. Scarring and pigmentary changes are the most common, especially in Fitzpatrick types IV to VI. Bacterial, fungal, and viral infection can also occur. Patients with a history of herpes simplex should be pretreated with the appropriate antiviral agent. Phenol-based peels pose systemic risk to those with hepatic, renal, and cardiac disease.

13. What kind of pigmentary changes can occur?

Pigmentary changes include hyperpigmentation, hypopigmentation, depigmentation, lines of demarcation, and nevi accentuation.

14. Should a patient with a history of herpes be given a face peel?

These patients should be pretreated with acyclovir (400 mg three times a day) 2 days before the peel. After the peel, acyclovir should be continued until epithelialization has occurred, and sun exposure should be strictly avoided.

15. What is dermabrasion?

Dermabrasion is performed with an abrasive wheel that is attached to an electrically driven handpiece. Layers of skin are literally "sanded off" to the proper depth for the clinical problem. An eschar forms over the dermabraded area. It takes several weeks for the eschar to detach and the underlying skin to heal.

16. What is a laser?

The term LASER is actually an acronym for *l*ight *a*mplification by *s*timulated *e*mission of *r*adiation. A laser is a light that is collimated (has parallel rays), coherent (has all waves of the same frequency and periodicity), and monochromatic (is a single wavelength). A laser may be used in a defocused mode to treat superficial lesions, or it may be used in a focused excisional mode much like a scalpel is used.

17. Define selective photothermal epidermolysis.

Selective photothermal epidermolysis refers to the ability of a laser to selectively destroy small layers of cells with little peripheral tissue damage. The most frequently used lasers for this purpose are the CO_2 laser and the flash pump dye laser.

18. What happens to the skin when it is treated with a CO_2 laser?

When the CO_2 laser contacts skin, it immediately boils intracellular water and leads to tissue vaporization. The effect of the laser depends on the anatomy, thickness of the skin, and dose of the laser. When eyelid skin is treated with 100 mJ/cm^2, there is complete loss of the epidermis, minimal coagulation of the papillary dermal collagen, and minimal degeneration of the necks of adnexal structures. The deep dermal layers are unaffected. When the tissue is treated with 200 mJ/cm^2, there is complete loss of the epidermis, moderate coagulation of the papillary dermal collagen, and moderate degeneration of the necks of adnexal structures. The deep dermal structures remain unaffected. When eyelid tissue is treated with 300 mJ/cm^2, there is complete loss of the epidermis and moderate to severe coagulation of the papillary and reticular dermis. At this dose, there is extensive degeneration of the adnexal structures and coarse cystic changes throughout the deeper dermis.

19. What is rhinophyma? How is it treated?

Rhinophyma is a form of rosacea that is caused by sebaceous hyperplasia. Common in elderly men, this hyperplasia leads to an erythematous, swollen, nodular nose. Currently, the CO_2 laser is the treatment of choice. It can be used much like a scalpel to sculpt the soft tissue, and it can be used more superficially to vaporize excess hypertrophic tissue. Re-epithelialization begins about 1 week after laser treatment.

20. How are injectable fillers used?

Fillers can be injected under the skin to elevate depressed scars or wrinkles. The most commonly used substance is bovine collagen. Unfortunately, the material can cause allergic reactions and requires a test dose several weeks prior to injection. Injectable fillers need to be reinjected at 6-month intervals to maintain the result.

CONTROVERSY

21. Is one method of skin resurfacing surgery better than another?

Each technique has its advantages and disadvantages. It is often difficult to achieve controlled results with dermabrasion. Chemical peeling around areas such as the eyelids can cause sensitivity problems. Some procedures are safer to do in combination with other aging-face procedures, such as blepharoplasty or facelift surgery.

BIBLIOGRAPHY

 1. Acland KM, Barlow RJ: Lasers for the dermatologist. Br J Dermatol 143:244–255, 2000.
 2. Aghassi D, Carpo B, Eng K, et al: Complications of aesthetic laser surgery. Ann Plast Surg 43:560–569, 1999.
 3. Alora MB, Anderson RR: Recent developments in cutaneous lasers. Lasers Surg Med 26:108–118, 2000.
 4. Dover JS, Hruza G: Lasers in skin resurfacing. Australas J Dermatol 41:72–85, 2000.
 5. Jacobson D, Bass LS, VanderKam V, et al: Carbon dioxide and ER:YAG laser resurfacing: Results. Clin Plast Surg 27:241–250, 2000.
 6. Kauvar AN: Laser skin resurfacing: Perspectives at the millennium. Dermatol Surg 26:174–177, 2000.
 7. Marcells GN, Ellis DA: Laser facial skin resurfacing: Discussion on erbium:YAG and CO_2 lasers. J Otolaryngol 29:78–82, 2000.
 8. Newman JP, Fitzgerald P, Koch RJ: Review of closed dressings after laser resurfacing. Dermatol Surg 26:562–571, 2000.
 9. Tayani R, Rubin PA: Laser applications in oculoplastic surgery and their postoperative complications. Int Ophthalmol Clin 40:13–26, 2000.
10. Weinstein C, Scheflan M: Simultaneously combined ER:YAG and carbon dioxide laser (derma K) for skin resurfacing. Clin Plast Surg 27:273–285, xi, 2000.

54. RHINOPLASTY

David A. Hendrick, M.D.

1. What is rhinoplasty?

Rhinoplasty is plastic surgery that involves the repositioning and/or refinement of the nasal skeleton and soft tissue. This surgery serves to improve function, facial aesthetics, or both. Obstruction is the most commonly addressed functional problem. Often, a septoplasty is incorporated into the surgery. Aesthetic concerns often focus on a dorsal nasal hump, a poorly defined nasal tip, or an acquired deformity from trauma.

2. What is the nasal valve?

The nasal valve is defined as the area inside the nose that lies just beneath the caudal edge of the upper lateral cartilage. Here the angle between the upper lateral cartililage and the septum is most acute (from 9 to 5 degrees) and the inferior turbinate significantly encroaches upon the airway. This area, which some have further defined as the *internal nasal valve,* is an important anatomic site for nasal obstruction.

3. What is alar collapse?

Alar collapse occurs when the sidewalls of the nostril, the ala, are too flimsy and collapse with inspiration, resulting in nasal obstruction. This area of collapse, involving the alar sidewalls, the caudal septum, the collumellar sidewalls, and the soft tissues around the piriform aperture, has been termed the external nasal valve by some. This is also an important anatomic site for nasal obstruction and, together with the internal nasal valve, constitutes the "flow-limiting segment" of the nose.

4. What is valvuloplasty?

A nasal valvuloplasty is a functional "tip" rhinoplasty designed to correct internal and/or external nasal valve obstruction. A careful preoperative assessment identifies the sites and causes of obstruction. Internal nasal valve collapse is classically corrected by cartilage **spreader grafts** to lateralize the upper lateral cartilages. External nasal valve collapse, or alar collapse, is typically corrected by cartilage alar **batten grafts** to stiffen and lateralize the lower lateral cartilage. Soft tissue stenosis problems are corrected by various excision or Z-plasty techniques.

5. What is the Frankfort horizontal plane? Why is it important?

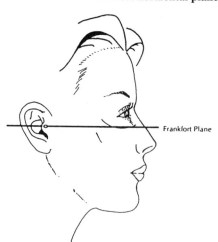

Frankfort Plane

The Frankfort plane. (From Powell N, Humphries B: Proportions of the Aesthetic Face. New York, Thieme-Stratton, 1984, p 8, with permission.)

On a radiograph, the Frankfort horizontal plane is a line drawn from the top of the bony external auditory canal to the bony infraorbital rim. On facial photographs, it is approximated as a line from the top of the tragus to the infraorbital rim. This line is important because it provides a good, reproducible reference plane for facial photography and analysis.

6. Describe the basic steps of nasal analysis.
- Assess the "fabric" of the nose—the skin quality (thickness, sebaceousness, color, etc.).
- Address the nose with respect to facial proportions (one-third the facial height, one-fifth the facial width are norms).
- Give the nose a one- to two-word summary description ("twisted," "big," "humped," etc.).
- Break the nose down into the following detailed views (in order): frontal view, base view, lateral or profile view, oblique or quarter view.
- Give a detailed description of the nose in each view.

7. What should be considered in a detailed nasal analysis?
A detailed nasal analysis should involve a systematic evaluation of the nose from each of the standard views of the nose: frontal, basal, lateral, and oblique.

Frontal:	Alignment (straight, twisted, C-shaped, angled)
	Widths (upper third, middle third, lower third)
	Tip (bulbous, bifid, asymmetric, etc.)
Base:	Triangularity (triangular or trapezoidal)
	Columellar-lobule ratio (2:1 is the norm)
	Nostrils (shape and size)
	Alar base width (intercanthal distance is the norm)
	Tip (symmetry, bifidity, boxiness, narrowness, etc.)
Lateral:	Profile (hump, saddle, tip-supratip relationship, double break, columellar show, etc.)
	Nasal length (long, short) and "starting point" (high, low)
	The angles (nasolabial, nasofacial, nasofrontal)
	Tip projection (Goode's ratio, Simon's ratio)
	Chin projection (is it balanced with the nose?)
Oblique:	What is the overview?

8. What is the sellion? How is this different from the nasion?
The sellion is a soft-tissue landmark representing the deepest point of the nasofrontal angle. The nasion is a bony landmark at the nasofrontal suture. It is usually slightly higher than the sellion. Other useful landmarks of the nasal profile include the rhinion, radix, and glabella. The **rhinion** is a point representing the bony-cartilaginous junction of the nasal dorsum. The **radix** is the region that is considered to be the "root" of the nose. This area contributes to the nasofrontal angle. The sellion and nasion exist within the radix. The **glabella** is a frontal prominence between the brows above the root of the nose. (See *top* figure, next page.)

9. What are nasal aesthetic units? What is their role in reconstructive rhinoplasty?
The complex contours of the nose can be divided into units based on natural boundaries of shadowed valleys and lighted ridges. Each unit is generally convex or concave. A defect in a given aesthetic unit is best reconstructed with skin from the same unit. Incisions that follow unit boundaries heal with the least perceptible scar, whereas incisions that cross unit boundaries heal with the most noticeable scars. When defects involve most of an aesthetic unit, it is best to resect and reconstruct the entire unit as a single entity. Aesthetic units include the sidewall, tip, columella, dorsum, alar-nostril sill, and soft triangle.

10. Describe the important incisions employed in rhinoplasty.
Several incisions are possible to gain access to the tip and dorsum. Most incisions in rhinoplasty are situated around the lower lateral cartilage. (See *bottom* figure, next page; also, answer continues on page 347.)

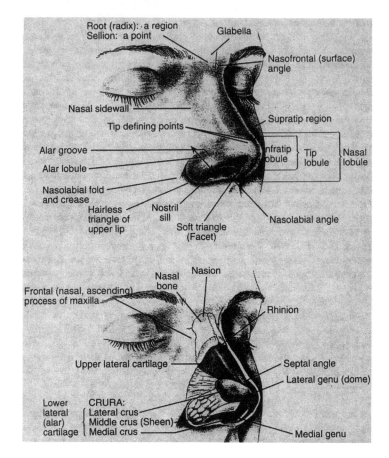

Landmarks and anatomy of the nose. (From Burget GC, Menick FJ: Aesthetic Reconstruction of the Nose. St. Louis, Mosby, 1994, p 7, with permission.)

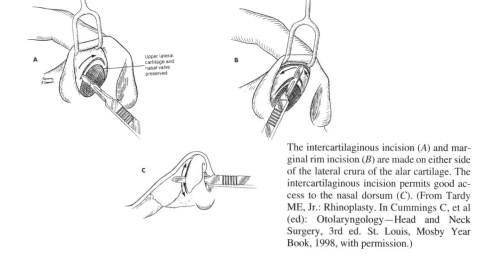

The intercartilaginous incision (A) and marginal rim incision (B) are made on either side of the lateral crura of the alar cartilage. The intercartilaginous incision permits good access to the nasal dorsum (C). (From Tardy ME, Jr.: Rhinoplasty. In Cummings C, et al (ed): Otolaryngology—Head and Neck Surgery, 3rd ed. St. Louis, Mosby Year Book, 1998, with permission.)

Transcartilaginous incision—This incision is made directly beneath the alar cartilage to "split" the cartilage. It is used only for conservative volume reduction of the lower lateral cartilage.

Intercartilaginous incision—This incision is made between the lower lateral and upper lateral cartilage to gain access to the nasal dorsum in closed rhinoplasty. It may be extended down onto the septum as a hemitransfixion or even full transfixion incision for access to the septum.

Marginal rim incision—This incision is made along the caudal edge of the lower lateral cartilage to gain access to the nasal tip. In closed rhinoplasty, where the lower lateral cartilage is "delivered" into direct view, this incision is combined with an intercartilaginous incision. In open rhinoplasty, in which the nose is to be degloved, this incision is combined with a transcolumellar incision.

Transcolumellar incision—This incision is made through the skin of the columella and extends up along both anterior edges of the medial crura of the lower lateral cartilage. Incisions then extend into marginal rim incisions to permit degloving the nose for open rhinoplasty. This technique is usually performed at the narrowest portion of the columella in a broken-line fashion (typically an upward directed dart of skin in the midline) for best cosmetic results.

11. Where is the "soft triangle" of the nose? What complication is associated with it?

The soft triangles are the apices of the nostrils beneath the lobules. Iatrogenic injury to these areas can result in notching of the nostril rim, which is exceedingly difficult to correct. These areas should not be violated, especially during marginal incisions, delivery of the lower lateral cartilages during closed rhinoplasty, or open rhinoplasty skin elevation.

12. Name the three major tip support mechanisms.

- Cartilage of the medial and lateral crura
- Attachments of the medial crura to the caudal septum (an overlapping connection)
- Attachments of the lateral crura to the upper lateral cartilage (a "scrolled" intercartilage connection)

Most tip rhinoplasty techniques deliberately alter one or more of these major tip supports. "Minor" tip support mechanisms that can be altered in rhinoplasty include: (a) interdomal ligaments, (b) dorsal cartilaginous septum, (c) attachments of the lower lateral crura to the piriform aperture (the "sesamoid complex," or "hinge" area), (d) attachments of the alar cartilage to the overlying skin and subcutaneous tissues, (e) membranous septum, and (f) nasal spine.

13. How is the nasal "tripod" used in planning tip rhinoplasty?

The nasal tripod is a model for the alar cartilage and tip support mechanisms. The middle leg represents the medial crura, and the two lateral legs the lateral crura. The tripod apex (which acts as a floating hinge) is the nasal tip. The tripod legs are held in place by the various forces of tip support described earlier. In this manner, one can analyze how altering some aspect of the tripod or its support will affect the nasal tip.

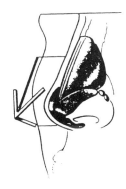

The nasal "tripod" (with a fourth leg depicted for the influence of the nasal dorsum on tip support). (From Toriumi DM, Johnson CM, Jr.: Open structure rhinoplasty. Fac Plast Surg Clin North Am 1(1):2, 1993, with permission.)

14. What is the most important technique for upward tip rotation?

Tip rotation involves movement of the tip either up or down along an arc such that the nasolabial angle is altered without a significant change in tip projection. The most dramatic amount of upward tip rotation is achieved by using tip suspension sutures to pull the alar cartilage lobules in the cephalic direction. More subtle rotation is achieved by simply resecting cartilage from the cephalic portion of the alar cartilage or from the caudal edge of the upper lateral cartilage. The key to this method of tip rotation is in understanding the dynamics of healing and scar contracture. Postoperative fibrosis will form in the resected void and contract to cause tip rotation in the cephalic direction. Finally, one can simply redefine the nasolabial angle and achieve tip rotation by resecting a wedge out of the caudal septum.

Besides actually rotating the tip, one can also create an illusion of tip rotation. Angulating the infratip lobule in a cephalic direction (i.e., enhancing the "double break") using tip grafts or blunting the nasolabial angle using "plumping" grafts can both achieve the illusion of upward tip rotation.

15. How is tip projection measured? What is the most important technique for increased tip projection?

Tip projection refers to the distance the tip projects from the face and can be measured in a number of ways. The **Simon method** is the simplest to remember, since it equates the projected length of the nasal base to the length of the upper lip (a 1:1 ratio). **Goode's method** is more exacting. By Goode's method, the length of nasal projection (from the alar groove to the nasal tip) should be related to nasal height (from the nasolabial angle to the nasal starting point) as a ratio. Most rhinoplasty techniques risk loss of projection through interruption of tip support mechanisms.

Tip projection is most effectively augmented using a **medial crural strut graft.** The use of various tip grafts can also enhance projection and may be necessary when using strut grafts to avoid a "tent pole" appearance to the projected tip.

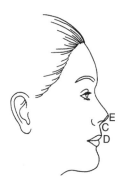

Measuring nasal tip projection. Simon's method simply notes that the length of the lower nasal contour (CE) and the length of the upper lip (CD) should exist in about a 1:1 ratio. (From Kridel RWH, Konior RJ: The underprojected tip. In Krause CJ, Pastorek N, Mangat DS (eds): Aesthetic Facial Surgery. Philadelphia, J.B. Lippincott, 1991, p 193, with permission.)

16. Describe the three basic methods for reducing alar cartilage volume (lobule modification).

Volume reduction of the lobules involves excising some portion of the cephalic border of the alar cartilage. This residual strip can be left intact as a **complete strip;** it can be cut strategically to create an **interrupted strip;** or it can be weakened in various ways to create a **weakened complete strip**. In general, the greater the resection is the more dramatic the tip narrowing and rotation up. Conversely, the greater the strip weakening (or interruption) is, the more severe the loss of tip support and the greater the potential for undesirable tip retrodisplacement or postoperative tip asymmetries. Most surgeons believe that a minimum of 4–8 mm of residual strip must be preserved to avoid significant loss of tip support.

17. How can the nasal base be reduced?

The nasal base may be narrowed through some form of wedge excisions of the alar base, such as the Weir incision. Most radically, this type of excision would be a Weir excision through the entire alar lobule. Most commonly, this reduction involves only a modest wedge excision of the vestibular floor of the nostril. These excisions can be fashioned in various ways, such that in addition to narrowing the alar base, the nostrils can be narrowed and/or the tip can be retrodisplaced.

18. What techniques can be used to shorten nasal length?

Nasal length is modified by causing the nasal tip to be rotated up or down. This maneuver can be performed with or without altering the nasolabial angle, depending on what is done with the caudal edge of the septum. The septum plays a major role in tip and columellar position. Tip rotation up will shorten the dorsum and increase the nasolabial angle. Resecting the caudal septum will change the columellar position, to alter or preserve the original nasolabial angle while permitting this dorsal shortening.

19. What other techniques can be used to alter the nasolabial angle?

Aside from the caudal septum resection techniques, the nasolabial angle can be changed through the use of caudal septal grafts, medial crura stay sutures, columellar strut grafts, or, for overly acute angles, "softened" through the use of "plumping" grafts anterior to the nasal spine. To make the angle more acute, resection of the procerus muscle and/or the nasal spine can be performed.

20. What are some important factors in determining how much dorsal hump to remove?

A straight nasal dorsum is the generic "unisex" norm. However, a slightly concave dorsum is considered a desirable feminine trait, whereas a slightly convex dorsum is considered a distinctive masculine characteristic. Long-term postoperative results may be slightly more concave than the intraoperative result. This phenomenon is due to the thinner skin overlying the middle one-third of the nose, which is more easily distorted with local anesthetic and edema. This distortion may take some time to resolve and must be considered when performing a dorsal reduction. In general, some amount of convexity to the cartilage and bone must be preserved to achieve a straight or concave dorsal profile.

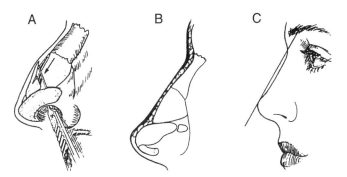

A, Reducing a cartilaginous dorsal hump. *B,* Nasal dorsal skin is thinnest over the rhinion. The bony-cartilaginous dorsum must still be convex to achieve a straight dorsum. *C,* In females, a slightly concave dorsum is aesthetically desirable. (Panel *A* from Tardy ME Jr: Rhinoplasty. In Cummings CW, et al (eds): Otolaryngology–Head and Neck Surgery, 3rd ed. St. Louis, Mosby 1998; Panels *B* and *C* from Gunter JP: Deformities of the nasal dorsum. In Krause CJ, Pastorek N, Mangat DS (eds): Aesthetic Facial Surgery. Philadelphia, J.B. Lippincott, 1991, p 342, with permission.)

21. What is a "pollybeak" deformity?

Pollybeak is a postsurgical convexity of the supratip relative to the rest of the nose, such that the lower two-thirds of the nose takes on the convex profile of a parrot's beak. It is classically a complication of over-resection of the nose. Over-resecting the nasal dorsum or the nasal tip supports can lead to relative protrusion of the supratip region. Paradoxically, over-resection of the supratip itself may lead to excessive "dead space," especially if the overlying skin is thick and inelastic. Subsequently, excessive scar tissue can lead to a supratip prominence. Corrective measures are directed at resecting the prominent tissues, grafting the nasal dorsum, augmenting tip support and projection, or a combination of these methods.

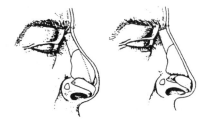

Correcting a pollybeak deformity by supratip excision of dorsal septal cartilage. (From Walter, C: Surgical approaches to problems of the nasal valve area and the extramucosal rhinoplasty. In Rees TD, Baker DC, and Tabbal N (eds): Rhinoplasty: Problems and Controversies. St Louis, C.V. Mosby Company, 1988, p 207, with permission.)

22. Why are osteotomies used in rhinoplasty?

It is important to free the nasal bones so that they can be manipulated into their desired positions. **Medial** osteotomies free the nasal bones from the nasal septum. **Lateral** osteotomies free the nasal bones from the maxilla. For example, once the dorsal hump has been removed, the nose has no anterior roof. Although it may look very straight on the patient's profile, the nose looks very broad and misshapen on the frontal view. With osteotomies, the nasal bones are surgically broken and bent medially so that they are once again in continuity with the midline.

23. How are splints used in the postoperative care of the rhinoplasty patient?

Both internal and external nasal splints may be used. External splints are placed over the nasal dorsum and may be constructed of a number of different materials. In general, splints for the nasal dorsum are first prepared using a skin prep solution such as benzoin. Tape is then applied to the nasal dorsum to protect the skin. The splint is shaped and placed over the tape. This splint is used to maintain the nasal bones in their desired position during early healing. The splint is usually removed about 7 days postoperatively. If a septoplasty has been performed, internal nasal splints are often placed along either side of the nasal septum. These are usually made of a flexible material such as Silastic and are usually held in place with sutures through the septum. The purpose of these splints is to maintain the septum in the midline and to assist in the prevention of a septal hematoma. They are also removed about 7 days postoperatively.

24. When is the rhinoplasty result in its final form?

The results should not be considered final until at least 6 months postoperatively. Although the bones may heal in about 6 weeks, the soft tissue swelling that is associated with rhinoplasty will take months to resolve completely. Swelling in the nasal tip is especially slow to dissipate. In fact, it has been said that after rhinoplasty, the nose continues to "heal " in small ways for "the rest of your life." Patients should be made aware of this fact preoperatively so that they are not disappointed by their immediate postoperative results. Also, if revisions are necessary, the surgeon should wait at least 6 months between operations.

CONTROVERSIES

25. Which surgical technique is superior, open or closed rhinoplasty?

Open rhinoplasty involves a transcolumellar incision to deglove the nose for optimal exposure of the nasal structures. Although exposure is superb, it requires more dissection trauma with more postoperative edema, and it results in an external scar that may or may not be easily visible on close inspection.

Closed rhinoplasty involves intranasal incisions (intercartilaginous, marginal, transcartilaginous) to gain access to the nasal structures through the nostrils. Exposure is limited and tip work requires "delivery" of the lower lateral cartilages into view. Although this method leaves no external scar, it does disrupt more of the nasal tip support mechanisms than does the open approach.

Most experienced rhinoplastic surgeons prefer (and preach) one approach over the other for general rhinoplasty. Nevertheless, few surgeons will argue against using the closed approach for addressing minimal defects and using the open approach for correcting significant, severe deformities of the nose.

26. What implant materials should be used in rhinoplasty?

Rhinoplasty frequently requires the implantation of materials to strengthen or augment the nasal structures. The patient's own cartilage and bone (**autogenous grafts**) is certainly the most biocompatible and perhaps most enduring material that can be used. However, harvesting autogenous graft material can be time-consuming and costly, and it risks morbidity to a separate operative site. Furthermore, available autogenous material may be limited, especially in the case of revision rhinoplasty, since septal or conchal cartilage may have already been harvested. Finally, autogenous material may be unsuitable for some applications because conchal cartilage and even septal cartilage or bone may have too much curvature or "memory" to provide a good long-term graft result.

Some surgeons have sought to circumvent these problems by using irradiated rib cartilage (**homograft**) or synthetic materials (**allografts**) such as silicone, Gore-Tex, and Medpore. These materials all represent compromises in terms of biocompatability and endurance but are faster and easier to use and capable of producing excellent postoperative results. However, the rate of graft infection (requiring removal), graft extrusion (a devastating complication), and graft resorption (requiring later revisions) for these materials continues to be a source of ongoing debate and investigations. The recent events surrounding silicone breast implants have caused many rhinoplastic surgeons to avoid the use of alloplastic implants completely.

RHINOPLASTY

Rhinoplasty was born of necessity in India. Susruta (78–144) developed a technique of nasal reconstruction to rehabilitate adultereers who had had their noses amputated for their crime. Tagliacozzi of Italy (1546–1599) learned of the work and developed it in Italy. Two hundred years later, Lucas (1703–1797) and Carpue (1764–1846) popularized the procedure in England and the West. The initial procedure, however, was for reconstruction of the missing member. The cosmetic procedure awaited Joseph's attention 100 years later.

~Weir N, Otolaryngology. An Illustrated History, 1990

BIBLIOGRAPHY

1. Burget GC, Nemick FJ: Aesthetic Reconstruction of the Nose. St. Louis, Mosby, 1992.
2. Farrior RT, Farrior EH: Special rhinoplasty techniques. In Cummings CW, et al (eds): Otolaryngology—Head and Neck Surgery. St. Louis, Mosby, 1998, pp 857–886.
3. Guyuron B: Dynamic interplays during rhinoplasty. Clin Plast Surg 23:223–231, 1996.
4. Guyuron B: The aging nose. Dermatol Clin 15:659–664, 1997.
5. Jones NS: Principles for correcting the septum in septorhinoplasty: Two-point fixation. J Laryngol Otol 113:405–412, 1999.
6. Larrabee WF Jr, Sherris DA: Principles of Facial Reconstruction. Philadelphia, Lippincott-Raven, 1995, pp 8, 68–69.
7. Lupo G: The history of aesthetic rhinoplasty: Special emphasis on the saddle nose. Aesthetic Plast Surg 21:309–327, 1997.

8. Madorsky SJ, Wang TD: Unilateral cleft rhinoplasty: a review. Otolaryngol Clin North Am 32:669–682, 1999.
9. Oneal RM, Beil RJ Jr, Schlesinger J: Surgical anatomy of the nose. Clin Plast Surg 23:195–222, 1996.
10. Pothula VB, Reddy KT, Nixon TE: Carotico-cavernous fistula following septorhinoplasty. J Laryngol Otol 113:844–846, 1999.
11. Rifley W, Thaller SR: The residual cleft lip nasal deformity: An anatomic approach. Clin Plast Surg 23:81–92, 1996.
12. Rohrich RJ, Adams WP Jr: Nasal fracture management: Minimizing secondary nasal deformities. Plast Reconstr Surg 106:266–273, 2000.
13. Schwab JA, Pirsig W: Complications of septal surgery. Fac Plast Surg 13:3–14, 1997.
14. Tardy ME Jr: Rhinoplasty: The Art and the Science. Philadelphia, W.B. Saunders, 1997.
15. Tebbetts JB: Rethinking the logic and techniques of primary tip rhinoplasty: A perspective of the evolution of surgery of the nasal tip. Clin Plast Surg 23:245–253, 1996.
16. Vuyk HD, Adamson PA: Biomaterials in rhinoplasty. Clin Otol Allied Sci 23:209–217, 1998.
17. Willett JM: How to assess the nose for rhinoplasty. J Otolaryngol 25:23–25, 1996.

55. BLEPHAROPLASTY

Bruce W. Jafek, M.D., FACS, FRSM

1. Define blepharoplasty.
Blepharoplasty is a facial plastic procedure intended to improve the eyelid appearance and/or function. When performed for cosmetic reasons, a blepharoplasty attempts to give the eyes a more youthful and attractive appearance. When the upper lids become so redundant that they actually drape over the upper lashes and obstruct the patient's view, the procedure is done to improve function, rather than appearance.

2. Which eyelid abnormalities can be corrected with a blepharoplasty?
In general, four abnormalities can be corrected with a blepharoplasty: blepharochalasis, dermatochalasis, pseudoherniation of fat, and orbicularis muscle hypertrophy. These may be isolated abnormalities, or they may be present in combination.

3. What is blepharochalasis?
Redundancy and draping of the eyelid skin that occurs in the aged face. This first occurs laterally where redundant skin becomes apparent only during animation (e.g., smiling). With time, this redundancy becomes a permanent feature, noticed even during repose. Blepharochalasis may progress such that skin actually drapes over the upper eyelashes and causes visual field defects in superior and superior-lateral gaze.

4. What is dermatochalasis?
Dermatochalasis refers to hereditary hypertrophy of skin and orbularis muscle that occurs in a young individual. It is thus unrelated to aging and occurs early in life. This hypertrophy results in a hooded appearance of the upper lid, and the upper lid fold is totally obscured.

5. What is the cosmetic effect of pseudoherniation of fat?
Pseudoherniation of orbital fat is a common cause of baggy lids and results from laxity in the orbital septum combined with continued gravitational forces on the orbital fat. The orbital fat then migrates anteriorly, causing a bulge that gives the appearance of a puffy or baggy lid. This may result in the objectionable look of sleepiness or weariness.

6. Is there any importance to orbicularis muscle hypertrophy?
The orbicularis muscle may become hypertrophied in the lower lid, adding to the bagginess associated with fat pseudoherniation. Unless recognized, this hypertrophy may result in residual bagginess after a blepharoplasty in which only the fat was addressed.

7. What tissues are excised during a blepharoplasty?
In both upper and lower lid blepharoplasty, three tissues need to be addressed: the skin, orbicularis muscle, and orbital fat. Depending on the pathology present, any combination of these three tissues may be excised.

8. Which features of the eyelid can be altered with a blepharoplasty?
Because a blepharoplasty addresses the skin, orbicularis muscle, and fat pockets of the upper and lower eyelids, only the features associated with these structures can be altered. Redundant skin (blepharochalasis or dermatochalasis) is usually the most obvious feature to be addressed. Redundant or hypertrophied orbicularis muscle (made obvious by having the patient squint) can also be resected. Lastly, pseudoherniation of fat in the upper and/or lower lid can also be corrected.

9. Which features of the eyelid cannot be altered with a blepharoplasty?

A patient may have complaints about some features around the eyelid that cannot be altered by a blepharoplasty alone; these must be pointed out and addressed during the preoperative visit. Problems that cannot be altered by a blepharoplasty alone include brow ptosis, lateral crow's feet, fine wrinkles of the lower lid, and cheek or malar bags.

10. What must the surgeon consider in the preoperative evaluation of a blepharoplasty candidate?

In addition to receiving a complete history and physical, each patient must be carefully evaluated for his or her particular aesthetic problem(s). The surgeon and patient must work together to ensure that both agree on what features are undesirable and how these can be corrected.

The surgeon must examine the skin of the eyelids, noting the presence of wrinkles, lesions, or abnormal pigmentations. Any asymmetries in the eyelids or palpebral fissures are noted and pointed out to the patient. These asymmetries may or may not be correctable. The eyes are examined for proptosis, and, if there is any doubt, the eyes are viewed from above and behind the patient in order to view both corneas as they relate to the upper lid margins. Next, the amount of excess skin in the upper and lower lids is estimated by pinching the skin together with blunt forceps until the lids are taut, but not so much so that complete eye closing is hindered. The snap test (see Question 11) gives an indication of excessive lid laxity and the need for lid-shortening procedures. The fat pockets are then examined individually, and the location and relative volume of each pocket are noted. Finally, the orbicularis muscle is examined while the patient squints, and any hypertrophy or "festooning" of the muscle is noted.

11. What is the snap test? How is it useful in the preoperative evaluation for blepharoplasty?

The snap test is a test for laxity in the lower lid. The patient looks directly forward, and the lower lid is grasped gently in the examiner's fingers. The lid is then pulled forward, off the globe, and then quickly released. The normal lid "snaps" immediately against the globe. A normal snap test is a reliable sign that the usual skin resection in a lower blepharoplasty will not result in scleral show or ectropion. If the lower lid remains off the globe for a few seconds or returns only after blinking, then a lid-shortening procedure may be indicated to avoid ectropion.

12. What should be included in the preoperative ophthalmologic evaluation?

A basic ophthalmologic examination is essential, including tests of visual acuity (both near and far vision), visual fields, and corneal protective mechanisms. These latter tests include checking for Bell's phenomenon (amount of corneal coverage as the eye is "rolled up"), lagophthalmos, facial nerve weakness, corneal sensitivity, and decreased tear production (Schirmer's test).

13. Describe the relationship of the brow to the upper eyelid.

The medial half of the brow normally lies at or just above the palpable superior orbital rim, and the lateral half lies slightly higher above the rim. The infrabrow skin differs from the delicate eyelid skin in that the infrabrow skin is thicker and more sebaceous.

14. How might the position of the brow affect your decision to perform a blepharoplasty>

The position of the eyebrows in relation to the superior orbital rim and upper eyelids is a *critical* factor in blepharoplasty planning. If brow ptosis goes unrecognized, the amount of skin excised in an upper blepharoplasty may be overestimated. This can lead to the reapproximation of delicate eyelid skin to the thicker and less pliable infrabrow skin, resulting in an unnatural appearance of the upper lid, and possibly even persistent lagophthalmos. In addition, uncorrected brow ptosis may result in a facial appearance dominated by the low-set brow, giving the face an angry or depressed look.

Therefore, the preoperative evaluation of the blepharoplasty patient must include palpation of the superior orbital rims and assessment of brow position. If brow ptosis is present, then it must be taken into account when planning the amount of skin excised and in deciding whether to combine the blepharoplasty with some type of brow lift.

15. What other factors must be considered in the decision to proceed with a blepharoplasty?

In addition to the technical details, the preoperative evaluation must also address psychosocial issues. These include the motivations of the patient as well as his or her psychological and medical background. Questionable motivations that should raise a "red flag" include early revision surgery to correct an unsatisfactory result, surgery at the insistence of a close family member or mate, sudden decisions, and a history of psychiatric illness. Medical factors that may influence the decision to proceed with surgery include a history of bleeding problems, history of ophthalmologic problems, any general or systemic disease, and alcohol and/or tobacco use.

16. Describe the anatomy of the upper eyelid.

To understand the steps in a blepharoplasty and to avoid injury to the lid levator mechanism, you must have a comprehensive understanding of the upper lid anatomy. In the lid, just deep to the skin, lies the orbicularis muscle, and just deep to this muscle lies the orbital septum (or *septum orbitale,* a fascial condensation extending from the periosteum of the inferior orbital rim to the tarsal plate). Orbital fat lies deep to the septum. This essentially describes the anatomy of the lower lid in its entirety, but in the upper lid, the levator mechanism is also present, making the anatomy more complicated.

In the upper lid, the levator muscle originates from the orbital periosteum and passes forward above the superior rectus muscle. As the levator approaches the lid, its fibers fan out to form the levator aponeurosis, which extends the full width of the lid. This aponeurosis then fuses with the orbital septum several millimeters above the superior margin of the tarsal plate. These fibers then continue forward to insert into the orbicularis muscle, subcutaneous tissue, and skin, forming the lid crease.

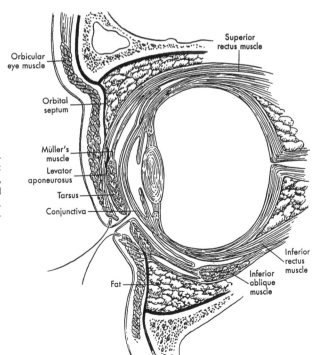

Cross section of orbit and eyelids. (From Colton JJ, Beekhuis GJ: Blepharoplasty. In Cummings CW, et al (eds): Otolaryngology–Head and Neck Surgery, 3rd ed. St. Louis, Mosby, 1998; with permission.)

17. What is Müller's muscle?

Müller's muscle is a smooth muscle that arises from the belly of the levator and inserts onto the superior border of the tarsal plate. This muscle receives sympathetic innervation off the oculomotor nerve and is responsible for the opening tone of the upper eyelid. Injury to either the levator or Müller's muscles may result in ptosis.

18. Describe the incision for an upper-lid blepharoplasty.

An upper blepharoplasty usually involves the excision of an ellipse of skin from the upper eyelid. The lower limb of this ellipse is placed horizontally in the upper lid crease. This crease represents the upper anatomic boundary of the tarsal plate, and it should be at least 8 mm above the upper lid margin. Medially, this incision ends 1–2 mm medial to the upper lid puncta. Carrying the incision more medially, into the concavity of the orbital rim or into the nasal skin, risks a webbed scar. Laterally, the incision is carried to the sulcus between the lateral orbital rim and lid. If there is redundant skin lateral to this point, the incision is extended lateral to this point and is angled upward.

The upper limb of the incision is then made such that it encompasses all of the redundant skin. This amount of skin is estimated by having the patient close his or her eyes; you then gently grasp the skin between the blades of a forceps, including enough skin so that the skin across the lid is tensed but the eyelid remains closed. This process is repeated medially and laterally so that the upper incision mimics the curvature of the lower incision.

Because the marks for these incisions are made with the patient in the supine position, care must be taken to push down gently on the brow during marking to mimic the effects of gravity in the upright position. If this is not done, the amount of skin excised may be underestimated.

19. Outline the steps in an upper-lid blepharoplasty.

Most surgeons prefer to perform a blepharoplasty under local anesthesia with intravenous sedation. The incisions are first marked with ink (see Question 18). The skin is then infiltrated with 1% lidocaine with 1:100,000 epinephrine. The outlined ellipse of skin is then sharply excised from the underlying muscle using a no. 15 blade. Some surgeons prefer to excise the skin and muscle as a single unit. Muscle is excised only if indicated, i.e., if it is redundant or if enhancement of the lid crease is desired.

If excision of pseudoherniated fat is indicated, this is performed next. Additional lidocaine (some surgeons prefer plain lidocaine here) is infiltrated into the orbital septum and anterior fat compartments. The orbital septum is then opened sharply, and the central and medial fat pads are dissected. Gentle pressure on the closed eyelid and upward traction on the medial brow will assist in exposing the medial fat pad. The superior oblique muscle must be identified prior to clamping the fat. Once the amount of fat to be removed has been teased into the field, the fat is clamped and excised. Prior to releasing the proximal stub of tissue, meticulous hemostasis is achieved. The central fat compartment is addressed in a similar fashion.

The skin is then draped over the wound, and any additional skin excision is performed so as to prevent any redundancy that may be apparent after the fat excision. The wound is then closed with a running subcuticular monofilament suture.

20. What techniques can be used for a lower-lid blepharoplasty?
- Skin-muscle flap technique
- Transconjunctival technique
- Skin flap technique

21. Describe the skin-muscle flap technique for a lower-lid blepharoplasty.

A subciliary incision is made 2–3 mm below the lashes and is extended laterally in a horizontal natural skin crease over the orbital rim. The initial incision is carried through the skin only, and a 3-mm-wide flap of skin is elevated inferiorly over the pretarsal portion of the orbicularis muscle. The incision is then carried through the orbicularis muscle, and a skin-muscle flap is elevated to the inferior orbital rim. This technique has the advantages that the plane of dissection behind the muscle is easy to identify and is avascular; there is minimal risk of button-holing the flap; and additional tightening of skin and muscle can be achieved by placing lateral suspension sutures. This is the preferred method when there is fat pseudoherniation with minimal skin excess.

22. Describe the skin flap technique for a lower-lid blepharoblasty.
The same incision is used, but the plane of dissection is between the skin and muscle all the way to the inferior orbital rim. This technique is advantageous when there is extremely wrinkled or redundant skin and when plication or resection of orbicularis muscle is desired.

23. When is the transconjunctival approach used for a lower-lid blepharoplasty?
In the transconjunctival approach, an incision is made in the conjunctiva on the inner aspect of the lower lid. This technique is useful when only fat removal is desired and there is no need for modification of the skin or muscle. Note that this is rarely the case.

24. How do the fat compartments of the upper and lower orbital compartments differ?
The orbital fat is located just deep to the orbital septum. There are three distinct compartments in the lower lid and two in the upper lid. In the **lower lid,** the *medial* and *central* compartments are separated by the inferior oblique muscle. Thus, this muscle must be identified prior to the cauterization or removal of fat from these compartments. The fat of the medial compartment is also lighter in color than that of the other compartments, which aids in its identification. The *lateral* pocket of the lower lid is separated from the central by a band of fascia.
In the **upper lid,** the *medial* and *central* compartments are separated by the superior oblique muscle, which also must be identified prior to fat removal. The lateral compartment in the upper lid is occupied by the lacrimal gland. During the removal of pseudoherniated fat from these compartments, hemostasis must be achieved prior to letting go of the remaining fat, as a bleeding vessel is difficult to isolate after the fat has retracted back into the orbit. An alternative to fat removal is simply to apply cautery to the orbital septum.

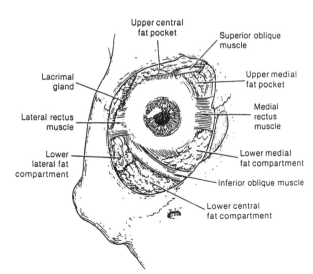

Fat compartments of right orbit and lacrimal gland. (From Colton JJ, Beekhuis GJ: Blepharoplasty. In Cummings CW, et al (eds): Otolaryngology–Head and Neck Surgery, 3rd ed. St. Louis, Mosby, 1998; with permission.)

Upper central fat pocket
Superior oblique muscle
Lacrimal gland
Upper medial fat pocket
Lateral rectus muscle
Medial rectus muscle
Lower lateral fat compartment
Lower medial fat compartment
Inferior oblique muscle
Lower central fat compartment

25. What is the most frequent complication of blepharoplasty? How is it treated?
Milia are the most frequent complication in blepharoplasty. These are white globular nodules that form along the suture tracks. They are easily and effectively treated with either pinpoint cautery or marsupialization with a knife.

26. What are some other possible complications of blepharoplasty?

Serious complications following blepharoplasty are rare. Lesser and usually self-limited complications are not so rare, but they can usually be managed simply, with local care measures and good communication with the patient. The more common complications include milia, scleral show or frank ectropion, hematoma, subconjunctival ecchymosis, chemosis, lagophthalmos, and ptosis. The unhappy post-blepharoplasty patient with lateral canthal dystopia, round eye, and scleral show presents perhaps the single greatest challenge. The problem may be as simple as a lax eyelid, which is inferiorly displaced by gravity, or as complex as an eyelid that has full-thickness vertical inadequacy in each of the three eyelid lamellae.

The transeyelid subperiosteal midface-lift with lower eyelid reconstruction is a reliable procedure for addressing full-thickness lower eyelid vertical tissue inadequacy, by totally reconstructing the lower eyelid with a three-layer reconstructive technique. Vertical and horizontal adequacy or inadequacy for each of the three eyelid layers is determined and then individually addressed in the total eyelid reconstruction. This procedure has the potential to fully reconstruct and reposition the lower eyelid and lateral canthus such that the final position, function, and appearance is as good or better than it was before the changes caused by time, gravity, and previous surgery.

27 How are scleral show and ectropion managed?

Scleral show is not uncommon following blepharoplasty and may be considered almost a normal variant in the postoperative period. It usually resolves as the edema and induration resolve in the first week or two.

Significant ectropion (the eversion or turning out of the lower lid) may be an indication of either too much skin excision or unrecognized lid laxity. Ectropion is first managed conservatively, with taping and eyelid massage. If it persists, either a lid-shortening procedure or a lower-lid skin graft, depending on the etiology, may be required.

28. How are hematomas, subconjunctival ecchymoses, and chemosis managed?

Hematoma is rare following blepharoplasty and must be differentiated from normal ecchymosis. If a hematoma is detected, it must be drained and the bleeding vessel cauterized.

Subconjunctival ecchymosis is a rare problem, the cause of which remains unexplained. Although it may be quite disturbing to the patient, it usually resolves completely in about 3 weeks. No treatment is necessary.

Chemosis is a marked swelling of the bulbar conjunctiva that may occur after a lower lid blepharoplasty. It also resolves on its own, but may take as long as 6 weeks to do so.

29. How are lagophthalmos and postoperative ptosis managed?

Lagophthalmos is the inability to close the eyelid completely, and it may follow upper lid blepharoplasty, especially secondary procedures. It is usually mild and is also temporary. Artificial tears and ointments may be necessary to protect the cornea until complete healing occurs.

Postoperative ptosis is due either to unrecognized preoperative ptosis or to injury to the levator mechanism during upper lid blepharoplasty. It is more common after procedures to elevate and deepen the upper lid fold. If it persists for > 6 months, surgical correction may be required.

30. What emergencies arise in the postoperative period?

The most common is **retrobulbar hematoma.** This rare complication is usually heralded by a sudden, intense increase in pain associated with lid swelling and proptosis. This bleeding is usually arterial and represents a surgical emergency. If not treated promptly, it can lead to increased intraocular pressure and blindness. Treatment consists of opening the wound to express any clots, lateral canthotomy to decompress the orbit, and emergent ophthalmologic consultation to measure intraocular pressure. The wound must be explored, and the bleeding vessel identified and controlled.

Another rare but potentially devastating problem is severe **dry eye syndrome.** This condition may be due either to unrecognized preoperative dry eyes or to lagophthalmos. If it occurs, it must be recognized and treated aggressively with lubricating drops and ointment.

Vision loss in the postoperative period is a very rare (1 in 25,000–50,000 patients) but very disturbing problem. Most commonly, it is related to a retrobulbar hematoma. In the absence of hematoma, vision loss is suspected to be related to unpreventable problems, such as idiopathic optic nerve atrophy or retrobulbar optic neuritis. To date, these problems have always been unilateral.

CONTROVERSIES

31. What is "westernization" of the Oriental eyelid?

The Oriental eyelid differs from the Western or occidental eyelid in that the Oriental upper lid lacks a lid crease and is more full, without a deep superior sulcus. In addition, the Oriental eye often has an epicanthal fold located medially. The absence of an upper lid crease is due to the levator aponeurosis fusing with the orbital septum below the superior tarsal border (whereas in occidentals, this fusion takes place a few millimeters above the superior tarsal border, creating the crease). The upper lid fullness is due to the presence of a thicker subcutaneous areolar layer as well as an additional layer of fat located between the orbicularis muscle and orbital septum.

Westernization of an Oriental eyelid involves the creation of an upper lid crease, thinning of the upper lid, and removal of the epicanthal fold. These three procedures may be performed together, singularly, or in any combination. These procedures are controversial because they may or may not be desired by a particular patient. *The patient should be the one to decide what is done.*

32. How is the laser used in blepharoplasty?

Cosmetic eyelid surgery has benefited from the use of the carbon dioxide laser. The short pulsed laser cuts through tissue with limited surrounding thermal damage, resulting in incisions that heal with minimal scarring comparable to traditional cold steel methods. The laser provides excellent hemostasis, which shortens surgical time and lessens postoperative bruising and swelling. It is quick, causes less sensory nerve stimulation, is less likely to damage the inferior oblique muscle, and has essentially no bleeding—and therefore, less ecchymosis—postoperatively.

In addition, the standard blepharoplasty yields little improvement in several of the major signs of periorbital aging, including: (1) wrinkling of the infrabrow and lower lid skin, (2) crow's foot wrinkles, (3) malar bags and wrinkles, (4) changes in the periorbital skin texture, (5) pigment spots and other actinic damage, (6) elongation of the apparent vertical height of the lower lid, and (7) loss of the gentle, indistinct transition between the lower lid and cheek skin. All of these indications can be improved by the combination of laser blepharoplasty and laser resurfacing of the periorbital region. This technique produces a high-quality result that maintains itself well over time, improves the signs of periorbital aging not treated by traditional blepharoplasty, and has a low rate of complication and high patient satisfaction.

BIBLIOGRAPHY

1. Biesman BS: Blepharoplasty. Semin Cutan Med Surg 18:129–38, 1999.
2. Biesman BS: Lasers play a useful role in periorbital incisional surgery. Derm Surg 26:883–6, 2000.
3. Black J. Complications following blepharoplasty. Plast Surg Nurs 18:78–83, 1998.
4. Bosniak SL: Cosmetic Blepharoplasty and Facial Rejuvenation. Philadelphia, Lippincott-Raven, 1999.
5. Callina TL, Hunts JH: Applications of CO2 laser in oculoplastic surgery. J Ophthal Nurs Technol 18:95–9, 1999.
6. Carruthers J, Carruthers A: The adjunctive usage of botulinum toxin. Derm Surg 24:1244–7, 1998.
7. Coleman WP III: Cold steel surgery for blepharoplasty. Derm Surg 26:886–7, 2000.
8. Edelstein C, Balch K, Shorr N, et al: The transeyelid subperiosteal midface-lift in the unhappy postblepharoplasty patient. Semin Ophthalmol 13:107–14, 1998.
9. Egan R, Rizzo JF III: Neuro-ophthalmological complications of ocular surgery. Int Ophthalmol Clin 40:93–105, 2000.
10. Goldberg RA, Edelstein C, Balch K, et al: Fat repositioning in lower eyelid blepharoplasty. Semin Ophthalmol 13:103–6, 1998.
11. Lessner AM, Fagien S: Laser blepharoplasty. Semin Ophthalmol 13:90–102, 1998.

12. Pastorek N: Blepharoplasty. In Bailey BJ (ed): Head and Neck Surgery–Otolaryngology, vol 2. Philadelphia, J.B. Lippincott, 1998.
13. Putterman AM (ed): Cosmetic Oculoplastic Surgery: Eyelid, Forehead, and Facial Techniques, 3rd ed. Philadelphia, W.B. Saunders, 1999.
14. Roberts TL III: Laser blepharoplasty and laser resurfacing of the periorbital area. Clin Plast Surg 25:95–108, 1998.
15. Zilkha MC, Bosniak SL: Cosmetic Blepharoplasty and Facial Rejuvenation. Philadelphia, Williams & Wilkins, 1999.

Mt. Rushmore

Some patients are not plastic surgery candidates.

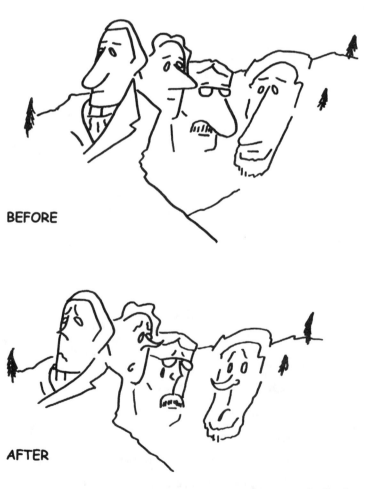

BEFORE

AFTER

Jim Gough

56. OTOPLASTY

David A. Hendrick, M.D.

1. What anatomic landmarks of the external ear are important in otoplasty?

The circumference of the external ear consists of the tragus, helix, and lobule. The inner folds of the ear consist of the antihelix and its two crura. Between the two crura lies the fossa triangularis. Between the helix and antihelix is the scaphoid fossa. The "bowl" of the ear is the concha. Most otoplasty techniques are designed to augment the antihelical folds and/or reduce the conchal bowl.

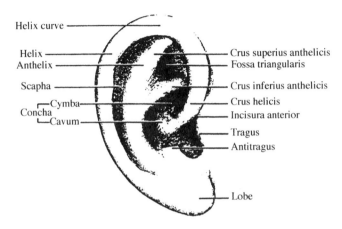

Important anatomic landmarks of the external ear. (From Siegert R, Weerda H, Remmert S: Embryology and surgical anatomy of the auricle. Fac Plast Surg 10:236,1994, with permission.)

2. What is the incidence of congenital ear deformities and malformations?

About 5% of live-born infants will have a diagnosable deformity of the external ear, ranging from "prominent" ears to microtia.

3. How are external ear malformations classified?

Various grading systems have been proposed for congenital malformations of the auricle. The best known system is Tanzer's five-stage system, ranging from stage I (complete anotia, or absence of the ear) to stage IV (prominent ear). The simplest system is Aguilar's three-stage system, in which stage I is normal, II is deformed, and III is microtia or anotia. The most comprehensive may be the three-stage Weerda system. Each stage is determined by the degree of surgical reconstruction required:

Weerda Stage I: First-degree dysplasia, in which most structures of the normal auricle are recognized. No additional skin or cartilage is needed for reconstruction. This category includes prominent ears, macrotia, minor deformities, and mild to moderate cup-ear deformities.

Weerda Stage II: Second-degree dysplasia, in which some structures of the normal auricle are recognized. Partial reconstruction requires additional skin and/or cartilage. Severe cup-ear and mini-ear are included in this category.

Weerda Stage III: Third-degree dysplasia, in which no structures of the normal auricle are recognized. Reconstruction is total, requiring additional skin and large amounts of cartilage. Microtia and anotia fall under this heading.

4. What is a "prominent" ear?

The normal ear has an angle between the auricle and head of 25–30 degrees. The helical rim extends < 20 mm from the mastoid, and a well-defined antihelical crus is present. The prominent or protruding ear is abnormal in one or more of these areas. Typically, the protruding ear has an auriculocephalic angle approaching 90 degrees, a helical rim > 20 mm from the mastoid, and a scaphoid fossa deficient in antihelical folds or crura.

5. When should prominent ears be corrected?

The best time to correct prominent ears is between the ages of 4 and 6 years. At this age, ear growth is nearly complete (seven-eights of ear growth is complete by age 7), and correction is completed prior to school age, when children become subject to peer ridicule. For the same reasons, 6 years is also the most appropriate age for microtia reconstruction.

6. When assessing an ear for otoplasty, what are the important considerations on antero-posterior or posteroanterior views?

When assessing an ear for otoplasty, the following deficiencies should be anticipated:
Poor antihelical fold
Deficient superior and inferior crus around the fossa triangularis
Abnormal scapha
Overdeveloped concha
Abnormal helix definition and curvature
The first four deficiencies involve assessment for a prominent ear. The last assessment involves ensuring that the helix is visible lateral to most of the antihelical fold and that the helix is an appropriate distance from the head. A horizontal line drawn through the inferior orbital rims should intersect the top of the two tragi (the "Frankfort horizontal plane"). A horizontal line drawn through the two pupils should pass through the maximum width of the auricles. A horizontal line drawn through the lateral brows should transect the upper helical rims.

7. When assessing an ear for otoplasty, how should the ear appear on the lateral view?

In general, the slope of the ear should approximate the slope of the nasal dorsum. More precisely, the "line of balance" of the auricle should be about 20 degrees from the vertical. The ear should sit slightly posterior to the midcoronal plane on the head, a distance said to be about one ear width from the lateral orbital rim. Ear width is normally about 60% of its height. Ear height in an adult is about 60 mm. Ear position with respect to the orbit, eye, and brow should be as described for the anteroposterior view.

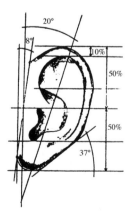

Proportions and angles of the aesthetic ear on lateral view. (From Tolleth H: Artistic anatomy, dimensions, and proportions of the external ear. Clin Plast Surg 5:338, 1978, with permission.)

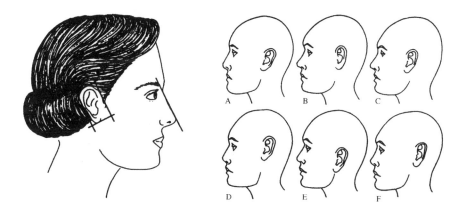

The angle of the external ear on the head should approximate the angle of the nasal dorsum. Schematic A demonstrates the proper location of the auricle on the side of the head. (Left panel from Ridley MB: Aesthetic facial proportions. In Papel ID, Nachlas NE (eds): Facial Plastic and Reconstructive Surgery. St. Louis, Mosby, 1992, p 107, with permission; right panel from Tolleth H: Artistic anatomy, dimensions, and proportions of the external ear. Clin Plast Surg 5:339, 1978, with permission.)

8. Describe the major goals of otoplasty.

The six major goals of otoplasty are described by McDowell:
- Correct protrusion of the upper one-third of the ear (the most critical portion).
- Allow helix to be visible beyond the antihelix on anteroposterior view.
- Give the helix a smooth contour.
- Avoid a decreased or distorted postauricular sulcus.
- Achieve appropriate distances from mastoid to helical rim.
- Achieve symmetry between the two ears within 3 mm at any given point.

9. The varied techniques of otoplasty can be divided into what general groups?
- Removal of postauricular skin
- Weakening of antihelical cartilage
- Shaping the antihelical cartilage into folds
- Reduction of the conchal bowl if indicated

Most otoplasty techniques can be grouped according to how the second and third steps are performed. Weakening of the antihelical cartilage can be achieved through scoring, thinning (e.g., drilling), or cutting. Shaping of the folds can be accomplished passively after weakening or actively through the use of mattress sutures.

10. What is the Mustardé technique of otoplasty?

The Mustardé technique was described in 1960 and again in 1963 with modifications. This method is the best known and perhaps easiest for correcting prominent ears. The technique essentially involves a postauricular skin excision and placement of permanent horizontal mattress sutures in the cartilage to shape the deficient antihelical fold. Suture placement is planned by using needles through the front of the auricle. When the ink-tipped needles are withdrawn from the cartilage, ink spots are left on the posterior side for suture placement. The primary disadvantages of the Mustardé technique are the possibility that the mattress sutures can become visible under the skin if they are poorly placed. The method also fails to address any excess of conchal bowl cartilage. Most surgeons also will do cartilage weakening techniques and conchal setback sutures (Furnas sutures) to correct the prominent ear more fully. (See figure on next page.)

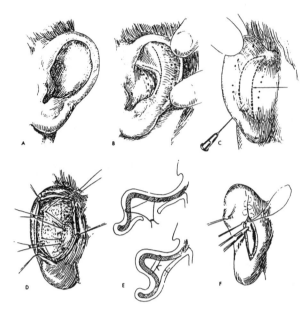

The Mustardé technique of otoplasty. (From Wood-Smith D: Otoplasty. In Rees TD (ed): Aesthetic Plastic Surgery. Philadelphia, WB Saunders Company, 1980, p 851, with permission.)

11. What are other popular methods of otoplasty?

Converse: This method creates an "island" of antihelical cartilage that sits anterior to the rest of the auricular cartilage. This method is technically more complicated than the Mustardé technique but is better suited for thicker cartilage.

Farrior: This method refines the "island" of cartilage. The cartilage island itself is scored to allow additional rolling of the cartilage. This method is technically complicated.

Furnas: This simple technique sets the conchal bowl back to the mastoid periosteum using sutures. It is often used in conjunction with other methods of otoplasty to fully correct the prominent ear. Its main disadvantage is the tendency for the conchal cartilage to protrude into the os of the external auditory canal. Resection of cartilage may be necessary.

12. How can auricular reduction be accomplished?

Auricular reduction is usually only employed when trying to match a smaller reconstructed ear on the opposite side. Such a reduction may be easier than trying to reconstruct the deficient ear to a larger size. Historically, many methods have been described for reducing the auricle. All of these methods involve a geometric excision and closure.

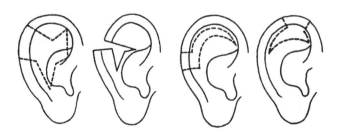

Resection methods for auricular reduction. (From Adamson PA, Tropper GJ, McGraw BL: Otoplasty. In Krause CJ, Pastorek N, Mangat DS (eds): Aesthetic Facial Surgery. Philadelphia, J.B. Lippincott, 1991, p 719, with permission.)

13. How can a protruding lobule be corrected?

The protruding lobule is usually a product of a flared caudal helical cartilage. Resecting this tail of cartilage will make the lobule less protruding. Excessive lobule skin can also be elipsed out on the postauricular side to further reduce the ear lobe. As with auricular reductions, very large lobules can be reduced with a geometric excision and closure of skin. Simple wedge excisions here can be associated with scar contracture and lobule notching.

14. How can a deeply cupped, protruding concha be managed?

An excessively large conchal cartilage must be reduced by removing a crescent of cartilage from the bowl. This can be done through the postauricular incision, or it may be done through a separate, anterior incision hidden in the crease of the antihelix. The protruding concha is laid back on the head using conchamastoid sutures.

15. How can a "cup ear" be corrected?

The cup ear has a constriction of the helix and scapha that requires helical rim unfurling, expansion, and redraping of skin over the expanded cartilage. Most authors describe techniques that involve dividing the helical-scaphoid cartilage into interdigitating fingers that can then be expanded open in a fanlike manner. Conchal cartilage can be used to stabilize the tips of the framework. Severe cases may require skin grafts or flaps to cover the expanded cartilage. Other techniques of correcting the cup ear deformity involve wedging open the cupped helical rim and rotating a composite flap of skin and cartilage into the opening from the postauricular area.

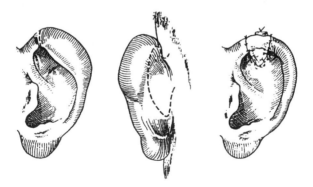

Correction of a moderate cup ear deformity using a pedicled post auricular composite flap. (From Walter C, Trenite JN: Revision otoplasty and special problems. Fac Plast Surg 10:303, 1994, with permission.)

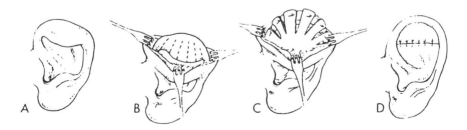

Correction of severe cup ear deformity. (From Converse JM: Congenital deformities of the auricle. In Converse JM (ed): Reconstructive Plastic Surgery 2nd ed. Philadelphia, WB Saunders Company, 1977, p 1708, with permission.)

16. What is a "telephone ear"?

Telephone ear is a deformity caused by overcorrecting the middle third of a prominent ear such that the ear takes on the appearance of a telephone on anteroposterior view. Such overcorrection can be due to excessive removal of postauricular skin or mastoid soft tissue or by overtightening conchamastoid sutures.

17. What is the temporal-parietal fascia flap? What is its role in ear reconstruction?

The temporal-parietal fascia flap is a thin vascularized fascia layer beneath the parietal scalp and overlying the temporalis muscle and is based on the distribution of the temporal artery and its superficial branches. Ear reconstruction requires the use of cartilage grafts and thin skin grafts to recreate the delicate ear structure. These transplanted tissues need a vascular supply to survive. As the closest vascularized, "flappable" tissue to the external ear, the temporal-parietal fascia flap is the primary means of covering auricular cartilage grafts with vascularized tissue. In this manner, thin skin grafts can then be successfully placed over the reconstructed framework.

18. Should a completed otoplasty be covered in dressings?

The completed otoplasty requires a soft cast to support and help define the remodeled cartilaginous folds. Cotton soaked in glycerol or antibiotic ointment will mold well for this purpose. A mastoid dressing should be applied over this cast and maintained for a week. After removal of this dressing, an elastic headband should be used to splint the ears back for an additional 4–6 weeks.

19. Describe the major early complications of otoplasty.

Hematoma is the most worrisome postoperative complication. Failure to investigate the persistent postoperative pain associated with otoplasty hematoma can lead to perichondritis and a disastrous loss of cartilage. Treatment is immediate evacuation of clot and débridement of necrotic tissue. Other early complications of otoplasty include skin hypersensitivity to pressure or temperature, dressing pressure necroses, and suture splitting.

20. What are the significant late complications?

The most common late complication is inadequate correction. Asymmetries and deformities may require revision otoplasty. Other late complications include scar hypertrophy and keloid formation.

21. What are the five stages of microtia reconstruction otoplasty?

Microtia reconstruction is a process requiring multiple surgeries over a protracted period of time. Although as many as a dozen procedures may be required in reality, the process is classically divided into five stages.

Stage I: **Auricular reconstruction**—Autogenous rib is harvested, fashioned into an auricular cartilage framework, and implanted beneath the skin of the scalp. Usually done at age 6.

Stage II: **Lobule transposition**—A pedicle of preauricular skin is rotated into position at the caudal end of the neoauricle. Done as an outpatient procedure about 2 months after stage I.

Stage III: **Atresia repair**—An otologist corrects the atretic external auditory canal for functional improvement. This stage follows the previous two stages to avoid compromising skin elasticity and vascularity for graft placement.

Stage IV: **Tragal reconstruction**—A composite graft of skin and cartilage is taken from the contralateral ear to create the tragus.

Stage V: **Auricular elevation**—A postauricular incision and skin graft are done to elevate the auricle away from the mastoid.

CONTROVERSY

22. How long should a head dressing remain on after an otoplasty?

A firm head dressing is usually applied after otoplasty. Some surgeons recommend that the patient wear this dressing for up to 10 days after surgery. However, these bandages are frequently displaced or come off. Patients complain of reduced hearing, itch, and the smell of old blood in the bandages. In a series of 52 patients undergoing bilateral otoplasty who had a head bandage on for only 24 hours, Bartley found only minor complications in two patients, with excellent preservation of the initial surgical correction. He concluded that a head bandage does not need to remain on for more than 24 hours after otoplasty. However, it is probably wise for the patient to wear a headband at night for 6–8 weeks to avoid accidental trauma while sleeping. Girls may also be able to wear this during the day.

NONSURGICAL CORRECTION OF LOP EAR

Kurozumi et al. presented a case in which the unusual congenital lop ear deformity was treated successfully by splinting with Reston foam. The deformity did not recur after an interval of 18 months, when it was reported. It is suggested that this method may be useful in the correction of similar deformities in very young infants in whom the ear cartilage is very soft, avoiding or simplifying subsequent otoplasty.

~Kurozumi, Br J Plast Surg 35:181, 1982

BIBLIOGRAPHY

1. Bartley J: How long should ears be bandaged after otoplasty? J Laryngol Otol 112:531–532, 1998.
2. Beasley NJ, Jones NS: Otoplasty: The problem of the deep conchal bowl. J Laryngol Otol 110:864–868, 1996.
3. Burres S: The anterior-posterior otoplasty. Arch Otolaryngol Head Neck Surg 124:181–185, 1998.
4. Caouette-Laberge L, Guay N, Bortoluzzi P, et al: Otoplasty: Anterior scoring technique and results in 500 cases. Plast Reconst Surg 105:504–515, 2000.
5. Connolly A, Bartley J: 'External' Mustarde suture technique in otoplasty. Clin Otol Allied Sci 23:97–99, 1998.
6. Converse JM: Congenital deformities of the auricle. In Converse JM (ed): Reconstructive Plastic Surgery, 2nd ed. Philadelphia, W.B. Saunders, 1977, pp 1707–1719. *(A classic)*
7. de la Torre J, Tenenhaus M, Douglas BK, et al: A simplified technique of otoplasty: The temporary Kaye suture. Ann Plast Surg 41:94–96, 1998.
8. Ducic Y, Hilger PA: Effective step-by-step technique for the surgical treatment of protruding ears. J Otolaryngol 28:59–64, 1999.
9. Foda HM: Otoplasty: A graduated approach. Aesthetic Plast Surg 23:407–412, 1999.
10. Hilger P, Khosh MM, Nishioka G, et al: Modification of the Mustarde otoplasty technique using temporary contouring sutures. Plast Reconstr Surg 100:1585–1586, 1997.
11. Lavy J, Stearns M: Otoplasty: Techniques, results and complications—a review. Clin Otolaryngol Allied Sci 22:390–393, 1997.
12. Lee D, Bluestone CD: The Becker technique for otoplasty: Modified and revisited with long-term outcomes. Laryngoscope 110:949–954, 2000.
13. Spira M: Otoplasty: What I do now—a 30-year perspective. Plast Reconstr Surg 104:834–840; discussion 841, 1999.
14. Vuyk HD: Cartilage-sparing otoplasty: A review with long-term results. J Laryngol Otol 111:424–430, 1997.
15. Zaoli G: Technical devices in otoplasty to obtain a natural appearance. Fac Plast Surg 13:197–205, 1997.

57. RHYTIDECTOMY

Richard Schaler, M.D., FACS

1. What is rhytidectomy?

Rhytidectomy, commonly but incorrectly called a "facelift," is the general name applied to a variety of surgical operations that seek to reduce or eliminate facial *rhytids,* or wrinkles, through the resuspension of the superficial fascia of the face.

2. Why do rhytids occur?

Facial rhytids are caused or worsened by a complex series of histologic, environmental, and personal factors. Superficial aging of the face may result from changes in three important components of the facial dermis: **collagen, elastin,** and **ground substance**. With age, the amount of type III collagen in the dermis increases, which may impair the synthesis of type I collagen and contribute to a thickening of the skin. As the amount of elastin begins to decrease in early middle age, skin fibers become increasingly lax. The glycosaminoglycans and proteoglycans of ground substance gradually diminish with age, prompting the formation of wrinkles.

Tobacco use and **sun exposure** are among the environmental factors that promote rhytid formation. Smoking may cause prolonged vasoconstriction of the facial vasculature, resulting in thinner skin. Sun-related damage produces both genetic and structural skin changes.

Naturally **fair or thin skin** increases the risk of rhytid formation. Wrinkles may be more severe in patients with animated facial expressions or in those who always sleep in the same position.

3. How does ultraviolet (UV) radiation affect the skin?

UVA is associated with actinic damage, and UVB is associated with DNA damage and skin cancer. Actinic damage is not simply an acceleration of the aging process. The dermis becomes thickened, and, overall, the amount of elastin increases. While there is a decreased amount of type I collagen, there is an increased amount of immature type III collagen. The histologic changes, referred to as **elastosis,** are the result of degraded elastic fibers, which accumulate and thicken the dermis. Common sources of UVA include sunlight, tanning lights, and fluorescent bulbs.

4. What are the indications for rhytidectomy?

Rhytidectomy has the potential to correct wrinkling in only the lower two-thirds of the face and the neckline. Significant wrinkling in these areas is an appropriate indication for rhytidectomy. Other procedures may be required to address rhytids elsewhere on the face, including brow lifts, submental and facial liposuction, laser-mediated skin resurfacing, and injection of botulinum toxin to weaken the musculature in the forehead that is responsible for wrinkling.

5. Who are the best candidates for rhytidectomy?

Patients who wish to seem "fresher" or less fatigued in appearance and those whose friends or relatives have successfully completed rhytidectomy are among the best candidates. Open and continued communication between the surgeon and the patient will promote an understanding of the benefits, risks, and limitations of the procedure and will permit patients to have reasonable and achievable expectations for rhytidectomy.

6. Is modern rhytidectomy one standard operation?

No. What was originally a procedure that did no more than remove excess wrinkled skin is now potentially one of several operations, all of which are generally known as rhytidectomy. The difference between these procedures is principally in the depth of the dissection in relation to the superficial musculo-aponeurotic system.

7. What is the superficial musculo-aponeurotic system (SMAS)?

The SMAS includes the platysma and risorius, triangularis, and auricularis posterior muscles and is connected to the dermis by fibrous septa. It is a fibrous dissectable layer that can be used to provide traction on facial tissues during rhytidectomy. Although there is some controversy, the SMAS is probably contiguous with the frontalis muscle and may insert into the nasolabial crease. The significance of this structure is its relationship to the nerves in the face, deeper facial motor nerves, and more superficial sensory nerves.

8. Why is the SMAS structurally important to rhytidectomy?

The SMAS is connected to the facial skin by a layer of fibrous septa that can be dissected away during rhytidectomy, allowing the skin to be resuspended to reduce the wrinkled appearance of the face. Because it is superficial to most of the sensory and motor nerves of the face, the surgeon can apply traction to the SMAS to tighten the facial skin.

9. What is a composite rhytidectomy?

The composite rhytidectomy is a combination of sub-SMAS dissection to the masseter and subcutaneous dissection anterior to the lateral border of the masseter to protect the facial nerve. The dissection of both subcutaneous and sub-SMAS planes allows the skin and SMAS to be redraped separately, providing multiple directions of pull. However, this technique does not provide the improved blood supply through the SMAS.

10. What are the variations and significance of the platysma muscle anatomy in the midline?

The anatomy of the platysma muscle in the anterior midline has three variations with respect to the decussation of its fibers. In general, fibers cross at the level of the thyroid cartilage, submentally, or at the mentum. The "turkey gobbler" appearance is caused by a laxity in the platysma that does not decussate across the midline.

11. How is the "turkey gobbler" appearance of the neck addressed?

Submental skin laxity is of particular aesthetic concern to many patients. Suspension of the anterior platysma and careful tightening of the preauricular skin may improve this condition. A T incision in the neck is used by some surgeons, with the advantage that redundant skin at the locus of the problem is directly excised, but the disadvantage that a more anterior scar may result.

12. Describe the anatomy of the nasolabial fold.

The nasolabial fold is formed by the insertion of muscles originating on the zygoma and the insertion of the thinned SMAS. This fold arises above the nasal ala and descends toward the mandible lateral to the parasymphysis. Of clinical significance, dissection anterior to the fold during facialoplasty produces little change in the contour of the nasolabial fold. Patients must be aware of this preoperatively.

13. What special challenges are presented by the nasolabial fold during rhytidectomy?

Dissection anterior to the nasolabial fold usually fails to improve wrinkles in that area. The judicious placement of processed collagen or artificial materials may improve the aesthetic outcome.

14. What are the osseocutaneous retaining ligaments in the face?

These are areas where the skin is attached to the underlying bone or fascia directly. The areas of the bony ligaments are the zygoma and the mandible at the parasymphysis. The ligaments to fascia are to the platysma, the platysma-auricular ligament, and the parotid and masseter area. The significance of these ligaments is that they must be released to adequately redrape the skin in a facialoplasty.

15. Describe the course of the frontal and mandibular branches of the facial nerve.

The facial nerve exits the stylomastoid foramen and enters the substance of the parotid gland, where it typically divides into five main branches: temporal, zygomatic, buccal, mandibular, and cervical. The *frontal branch* traverses the zygoma deep to the SMAS and through the temporal region on the temporoparietal fascia deep to the superficial temporal fascia. The nerve usually lies within 2 cm of the lateral brow and enters the frontalis muscle on the deep surface.

The *mandibular branch* courses within 1 cm of the inferior border of the mandible, posterior to the facial artery. This relationship changes when the head is turned away, as in surgery, and the nerve may be as far as 3–4 cm below the mandible. The mandibular branch is at risk during an anterior dissection deep under the skin flap because it becomes more superficial. This nerve lies deep to the platysma and superficial to the facial artery.

16. Which nerve is injured most commonly in a rhytidectomy?

The greater auricular nerve, which supplies sensation to the skin of the ear and nearby skin, is most commonly injured. The nerve lies deep to the SMAS about 6.5 cm inferior to the external auditory canal in close proximity to the external jugular vein. After emerging from the posterior border of the sternocleidomastoid muscle, it lies on the surface of this muscle.

17. How should nerve injury be treated?

If the injury is noted *intraoperatively,* the nerve, whether the greater auricular or a facial nerve branch, should be repaired under appropriate magnification. The patient who is recognized *postoperatively* to have a facial nerve injury (delayed) should be observed for spontaneous recovery, as the nerve was not transected. Recovery may occur in weeks to months, depending on whether the injury is partial and whether it occurs from traction or cautery.

18. Discuss some of the advantages and disadvantages of rhytidectomy techniques.

The subcutaneous, or **superficial plane rhytidectomy,** lifts the skin only, which is then safely dissected beyond the nasolabial fold. This technique is one of the oldest and most reliable. This technique provides versatility of access to the SMAS for adjunctive procedures with little risk to the facial nerve. However, it does not provide the improved blood supply to the skin via the SMAS. In addition, the vectors of pull are limited.

The **sub-SMAS technique** offers improved blood supply to the skin, which may be an advantage to smokers. However, the facial nerve is at greater risk, the nasolabial fold is not addressed, and the vectors of pull are limited.

The **subperiosteal dissection** provides vertical lift, redraping of the periorbital area, and good blood supply, and it preserves the relationships between tissues. However, this lifting is less effective in the lower face and does not address the jowls. The subperiosteal procedure can be combined with a cervicoplasty to address these issues.

19. What is the most common complication of rhytidectomy?

Damage to the greater auricular nerve may occur in as many as 5% of cases and produces parasthesias, or numbness, of the skin of the ear. Although deep to the SMAS, such injury may occur in superficial plane rhytidectomy secondary to traction. Less commonly, the nerve may be damaged by sharp dissection or cautery.

If injury has occurred as the result of traction alone, the nerve will often recover without treatment in weeks to months. Unnoticed transection at operation may lead to permanent loss.

20. What is the most feared complication of rhytidectomy?

Facial nerve weakness or paralysis occurs in 1–2% of cases and can occur even in superficial plane dissections. If intraoperative injury is observed, repair of the nerve is undertaken at once. Injury that is unrecognized during surgery is likely to be the result of traction on the nerve. Most traction-induced insults to the nerve resolve spontaneously, but the patient may report weakness on the affected side for as long as 1 year before recovery is complete.

21. What are some other common complications of rhytidectomy?

Hematomas and seromas occur in 4–5% of cases and may often be prevented by the placement of an appropriate vacuum drain for about 24 hours. Hematomas that present despite vacuum drain placement or after the drain is removed must be evacuated under sterile conditions. Small hematomas can be aspirated by syringe, and small infections can be drained locally.

Skin slough near the auricular incisions may occur in 3–4% of cases and is not usually severe. Modest débridement may be required, but slough is often treated expectantly by minimal débridement, as the eschar separates to allow maximal wound contraction and re-epithelialization.

Alopecia near the hairline occurs in less than 2% of cases and may be difficult to treat without additional surgery.

Infection of significance is a rare complication of rhytidectomy, owing to the good blood supply of the face.

22. What are the special risks associated with liposuction during rhytidectomy?

Although suction lipectomy may have a role in sculpting the submental area and the supraplatysmal plane below the mandible, it must be used cautiously—if at all—elsewhere. Fat excision in the cheeks may lead to a sunken appearance as the natural atrophy of the fat pads progresses over time. Lipectomy deep to the platysma may threaten the mandibular branch of the facial nerve or may produce unwarranted bleeding. It has been useful in the supraplatysmal plane below the mandible to de-fat the anterior neck and improve the cervicomental angle. This can be done through a small submental incision as well as from a lateral approach under the skin flaps. Deep to the platysma, fat excision is dangerous, owing to the location of the mandibular branch of the facial nerve and vascular structures.

23. What additional complications are reported in endoscopic facial plastic surgery?

Recurrence of the ptotic deformity has been reported in endoforehead lifts due to excessive skin and galea redundancy or inadequate fixation. Full-thickness skin burns from the use of cautery during endoscopic surgery and injury from the light source have also been reported.

24. What are reasonable goals of rhytidectomy?

Rhytidectomy addresses only the lower two-thirds of the face and neckline. Skin redundancy in the lower face, jowls, laxity of the neck, turkey gobbler deformity, and an obtuse cervicomental angle are all improved. Adjunctive procedures, such as forehead-plasty, blepharoplasty, and skin resurfacing, can often be done in conjunction with rhytidectomy for more complete facial rejuvenation.

25. Describe the indications for brow lift.

Brow-lifting is used in patients with eyebrows that are ptotic and to improve lateral upper lid ptosis. The glabellar and transverse frown lines that cause a stern appearance are also improved. Blepharoplasty is frequently performed in conjunction with a brow lift. However, the blepharoplasty must be done after the brow lift to avoid overresection of upper lid skin, leading to lagophthalmos and corneal exposure.

26. Describe the incision and dissection for brow-lifting.

A coronal incision is placed just anterior to the ear and is carried across the top of the head to the opposite side. In variations, the incision follows along the hairline or just posterior to it. The dissection is carried in the subgaleal plane down to 2 cm above the orbital rim. Here, the plane is deepened to the subperiosteal plane to protect the frontal branch of the facial nerve. The dissection is carried over the orbital rim and, on occasion, onto the dorsum of the nose. The frontalis, corrugator supercilii, and procerus are thus exposed and resected as needed. Muscle resection will weaken the forces that contribute to the wrinkling. It also creates a raw surface that can adhere to the periosteum, fixing the flap in position.

27. What is the ideal position of the eyebrows in women? In men?

The ideal brow level in women lies just above the superior orbital rim. The shape of the brow individually varies but tends to be a gentle arc with the apex corresponding to the lateral aspect of the limbus. The horizontal level, both medially and laterally, is even.

In men, the brow is similar in shape but lies over, not above, the orbital rim.

28. Are there alternatives to the coronal approach to brow rejuvenation?

Direct full-thickness skin and galea excision can be done on the forehead within the wrinkle lines, but these procedures may leave prominent scars. The glabellar area muscles are accessible through upper blepharoplasty incisions when the indications are hyperactivity of the corrugator supercilii and procerus. A new alternative, endoscopic brow-lifting, appears promising. This may be the procedure of choice for balding men and, as experience grows, may be as versatile as current conventional brow lifts.

29. What is the role of brow lift in rhytidectomy? How is it performed?

Brow lift does not significantly increase surgery time and may limit the amount of periorbital wrinkling after rhytidectomy. Standard coronal approaches to the brow lift may increase the risk of hair loss. Although associated with less risk of alopecia, endoscopic brow lift is reportedly complicated by a more frequent recurrence of the ptotic deformity. Preoperative injection of the forehead with botulinum toxin may reduce the risk of insufficient elevation.

30. Are there special considerations in the concomitant performance of blepharoplasty and rhytidectomy?

If blepharoplasty is indicated, simultaneous performance of both operations may allow a more uniform and more natural postoperative appearance of the malar fat pad.

31. What are some of the major issues that should be carefully reviewed during the surgical consent for rhytidectomy?

Every patient must understand the **limitations** of the surgery, particularly as they relate to the nasolabial folds, rhytids that surround the mouth, and wrinkling of the forehead.

Every patient must be aware of the **potential for nerve injury** and must be told that such injury could be permanent. A specific discussion of the possibility of facial nerve weakness or paralysis is mandatory.

Patients who plan a campaign of major **weight loss** should be counseled to defer rhytidectomy until after that weight loss has been completed. The outcome of rhytidectomy can be significantly altered by dramatic weight changes.

Patients must understand that tobacco use for several weeks before or after surgery can dramatically increase the risk of **skin sloughing** secondary to the impairment of skin oxygenation. Many surgeons decline to perform rhytidectomy for patients who continue to smoke.

Surgeons may tend to focus on the complications of rhytidectomy itself, at the expense of the consideration of general surgical risks. Although most patients can proceed to rhytidectomy safely in either the hospital or the properly equipped and staffed ambulatory surgery suite, due consideration must given to the patient's general medical condition, especially if the patient presents with diabetes, hypertension, or other cardiovascular diseases. Aesthetic surgeons who do not wish to do so themselves should ask the patient's primary care physician or another appropriate provider to screen the patient preoperatively for surgical risks.

32. What is the importance of smoking cessation in the prospective facial plastic surgery patient?

The rate of skin slough in patients who smoke has been reported to be 12 times that in non-smokers. The effects of nicotine have been studied experimentally and clinically. Nicotine triggers the release of epinephrine and increases platelet adhesiveness, leading to vasospasm and microclots. Cigarette smoke contains carbon monoxide, which impairs oxygen delivery, and hydrogen cyanide, which inhibits oxidative metabolism and oxygen transport. Many surgeons require that a patient abstain from smoking for 2 or more weeks before and after facial plastic surgery.

CONTROVERSIES

33. What are the emotional and social considerations when evaluating a patient for rhytidectomy?

Several books have been written on the psychological aspects of aesthetic plastic surgery, as many psychological considerations accompany this field. The surgeon must assess the patient's motivation for and expectations of surgery. Patients with recent dramatic life changes, such as marital separation, loss of a loved one, or children leaving home, can have unreasonable expectations about what the surgery will do for them. Beware of patients with a long history of plastic surgery. You should also be cautious of patients who denigrate the previous surgeon while praising the current surgeon.

34. What is the future of rhytidectomy?

The treatment of significant rhytids attempted solely by the application of laser light appears to be much less effective than rhytidectomy. It is expected that laser-mediated facial resurfacing will continue as an adjuvant treatment for wrinkling. Deep plane and endoscopic techniques are gaining favor in rhytidectomy. The direct vision afforded by endoscopic surgery may lessen the likelihood of neurovascular injury.

35. What is the "best" approach to rhytidectomy?

There is considerable disagreement about the "best" approach to the operation. Superficial plane rhytidectomy is the oldest, most common, and, in the minds of many surgeons, safest type of facelift because it poses a limited risk to the facial nerve.

The sub SMAS dissection technique allows preservation of a better blood supply to the facial skin but increases the likelihood of facial nerve injury and, in the opinion of some surgeons, limits the degree to which nasolabial rhytids can be lessened.

Subperiosteal dissections allow for preservation of the blood supply but are arguably less effective than other approaches to address the lower face. Subperiosteal dissections are usually combined with cervicoplasty to reduce this concern.

The type of rhytidectomy performed in individual cases may be more a matter of individual preference than any other factor.

36. Can laser facial resurfacing be safely undertaken with rhytidectomy?

Many surgeons now routinely perform both operations safely. A short-flap rhytidectomy may lessen the potential for preauricular skin sloughing when the procedures are performed together.

SURGERY IN THE MIDDLE AGES

Surgery in the Middle Ages was practiced by individuals belonging to a guild of barbers, with no basic medical education. The transformation into a scientific branch of medicine began in the 16th century. In this process, a great role was the one played by Leonardo Fioravanti. He was an MD from the University of Bologna. A controversial man, he was also innovative in many fields of medicine, such as prevention of diseases, pharmacology, therapy, and so on, and he was a surgeon himself. On the way back from one of the last Crusades, he visited the Vianeos brothers in Calabria, and he was able to learn from them the technique for reconstructing the nose that had been devised by

Antonio Branca in the previous century and still practiced only by barber-surgeons. He published his experience in a book that probably inspired his contemporary, Gaspare Tagliacozzi, Professor at the University of Bologna, and allowed him to become acquainted with this kind of reconstructive surgery. Tagliacozzi understood the value of the method described by Fioravanti and transformed a barber-surgery technique into a remarkable chapter of scientific surgery by divulging in the academic circles the principles of the pedicled flap, which have been the basis for development of modern plastic surgery.

~Santoni-Rugiu P, Plast Reconst Surg 99:570, 1997

BIBLIOGRAPHY

1. Brandt FS, Bellman B: Cosmetic use of botulinum A exotoxin for the aging neck. Dermatol Surg 24:1232–1234, 1998.
2. Campanile G, Hautmann G, Lotti T: Cigarette smoking, wound healing, and face-lift. Clin Dermatol 16:575–578, 1998.
3. Dover JS, Hruza G: Lasers in skin resurfacing. Australas J Dermatol 41:72–85, 2000.
4. Fagien S: Facial soft-tissue augmentation with injectable autologous and allogeneic human tissue collagen matrix (autologen and dermalogen). Plast Reconst Surg 105:362–373; discussion 374–375, 2000.
5. Formica K, Alster TS: Cutaneous laser resurfacing: A nursing guide. Dermatol Nurs 9:19–22, 1997.
6. Ghali GE, Smith BR: A case for superficial rhytidectomy. J Oral Maxillofac Surg 56:349–351, 1998.
7. Horton S, Alster TS: Preoperative and postoperative considerations for carbon dioxide laser resurfacing. Cutis 64:399–406, 1999.
8. Kennedy BD, Pogue MD: Fixation techniques for endoscopic browlift. J Oral Maxillofac Surg 57:588–594, 1999.
9. Klein AW, Wexler P, Carruthers A, et al: Treatment of facial furrows and rhytides. Dermatol Clin 15:595–607, 1997.
10. Krauss MC: Recent advances in soft tissue augmentation. Semin Cutan Med Surg 18:119–128, 1999.
11. Manaloto RM, Alster TS: Periorbital rejuvenation: A review of dermatologic treatments. Dermatol Surg 25:1–9, 1999.
12. Matarasso A: Facialplasty. Dermatol Clin 15:649–658, 1997.
13. Michelow BJ, Guyuron B: Rejuvenation of the upper face: A logical gamut of surgical options. Clin Plast Surg 24:199–212, 1997.
14. Miller AJ, Graham HD 3rd: Comparison of conventional and deep plane facelift. J La State Med Soc 149:406–411, 1997.
15. Pitanguy I, Radwanski HN: Rejuvenation of the brow. Dermatol Clin 15:623–634, 1997.
16. Rohrich RJ, Beran SJ: Evolving fixation methods in endoscopically assisted forehead rejuvenation: Controversies and rationale [see comments]. Plast Reconstr Surg 100:1575–1582; discussion 1583–1584, 1997.
17. Ross EV, McKinlay JR, Anderson RR: Why does carbon dioxide resurfacing work? A review. Arch Dermatol 135:444–454, 1999.
18. Salisbury CC, Kaye BL: Complications of rhytidectomy. Plast Surg Nurs 18:71–77, 89, 1998.
19. Sherris DA, Larrabee WF Jr: Anatomic considerations in rhytidectomy. Fac Plast Surg 12:215–222, 1996.

58. HAIR TRANSPLANTATION

James A. Harris, M.D., FACS

1. Which androgen is implicated in androgenetic alopecia (AA)? What is the physiologic basis for the treatment of this condition?

Dihydrotestosterone (DHT), produced by the conversion of testosterone by 5α-reductase (5α-R), seems to be the responsible androgen. Men who have a genetic abnormality resulting in a deficiency of DHT are protected against AA. The drug finasteride binds to 5α-R (Type II) and reduces the amount of DHT produced, thus slowing hair loss.

2. What is the Norwood classification of male pattern baldness?

A refinement of the classification system first proposed by Hamilton in 1951. Norwood evaluated 1000 men to develop the current classification scheme.

Norwood classification of the most common types of male pattern baldness. (From Norwood OT, Schiell R (eds): *Hair Transplant Surgery*, 2nd ed. Philadelphia, Charles C. Thomas, 1984; with permission.)

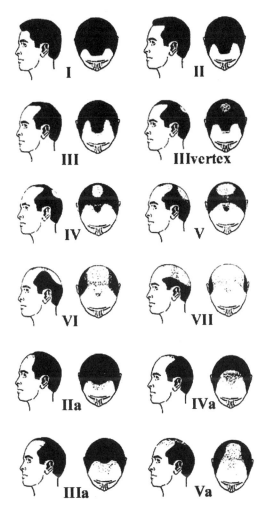

3. What percentage of the scalp is considered the "permanent" donor area?

Twenty-five percent of the scalp represents the permanent area. This is approximately 25,000 hairs.

4. When considering the donor area, what is considered the "safe" zone?

The safe zone is that area of the scalp from which donor tissue may be harvested and considered to be permanent, with a relative degree of certainty. A conservative estimate, proposed by Alt, and a more aggressive stance by Unger, is illustrated below.

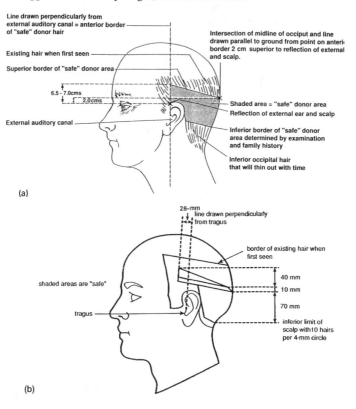

(a) Alt's safe donor area. (b) Unger's safe donor site for 80% of patients under age of 80 years, as determined from studies of 328 men aged 65 years or older. (From Unger WP (ed): Hair Transplantation, 3rd ed. New York, Marcel Dekker, 1995; with permission.)

5. Which harvesting technique allows for the least damage to hair follicles?

The primary harvesting methods are the single-strip harvest and the multibladed knife. The **single-strip harvest method** limits the blind cuts to the periphery of the donor strip and results in the least amount of trauma to the follicles. The multibladed knife technique allows for the rapid generation of narrow strips of skin and allows for a more rapid dissection. However, each incision by an individual blade is made blind, and follicle transection is increased.

6. What is a follicular unit?

It is an anatomic and physiologic entity that consists of 1 to 4 (occasionally 5) hair follicles, 1 or 2 vellus follicles, the insertion of the arrector pili muscles, sebaceous glands, and the surrounding adventitial collagen (the perifolliculum). A follicular unit is a natural grouping of hair in which the distance between the follicular units is greater than the width of the follicular unit.

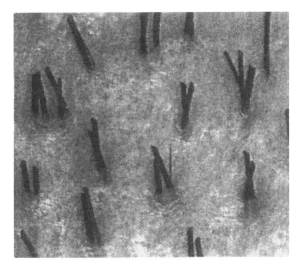

Natural follicular unit groupings. (From Bernstein RM, Rassman WR: Follicular transplantation, patient evaluation, and surgical planning. Dermatol Surg 23:771–784, 1997; with permission.)

7. What are the criteria defining follicular unit transplantation (FUT)?

A method of hair transplantation in which the graft is a naturally occurring, individual follicular unit. The requirements are single-strip harvesting, stereo-microscopic dissection, and placement into small recipient sites (usually < 1.8 mm).

8. Define mini- and micrografts. Describe the characteristics of the mini-micrograft technique of hair transplantation.

A micrograft is a 1- or 2- hair graft that may be a follicular unit or may be produced by dividing larger follicular units. A minigraft is a 3- to 6-hair graft that may consist of intact follicular units, multiple follicular units, or multiple partial follicular units.

The technique uses grafts having 1–6 hairs that meet the above criteria, and places them at recipient sites that can be incisions, excisions (round punch holes or slots), or both. The micrografts are placed at the hairline to allow a more natural appearance.

9. What are the relative advantages and disadvantages of FUT versus mini-micrografting?

FUT proponents state that the methodology decreases trauma to the follicles, which in turn promotes better hair growth. The very small incisions limit scarring and trauma to the scalp and allow for close placement of grafts. By employing nature's "building blocks" for a hairy scalp, a more natural density and distribution of hair is obtained. Multiple sessions are only needed to increase the desired density or to cover a new area, never to make the area appear more natural. The arguments against the procedure are the possibility that the handling and the increased risk of desiccation of the grafts may actually decrease the hair yield. Moreover, the additional technician time to produce the grafts and implant them is not warranted based on the final results.

Supporters of the mini-micrografting method feel that the results of this technique can be as natural as FUT after three to four sessions, without the added time in surgery and expenditures for the equipment required for FUT. Larger grafts may also resist the influence of graft handling and drying better than follicular unit grafts, thereby resulting in improved growth. Detractors of this method note that multiple sessions are the rule; the results are not as natural (i.e., pluggy and detectable); complications (see Question 11) are more common; and there is a more rapid depletion of the donor area.

10. What is alopecia reduction? What are the arguments for and against this procedure?

It is the surgical excision of "redundant" tissue from one or more areas of the scalp to reduce the "bald" area.

Those *in favor* of this procedure state that there is the ability to decrease the bald area while conserving the donor area, implying a change in the supply to demand ratio.

Those *not in favor* of this procedure cite numerous problems: the creation of scars which will require transplants to hide them, misdirection of hair as the fringes are pulled to the midline, "stretch-back" of the tissue resulting in less gain than originally thought, and stretching of the donor area which will limit the ability to harvest additional grafts in the future (i.e., *no* change in the supply to demand ratio).

11. List the most common complications of hair transplantation surgery.

- Ingrown hairs/foreign body reactions (implanted hair spicules) affect about 20% of patients at 8–10 weeks following surgery.
- Cobblestoning can occur with minigrafts or standard grafts (4–4.5 mm) when the graft is elevated above the recipient surface; 5% of patients are affected.
- Complications occurring less than 1%: epidermal cysts from the presence of bald skin in a recipient site, bleeding, infection, A-V fistula, wound dehiscence, chronic folliculitis, and hyperfibrotic healing.

12. Approximately what percentage of the hair can be removed from any area before there is apparent thinning on visual examination?

Fifty percent.

13. Describe a Juri flap.

It is a delayed temporoparieto-occipital pedicled flap (25 cm × 4 cm) based on the superficial temporal artery. The primary indication is fronto-parietal alopecia.

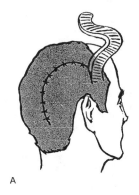

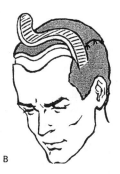

A   B

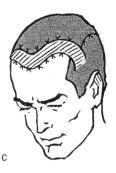

C

Juri flap. (A) Closure of the donor wound following undermining. (B) Resection of the glabrous zone. (C) Placing and suturing of the flap. (From Unger WP (ed): *Hair Transplantation,* 3rd ed. New York, Marcel Dekker, Inc., 1995; with permission.)

14. What are the advantages and disadvantages of flap procedures?

The advantages are immediate, continuous, and dense growth of hair after the transposition. Disadvantages include hair growth in the opposite direction of the natural pattern, hair growth in bands or strips, and hair growth at the original donor density, which diminishes available hair for transplantation in other areas.

15. What is miniaturization? What does it imply?

This is a decrease in the hair shaft diameter and length due to the effect of androgens. In a "normal" area of the scalp, the miniaturization is typically < 20%. Areas where it exceeds 35% are at risk for becoming bald.

16. What is meant by diffuse pattern alopecia (DPA) and diffuse unpatterned alopecia (DUPA)?

DPA is adrogenetic alopecia characterized by diffuse thinning in the front, top, and vertex, but with a stable or full-density permanent zone. DUPA is similar to DPA except that the permanent zone has thinned significantly and almost appears transparent. This patient is not a candidate for hair transplantation as the donor area is not stable.

17. List favorable hair characteristics.

- Lighter hair color (blonde, red, gray) reflects light and decreases the contrast between the skin and hair.
- Wavy or curly hair provides better coverage, as more hair volume is provided for any given distance from the scalp.
- Higher hair density (number of hairs/follicular unit) means more hair per graft.
- Wide hair shaft diameter increases the volume of hair. The volume of hair increases to the square of the radius, therefore shaft diameter has a more significant visual impact than does the absolute number of hairs.

18. Why are women frequently not candidates for hair transplantation procedures?

Many women with hair loss lose hair in a fashion similar to diffuse unpatterned alopecia, with retention of the frontal hairline. Unfortunately the donor area loses as much hair as the remaining scalp and it cannot provide the amount of hair necessary to make a significant cosmetic impact on the thinned areas on top.

19. What is postoperative effluvium? What types are encountered after a transplant?

Effluvium is the shedding of hair. The newly implanted hairs will undergo an **anagen (growth phase) effluvium.** The normally rapidly dividing cells are interrupted as a result of the traumatic move. The loss of hair in the recipient area undergoes a **telogen (resting phase) effluvium** and usually occurs after a 2–3 month delay.

20. What is the equation to predict future hair loss in any given male individual?

The *hair loss equation* is:

Future hair loss = Current hair loss + Lots more hair loss

This tongue-in-cheek relationship, elucidated by Dr. Emanuel Marritt, underscores the fact that male pattern baldness is a relentless, progressive, unpredictable process that should be treated in a conservative fashion, always assuming the patient will lose more hair than planned. Intervention must always be consistent with the long-term interest of the patient in mind.

BIBLIOGRAPHY

1. Bernstein RM, Rassman WR: Follicular transplantation, patient evaluation, and surgical planning. Dermatol Surg 23:771–784,1997.
2. Bernstein RM, Rassman WR, Seager D, et al: Standardizing the classification and description of follicular unit transplantation and mini-micrografting techniques. Dermatol Surg 24:957–963, 1998.
3. Konior RJ, Rousso DE (eds): Hair replacement surgery. Facial Plast Surg Clin North Am 2(2), 1994.
4. Marritt E, Dzubow L: A redefinition of male pattern baldness and its treatment implications. Dermatol Surg 21:123–135,1995.
5. Marritt E, Konior RJ: Patient selection, candidacy, and treatment plan for hair replacement surgery. Facial Plast Surg Clin North Am 7(4):537–562, 1999.
6. Norwood OT, Schiell R (eds): Hair Transplant Surgery, 2nd ed. Philadelphia, Charles C. Thomas, 1984.
7. Unger WP (ed): Hair Transplantation, 3rd ed. New York, Marcel Dekker, Inc., 1995.

VIII. Trauma and Emergencies

59. PRINCIPLES OF TRAUMA

Kjell N. Lindgren, M.S., and Bruce W. Jafek, M.D., FACS, FRSM

1. What is meant by the trimodal distribution of death?
Death from trauma generally occurs in one of three time frames:
- Within seconds to minutes after the injury: These patients die as a result of overwhelming trauma and/or head and brain injury. They can rarely be saved.
- From minutes to hours after the injury: This period is known as the "golden hour," and modern trauma care focuses on these victims.
- From days to weeks after injury: These patients often succumb to progressive organ failure or sepsis.

2. In general, what activities are undertaken in the effective evaluation and management of the trauma patient?
The initial management of the trauma patient begins with the **primary survey.** This first step identifies life-threatening conditions, which must be immediately addressed. The **resuscitation phase** begins with the management of any problems identified in the primary survey or during subsequent evaluation. As such, the resuscitation phase can run concurrently with the primary and subsequent surveys. During this phase, in addition to immediate life-saving therapies, the patient also receives intravenous fluids, a nasogastric tube, cardiac monitors, necessary radiographic studies, a urinary catheter, and laboratory studies. The **secondary survey** can be initiated once the primary survey has been performed and the indicated therapies initiated. The secondary survey is a quick head-to-toe examination aimed at identifying further injury. The patient's disposition may be determined once the primary and secondary surveys have been completed. Options might include transfer, admission, or a trip to the operating room.

3. What is the primary survey?
The primary survey involves the rapid identification and treatment of life-threatening injuries. Every trauma case should begin with a primary survey, which involves an evaluation of the ABC's (airway, breathing, and circulation). It should be emphasized that the most interesting or spectacular injury is not always the most life threatening. The reduction of a compound lower leg fracture will yield little long-term benefit to a patient struggling with a tension pneumothorax. Additionally, the presence of one life-threatening injury in no way rules out a second or third. The primary survey must be quick but also complete.

4. What specific lethal conditions should be identified immediately during the primary survey?
Airway obstruction, tension or open pneumothorax, flail chest, massive hemorrhage, and cardiac tamponade.

5. What are the ABC's (ABCDE's)?
A—Airway
B—Breathing

C—Circulation

D—Disability (Some use this for **D**rugs [What is patient taking, as well as what should be given?])

E—Exposure (Some use this for **E**verything **E**lse)

6. What is meant by "airway" in ABCDE?

The first step in managing the trauma patient involves airway assessment and stabilization. This step is accomplished while maintaining positive control of the cervical spine to avoid exacerbating any existing cord injury. Like any part of the trauma evaluation, airway management is a dynamic process, requiring constant monitoring and adjustment as needed.

7. What are common causes of airway obstruction?

Blood, emesis, posterior displacement of the tongue, dentures, and occluding neck or facial trauma can all cause airway compromise. Other reasons for initiating active airway management include decreased level of consciousness and head injury (patient may require hyperventilation for brain edema).

8. Describe the most common, nonsurgical ways to manage the airway.

Chin lift—The mandible is lifted to bring the chin anteriorly.

Jaw thrust—The entire mandible is displaced forward by applying pressure behind the angle of the jaw bilaterally. This maneuver is favored over the chin lift in patients with suspected cervical spine injuries. This method is especially suited to ventilation with a facemask and an Ambu bag.

Oropharyngeal airway—This tube is inserted either by using a tongue blade or by inserting it upside down and rotating it 180 degrees. It should never be inserted and rotated in children because of the risk of extensive soft tissue injury.

Nasopharyngeal airway—This method is very well tolerated in the conscious patient.

Orotracheal intubation—This is the most common way to definitively manage the airway. Spinal immobilization must be maintained during intubation.

Nasotracheal intubation—This method involves placement of a soft, pliable tube through the nose and into the pharynx and is useful in patients with known cervical spine injuries but should not be used in patients with extensive midface fractures.

9. Describe two common surgical ways to manage the airway.

Needle cricothyroidotomy—A large-bore intravenous catheter (12–14 gauge) is inserted into the cricothyroid membrane. After insertion, high-pressure oxygen is used to ventilate and oxygenate the patient. This procedure is preferred in children under age 12, as surgical cricothyroidotomy can easily damage the larynx.

Surgical cricothyroidotomy—This procedure is always preferred over the needle technique in patients over age 12, because a greater diameter airway can be established. A vertical skin incision is made to expose the cricothyroid membrane. The cricothyroid membrane is then perforated with an incision perpendicular to the skin incision. The knife handle or a hemostat can then be used to widen the cricothyroid opening and a tracheostomy tube is inserted. A cricothyroidotomy should be converted to a tracheotomy within 24 hours to prevent possible damage to the larynx, although the timing remains somewhat controversial.

10. What is meant by "breathing" in ABCDE?

Breathing refers to maintenance of ventilation and oxygenation. Breathing should be supported with 100% high-flow oxygen through a tight-fitting reservoir mask to provide the highest partial pressure of oxygen possible. A nasal cannula alone is not sufficient. The patient should be examined for signs of compromised lung or chest wall integrity (tracheal deviation, subcutaneous emphysema, crepitus, flail segment, paradoxical movement) or restricted chest wall mobility (circumferential burn). Breath sounds should be auscultated bilaterally to ensure good air flow. Necessary interventions may include the need for needle thoracocentesis followed by chest tube placement, mechanical ventilation, or repositioning of the endotracheal tube.

11. What is meant by "circulation" in ABCDE?

Circulation refers to the recognition of shock, identification of its probable cause, and the subsequent treatment. Shock is defined as inadequate perfusion of end organs. In the trauma patient, shock is almost always caused by hemorrhage. If an obvious source of bleeding is not found in a patient suffering with shock, an undiagnosed source should be sought.

12. Name four body cavities into which significant volumes of blood can collect.

Thorax, abdomen, retroperitoneum, and muscle compartments (thighs).

12. How is organ perfusion assessed in the acutely injured patient?

In the acutely injured patient, pulse, blood pressure, urinary output, skin color, and mental status reflect organ perfusion.

13. Should central venous pressure (CVP) monitoring be used in the acutely injured patient?

Although CVP monitoring is extremely useful when evaluating patients hemodynamically, it should not be used routinely in the initial management of a trauma patient. In certain settings, CVP line placement may be reasonable. For example, when peripheral access is unavailable, a CVP line can permit rapid intravenous infusion as well as CVP monitoring.

14. What are the different classes of blood loss? What do they mean?

Blood loss can be classified as class I through IV.

Class I	15% of total blood volume
Class II	15–30% of total blood volume
Class III	30–40% of total blood volume
Class IV	> 40% of total blood volume

It is important to recognize that internal bleeding can result in significant depletion of intravascular volume. A young, previously healthy patient can lose 15–30% of their blood volume to internal bleeding with minimal symptoms. Serial evaluation of vital signs and a heightened index of suspicion are needed to recognize occult hemorrhage.

15. How do you treat shock?

The cornerstone to management is vascular access and rapid infusion of warm, isotonic, crystalloid fluids. Two large-bore (18-gauge or larger) lines should be established. In adults, 1–2 liters of intravenous fluid is the usual initial dose, with 20 mL/kg being the initial dose for pediatric patients. Acutely, it takes approximately 3 mL of crystalloid to replace each 1 mL of blood loss. The exact amount of blood loss is not usually known however, so fluids are usually run at a maximum rate and adjusted according to the patient's vital signs and overall condition. If more fluid is required, a careful search should be made for a previously unnoticed injury.

Patients with class III and IV blood loss often require blood transfusions.

16. Should colloids or crystalloids be used in initial fluid resuscitation?

Colloid-containing fluids such as albumin or hetastarch have been used with the thought that they provide more rapid intravascular expansion and protect against pulmonary edema. Several studies were unable to support these claims and further found no significant difference in mortality between colloid- and crystalloid-treated groups. Crystalloid solutions, either normal saline or lactated Ringer's solution, are generally preferred for initial volume replacement in the trauma patient, because they are as safe and efficacious as colloid and are not as expensive.

17. When should a transfusion be considered?

As a general guide, consider giving blood products if the patient hasn't hemodynamically stabilized after receiving 2–3 L, or 40–50 mL/kg, of crystalloid.

18. What kind of blood should be given?

There are three general "flavors" of blood available, A, B, and O. Type O blood, the so-called "universal donor," should be used as a last resort in the face of exsanguinating hemorrhage. Specific blood (i.e., B, O, AB, rH+, or rH−) is available in < 15 minutes in most hospitals and is usually the best choice. Fully typed and cross-matched blood most closely resembles the patient's own blood. However, typing and crossing can be a time-consuming task (>1 hour in many institutions).

19. How is the electrocardiogram (ECG) used in the trauma patient? What should you look for?
All trauma victims should have an ECG acutely. Cardiac contusions can result in a myriad of dysrhythmias, including premature ventricular contractions, atrial fibrillation, and ST-segment changes. Electromechanical dissociation can result from a tension pneumothorax, cardiac tamponade, or severe hypovolemia.

20. What is meant by "disability" in ABCDE?
After the airway, breathing and circulation have been addressed, it is appropriate to quickly evaluate for disability by doing a quick neurologic exam. Motor function and pupil size/reactivity should be noted. The patient's level of consciousness can be quickly assessed using the AVPU method:
A—*a*lert
V—responds to *v*erbal stimuli
P—responds to *p*ainful stimuli
U—*u*nresponsive
The patient's level of consciousness should also be assigned a Glasgow Coma Scale score. As with any part of the primary survey, the patient's neurologic status should be constantly reassessed for any deterioration.

21. How is the Glasgow Coma Scale score measured?
The Glasgow Coma Scale is a standardized assessment of the neurologic impairment of a patient. It assigns a number to a patient's level of consciousness, ranging from 3 (no response) to 15 (best response). This score provides a way to communicate important information quickly and objectively. Furthermore, it permits rapid identification of trends and changes in mental status. It is the sum of the best verbal, eye opening, and motor scores. Scores of < 8 suggest severe head injury/coma, 9–12 moderate head injury, and > 13 mild head injury.

Eye Opening
4   Normal
3   Responds to speech
2   Responds to pain
1   No eye opening
Verbal
5   Oriented
4   Confused
3   Inappropriate words
2   Incomprehensible sounds, grunts, groans, etc.
1   None
Motor (measured in best extremity)
6   Moves best extremity to command
5   Localizes best extremity to pain
4   Withdraws best extremity from pain
3   Decorticate posturing
2   Decerebrate posturing
1   No movement

22. What is meant by "exposure" in ABCDE?
The patient should be completely undressed to permit a complete examination for any pre-

viously unrecognized injuries. When possible, the patient should be logrolled (while someone maintains cervical spine alignment) to allow for an examination of the thoracolumbar spine and posterior chest. The buttocks and gluteal cleft should also be examined.

23. When should monitors be applied and nasogastric tubes and urinary catheters placed? When should they not?

The placement of catheters and monitors (ECG leads, pulse oximeter) should be done as a routine part of the resuscitation. The initial assessment (ABCDEs) and resuscitation (intravenous fluids, airway control, and monitors) should proceed simultaneously. Urinary catheters should also be placed unless there is evidence of urethral injury. Evidence of blood at the meatus, blood in the scrotum, and a high-riding or nonpalpable prostate are contraindications to catheter placement. If a cribriform plate fracture or severe midfacial fractures are present, a nasogastric tube should not be placed.

24. In general, what laboratory tests are useful in the management of blunt trauma?

Complete blood cell count, electrolytes, blood urea nitrogen, creatinine, and prothrombin and partial thromboplastin times. Consider sending blood for typing and screening for patients with serious injuries, and typing and matching for patients with active or imminent severe hemorrhage.

25. At a minimum, which radiographic views should be obtained in a blunt trauma victim?

Anteroposterior chest, lateral cervical spine, and anteroposterior pelvis views are considered the "Big Three" and should be obtained as early as possible. Other films should be ordered as the mechanism of trauma suggests. However, no radiographic study should interfere with the resuscitation of the patient.

26. What should you do when a previously stabilized patient begins to deteriorate?

Go back to your ABCDEs. Often, an injury is unrecognized, or a previously treated injury remanifests itself. For example, even if a patient did not have a clinically significant pneumothorax on admission, such an injury could declare itself hours later and compromise the patient's life.

CONTROVERSY

27. What types of diagnostic studies are useful in a patient with suspected blunt abdominal injury?

Abdominal computed tomography (CT), diagnostic peritoneal lavage (DPL) and ultrasonography (US) have all been used to evaluate the abdomen for traumatic injury. Each modality has its advantages and disadvantages. DPL and US are similar in that they can identify the presence of hemoperitoneum but cannot define the cause of the bleed. Evidence for the use of DPL and US are largely derived from case control or cohort studies and suggest sensitivities of 94–96% and 81–90%, respectively. Though rapid, safe, and inexpensive, DPL is an invasive procedure, conducted by introducing a catheter into the abdomen. Aspiration of more than 10 mL of free-flowing blood constitutes a positive tap. Saline can be introduced into the peritoneal cavity and drained by gravity to further identify hemorrhage.

Abdominal CT can identify organ-specific injury but involves radiation exposure and may require the use of oral contrast. Although it is a sensitive and specific study, CT is not an option in a hemodynamically unstable patient, as it requires the displacement of the patient to the radiology suite.

US, long used in Europe, is gaining favor in the United States. US is rapid, noninvasive, and inexpensive and can be repeated as often as needed. The literature supports its use in the unstable patient for a determination of the need for laparotomy, or to look elsewhere for hemorrhage.

—➤●◄—

ARE CERVICAL SPINE RADIOGRAPHS MANDATORY
IN ALL BLUNT TRAUMA PATIENTS?

Pain and/or tenderness in the cervical region are valid criteria with regard to the timely diagnosis of cervical spine injuries. Therefore, routine cervical spine radiographs may be unnecessary for those blunt trauma patients who are conscious, fully orientated, cooperative, and non-intoxicated, who exhibit no neurologic deficits and do not have neck pain or tenderness. Omitting the cervical radiographs speeds up patient evaluation, protects the emergency department staff from unnecessary exposure to ionizing radiation, and mitigates treatment costs, while maintaining the quality of the health care provided.

~Ersoy, Eur J Emerg Med 2:191, 1995

—➤●◄—

BIBLIOGRAPHY

1. American College of Emergency Physicians: Clinical policy for the initial approach to patients presenting with acute blunt trauma. Ann Emerg Med 31:422–454, 1998.
2. Amoroso TA: Evaluation of the patient with blunt abdominal trauma: An evidence based approach. Emerg Med Clin North Am 17:63–75, 1999.
3. Bunn F, Lefebvre C, Li Wan Po A, et al: Human albumin solution for resuscitation and volume expansion in critically ill patients. The Albumin Reviewers. Cochrane Database of Systematic Reviews [computer file]. (2):CD001208, 2000.
4. Choi PL, Yip G, Quinonez LG, et al: Crystalloids vs. colloids in fluid resuscitation: A systematic review. Crit Care Med 27:200–210, 1999.
5. Cornwell EE: Initial approach to trauma. In Tintinalli JE (ed): Emergency Medicine: A Comprehensive Study Guide, 5th ed. New York, McGraw-Hill, 2000, pp 1609–1614.
6. Erstad BL: Concerns with defining appropriate uses of albumin by meta-analysis. Am J Health Syst Pharm 56:1451–1454, 1999.
7. Erstad BL: Venous thromboembolism in multiple trauma patients. Pharmacotherapy 18:1011–1023, 1998.
8. Gin-Shaw SL, Jorden RC: Clinical management of trauma. In Rosen P (ed): Emergency Medicine: Concepts and Clinical Practice, 4th ed. St Louis, Mosby-Year Book, 1998, pp 355–368.
9. Jurkovich GJ, Carrico CJ: Initial management of the acutely injured patient. In Sabiston DC (ed): Textbook of Surgery, 15th ed. Philadelphia, W.B. Saunders, 1997, pp 296–298.
10. Pearl WS, Todd KH: Ultrasonography for the initial evaluation of blunt abdominal trauma: A review of prospective trials. Ann Emerg Med 27:353–361, 1996.
11. Schierhout G, Roberts I: Fluid resuscitation with colloid or crystalloid solutions in critically ill patients: A systematic review of randomised trials. Br Med J 316:961–994, 1998.
12. Schierhout G, Roberts I: Mannitol for acute traumatic brain injury. Cochrane Database of Systematic Reviews [computer file]. (2):CD001049, 2000.
13. Schierhout G, Roberts I: Hyperventilation therapy for acute traumatic brain injury. Cochrane Database of Systematic Reviews [computer file]. (2):CD000566, 2000.

60. EPISTAXIS

Amir A. Rafii, M.S. IV, and Bruce W. Jafek, M.D., FACS, FRSM

1. What percentage of the U.S. population has had at least one serious episode of epistaxis in their lifetime?
About 11%. It affects all age groups without a predilection for sex.

2. How does epistaxis generally differ in younger and older populations?
Children and young adults tend to bleed from the anterior nasal cavity, commonly from an area called Kiesselbach's plexus. Posterior epistaxis is most often seen in older patients, in whom arteriosclerosis and hypertension may play a role.

3. Describe the relationship between respiratory microanatomy and epistaxis.
Respiratory epithelium consists of pseudostratified columnar ciliated epithelium, along with interspersed goblet cells. These cells are covered by a protective layer of mucous, continuously circulated via ciliary activity. A rich network of blood vessels fills the lamina propria, which lies just below the basement membrane. Any process that interferes with mucus production or ciliary function can cause drying and ulceration of the underlying mucosa, exposing the rich underlying vascular plexus.

4. What is Kiesselbach's plexus? Where is it located?
Kiesselbach's plexus is a confluence of vessels arising from both the internal and external carotid artery systems. It supplies an area on the anteroinferior septum known as Little's area, a common site for epistaxis. Although this area is easily irritated (via digital trauma, cold, dry air, cigarette smoke, etc.), it is also easier to access and treat than sites of bleeding deeper in the nasal cavity.

5. Which blood vessels supply the nasal mucosa?
The nasal mucosa is supplied by both the internal and external carotid arteries: The internal carotid artery gives rise to the **ophthalmic artery,** which branches into the **anterior** and **posterior ethmoid arteries.** These supply the anterior and posterior superior nasal cavity and septum.
The external carotid artery contributes blood via the **internal maxillary** and **facial arteries.** The internal maxillary artery divides into several branches, including the **greater palatine** and **sphenopalatine** arteries. The greater palatine artery contributes to Kiesselbach's plexus, whereas the sphenopalatine artery supplies the posterolateral nasal wall and is a main source of posterior epistaxis. The facial artery gives rise to the superior labial artery. The nasal branch of the superior labial artery contributes to Kiesselbach's plexus.

6. What are the causes of epistaxis?
Local factors:
Trauma, the most common being nose-picking and accidental injury.
Nasal septal deviation, spurs, and perforations cause turbulent airflow, which may lead to mucosal drying and bleeding.
Iatrogenic, following septal, nasal, sinus, turbinate, or orbital surgery.
Inflammation (due to upper respiratory infections, sinusitis, allergies, chemical irritation). It has been established that recurrent epistaxis is more frequent in patients with rhinitis.
Foreign body. Patients present with unilateral foul discharge and occasional epistaxis.
Environmental factors: Cold, dry air (especially in winter months due to the drying effects of most central heating systems) and temperature (nasal ciliary action decreases as temperature drops).

Malignant or benign neoplasms: Melanoma, squamous cell carcinoma, adenoid cystic, inverted papillomas. In the pediatric population, consider polyps, meningoceles, encephaloceles, or gliomas.

Systemic disorders: Arteriosclerosis and hypertension (implicated in older patients with posterior bleeds). Blood dyscrasias include Von Willebrand's disease, malignant tumors, liver disease, hemophilia, thrombocytopenia, chemotherapy, and use of aspirin, coumadin, and nonsteroidal anti-inflammatory drugs (NSAIDs).

7. Which genetic disorder predisposes patients to severe recurrent nosebleeds?

Osler-Weber-Rendu disease is an autosomal dominant disorder in which vessel walls lack contractile elements and mucosal telangiectasias are present throughout the respiratory and gastrointestinal systems. Since coagulation parameters of affected individuals are normal, diagnoses is made via a family and clinical history in patients with multiple telangiectasias. This condition requires repeated laser coagulation treatment of vessels, or skin grafting of the nasal cavity.

8. When a patient presents with epistaxis, what are the key questions in your history?

- On which side did the bleeding begin? (In children, suspect digital trauma if anterior epistaxis occurs on the side of dominant hand).
- How did the patient first notice the bleeding? (Initial awareness in the back of the throat indicates a posterior bleed).
- What is the amount and duration of bleeding? How many soaked towels?
- Has the patient had any past episodes of epistaxis? How were they treated?
- Does the patient have any significant medical problems or blood dyscrasias? (Heart disease, diabetes, and alcohol abuse may influence management).
- Does the patient take aspirin, warfarin, or NSAIDs?

9. Which laboratory tests should be performed to evaluate the condition of the bleeding patient?

You should obtain a complete blood cell count, prothrombin time, and partial thromboplastin time and rule out hematopoietic malignancies or blood dyscrasias. You should also type and cross the patient's blood. You may need to order additional tests if a coagulation disorder is suspected (bleeding time, liver function tests, thyroid function tests, fibrinogen, fibrin split products, d-dimer, von Willebrand's factor)

10. How can imaging studies help in the diagnosis?

Radiographs and **computed tomographic (CT) scans** will help evaluate bone integrity and erosion.

Magnetic resonance imaging (MRI) and **CT scans with contrast** will visualize soft tissue anomalies or nasopharyngeal neoplasms.

Angiography can delineate the vascular nature of the problem or the source of the hemorrhage.

11. The patient is bleeding profusely. How do you determine the origin of hemorrhage?

Initial clinical assessment should include the ABCs (airway, breathing, circulation) with correction of hypovolemia. By history, did the blood exit anteriorly (suspected anterior bleeding site) or posteriorly, down the throat (suspected posterior bleeding site). For the examination, you will need adequate lighting, a nasal speculum, Frazier and Yankauer suction tips, bayonet forceps, and gloves, facemask, and eye protection. A 0- to 30-degree telescope or nasopharyngoscope, along with suction, is helpful to assess the source of subtle bleeding, especially in the posterior and superior nasal cavity. With a posterior bleed, the examination should reveal little bleeding from the nostrils and more blood along the posterior pharynx, although severe bleeding may preclude a specific assessment, since the blood exists anteriorly and posteriorly.

12. What should you watch for on physical examination?

Vasovagal syncopal attacks. It is a good idea to have smelling salts and an assistant.

13. How would you manage bleeding localized to the anterior septum?

Pinch the nose! The majority of anterior bleeds respond to local finger compression anterior to the frontal process of the maxilla, for 10–12 minutes. Application of a topical vasoconstrictor (such as pseudoephedrine or 4% cocaine hydrochloride) will also help decrease edema and slow active bleeding. If bleeding persists, chemical cautery of the site with silver nitrate applicator sticks may be effective. You should apply the applicator stick specifically to the bleeding site, trying carefully not to cauterize uninvolved mucosa, until a gray residue appears. Avoid cauterizing both sides of the septum, as this may lead to septal perforations. If the bleeding is more profuse, or pulsatile, electrocautery may be helpful in producing a deeper burn.

14. Compression and cautery did not work. What next?

Consider placing an **anterior nasal pack.** Classic anterior packs are composed of Vaseline gauze, coated with antibiotic ointment (other options for packing include merocel sponge packs that expand when moistened or balloon packing). The entire 72-inch length of a 1/2-inch Vaseline gauze may be used. Using bayonet forceps, the pack is layered from top to bottom and from the back of the nose forward, until sufficient pressure exists to tamponade the bleeding. **Systemic anti-staphylococcal antibodies** should be considered to reduce the incidence of toxic shock syndrome.

15. When is a posterior pack indicated?

A posterior pack is indicated for posterior bleeds, which are diagnosed when:

The chief complaint is bleeding into the throat.

A posterior nosebleed is visualized.

Bleeding cannot be controlled with a well-placed anterior pack.

16. How do you construct and place a posterior pack?

First, secure three 2–0 silk sutures to the center of a finely rolled piece of gauze or vaginal tampon (1-inch long, 1/2- to 3/4-inch diameter). Next, pass a 14-French catheter through the affected nostril into the nasopharynx and subsequently into the mouth. Secure two of the three silk ties to the end of the catheter in the mouth. Now, when the catheter is withdrawn, the pack will be lodged in the affected choana. The nasal sutures should be secured with a dental roll at the nostril. They should not be tied across the columella, as this may lead to disfiguring pressure necrosis. The third suture (protruding from the mouth) may be taped to the cheek for easy pack removal.

Alternatively, a 14 French Foley catheter with a 30 mL balloon my be used. It should be inflated with 10–15 mL of saline (air leaks and is ineffective). Although a balloon catheter is easier to place and is better tolerated than the standard pack, it is usually less effective in controlling the bleeding.

17. How long should a posterior pack be left in place?

For 3–5 days.

18. What are the complications of posterior nasal packs?

In addition to pain and discomfort, there are significant complications associated with posterior nasal packs:

- Cardiopulmonary failure secondary to hypoxia—although this is the most significant complication, supplemental oxygen should be used cautiously, as it may depress the patient's respiratory drive.
- Pharyngeal fibrosis or stenosis secondary to pressure necrosis by the pack
- Alar or septal necrosis due to local ischemic changes
- Sinusitis due to the blockage of the osteomeatal complex on the affected side

- Toxic shock syndrome
- Aspiration

Thus, patients should be admitted to the hospital for oxygen saturation monitoring and systemic antibiotics.

19. Unfortunately, despite all packing measures, epistaxis persists in an otherwise healthy patient. What are your options now?
Arterial ligation, embolization, and endoscopic cauterization.

20. You decide to proceed with arterial ligation. Which vessels will you approach and how?
If the patient is bleeding from the superior nasal vault, it is appropriate to ligate the anterior and posterior ethmoidal arteries. Access is gained through an incision near the medial canthus. The angular veins should be ligated to prevent bleeding. Next, the periosteum of the ascending process of the maxillary bone and anterior lacrimal crest is elevated. Following retraction of the lacrimal sac and periosteum, the vessels may be visualized and clipped along the frontoethmoidal suture. The landmarks are the anterior ethmoid artery ~1 cm posterior to posterior lacrimal crest, the posterior ethmoid artery ~2 cm posterior, and the optic nerve (where you *really don't want to be!*) ~3 cm posterior.

If the patient is bleeding from a posterior location, it is appropriate to ligate the internal maxillary artery (in severe cases, ligation of the external carotid artery is also possible). Traditionally, a transantral, or Caldwell-Luc approach is used. First, an incision is made in the gingivobuccal sulcus. The surgeon proceeds to elevate soft tissue and periosteum from the maxilla, thus exposing the canine fossa. Carefully avoiding the infraorbital nerve and vessels, the surgeon opens the maxillary antrum. Next, an opening is made into the pterygopalatine fossa, on the posterior wall of the antrum, for visualization of the vessels. A blunt, right-angle hook may be used to elevate the vessels, which are subsequently clipped. This approach is technically difficult.

21. What are the pros and cons of embolization?
Embolization is an alternative to surgical ligation in patients unable to tolerate general anesthesia, or patients with unfavorable anatomy. In addition, more selective blockade of smaller vessels can be achieved. It is up to 96% effective. However, it is limited by availability of an experienced interventional radiologist. A potential for strokes (6%) also exists because of dislodged carotid artery plaques.

CONTROVERSIES

22. When should endoscopic cauterization be performed?
Endoscopic cautery is usually attempted once control of epistaxis fails, despite posterior pack placement. In these patients, the packs are usually removed under general anesthesia, and suction cautery is applied to address the source of bleeding. However, given the risks of posterior packs—along with the necessary hospitalization of these patients—many physicians prefer endoscopic evaluation under anesthesia and cautery over posterior pack placement. In addition to reducing the hospital stay, endoscopic cautery also eliminates cardiopulmonary complications and prolonged discomfort. A posterior pack can still be placed if endoscopic cautery is unsuccessful.

23. What is the role of hypertension in epistaxis?
Hypertension is often cited as a significant contributing factor to epistaxis, especially in the elderly. However, many studies have failed to demonstrate a higher rate of underlying hypertension among patients with epistaxis, when compared to the general population. Thus, hypertension at the time of epistaxis may be related to patient anxiety. Often, the patient is reassured as the bleeding is controlled, and blood pressure returns to normal. Keep in mind, however, that a thorough medical evaluation is warranted to rule out underlying hypertension. Adults may require

long-term treatment, and hypertension in children could be the manifestation of more serious conditions such as aortic coarctation, renal disease, and renal artery stenosis.

BIBLIOGRAPHY

1. Adornato SG: A new ligation approach to the management of chronicepistaxis. Ear Nose Throat J 79:721–728, 2000.
2. Alvi A, Joyner-Triplett N: Acute epistaxis. Postgrad Med 99(5):83–96, 1996.
3. Ballenger JJ, Snow JB Jr (eds): Diseases of the Nose, Throat, Ear, Head, and Neck, 15th ed. Philadelphia, Lea & Febiger, 1996.
4. Bergler W, Gotte K: Hereditary hemorrhagic telangiectasias: A challenge for the clinician. Eur Arch Otorhinolaryngol 256:10–15, 1999.
5. Bird D: Managing epistaxis in A&E. Emerg Nurse 7:10–13, 1999.
6. Chopra R: Epistaxis: A review. J R Soc Health 120:31–3, 2000.
7. Manning SC, Culbertson MC: Epistaxis. In Bluestone CD, Stool SE, Kenna M (eds): Pediatric Otolaryngology, 3rd ed. Philadelphia, W. B. Saunders, 1996.
8. Marple BF: Epistaxis. In Cotton RT, Myer CC (ed): Practical Pediatric Otolaryngology. Philadelphia, Lippencott-Raven, 1999.
9. O'Flynn PE, Shadaba A: Management of posterior epistaxis by endoscopic clipping of the sphenopalatine artery. Clin Otolaryngol 25:374–377, 2000.
10. Peyvandi F, Mannucci PM: Rare coagulation disorders. Thromb Haemost 82:1207–1214, 1999.
11. Pfaff JA, Moore GP: Eye, ear, nose, and throat. Emerg Med Clin North Am 15(2) 327–341, 1997.
12. Tan LKS, Calhoun KH: Epistaxis. Med Clin North Am 83:43–56, 1999.
13. Valavanis A, Christoforidis G: Applications of interventional neuroradiology in the head and neck. Semin Roentgeno 35:72–83, 2000.

61. NASAL TRAUMA

Bruce W. Jafek, M.D., FACS, FRSM

1. Which bone in the body sustains the most fractures?
Studies place the clavicle, wrist, and nasal bones as the top three.

2. What are the key questions to be asked during the history in evaluating nasal trauma?
- *When* did the trauma occur?
- What was the *mechanism*?
- Did the patient experience *epistaxis*?
- Has the appearance of the nose *changed*?
- Is the patient experiencing any new onset of nasal airway *obstruction*?
- Was the patient *unconscious*?
- Are there any *vision* changes (e.g., diplopia)?

3. What should you evaluate on the physical exam?
Evaluate the nose, both internally and externally. Proper lighting (i.e., fiberoptic headlight) and suction are usually necessary. It is best to anesthetize and decongest the mucosa prior to the examination. Examine the septum for fractures, deviation, perforation, hematoma, and mucosal tears. Check the lateral nasal wall in the same manner. Also examine the external nose in a systematic approach. Note any new nasal deviation. Palpate the nasal bones for any instability, motion, or crepitus. A recent photograph of the patient (e.g., driver's license, if this is the only one available) is helpful for pre-trauma comparison.

4. How do you confirm the presence of a septal hematoma?
A septal hematoma has a bluish or reddish hue. If someone is not familiar with intranasal exams, it can be easily confused with a deviated septum. A cotton-tipped swab is used to blot the suspected hematoma. A hematoma will blot; a deviated septum will not. If there is still doubt, the swelling can be aspirated to confirm the presence of blood.

5. How do you treat a septal hematoma?
The nasal mucosa is first anesthetized. A scalpel then is used to widely open the hematoma, and the hematoma is drained. A rubber band drain is inserted, and the mucosa is reapproximated with a 4–0, plain-gut, quilting stitch. The suture can be omitted if the nose is packed bilaterally with Vaseline gauze. If a drain is used, it is removed 24–72 hours after insertion.

6. What else should the physician be alert for in a patient with a nasal fracture?
If trauma to the face is sufficient to fracture the nasal bones, it can also injure surrounding structures. The eye, lacrimal system, paranasal sinuses, teeth, and oral cavity should also be examined. The possibility of a CSF leak should not be overlooked.

7. When should a nasal fracture be reduced?
Most agree that nasal fractures can be reduced in the first few hours after injury. After this, edema makes accurate judgment of the degree of deformity difficult. The next window of opportunity occurs after the edema has resolved but before bony healing has started, generally 3–14 days.

8. What is a closed nasal reduction? How is it performed?
A closed reduction is generally reserved for simple fractures with only minimal displacement. This procedure may be performed in the clinic. After the nose is anesthetized, the surgeon

uses a blunt instrument to lift the displaced nasal bones. The bones are then reset into their normal anatomic position. A splint is applied to the dorsum of the nose, and Vaseline-impregnated gauze packing stabilizes the nasal cavity internally.

9. When is a closed reduction inadvisable?

If there is severe deformity of the nose. In these cases, an open reduction may be necessary. Likewise, a fractured, displaced septum may best be treated with open reduction and septoplasty.

10. How is an open reduction performed?

An open reduction is performed in the operating room. The septum is addressed first, and then the nasal pyramids. With the patient under local or general anesthesia, the surgeon makes a **hemi-transfixion incision** (an incision along the caudal edge of one side of the septum), and a mucoperichondrial flap is elevated. The bony and cartilaginous septum are exposed and reduced. If the fragments are not reducible and protrude into the airway, the fragments may need to be removed. However, the surgeon should be very conservative when removing any cartilage or bone. At this point, the surgeon should attempt a closed reduction of the nasal pyramid.

If the nasal pyramid is not amenable to a closed reduction, then an open reduction is required. This procedure is similar to a normal rhinoplasty. **Intercartilaginous incisions** (between the upper and lower lateral cartilages) are made, and the periosteum over the dorsal nasal bones is elevated. **Stab incisions** are made laterally at the tips of the inferior turbinates, and the lateral periosteum is similarly elevated. The surgeon again attempts to reduce the nasal pyramid. If adequate reduction is not obtained, then formal medial and lateral **osteotomies** are performed. Osteotomies should free up the fragments adequately to allow proper reduction. When adequate reduction is obtained, the nose is splinted and packed with Vaseline-impregnated gauze.

11. A patient sustained an injury over 2 weeks ago. He now comes to your office desiring reduction. What is your next step?

First, examine the injury as you would a new fracture. Direct careful attention to the septum to rule out a septal abscess. These patients usually cannot be adequately reduced at this time. Definitive management, usually a formal septorhinoplasty, should be considered but should not be performed for at least 6–12 months to allow for healing maturation.

12. How do pediatric fractures differ from adult ones?

It is often necessary to reduce pediatric nasal fractures with the child under a general anesthetic. Pediatric fractures begin to heal more quickly than adult fractures, and reduction becomes difficult in 5–7 days. Injury to growth centers in the nose may become compromised by either the fracture itself or poor surgical management. *Conservative management* is the key to pediatric injuries. The mechanism of injury should be thoroughly investigated. Do not overlook child abuse.

13. List some late complications of nasal fractures.

- Airway obstruction
- Nasal deformity (secondary to scar contracture/formation, altered growth centers, "saddle nose" resulting from a missed septal hematoma, or poor reconstitution of septal blood flow with resulting necrosis of septal cartilage)
- Septal perforation
- Recurrent epistaxis
- Recurrent sinusitis secondary to intranasal anatomic abnormalities

14. What are the most important outcomes in the management of nasal fractures?

- Good cosmetic result
- Good nasal airway
- Normal nasal growth and development in pediatric patients

15. What is a septal abscess?

If a patient develops a hematoma that goes untreated, it may become infected and form an abscess in as little as 24 hours. The cartilage can rapidly die and be reabsorbed, resulting in loss of dorsal support and a saddle-nose deformity. The best way to prevent this complication is to evaluate and treat septal hematomas aggressively before they progress.

16. How do you treat a septal abscess?

Like any other abscess. It is opened and drained just as a septal hematoma would be. A drain may or may not be used. Antibiotics may be indicated, but some clinicians avoid them (except in the obviously infected cases) to avoid overgrowth of resistant strains of bacteria.

17. Which organisms most commonly cause a septal abscess?

The most common pathogen reported is *Staphylococcus aureus*. Group A streptococci, *Staphylococcus epidermidis, Streptococcus pneumoniae, Haemophilus influenzae,* and anaerobes have also been reported.

18. What is a good choice for antibiotic coverage in a septal abscess?

When selecting an antibiotic, it is important to consider the initial Gram stain. Because staphylococci are the most commonly encountered organisms, staph coverage is vital. A first-generation cephalosporin provides good coverage, even for penicillin-resistant strains. Obviously, the antibiotic should be altered according to the final microbiology report.

19. A little pus in the septum doesn't sound too bad. Can it really lead to serious complications?

Yes. Meningitis, brain abscesses, subarachnoid empyema, cavernous sinus thrombosis, and orbital abscesses have all been reported as complications of septal abscesses. Intercranial extension is believed to result from communication of the anterior septal veins with the veins of the upper lip and palate. In turn, these veins communicate with the facial angular and ophthalmic veins, which communicate with the cavernous sinus. The ethmoidal veins may also contribute with communication to the sagittal sinus.

CONTROVERSIES

20. Should plain films of the nasal bones be ordered?

Studies have shown that plain films of the nasal bones often do not add to or change the management of nasal fractures. In fact, they may be misleading. On the other hand, they may be of medicolegal importance when documenting an injury. Photographs of the nose are very helpful in documenting the nasal appearance before the nose is reduced or surgically modified.

21. Should antibiotics be prescribed for nasal fractures?

There is no evidence to support the routine use of prophylactic antibiotics, although some use antibiotics if the nose is packed. The antibiotic theoretically prevents toxic shock syndrome, although no studies have proven this. The excellent vascular supply to the nose, in combination with a competent immune system, is usually sufficient to prevent infection.

22. How can you minimize the likelihood of late post-traumatic nasal deformity?

Current management techniques for acute nasal fractures result in a high incidence of post-traumatic nasal deformity (14–50%). Associated traumatic edema, unrecognized pre-existing nasal deformity, and occult septal injury account for most of these acute reduction failures. Rigid nasal endoscopy, the use of general anesthesia, and primary septal reconstruction in cases with severe septal fracture dislocation should reduce the incidence of post-traumatic nasal deformity in severely injured cases.

BIBLIOGRAPHY

1. Alvarez H, Osorio J, De Diego JI, et al: Sequelae after nasal septum injuries in children. Auris Nasus Larynx 27:339–42, 2000.
2. Druelinger L, Guenther M, Marchand EG: Radiographic evaluation of the facial complex. Emerg Med Clin North Am 18:393–410, 2000.
3. Ehrlich A: Nasal septal abscess: An usual complication of nasal trauma. Am J Emerg Med 11: 149–150, 1993.
4. Escada P, Penha RS: Fracture of the anterior nasal spine. Rhinol 37:40–42, 1999.
5. Haug RH, Foss J: Maxillofacial injuries in the pediatric patient. Oral Surg Oral Med Oral Pathol Oral Radiol Endod 90:126–34, 2000.
6. Rhea JT, Rao PM, Novelline RA: Helical CT and three-dimensional CT of facial and orbital injury. Radiol Clin North Am 37:489–513, 1999.
7. Rohrich RJ, Adams WP Jr: Nasal fracture management: minimizing secondary nasal deformities. Plast Reconst Surg 106:266–273, 2000.
8. Rubinstein B, Strong EB: Management of nasal fractures. Arch Fam Med 9:738–742, 2000.
9. Sadrian R, Rappaport NH: An overview of maxillofacial trauma for nurses. Plast Surg Nurs 18:177–181, 1998.
10. Stanley RB: Maxillofacial trauma. In Cummings CW, et al (eds): Otolaryngology–Head and Neck Surgery, 3rd ed. St Louis, Mosby, 1998.
11. Tesini DA, Soporowski NJ: Epidemiology of orofacial sports-related injuries. Dent Clin North Am 44:1–18, 2000.
12. Waldron J, Mitchell DB, Ford G: Reduction of fractured nasal bones; Local vs. general anesthesia. Clin Otolaryngol 14:357–364, 1989.

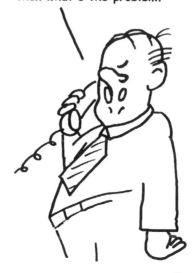

"So if he sewed it back on, then what's the problem."

Jim Gough

62. PENETRATING NECK AND FACIAL TRAUMA

Kjell N. Lindgren, M.S., M.S. IV and Bruce W. Jafek, M.D., FACS, FRSM

1. What is the incidence of penetrating neck injury among all trauma victims? What mortality rates are associated with penetrating neck trauma?

Penetrating neck trauma accounts for 5–10% of all injuries suffered by trauma victims. Mortality rates for penetrating neck trauma range from 2% to 6%, with some authors suggesting rates as high as 11%. Acute demise is usually a result of exsanguinating hemorrhage, but is also caused by spinal cord injury, cerebral ischemia/infarct, air embolism, or pulmonary embolism.

2. List three general causes of penetrating neck/facial injury.

- Gunshot—This mechanism has the greatest potential for serious injury. Low-velocity handgun rounds are associated with a mortality rate of 5–12%, while high-velocity shotgun pellets and rifle rounds have reported mortality rates up to 50%.
- Stab—These injuries yield mortality rates of 1–2%
- Other—This category includes glass, shrapnel, etc.

3. What initial steps should be taken in the management of a victim with face and neck trauma?

As with any trauma victim, the initial management of a patient with neck or facial trauma involves a complete primary survey. This rapid exam should address the ABCDE's (airway, breathing, circulation, disability, and exposure) and lead to the identification and treatment of any life-threatening conditions.

4. How should the airway be managed in a patient with penetrating neck or facial injuries?

There is some controversy as to the proper management of patients with this difficult clinical presentation. In penetrating neck and facial injuries, distorted neck anatomy, excessive secretions, and expanding hematomas can lead to rapid airway compromise. For this reason, some clinicians believe that all patients with penetrating neck/facial trauma should be intubated prophylactically, regardless of their presenting airway status. Many others believe that airway support can usually be reserved until it is clearly indicated. In general, patients should be intubated at the first sign of airway compromise.

Some controversy exists as to which airway technique is best suited in the penetrating neck trauma victim. Nasotracheal intubation is not recommend due to poor airway visualization and a greater frequency of complications. Surgical airways should be used as a last resort, since the patient often has distorted anatomical landmarks, and since a tissue incision could potentially release a tamponading hematoma. In some cases, the patient can be directly intubated through the wound. When possible, **endotracheal intubation** is the preferred method for securing the airway in this special class of trauma patient. While some authors suggest that the use of paralytics can cause airway collapse in an already compromised patient, Mandavia et al. found rapid sequence intubation to be a safe and effective method for gaining airway control.

5. Describe the anatomic divisions of the face.

- Area 1—superior to the supraorbital rim; contains the forehead
- Area 2—from the commissary of the lips to the supraorbital rim
- Area 3—from the hyoid to the commissure of the lips

Some authors favor a two-zone classification that groups injuries into either a *midface* or *mandibular* category. This system lends itself particularly well to gunshot wounds, as the injury patterns in these two zones are distinct. For example, midfacial gunshot injuries have a high incidence of vascular injury, globe injury, intracranial penetration, and facial fracture.

6. Define the mandibular angle plane.

The mandibular angle plane (MAP) is an imaginary vertical plane that runs through the angle and neck of the mandible and through the base of the skull. Any injuries that cross this plane must be assumed to involve the carotid sheath.

7. In facial trauma, how are area 1 injuries evaluated and treated?

After a neurologic exam, a CT scan best evaluates damage to the brain and frontal sinus. Depending on the injury, craniotomy and/or a frontal sinus procedure (obliteration, cranialization, or repair) may be necessary.

8. In facial trauma, how are area 2 injuries evaluated and treated?

After a neurologic, ophthalmologic, and oropharyngeal exam, a head CT should be obtained to evaluate for any disruption of the brain, orbits, or sinuses. Orbital involvement requires an ophthalmology consult. Involvement of the maxilla may require surgical exposure and debridement. Severe maxillary involvement may require rigid fixation with plates and/or intermaxillary fixation. Injuries that cross the MAP need to be evaluated with an arteriogram. Facial nerve function should also be carefully documented.

9. How should injury to the parotid duct be managed?

The two ends of the severed duct should be repaired over a small catheter. The catheter should be left in place as a stent for 10–14 days.

10. What treatment is required for transection of the facial nerve?

In a stable patient, facial nerve injury located lateral to the lateral canthus of the eye can be addressed with local exploration and primary repair of the transected nerve. Sensory deficits caused by nerve lesions medial to the lateral canthus often recover through nerve regeneration or cross innervation.

11. In facial trauma, how are area 3 injuries evaluated and treated?

After a complete oropharyngeal and neck exam, triple endoscopy should be performed. Again, injuries crossing the MAP need to be evaluated with an angiogram. Mandibular injuries are treated with either intermaxillary fixation or open reduction/internal fixation. A panoramic view (Panorex) is the single best plain film to diagnose mandibular injuries.

12. What are two general indications for angiography in a penetrating facial wound?

Remember the 2 P's: A patient with a wound path or foreign body that lies in close *proximity* to a major vascular structure or *penetrates* the mandibular angle plane should undergo angiography.

14. What systems are at risk in a penetrating neck injury?

Vascular—Injuries may include the internal, external, and common carotids; vertebral and subclavian arteries; and the internal and external jugular veins. Vascular injuries occur in 25% of penetrating neck trauma cases. Signs of vascular injury include external hemorrhage, expanding hematoma, shock, neurologic deficit, and diminished carotid pulses.

Pharyngoesophageal—These injuries occur in about 5% of penetrating neck trauma. While the presence of dysphagia, odynophagia, hemoptysis, or subcutaneous emphysema are important signs of a digestive tract lesion, these injuries are often difficult to detect. A high index of suspicion is required, as missed injuries can result in serious complications, such as mediastinitis or sepsis.

Laryngotracheal—These injuries are often accompanied by dyspnea, stridor, hoarseness, and subcutaneous emphysema. The airway is affected in about 10% of penetrating neck injuries, with a mortality rate up to 20%.

CNS (spinal cord) — In general, the risk of spinal cord injury is minimal. If an injury exists, it is due to direct insult and not cervical instability.

15. In general, how should vascular injuries be addressed?
External hemorrhage often responds to the application of direct pressure. No attempt should be made to blindly clamp bleeding vessels, as this only results in greater tissue damage and may dislodge hemostatic clots. Intravascular access should be established in a vein contralateral to the wound site, so that administered fluid is not immediately extravasated. Ultimately, any patient with hemodynamic instability and incomplete hemostasis should be managed in the OR.

16. What are the anatomic divisions of the neck?
There are two classification systems. The *anterior/posterior* divisions are more descriptive than clinically pertinent, and simply use the traditional anatomic triangles of the neck:
Anterior triangle—This area is described by the sternocleidomastoid posteriorly, the mandible superiorly, and the neck midline anteriorly. Injuries to this region are associated with significant vascular and aerodigestive injuries. The larynx, trachea, pharynx, esophagus, thyroid, vagus, and major vessels all traverse the anterior triangle.
Posterior triangle —This region lies posterior to the sternocleidomastoid and contains axial musculature, the spinal accessory nerve, and spinal cord.
The *three-zone* classification provides a basis for clinical management and prognosis:
Zone 1 involves the base of the neck and the thoracic outlet. It extends from the clavicles to the inferior aspect of the cricoid cartilage. Injuries to this region have the highest mortality.
Zone 2 is the most commonly injured region. Traumatic injuries to this zone are associated with the lowest mortality, however, due in large part to their greater accessibility. This zone is bounded by the cricoid cartilage inferiorly and the angle of the mandible superiorly.
Zone 3 extends from the mandibular angle to the base of the skull.

17. How are superficial neck injuries differentiated from more serious penetrating injuries?
The platysma muscle plays an important role in the evaluation of neck injuries. Any injury that penetrates the platysma must be considered serious, requiring at least admission and observation for 24 to 48 hours. Injuries that remain superficial to the platysma require only local repair.

18. Which diagnostic test is used to evaluate zone 1 injuries of the neck?
All zone 1 injuries require mandatory evaluation for vascular and esophageal injury. Control of zone 1 bleeding is generally obtained in the superior thorax. **Angiography** permits visualization of the aorta and great vessels of the mediastinum and lower neck, to evaluate the need for midline sternotomy or thoracotomy. Esophageal injuries, while uncommon, are often occult, with up to a third remaining clinically silent until the patient becomes septic. While these injuries are difficult to diagnose, the complementary use of both **esophagoscopy** and **esophagography** has a sensitivity of almost 100%

19. How should symptomatic patients with zone 2 neck injuries be managed?
These patients should be taken to the OR for surgical exploration. Examples of signs that require immediate exploration include: hypotension, active arterial bleeding, decreased carotid pulse, hemoptysis, hematemesis, and expanding hematoma.

20. Can zone 2 neck injuries be treated without surgery?
These patients can be managed either operatively or nonoperatively. Nonoperative management consists of panendoscopy, angiography, and possibly esophagography. Otherwise, surgical exploration of the penetrating wound tract is performed. If the facilities to image the neck are not available, the wound should be explored, the patient's condition stabilized, and then the patient

transferred to another facility. Soft tissue films of the neck are also helpful. Air in the tissues may suggest injury to the aerodigestive tract. Radiopaque foreign bodies, such as bullets, can also be identified. Their location, in conjunction with the site of the entry wound, can be used to hypothesize the missile tract. (See "Controversy.")

21. In neck trauma, how are zone 3 injuries evaluated and treated?

Exposure and control of bleeding posterior to the mandible and at the base of the neck is difficult. Therefore, all penetrating zone 3 injuries require evaluation with angiography. In some cases this diagnostic procedure can become therapeutic if interventional radiology is able to embolize the offending vessels. Otherwise, proximal control of zone 3 hemorrhage can often be obtained in zone 2.

22. What routine lab tests/imaging/procedures should be performed in the event of penetrating neck or facial trauma?

The facial trauma patient should have anteroposterior (AP) and lateral skull x-rays taken. The neck trauma patient requires an AP and lateral of the neck. Both types of patients should have a lateral neck and chest film taken. Baseline labs should be obtained, including a blood type and cross. A Foley catheter should be placed if possible. A nasogastric tube should *not* be routinely placed, because it can directly and indirectly (through stimulation of retching) cause disruption of a hematoma.

23. Name some common mechanisms for blunt trauma to the neck.

Automobile, bicycle, motorcycle, and snowmobile accidents; assaults; and hanging or strangulation attempts.

24. What are some signs and symptoms of blunt laryngeal trauma?

Hoarseness, stridor, voice change, airway obstruction, cough, subcutaneous emphysema, and hemoptysis are often associated with blunt laryngeal trauma. Such trauma may also be associated with loss of the thyroid prominence and loss of the normal crepitus of the laryngeal framework.

25. How is blunt laryngeal trauma diagnosed?

Flexible fiberoptic laryngoscopy and CT scanning of the laryngeal framework are the mainstays of evaluation in these situations. Careful attention should be given to a posteroanterior and lateral chest film and to the anteroposterior and lateral soft tissue neck films. Rigid laryngoscopy and an esophagogram may also be indicated.

26. How is mild blunt laryngeal trauma managed?

Patients with mild cases of blunt laryngeal trauma, which involve only edema or simple mucosal lacerations, can be observed if they are in a monitored hospital bed. Treatment includes humidified air or oxygen, steroids, a soft diet, and frequent evaluations.

27. How is severe blunt laryngeal trauma managed?

Severe cases may require that the airway be secured with a tracheostomy. Intubation and cricothyrotomy may further compromise the airway. Open exploration is then undertaken. Thyroid cartilage fractures can be reduced and wired or sutured in place. If there is gross displacement of the vocal cords, the lumen should be explored either via the fracture itself or a midline laryngofissure. The mucosa should be repaired, the cartilage reapproximated, and the external perichondrium closed. Fracture of the cricoid cartilage is managed by reducing and securing the cartilage and then closing the external perichondrium. If the cricoid ring is too unstable, a stent may be necessary. Rarely, a formal laryngotracheoplasty using rib or auricular cartilage is required.

CONTROVERSY

28. In asymptomatic patients, should zone 2 injuries of the neck be explored routinely or selectively?

Routine exploration: Popularized during World War II, mandatory exploration is advocated by some clinicians for the management of all asymptomatic patients with penetrating zone 2 injuries. Proponents of this policy cite the poor reliability of the clinical exam, and suggest that a negative exploration is far more desirable than a missed injury.

Selective exploration: Opponents of mandatory exploration cite the high rate of negative exploration (30–89% in some reports). They suggest that the application of an established physical exam protocol can be used to direct further diagnostic tests, such as angiography, color flow Doppler, esophagoscopy, and bronchoscopy. These tools can better identify candidates for surgical exploration. Benefits of this approach include fewer unnecessary operations, shorter hospitalizations, and decreased medical expense.

Ultimately, both of these methods have been proven safe and effective. The choice of approach often depends on staff expertise and the availability of the necessary diagnostic tools.

BIBLIOGRAPHY

1. American College of Emergency Physicians: Clinical policy for the initial approach to patients presenting with penetrating extremity trauma. Ann Emerg Med 33:612–636, 1999.
2. Baron BJ: Penetrating and blunt neck trauma. In Tintinalli JE (ed): Emergency Medicine: A Comprehensive Study Guide, 5th ed. New York, McGraw-Hill, 2000, pp 1669–1675.
3. Demetriades D: Complex problems in penetrating neck trauma. Surg Clin North Am 76:661–683, 1996.
4. Howes DS, Dowling PJ: Triage and initial evaluation of the oral facial emergency. Emerg Med Clin North Am 18:371–378, 2000.
5. Jorden RC: Penetrating trauma. In Rosen P (ed): Emergency Medicine: Concepts and Clinical Practice, 4th ed. St Louis, Mosby-Year Book, 1998, pp 505–509.
6. Jurkovich GJ, Carrico CJ: Recognition and management of specific injuries: Neck. In Sabiston DC (ed): Textbook of Surgery, 15th ed. Philadelphia, W. B. Saunders Company, 1997, pp 300–303.
7. Kendall JL: Penetrating neck trauma. Emerg Med Clin North Am 16:85–105, 1998.
8. Mandavia DP: Emergency airway management in penetrating neck injury. Ann Emerg Med 35:221–225, 2000.
9. Stewart MG: Penetrating face and neck trauma. In Bailey BJ: Head and Neck Surgery–Otolaryngology, 2nd ed. Philadelphia, Lippincott-Raven Publishers, 1998, pp 1033–1042.

63. UPPER AIRWAY OBSTRUCTION

Gresham Richter, M.D., and Tyler M. Lewark, M.D.

1. Briefly describe the anatomy that defines the upper airway.

The nasal and oral cavities as well as the pharynx and larynx make up the upper airway. It is divided into the **nasopharynx** (pharynx above the soft palate and posterior to the nasal turbinates), **oropharynx** (pharynx from the hard palate downward to the tip of the epiglottis), and **hypopharynx** (pharynx [behind the larynx] from the tip of epiglottis to the bottom of the pyriform sinuses—approximately the level of the cricoarytenoid joint). The oropharynx has two divisions; retropalatal (hard palate to superior portion of soft palate) and retroglossal (superior soft palate to base of epiglottis). The larynx is further subdivided into supraglottic (above the vocal folds), glottic (area comprising vocal folds), and subglottic (below vocal folds) regions.

2. What is the differential diagnosis of upper airway obstruction?

The causes of upper airway obstruction can be best classified by anatomic site (see Table). Obstruction may occur anywhere from the nose to the carina.

Origins of Upper Airway Obstruction by Anatomic Site

Nasal airway obstruction	**Pharyngeal obstruction**
Upper respiratory infections (bacterial, viral)	Infectious (tonsillitis, pharyngitis, parapharyngeal
Allergy	space abscess, peritonsillar abscess)
Rhinitis medicamentosum	Ludwig's angina
Sinusitis	Foreign bodies
Granulomatous diseases	Pharyngeal tumors (benign, malignant)
Deviated nasal septum	Allergic reactions, angioedema
Nasal trauma (sepal hematoma)	**Laryngeal and tracheal airway obstruction**
Foreign bodies	Infectious (epiglottitis, laryngitis, croup, tracheitis,
Nasal tumors (malignant, benign)	bronchitis)
Choanal atresia	Trauma
Nasopharyngeal obstruction	Foreign bodies
Adenoid hypertrophy/adenoiditis	Laryngeal tumors (benign, malignant)
Infectious (tuberculosis, mononucleosis,	Subglottic stenosis
syphilis)	Congenital lesions (laryngotracheal malacia)
Nasopharyngeal tumors (benign, malignant)	Gastroesophageal reflux
Cysts (Thornwaldt's, encephalocele)	Tracheal compression
	Vocal cord paralysis

From Josephson GD, Josephson JS, Krespi YP, et al: Airway obstruction: New modalities in treatment. Med Clin North Am 77:540, 1993, with permission.

3. Describe the symptoms of upper airway obstruction.

Common symptoms of acute upper airway obstruction include dyspnea, dysphagia, local pain, coughing, choking, and voice change. Progressive dyspnea suggests an increasing degree of obstruction. Few symptoms may exist except progressive dyspnea with nearly complete airway obstruction.

4. List the signs of upper airway obstruction.

Stridor, or noisy respiration due to obstruction of airflow, is the hallmark finding. Stridor due to obstruction above the glottis is usually inspiratory, whereas distal obstruction is often expiratory, and midtracheal (glottic) involvement may be biphasic.

Suprasternal retractions may be evident. Retractions at the sternal notch and midline neck as well as accessory muscle activity of the sternocleidomastoid suggest obstruction of the upper airway.

Voice changes may be present. **Hoarseness** suggests laryngeal involvement, and a **muffled**

401

voice may be due to supraglottic obstruction. Lack of a cough or a weak cry implies vocal cord paralysis.

Fever suggests an infectious cause.

Restlessness and agitation are often signs of airway obstruction with resultant hypoxia.

Drooling may occur with epiglottitis or decreased function of the pharyngeal muscles when traumatized or infiltrated with blood.

Bleeding is a sign of mucosal disruption.

Subcutaneous emphysema, or air in the soft tissues, is diagnostic of a rupture in the continuity of the aerodigestive tract.

Palpable fracture involving any portion of the laryngeal or tracheal cartilage or facial skeleton may be present with trauma.

Swelling is often associated with the site of obstruction.

5. What is Ludwig's angina? How is it treated?

Ludwig's angina is cellulitis of the submandibular space and floor of the mouth or sublingual space. It presents as bilateral submandibular swelling with posterior and superior displacement of the tongue. It can rapidly result in complete upper airway obstruction, with symptoms of airway compromise occurring in 25% of patients. Additional symptoms include neck swelling with restricted neck movement, neck pain, and, sometimes, trismus. Poor dental hygiene (anaerobes) is the most common predisposing condition. Treatment includes management of the airway, antibiotics, and surgical exploration with drainage when indicated.

6. What is angioedema? What causes it? How is it treated?

Angioedema can result in life-threatening upper airway obstruction. It is characterized by transient episode of painless, well-demarcated, nonpitting, asymmetric edema of the face, lips, tongue, mucous membranes, and eyelids. About 20% of patients with angioedema suffer severe upper airway obstruction. Angioedema may be idiopathic or caused by allergic IgE-mediated reactions, hereditary angioneurotic edema, acquired deficiency of C1 esterase inhibitor, and prescription drugs (e.g. angiotensin-converting enzyme [ACE] inhibitors). Treatment includes airway management (e.g., racemic epinephrine, systemic steroids) and subsequent therapy directed toward the underlying cause (e.g., avoidance of allergens, discontinuing ACE inhibitors, etc.).

7. What is the definitive diagnostic tool for evaluating upper airway obstruction?

Abnormalities of the entire upper airway can be best evaluated by endoscopy. **Nasopharyngoscopy** can assess the airway from the nasal alae to the subglottic larynx. **Bronchoscopy** allows evaluation of the hypopharynx, larynx, trachea, and bronchi. A flexible bronchoscope can best assess the mobility of the upper airway, whereas the rigid bronchoscope permits active intervention in cases such as foreign body removal.

8. Which studies are commonly ordered to evaluate upper airway obstruction?

Complete blood cell count, chemistry panel, arterial blood gases, anteroposterior and lateral neck radiographs, chest radiograph, and spirometry are commonly ordered during upper airway obstruction. Sleep studies (polysomnographic recording) are employed in patients with suspected sleep apnea.

9. What is the role of blood gases in evaluating a patient with suspected upper airway obstruction?

Blood gases may illustrate the degree of hypoxia or identify an acid-base disorder. However, the decision to intubate should be determined clinically, as a patient with near-obstruction can have normal-appearing blood gases.

10. Are plain film radiographs helpful when evaluating upper airway obstruction?

Yes. they may identify tracheal deviation, airway compression, foreign bodies, or vascular abnormalities. The condition of the cervical spine can also be determined before you make decisions regarding head positioning for intubation or tracheotomy. Inspiratory films may help identify croup ("steeple sign") and epiglottitis ("thumb-print sign" of a thickened epiglottitis). Lateral soft tissue films of the neck may help to identify supraglottic lesions and edema. Anteroposterior neck films will better illustrate subglottic pathology. Facial images are useful in patients with airway obstruction associated with facial trauma.

11. Which causes of upper airway obstruction may be identified with computed tomography (CT)?

CT scan can help evaluate the airway and mediastinum for suspected tumors, deep abscesses, or other compressive lesions. Contrast enhancement can assist in defining obstructive vascular anomalies (vascular slings). However, CT is unable to image the trachea along its long axis, and magnetic resonance imaging (MRI) shows better resolution of vascular abnormalities.

12. When does spirometry play a role in the evaluation of upper airway obstruction?

Spirometry is often one of the first tests ordered when evaluating chronic upper airway obstruction electively. However, because of its relatively insensitivity, it does not play a significant role in managing patients with acute respiratory distress. Luminal obstruction of $> 80\%$ is often necessary before an abnormality is detected on a flow-volume loop. Nonetheless, spirometry may suggest the cause or functional severity of an obstruction. A **sawtooth** appearance in a flow volume loop is a nonspecific sign of upper airway obstruction in neuromuscular diseases, Parkinson's disease, laryngeal dyskinesia, and upper airway burns. A **double-hump pattern** in the expiratory portion of the loop may also indicate an obstructing lesion with a juggling intrathoracic and extrathoracic location that varies with expiration or neck flexion and extension.

13. What options are available for treating acute upper airway obstruction?

Clinically stable (nonadvancing), mild to moderate airway obstruction can be treated with **observation** alone. However, **medical therapy** and observation are often required during progressive or severe symptoms. Thus, observation must occur in an intensive care unit (ICU) personnel present who can capably assess the airway and intervene. **Artificial airways** (see Question 16) are often quite useful. However, **endotracheal intubation** may be necessary when these measures fail. If intubation is unsuccessful, an emergent **surgical airway** is necessary to insure adequate ventilation.

14. What medical treatments are used in upper airway obstruction?

First and foremost, **oxygen** with or without humidification is administered via face mask or artificial airway. **Humidification** may help to liquefy secretions and improve clearance of partially obstructing secretions.

Racemic epinephrine can decrease mucosal edema (via vasoconstriction) and has been shown to decrease morbidity, mortality, and length of hospital stay in croup patients. Nonetheless, racemic epinephrine is usually not effective and may be deleterious in treating epiglottitis. Some clinicians also use this drug as empiric treatment in laryngeal edema.

Corticosteroids are often used to reduce airway swelling during croup and postextubation laryngeal edema. However, controversy exists surrounding the benefit of routine steroid use in preventing postextubation laryngeal edema.

Antibiotics should be administered with evidence of infection or transmucosal injury.

15. Describe helium-oxygen treatments in upper airway obstruction.

Helium-oxygen treatments involve administering an 80% helium/20% oxygen mixture to the patient with upper airway obstruction. The lowered density of this mixture reduces airway resistance to turbulent flow and thus decreases flow-resistive work. In addition, the decreased pressure gradient required to produce a specific flow may decrease the tendency of the airway to collapse distal to the obstruction. These treatments have been used in several upper airway conditions, including postextubation stridor, tracheal stenosis or compression, status asthmaticus, and angioedema. Helium-oxygen treatments serve as a temporizing measure before definitive intervention can be employed and can be extremely helpful in "buying some time" in the emergency setting.

16. List the available types of artificial airways and their indications.

The **oral airway** is a curved, semirigid plastic device that is inserted into the oropharynx and prevents ventilatory obstruction from a relaxed tongue. It can be used to bypass an obstruction in the nose or mouth but is not well tolerated and is easily dislodged by awake patients.

The **nasopharyngeal airway** is a soft hollow trumpet-shaped device that fits easily into the nares and is used for maintaining an airway in the patient recovering from general anesthesia or obtunded after a mild to moderate head injury. It is more readily tolerated by patients than the oral airway. It can bypass oral, nasopharyngeal and oropharyngeal obstruction.

The **esophageal airway** is a tube inserted blindly into the esophagus where a balloon is distended and guides insufflated air into the hypopharynx. Inappropriate placement can lead to complete airway obstruction, injury to the esophagus, or worsening of evolving supraglottic edema.

17. What are the indications for endotracheal intubation?

Endotracheal intubation is indicated to improve respiratory toilet, assist ventilation, bypass obstruction, and prevent aspiration in cases of emergent or potentially prolonged airway compromise. Although it may be used for extended periods in neonates and burn patients, it should be considered a short-term solution. To prevent damage to the larynx and trachea, tracheotomy should be performed if ventilatory support is needed longer than 2 weeks.

18. What are the contraindications to endotracheal intubation?

The presence of a **cervical spine fracture** is a relative contraindication to transoral intubation because neck hyperextension during intubation may complete an unstable neurologic injury. **Laryngeal trauma** is also a relative contraindication, as passage of the tube through an injured larynx may aggravate the injury. Also, **severe facial or oral trauma** may obscure an adequate view of the vocal anatomy for appropriate placement.

19. What are the advantages and disadvantages of orotracheal intubation?

Advantages: This procedure allows full control of ventilation and prevents aspiration.

Disadvantages: It requires expertise and proper expensive equipment. It may cause injury to the larynx and/or pharynx.

20. How is orotracheal intubation performed?

This procedure requires endotracheal tubes of varying sizes, a stylet to give rigidity to the tip of the tube, adequate suction, and a laryngoscope. Ideally, the patient is placed in the **"sniffing position,"** with the neck flexed slightly on the chest and the head extended slightly on the neck. A right-handed clinician uses the left hand to direct the laryngoscope into the right aspect of the mouth while pushing the tongue to the left. The curved-blade laryngoscope (MacIntosh) is directed into the vallecula, and the larynx is lifted anteriorly or ventrally to expose the glottis. The clinician introduces the straight-blade laryngoscope (Miller) under the epiglottis, fixing the larynx at the petiole of the epiglottis and lifting the larynx anteriorly to expose the glottis. The endotracheal tube is inserted with the right hand and the stylet removed. An assistant can provide slight cricoid pressure to help visualize the vocal cords and prevent the patient from aspirating gastric contents.

21. What are the advantages and disadvantages of nasotracheal intubation?

Advantages: Nasotracheal intubation maintains the airway, facilitates suctioning, is simple to perform, and is well tolerated by alert patients.

Disadvantages: It can cause epistaxis, and it requires normal ventilatory support.

22. What are the indications for nasotracheal intubation?

Nasotracheal intubation is used when:

It is important to leave the oral cavity clear of obstruction for operative procedures.

Cervical spine injury is suspected.

Prolonged intubation is expected.

Orotracheal intubation is impossible.

23. How is nasotracheal intubation performed?

The nasal cavity is topically anesthetized and decongested. Dilatation of the nasal cavity is performed with progressively larger nasal airways, which are coated with viscous lidocaine. The tube is then introduced transnasally into the pharynx, and a laryngoscope is inserted through the mouth. Magill forceps are then used to grasp the tube and insert it through the glottis.

If a difficult intubation is expected, intubation over a fiberoptic bronchoscope may be attempted. In these cases, the nose is prepared as described, and topical anesthesia may be applied to the larynx and pharynx. The bronchoscope, with the endotracheal tube slid up to the observer port, is introduced through the tube and into the nose, larynx, and cervical trachea. The endotracheal tube is advanced over the bronchoscope and into the trachea with subsequent withdrawal of the bronchoscope.

Blind nasotracheal intubation may be attempted in patients with suspected cervical spine injury or those who are awake if there is not enough time to anesthetize the patient. This approach is difficult, however, and should be left to an experienced anesthesiologist.

24. What are the acute complications of endotracheal intubation?

Acute pulmonary edema is seen when obstruction is relieved by endotracheal intubation in a patient who has labored under partial upper airway obstruction for an extended period of time. This is thought to be due to the sudden loss of highly negative intrathoracic pressures during inspiration and positive pressures during expiration. The subsequent rapid increase in systemic venous return and pulmonary hydrostatic pressure creates an imbalance in pressure gradients across the alveolar membrane. Frothy fluid from the endotracheal tube or hypoxia with inadequate ventilation may be seen in the recovery room. Diuretics with institution of mechanical ventilation and positive end-expiratory pressure are the treatment for this complication. This is considered further in Chapter 68.

Improper tube placement is another potential complication of endotracheal intubation. An endotracheal tube may be inadvertently placed into the esophagus, through the pyriform sinus, or too far inferiorly into the right mainstem bronchus.

25. List the complications of long-term endotracheal intubation.

Laryngeal stenosis may result from long-term endotracheal intubation, and most clinicians opt for timely tracheotomy to avoid this complication. Tube motion, infection, and high cuff pressures predispose to this injury. To minimize the chance of laryngeal stenosis, the smallest tube that maintains adequate ventilation should be used, while the cuff is inflated to the minimal occlusion volume.

Tracheoesophageal fistula may also develop during chronic intubation. The concomitant presence of endotracheal and nasogastric tubes increase the incidence of this complication.

Recurrent laryngeal nerve injury may occur from long-term intubation. The occurs as the nerve is pinched by the tube at its location near the articulation of the cricoid and thyroid cartilages.

Sinusitis is also common in patients who are *nasotracheally* intubated for more than several days. Obstruction at the normal drainage site of the paranasal sinuses by this tube predisposes to the development of purulent sinusitis.

26. Your patient has upper airway obstruction and life-threatening hypoxia. You are unable to secure an endotracheal tube. What do you do?

This patient requires a **surgical airway** to ensure adequate ventilation and relieve the hypoxia. **Transtracheal needle ventilation** is useful in the emergency setting and provides rapid ventilatory control while a patient is being stabilized prior to more definitive measures (see figure). A large-bore needle is directed through the cricothyroid membrane and attached to an oxygen line under pressure. The patient may be ventilated for at least 30 minutes.

Cricothyroidotomy is the procedure of choice with total upper airway obstruction. A horizontal or vertical incision is made through the cricothyroid membrane, and a tracheotomy tube is inserted into the trachea. The cricothyroidotomy should be converted to a formal **tracheotomy** at a later time if prolonged intubation is anticipated. Urgent tracheotomies should be performed by the most experienced surgeon available.

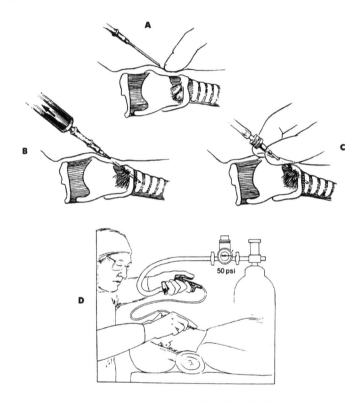

Transtracheal needle ventilation. *A,* Area of penetration identified. *B,* Sheathed needle inserted through cricothyroid membrane; trachea identified when air is aspirated. *C,* Needle removed; plastic cannula attached to jetting device; stabilized by hand. *D,* Transtracheal ventilation monitored by observing chest wall excursion. (From Weymuller EA: Airway management. In Cummings CW, et al (eds): Otolaryngology—Head and Neck Surgery, 3rd ed. St. Louis, Mosby, 1998, with permission.)

CONTROVERSIES

27. What options are available to obtain an immediate airway in a patient with laryngeal obstruction by a malignant tumor?

Five percent of patients with new laryngeal cancers will present with laryngeal obstruction and severe dyspnea and require an immediate airway. Three options are available to control the airway: **tracheostomy, emergency laryngectomy,** and **endotracheal intubation with tumor debulking.** Emergent tracheostomy has been associated with tumor seeding and increased stromal recurrences. Thus some authors propose emergency laryngectomy to minimize tumor seeding. However, inadequate metastatic and tumor work-up, poor patient nutritional and psychological preparation, and poor patient expectations have been criticisms of this approach. Recently, tumor debulking by CO_2 laser therapy has proven to be the simplest, safest, and most effective procedure in securing an airway in laryngeal cancer patients with severe dyspnea.

28. When is the placement of an airway stent necessary?

Current indications for laryngeal, tracheal, and bronchial stent placement include long term airway management of extrinsic malignant obstruction or benign stricture where current treatments have failed; tracheobronchial malacia; and malignancy-associated tracheobronchial and bronchoesophageal fisutulae. It may also be performed following laryngeal or tracheal stenosis reconstruction and acute traumatic injury.

Stenting is performed to provide palliative airway dilatation, support airway healing, and oppose scar contracture. Although many practitioners advocate the use of stents in these circumstances, secondary trauma to the airway from stenting has made this procedure still controversial. Various metallic and plastic stents are available, but the appropriate stent type and duration of stent use in each case also remains unclear.

BIBLIOGRAPHY

1. Bradley PJ: Treatment of the patient with upper airway obstruction caused by cancer of the larynx. Otolaryngol Head Neck Surg 120:737–741, 1999.
2. Chen K, Varon J, Wenker OC: Malignant airway obstruction: Recognition and management. J Emerg Med 16:83–92, 1998.
3. Dark A, Armstrong T: Severe postoperative laryngeal oedema causing total airwayobstruction immediately on extubation. Br J Anaesth 82:644–646, 1999.
4. Drake AF: Controversies in upper airway obstruction. In Bailey BJ (eds): Head and Neck Surgery—Otolaryngology. Philadelphia, J.B. Lippincott, 1998, pp 885–895.
5. Drazen JM: Leukotrienes as mediators of airway obstruction. Am J Respir Crit Care Med 158(5 Pt 3):S193–200, 1998.
6. Fu A, Kopec A, Markham M: Heliox in upper airway obstruction. CACCN 10:12–13; quiz 14–15, 1999.
7. Jones LM, Mair, EA, Fitzpatrick TM, et al: Multidisciplinary airway stent team: A comprehensive approach and protocol for tracheobronchial stent treatment. Ann Otol Rhinol Laryngol 109:889–898, 2000.
8. Lee RB: Surgical palliation of airway obstruction resulting from lung cancer. Semin Surg Oncol 18:173–182, 2000.
9. Lerner DL, Perez Fontan JJ: Prevention and treatment of upper airway obstruction in infants and children. Curr Opin Pediatr 10:265–270, 1998.
10. Levy RJ., Helfaer MA: Managing the airway in the critically ill patient. Crit Care Clin 16:1–14, 2000.
11. Rencken I, Patton WL, Brasch RC: Airway obstruction in pediatric patients. From croup to BOOP. Radiol Clin North Am 36:175–187, 1998.
12. Schwab RJ, Goldberg AN: Upper airway assesment. Otolaryngol Clin North Am 31:939–960, 1998.
13. Sonett JR: Endobronchial stents: Primary and adjuvant therapy for endobronchial airway obstruction. Md Med J 47:260–263, 1998.
14. Stohr S, Bolliger CT: Stents in the management of malignant airway obstruction. Monaldi Arch Chest Dis 54:264–268, 1999.
15. Weissler MC: Tracheotomy and intubation. In Bailey BJ (ed): Head and Neck Surgery—Otolaryngology. Philadelphia, J.B. Lippincott, 1993, pp 711–724.
16. Weymuller EA: Airway management. In Cummings CW, et al (eds): Otolaryngology—Head and Neck Surgery. St. Louis, Mosby, 1986, pp 2417–2432.
17. Woodson GE: Upper airway anatomy and function. In Baily B, Calhoun K (eds.): Head and Neck Surgery—Otolaryngology, 2nd ed. Philadelphia, Lippincott-Raven Publishers, 1998, pp 579–586.

64. THE MANDIBULAR FRACTURE

Steven B. Aragon, M.D.,D.D.S and Kent E. Gardner, M.D.

1. How are mandibular fractures classified?

- Anatomic location of the fracture
- Condition and position of the teeth relative to the fracture
- The "favorability," or displacement, of the fracture
- Type of fracture (e.g. greenstick, simple, compound, comminuted)

Each of these factors plays a role in choosing an approach to treatment.

2. Describe the anatomic classification of mandibular fractures.

The anatomic components of the mandible include the body, angle, ramus, coronoid process, condyle, alveolar process, and symphysis/parasymphysis. **Symphyseal or parasymphyseal fractures** occur anteriorly between the two lower canine teeth. **Body fractures** occur between the distal aspect of the canines and a hypothetical line which corresponds to the anterior attachment of the masseter. This anterior border of the masseter is located at approximately the second or third molar. **Angle fractures** occur in a triangular region located between the anterior border of the masseter and the posterosuperior insertion of the masseter, which is distal to the third molar. **Ramus fractures** occur between the angle and the sigmoid notch. **Coronoid fractures** simply involve the coronoid process. **Condylar fractures** may involve the intracapsular portion of the condylar head, within the temporomandibular joint (TMJ), or the neck of the condyle, also known as the subcondylar region. **Alveolar process fractures** are isolated to the teeth-bearing portion of the mandible.

3. What are the most commonly fractured sites of the mandible?

Weak areas of the mandible include the angle, especially when impacted third molars are present; the anterior body or parasymphyseal area, where the mental foramen exists; and the neck of the condyle, the subcondylar area, due to the small bone mass in this area. In order of decreasing frequency, the most common sites for fracture are subcondylar (36%), body (21%), angle (20%), parasymphysis (14%), ramus (3%), alveolar process (3%), coronoid process (2%), and symphysis (1%).

4. How does the presence of teeth in the fracture segments affect treatment?

Teeth are important because they are the key to reduction, stabilization, and immobilization in fracture repair. In 1949, Kazanjian and Converse classified mandibular fractures according to the presence or absence of teeth in the fractured segments:

- **Class I fractures** have teeth present in the segments on both sides of the fracture and are therefore amenable to closed reduction with maxillo-mandibular fixation.
- **Class II fractures** have teeth in only one of the two fracture segments. While the teeth can be used for fixation of that particular segment, the edentulous segment may require a splint or internal fixation if unstable.
- **Class III fractures** occur in edentulous patients and are always treated with either open reduction with internal fixation or closed reduction with splints (e.g., dentures).

5. What muscles insert into the mandible? What is the action of each muscle?

Muscles that insert into the mandible can be divided into anterior and posterior groups. The **anterior group** consists of the mylohyoid, geniohyoid, genioglossus, platysma, and the anterior belly of the digastric. The anterior muscles depress and retract the mandible.

The **posterior muscles** are the major muscles of mastication, including the temporalis, masseter, and the medial and lateral pterygoids. The lateral pterygoid muscle inserts into the TMJ capsule and condylar neck. This muscle protrudes and depresses the mandible and causes the mandible to move toward the opposite side. The medial pterygoid inserts into the medial ramus. It raises and protrudes the mandible and also causes the mandible to move toward the opposite side. The masseter inserts into the lateral ramus and coronoid process, and raises and retracts the mandible. The temporalis inserts into the coronoid process and anterior border of the ramus. It also raises and retracts the mandible.

Each of the anterior and posterior muscles can cause the distraction of fracture segments in unfavorable fractures (see Question 6).

6. Contrast favorable and unfavorable mandibular fractures.

Mandible fractures are described as favorable when muscles tend to draw the bony fragments together. They are unfavorable when the fragments are distracted or displaced by muscle forces. Fractures may be vertically or horizontally unfavorable. *Vertically unfavorable* fractures allow fracture segments to be distracted in a horizontal direction. *Horizontally unfavorable* fractures allow fracture segments to be distracted in a vertical direction. Favorable fractures can be treated with closed reduction, while unfavorable fractures tend to need open reduction with internal fixation.

Almost all fractures of the angle are unfavorable because of the action of the masseter, temporalis, and medial pterygoid, which distract the proximal segment superomedially. Subcondylar fractures tend to be unfavorable due to the action of the lateral pterygoid, which distracts the condyle anteromedially. Most vertically unfavorable fractures tend to occur in the body and symphysis-parasymphysis region. The anterior segments of vertically unfavorable body and symphysis fractures are displaced posteromedially by the mylohyoid and other suprahyoid muscles.

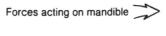

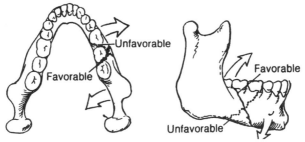

Forces acting on the mandible. *Left,* vertical plane; *right,* horizontal plane. (From Lowlich RA, Goodwin WJ: Facial and airway trauma. In Lee KJ (ed): Essential Otolaryngology, 6th ed. Norwalk, CT, Appleton & Lange, 1995, with permission.)

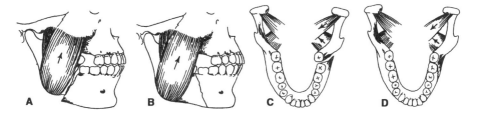

Mandibular fracture angulations and their relationship to muscle pulls. *A,* Horizontally unfavorable; *B,* horizontally favorable; *C,* vertically unfavorable; *D,* vertically favorable, (From Stanley RB: Pathogenesis and evaluation of mandibular fractures. In Mathog RH (ed): Maxillofacial Trauma. Baltimore, Williams & Wilkins, 1984, with permission.)

7. Describe the course of the inferior alveolar nerve.

The mandibular nerve is the third division (V3) of the trigeminal nerve, which exits the base of the skull through the foramen ovale. It then branches into the lingual and inferior alveolar nerves. The inferior alveolar nerve enters the mandible through the mandibular foramen near the lingula on the medial aspect of the ramus. It courses through the mandible and exits anteriorly through the mental foramen. The mental foramen is located just below the first or second bicuspids. After exiting the foramen, the nerve is referred to as the **mental nerve.** The mental nerve supplies sensation to the lower lip and chin.

8. What is the angle classification of occlusion?

The angle classification describes the dental relationship between the maxillary and mandibular first molars. In the **Class I** relationship, the mesiobuccal cusp of the maxillary first molar lies in the buccal groove of the mandibular first molar. This is accepted as the desired or normal occlusion. **Class II** occlusion is present when the maxillary cusp is anterior to the mandibular buccal groove and the maxilla protrudes anteriorly more than the mandible, *an overbite*. This malocclusion may be due to a protrusive maxilla, a retrognathic mandible, or a combination of both. In **Class III** occlusion, the mesiobuccal cusp of the maxillary first molar is posterior to the buccal groove of the mandibular first molar, and the maxilla is positioned more posteriorly than the mandible, *an underbite*. This occlusion may be due to a retrognathic maxilla, a prognathic mandible, or a combination of both.

9. What are the most common signs and symptoms of mandibular fractures?

Pain

Malocclusion

Paresthesia in the distribution of the mental nerve

Mucosal lacerations

Trismus

Fracture step-off or crepitance

Floor of the mouth hematoma (symphyseal fractures)

Impaired translational mobility or protrusion of mandible (condylar fractures)

Unilateral or bilateral open bite (unilateral or bilateral posterior mandibular fractures)

Bloody otorrhea due to external auditory canal laceration*

10. Do patients with mandibular fractures need antibiotics?

Any fracture that communicates with the oral cavity via a laceration, or that is in contact with an erupted tooth, is considered to be a compound fracture. Such fractures are contaminated and require antibiotic therapy. Penicillin or other antibiotics that cover the oral flora are the usual choice. Antibiotic therapy should be continued until the gingiva, periodontia, and mucosa have completely healed.

11. What x-rays should be taken if a mandibular fracture is suspected?

Traditionally, the mandibular series has included several views of the mandible to view the entire mandible adequately. These have included anteroposterior and bilateral oblique views to assess the symphysis, parasymphysis, body, angle, and ramus. Special views (Towne projection) are often required to assess the medial or lateral displacement of the condyle. Currently, the panoramic view (Panorex) has become the single most useful radiograph for assessment of the entire mandible. However, while a good panoramic radiograph will show the anterior displacement of the condyle, it may not reveal medial displacement, which is seen more easily on the Towne view.

12. What techniques are used in the closed reduction and fixation of mandibular fractures?

Many techniques of closed reduction have been employed. Closed reduction techniques assume that a fracture is reduced when a patient is placed into normal occlusion. Fixing the teeth

---

*Remember that the TMJ is just anterior to the external auditory canal.

into their normal occlusion is known as **maxillomandibular fixation** (MMF), formerly known as intermaxillary fixation.

One common technique to achieve MMF involves Erich arch bars, which are stainless steel bars with small blunt hooks. The bars are applied to both the mandible and maxilla by a series of stainless steel wires that are wrapped around each of the patient's teeth. The upper and lower arch bars are then solidly fixed to each other by elastics or stainless steel wires.

Other techniques used to achieve MMF include the use of wires without arch bars (e.g., Ivy loops, Risdon wires), dental splints, and dentures. Dentures are fixed to the mandible and maxilla with wires or screws and then are fixed to each other.

13. What techniques are available for open reduction and internal fixation (ORIF) of mandibular fractures?

When performing ORIF, the surgeon uses metal plates with screws, interosseous wires, and lag screws. When using **metal plates with screws,** the surgeon first places the patient in MMF to reduce the fracture and obtain proper occlusion. Next, an intraoral or external approach is used to expose the fracture, and metal plates are used to stabilize the fracture line.

The mandible has complex stresses (compression and tension) due to its unique articulation to the skull at the TMJs and the effects of the muscles of mastication. In general, both compression and tension forces must be addressed to stabilize the fracture adequately. For example, in mandibular body fractures, **compression** stresses occur along the inferior border of the mandible. They are managed by placing one plate across the inferior aspect of the fracture; it must conform perfectly to the contour of the mandible and (ideally) lie at a right angle to the direction of the fracture. A variety of plates are available, including compression and noncompression plates. **Tension,** in body fractures, occurs along the superior border of the mandible and tends to cause distraction or separation of the fracture segments superiorly. Thus, a body fracture repaired with a plate inferiorly will also need superior fixation to stabilize the fracture. This tension stabilization can be addressed with bone plates, wires, or an arch bar.

When using **intraosseous wiring,** the surgeon threads stainless steel wire through holes that are drilled in the bone segments on either side of the mandibular fracture. This wire is then twisted onto itself until the fracture segments are held in close approximation. Interosseous wires do *not* provide rigid internal fixation and total stability of the fractured segment. Therefore, patients require additional stabilization and immobilization, which can be provided with MMF or splints, for 4–6 weeks.

14. How are lag screws employed?

Lag screws are long, bicortical screws that are placed through the superficial cortex of one fracture segment, across the fracture line in an oblique direction, and into the deep cortex of the opposite fracture segment. The proximal segment and cortex are overdrilled so that the diameter of the hole is larger than the threaded part of the screw. The threads of the lag screw then engage the distal fragment only. As the screw is tightened, the distal segment is drawn into tight approximation with the proximal segment. Often, more than one lag screw is used to avoid rotation of the fracture line. Patients do not require additional periods of MMF (as with interosseous wiring) because lag screws provide rigid internal fixation and total stabilization, preventing interfragment mobility. Lag screws are best used in oblique fractures, which may occur in the symphysis, parasymphysis, and anterior body of the mandible.

15. When are lag screws used?

Parasymphaseal fractures are ideally suited for lag screw fixation. They may also be used for the body and angle regions. Often, more than one lag screw is necessary.

16. What are the contraindications to the lag screw technique?

Comminution of the fracture, bone loss in the fracture gap, and oblique fractures are contraindicated in the lag screw technique. The lag screw technique in these situations may result in shortening of the bony segment and severe malocclusion in the dentate arch.

17. What techniques are used to treat mandibular symphaseal, body, and angle fractures?

Closed reduction can be accomplished with maxillomandibular fixation (MMF) and lingual splints. Nonrigid open reduction may be achieved with wire osteosynthesis, and rigid open reduction and stabilization with reconstruction plates, compression and noncompression plates, and lag screws.

18. How do you treat a patient with a ramus fracture?

Fractures of the ramus are uncommon. They are usually nondisplaced due to the protective and splinting effect of the pterygoid and masseter muscles. Generally, these fractures can be managed with closed reduction. However, open reduction may be employed if multiple fragments or marked displacement is present.

19. How do you treat a coronoid process fracture?

Patients with isolated fractures of the coronoid process require only pain medication, a soft diet, and stretching exercises. Such exercises are used to prevent trismus from scar tissue formation. Occasionally, patients with severe trismus that does not respond to physical therapy require resection of the coronoid. Rarely, the fractured coronoid segment can cause a physical obstruction to mandibular movement and thus require removal.

20. How is a condylar fracture treated?

A patient with a nondisplaced or minimally displaced, unilateral condylar fracture with normal occlusion may be managed with a soft diet and close observation. A patient with a nondisplaced, bilateral condylar fracture or a unilateral fracture with significant displacement can be managed with intermaxillary fixation (IMF) for 2–3 weeks, followed by physiotherapy for jaw mobility. Early jaw mobility is essential to avoid ankylosis of the TMJ. When the patient is taken out of IMF, the arch bars are left in place for approximately 3 more weeks. During this time, the patient can be placed in fixation at night with elastics, if necessary.

21. Why is the treatment of mandibular fractures in children more complicated?

A child's mandible has tooth buds and growth regions that can be damaged during the treatment of a mandible fracture. For this reason, mandibular fractures in children are treated conservatively. The last deciduous tooth appears at 20–30 months of age. This deciduous dentition continues until about 6 years of age. Children under 6 years of age are treated with closed reduction techniques. ORIF in this age group puts developing tooth buds at risk. From age 6 until 12, a child has a mixed dentition of deciduous and permanent teeth. After age 12, only permanent teeth are generally present. In children with mixed and permanent dentition, ORIF with miniplates can be considered, due to the increase in distance from the inferior border of the mandible to the tooth buds. Mandible growth occurs because of elongation in the condylar region and remodeling and growth in the region of the ramus and body. Injuries in the condylar region are particularly concerning because they can affect mandible growth and lead to facial asymmetry.

22. How are condylar fractures managed in children under age 12?

Children with condylar fractures who are under age 12 and exhibit no malocclusion are treated with analgesics and a liquid or soft diet. They are closely observed for the development of malocclusion. Children with malocclusion require a short period of immobilization followed by soft diet, physiotherapy, and close observation. The condyles of children undergo rapid healing and remodeling; with closed management, very few long-term sequelae are reported. ORIF of condylar fractures in children is rarely indicated and should only be considered when closed reduction is not possible. If indicated, children over age 12 can be considered for ORIF.

CONTROVERSIES

23. How should the edentulous patient with a mandibular fracture be managed?

There is no uniform approach to treatment of the edentulous mandibular fracture. Problems include decreased osteogenesis; atrophic, dense cortical bone; and compromised blood supply. Treatment options include closed reduction with Gunning splints, dentures, and external pin fixation. Open reduction techniques include extraoral or intraoral bone plates and lag screws.

24. Contrast the advantages and disadvantages of open and closed reduction of mandibular fractures.

Much controversy exists over open versus closed reduction techniques for mandible fractures. Traditionally, MMF has been the workhorse of mandibular fracture repair. However, plating techniques and materials have improved, and the indications for open reduction are evolving. The advantages of **closed reduction** include proven efficacy, low complication rate, and short operating time. The disadvantages include fixation in MMF for 2–8 weeks, difficulty in maintaining adequate nutrition, risk to airway, and the possibility of TMJ ankylosis. Advantages of **ORIF** include more exact bone-fragment reapproximation and early mobilization. Disadvantages include cost, time in the operating room, and a higher reported complication rate.

25. Which condylar fractures should be managed with ORIF?

The controversial indications for open surgical treatment of condylar fractures have been argued in the literature for over 50 years. The desired results after treatment of a condylar fracture include lack of pain, good interincisal opening, functional jaw movement in all directions, stable TMJs, and facial symmetry. Most of the time, good results are obtainable with closed treatment of condylar fractures. The difficulty lies in determining which patients will have a poor outcome without an open reduction. Zide and Kent have proposed that open reduction is absolutely indicated if:

* The condyle is displaced into the middle cranial fossa.
* Lateral extracapsular displacement of the condyle is present.
* Good occlusion cannot be obtained with closed techniques.
* A foreign body in the TMJ is present.

Other indications might include:

* Bilateral condylar fractures with an associated comminuted, unstable midfacial fractures
* Bilateral condylar fractures in an edentulous patient when a splint is unavailable or the alveolar ridge is atrophic
* Unilateral or bilateral fractures when closed reduction is not indicated for medical reasons.

26. What should be done with a tooth that is located in the fracture line?

In the preantibiotic era, most teeth located in a fracture line became infected. However, with proper antibiotic therapy, many of these teeth can be retained, and some retained teeth may even be useful in reduction and stabilization of the fractured segments. Teeth should be removed if they have significant periodontal disease, are grossly carious with periapical pathology, or interfere with proper reduction and stability of the fractured segments.

FRACTURES OF THE ANGLE OF THE MANDIBLE

Fractures of the mandibular angle have the highest rate of complication of mandibular fractures. Possible treatment includes closed reduction or intraoral open reduction and non-rigid fixation; extraoral open reduction and internal fixation with a reconstruction bone plate; intraoral open reduction and internal fixation using a solitary lag screw; intraoral open reduction and internal fixation using mini-dynamic compression plates; intraoral open reduction and internal fixation using two 2.4 mm mandibular dynamic compression plates; intraoral open reduction and internal fixation using two non-compression miniplates; intraoral open reduction and internal fixation using a single non-compression miniplate; and intraoral open reduction and internal fixation using a single malleable non-compression miniplate. Both the extraoral open reduction and internal fixation with the AO/ASIF reconstruction plate, and the intraoral open reduction and internal fixation using a single miniplate, appear to be associated with the fewest complications.

~Ellis III, Int J Oral Maxillofac Surgery 28:243, 1999

BIBLIOGRAPHY

1. Clark WD: Management of mandibular fractures. Am J Otolaryngol 13:125–132, 1992.
2. Leach JL, Dierks EJ: Mandibular fractures. In Bailey BJ (ed): Head and Neck Surgery–Otolaryngology, 2nd ed. Philadelphia, Lippincott, 1998.
3. Ellis E III: Treatment methods for fracture of the mandible. J Cranio-Max Trauma 2:28–36, 1996.
4. Ellis E III: Treatment methods for fractures of the mandibular angle. Int J Oral Maxillofac Surg 28:243–52, 1999.
5. Hall MB: Condylar fractures: Surgical management. J Oral Maxillofac Surg 52:1189–1192, 1994.
6. Hayward JR, Scott RF: Fractures of the mandibular condyle. J Oral Maxillofac Surg 51: 57–61, 1993.
6a. Kazanjian VH, Converse JM: The Surgical Treatment of Facial Injuries, 3rd ed. Baltimore, Williams & Wilkins, 1974.
7. Lowlicht RA, Goodwin WJ: Facial and airway trauma. In Lee KJ (ed): Essential Otolaryngology, 6th ed. Norwalk, CT, Appleton & Lange, 1995.
8. Luhr HG, Reidick T, Merten HA. Results of treatment of fractures of the atrophic edentulous mandible by compression plating: A retrospective evaluation of 84 consecutive cases. J Oral Maxillofac Surg 54:250–254, 1996.
9. Manson PN, Clark N, Robertson B, et al: Subunit principles in midface fractures: The importance of sagittal buttresses, soft-tissue reductions, and sequencing treatment of segmental fractures. Plast Reconst Surg 103:1287–1306; quiz 1307, 1999.
10. Newman J: Medical imaging of facial and mandibular fractures. Radiol Tech 69:417–435; quiz 436–438, 1998.
11. Sykes JW, Smith BR, Mukherjee DP: An in vitro study of the effect of bony buttressing on fixation strength of a fractured atrophic edentulous mandible model. J Oral Maxillofac Surg 58:56–61, 2000.
12. Walker RV: Condylar fractures: Nonsurgical management. J Oral Maxillofac Surg 52: 1185–1188, 1994.
13. Yen SL: Distraction osteogenesis: Application to dentofacial orthopedics. Semin Orthodont 3:275–283, 1997.
14. Zide MF, Kent JN: Indications for open reduction of mandibular condyle fractures. J Oral Maxillofac Surg 41:89–98, 1983.

65. ZYGOMATIC, MAXILLARY, AND ORBITAL FRACTURES

Brennan T. Dodson, M.S. IV

1. What is the most common cause of facial fractures in the adult patient? In the pediatric patient?

Motor vehicle collision (especially unrestrained) is the most common cause in the adult. Pediatric facial trauma is rare, comprising less than 10% of all cases. **Falls** are typically blamed for most pediatric facial fractures. Always be careful to investigate for child abuse or neglect.

2. What is the most commonly fractured bone(s) in the face?

The **nasal bones.** A look at the required force of gravity (Table 1) to fracture various facial bones explains the decreasing incidence of fracture with increasing fracture force requirement.

Force Required for Facial Bone Fracture

BONE	FORCE OF GRAVITY (G)
Nasal bones	30
Zygomatic bone	50
Angle of mandible	70
Frontal-glabellar region	80
Midline maxilla	100
Midline mandible (symphysis)	100
Supraorbital rim	200

Modified from Rosen P, Barkin R, Danzl F, et al: Emergency Medicine: Concepts and Clinical Practice, 4th ed. St. Louis, Mosby-Year Book, Inc., 1998. p 457.

3. Which region should be included during CT scanning of facial fractures?

The cervical spine. In patients who incur facial fractures from motor vehicle collision, some 5–6% have concomitant c-spine injury. *A cervical spine fracture must be ruled out before the head is flexed or taken out of a cervical collar.* Posterior neck pain on palpation, lower extremity paresthesias, and respiratory failure may be signs of c-spine fracture and/or spinal cord compression.

4. Which imaging technique is best in maxillofacial trauma?

CT is the superior modality for evaluating facial trauma patients because it can: better determine fracture stability or instability; be used in planning reconstructive surgery; and determine the degree of displacement or rotation of the major bony fragments. The widespread availability of CT has dramatically reduced the price to less than half the cost of plain-film facial trauma x-ray series. CT can produce three-dimensional (3-D) reconstructions of the face, an invaluable tool for conceptualizing the extent of fracture and for use in surgical planning. In evaluating facial trauma, **helical CT,** if available, is superior to conventional CT because it is faster and produces less motion artifact in planar and in 3-D reconstructions.

Physical examination remains a sensitive and specific way of determining which patients need only a simple, plain-film x-ray (e.g., simple nasal bone fracture, simple mandibular fracture) and which need conventional CT or helical CT with 3-D reconstruction of the face (e.g., multiplane fractures of the mid-face, mixed Le Fort types, concomitant blowout fracture).

5. Describe the employment of computed tomography (CT) in maxillofacial trauma.

When performing CT in orbital trauma, use bone window and soft tissue settings to evaluate intraorbital contents. Use *coronal imaging* for orbital studies, but only when c-spine injury has been completely ruled out with axial imaging. Coronal imaging is useful for evaluating horizontal structures, such as the hard palate, orbital floor and roof, and cribriform plate. *Axial imaging* is useful for evaluating the zygomatic arch and pterygoid plates, as well as the cervical spine. In general, both coronal and axial images are obtained with any complex facial fracture.

6. How are plain-film x-rays used in maxillofacial trauma?

Plain films have traditionally been used to evaluate the facial trauma patient. However, the superimposition of multiple facial planes (and their associated fractures) in plain-film x-ray can make accurate assessment of facial trauma difficult. Additionally, at most medical centers, the cost of a plain-film series for facial trauma exceeds the cost of CT, even adding in the cost of 3-D reconstruction. Often, a series of plain-film x-rays is taken and then shown to be inadequate for evaluation of fracture stability, necessitating the added cost of a full imaging series with CT. Many authors advocate the need to proceed directly to CT, if available, in the case of potentially complex facial fractures.

Traditional plain-film x-ray views include the Waters, Caldwell posteroanterior, and lateral facial views. The submental vertex and "jug-handle" views are frequently added as part of the traditional series, but should be obtained only after c-spine injury has been ruled out.

7. What is the buttress system of the mid-face?

The vertical and horizontal mid-face buttresses are bony superstructures that add strength and structural integrity to the middle one-third of the facial skeleton.

The **vertical buttresses** maintain the vertical dimensions of the mid-face and, due to their role in bearing vertical mastication forces, are quite strong. These vertical buttresses are composed of the nasomaxillary, zygomaticomaxillary, and pterygomaxillary components.

The weaker **horizontal buttresses** maintain the horizontal dimensions (i.e., projection) of the mid-face and absorb horizontally directed forces. The horizontal buttresses function primarily as bridging supports between the stronger vertical buttresses; this horizontal system is weak, because, unlike the vertical system, it does not incur large daily force loads. The components of the horizontal buttresses are the frontal bar, inferior orbital rims, maxillary alveolus and palate, zygomatic process of the temporal bone, greater wing of the sphenoid, and medial and lateral pterygoid plates.

8. Why is the buttress system important?

The buttress system is important because the *disruption of a single buttress component may weaken the entire superstructure* and lead to failures in other buttress components; this may lead to a widespread collapse of the midface skeleton. The structural relationship and anatomical orientation between buttress components becomes important in identification, reconstruction, and repair of mid-face fractures. To maintain the overall integrity of the buttress system, the original anatomic dimensions and structure of the midface skeleton must be reconstructed accurately. Modern reconstruction techniques use titanium "plates" and screws to precisely re-approximate facial fractures and provide structural support until bony healing can occur.

9. What are Le Fort fractures?

The French surgeon Rene Le Fort (ca. 1901) used low-velocity impact forces directed against fresh cadavers to ascertain the **"great lines of weakness in the face."** He observed that facial fractures occurred in three typical patterns, were often bilateral, and could be "mixed" (the right or left face suffers a different Le Fort fracture than its contralateral side). All three types, however, involve a fracture of the pterygoid plates.

Le Fort I fracture: palate-face disjunction. These fracture lines pass transverse through the pyriform aperture above the alveolar ridge and above the floor of the maxillary sinus, extending posterior to involve the pterygoid plates. This fracture *allows the lower maxillae and hard palate to move separately* from the face, as a single detached block.

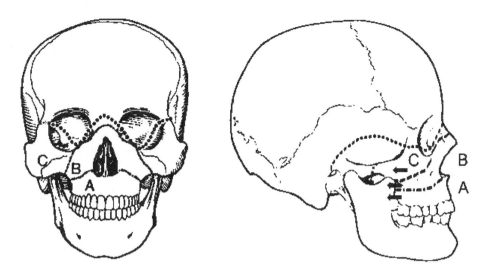

Le Fort I, II, and II fractures. *Line A* represents Le Fort I; *line B* represents Le Fort II; *line C* represents Le Fort III. The *arrows* indicate the potential for posterior displacement and airway obstruction by the Le Fort fracture components. (From Gotta AW: Maxillofacial Trauma: Textbook of Trauma Anesthesia and Critical Care. St. Louis, Mosby Year-Book Inc., 1993, pp 529-539; with permission.)

Le Fort II fracture: pyramidal disjunction. At its superior extent, the fracture line traverses the nasal bones or causes diastases of the nasofrontal sutures, extends laterally through the lacrimal bones and lamina papyracea of the ethmoid bone, across the floor of the orbit fracturing the medial and inferior orbital rims, and fracturing the pterygoid plates posteriorly. This fracture preserves the attachment of the zygomatic bones to the skull at the lateral orbital rims and at the zygomatic arches, while the *maxillary and nasal regions are movable* relative to the rest of the mid-face and skull.

Le Fort III fracture: craniofacial disjunction. This fracture line involves all of the buttresses linking the maxilla to the skull. In this type, trauma causes fractures across the nasal bones or diastases of the nasofrontal suture, across the frontoethmoidal suture and superior orbit, involves the frontozygomatic suture, extends through the root of the zygomatic bone, and crosses the temporal fossa to involve the pterygomaxillary space. The pterygoid plates are usually fractured free from the base of the skull. This fracture allows the *entire upper face (nasal, maxillary, and zygomatic regions) to move* relative to the skull.

10. What is the key physical finding common to *all* the Le Fort fractures?
    A mobile palate. A maxillary (includes palate) region that is mobile relative to the rest of the mid-face and skull is the key to diagnosing a Le Fort fracture; you must have a fracture of the pterygoid plates (the fracture common to all three Le Fort types) to have a mobile maxillary region. To examine for a mobile palate, the examiner stabilizes the forehead with one hand while attempting to move the palate and upper teeth with the other hand. Additionally, facial edema, ecchymosis, and malocclusion are commonly associated with Le Fort fractures. A patient may also exhibit epistaxis, bony "step-offs" along surfaces in the facial skeleton, and mid-face elongation or compression. Severe manifestations of a Le Fort fracture may include blindness, CSF rhinorrhea, and airway obstruction. Airway obstruction is more common to Le Fort II and III fractures.

11. Describe the physical signs of each Le Fort fracture.
    Le Fort I: maxillary alveolar bone and hard palate move as a single detached block relative to the mid-facial skeleton.

Le Fort II: maxillary and nasal regions move relative to the rest of the face and skull; airway obstruction (occasionally) and blindness (rarely; 0.6%) may result.

Le Fort III: movement of entire upper face (nasal, maxillary, and zygomatic regions) relative to skull; occasionally, airway obstruction and CSF rhinorrhea; rarely blindness (2.2%).

12. What is a tripod fracture?

A tripod fracture, also called a **zygoma complex fracture,** is the most common fracture of the zygomatic bone. The tripod fracture involves the three supporting "legs" of the zygomatic bone; these are the zygomaticofrontal suture (or may involve the frontal process of the zygoma), the zygomaticomaxillary suture inferomedially, and the zygomatic arch laterally. Commonly overlooked fourth and fifth components are fractures of the orbital floor and lateral orbital wall, and the anterior and lateral maxillary sinus walls. Typically, traumatic blows that produce a tripod fracture displace the zygomatic bone medially and posteriorly (clinically seen as a flattened malar eminence) with some degree of rotation. If the lateral orbital rim (containing the attachment of the lateral canthal tendon) is displaced inferiorly with the zygoma complex, an oblique slant of the palpebral fissure is seen.

3-D CT reconstruction can be helpful in surgical planning by characterizing the degree of displacement and rotation of the zygoma complex. Surgery is indicated if there are complications and/or the fracture is unstable; additionally, if the orbital volume is affected, reduction and fixation are indicated.

13. Describe the surgical approaches used to repair tripod fractures.

Modern surgical approaches to tripod fractures involve fracture **reduction and internal fixation under direct visualization;** this allows accurate reduction and fixation placement. Since the tripod fracture involves several different fracture sites, several separate incisions are needed to visualize these fracture lines. At least two fracture lines must be visualized to obtain adequate reduction and stabilization of the fracture complex:

- Lateral brow incision (along the inferior border of the lateral eyebrow) or an upper blepharoplasty incision for visualization of the zygomaticofrontal suture
- Subciliary or transconjunctival incision for visualization of the inferior orbital rim and orbital floor
- Upper gingival-buccal sulcus incision (under the upper lip) for visualization of the face of the maxilla
- Bicoronal approach for visualization of the lateral orbital rim and zygomatic arch.

The location and severity of the fractures determines which and how many incisions are necessary, keeping in mind, however, that incisions are made to ensure precise reduction of the zygomatic complex fragments. After proper reduction, fracture fixation is achieved by placing miniplates, microplates, and screws; these help resist torsional rotation and masticatory distraction, allowing bony healing to occur.

14. List the seven bones that compose the orbit. Which one is the weakest?

The **frontal, lacrimal, ethmoidal, zygomatic, maxillary, sphenoidal, and palatine** bones compose the orbit. The weakest bone is the **lamina papyracea of the ethmoid bone.** Fractures of the lamina papyracea are common in the realm of injury from traumatic (e.g., blowout fracture) or iatrogenic causes (e.g., penetration of the orbit during endoscopic sinus surgery).

15. What is a blowout fracture?

A blowout fracture is an **out-fracture of the orbital wall** caused by a blunt, non-penetrating force that impacts the eye and suddenly increases intraorbital pressure. In order to miss the orbital rim and directly impact the globe, the missile must be < 5 cm in maximum diameter; common missiles include baseballs, fists, hockey pucks, and champagne corks. Typically, there is an inferior displacement of the orbital floor into the maxillary sinus and a medial displacement of the medial orbital wall into the ethmoid sinus. Orbital fat, which serves to protect the ocular globe, may extrude through the orbital floor defect and into the maxillary sinus; additionally, the inferior rectus muscle may extrude and become entrapped. Small blowout fractures often cause entrapment; large fractures cause enophthalmos. Axial and coronal CT is necessary for accurate characterization of blowout fractures and surgical planning.

16. How do pure and impure blowout fractures differ?

A *pure* blowout fracture involves a downward displacement of any part of the orbital floor without damage to the orbital rim. The patient may present with pain that is confined to the orbit, ecchymosis, enophthalmos, and/or diplopia. *Impure* blowout fractures, also known as **rim fractures,** differ by their involvement of the inferior orbital rim in addition to the floor of the orbit. Typically, impure fractures are the result of a motor vehicle collision in which the passenger's face strikes the dashboard. These fractures typically present with a palpable step-off deformity in addition to diplopia (if entrapment is present), and/or regional anesthesia (if the infraorbital nerve is involved).

17. When is forced duction testing used?

Forced duction testing is used to examine for extraocular muscle entrapment in blowout fractures; it measures the freedom of movement of the extraocular muscles. After the conjunctiva is topically anesthetized, fine-toothed forceps are used to grasp the episcleral tissues near the insertion of the inferior oblique muscle; the examiner then attempts to rotate the globe superiorly. Similarly, this method can be used to test for entrapment of the medial oblique muscle. When complete restriction of passive motion exists, this is called a "4+" positive forced duction test; in this case, there is a high likelihood of muscle entrapment. Complete freedom of motion is a negative result, indicating no entrapment. Forced ductions are performed in the operating room after repair of a blowout fracture to determine if adequate reduction of the prolapsed orbital contents has been achieved.

18. What is the teardrop sign?

The teardrop sign is the presence of a teardrop-shaped opacity seen hanging from the roof of the maxillary sinus on Waters view plain-film x-ray. The opacity contains orbital contents (i.e., fat and/or extraocular muscle) that have herniated inferiorly into the maxillary sinus; it is an **indication of an orbital blowout fracture.** However, often the Waters view may simply show complete opacification of the maxillary sinus, and you cannot tell if this opacification is herniated orbital fat or accumulated blood from a mucosal tear. Axial and coronal CT is superior to plain-film x-ray and is necessary for definitive diagnosis and surgical planning.

19. What does enophthalmos indicate?

Enophthalmos (the appearance of a sunken-in globe) indicates **a blowout fracture** has occurred. However, a blowout fracture may be present without enophthalmos; this is seen in small blowout fractures and in large blowout fractures with orbital rim fracture and a medially displaced intact zygoma. In the latter case, the blowout fracture is masked by the medial displacement of the intact zygoma in compensating for lost orbital volume. As soon as the zygomatic component of the fracture is repaired, it unmasks the blowout fracture, and the patient exhibits enophthalmos. Similarly, swelling associated with an acute blowout fracture may mask enophthalmos. As the swelling subsides, the enophthalmos becomes apparent and may necessitate surgical correction. Enophthalmos is one of the most difficult surgical repairs in a blowout fracture.

20. How do you repair a blowout fracture?

After the herniated orbital contents are reduced into the intraorbital space, the **orbital floor is reconstructed.** A thin piece of autogenous or exogenous implant material is inserted between the orbital floor bone and orbital floor periosteum. This inserted material acts as a barrier to prevent further herniation of the orbital contents. The composition of the inserted material can be autogenous bone (from the anterior maxilla or outer table of the calvarium), autogenous cartilage (from nasal septum or conchal bowl), or an exogenous implant (Gelfilm, Silastic, Marlex mesh, or titanium mesh).

21. What is the most common error in orbital wall reconstruction?

Failing to repair the posterior orbital floor. Defects in the orbital floor can extend as much as 40 mm posterior to the inferior orbital rim. If you fail to explore the entire defect and identify a posterior edge of stable bone, the defect may not be adequately repaired, and orbital contents may continue to herniate, causing persistent enophthalmos. Proceed with the repair, but be aware that the optic nerve is approximately 50 mm posterior to the inferior orbital rim at the infraorbital grove. An outer-table, calvarial bone graft is ideally suited for reconstructing large orbital floor defects, as a large graft can be harvested and secured with miniplates and screws to the reconstructed orbital rim.

22. What is the most common complication of maxillary fracture repair? What are some other complications of maxillary and periorbital fracture repair?

Malocclusion is the most common complication in maxillary fracture repair. Additional complications of maxillary and periorbital fracture repair include: facial asymmetry, increased scleral show or gross ectropion, lip distortion, damage to the globe or optic nerve and/or blindness, forward positioning of globe by an oversized implant (causing an acute increase in intraorbital pressure), and lid distortion (due to plating on the inferior orbital rim).

23. What is the medial canthal tendon (MCT)?

Located in the naso-orbito-ethmoid (NOE) region, the MCT protects and supports the globe and assists in pumping tears from the lacrimal sac. Additionally, the MCT adds important cosmetic structure by shaping the medial aspect of the palpebral opening. The MCT is attached to the medial orbital wall in three places: the anterior horizontal, anterior vertical, and posterior horizontal attachments. As each of these three attachments is disrupted, the intercanthal distance increases, increasing the apparent deformity. Avulsion of the MCT disrupts its pumping of the lacrimal sac and may lead to epiphora. Signs of an MCT disruption include telecanthus, narrowing of the palpebral fissure (distance from the medial canthus to the lateral canthus), and epiphora. Failure to diagnose and repair a MCT disruption during the initial fracture repair leads to functional and cosmetic complications that are difficult to repair secondarily.

24. What degree of telecanthus is diagnostic of an NOE fracture?

Telecanthus (an intercanthal distance greater than half the interpupillary distance) of > 35 mm suggests a displaced NOE fracture, while an intercanthal distance of > 40 mm is usually diagnostic. Diagnosis of telecanthus is important because it is the most compelling reason for an open NOE repair. Edema may cause blunting of the medial palpebral fissure and/or epiphora, and thereby complicate the diagnosis of MCT disruption. Measurement of the intercanthal and interpupillary distances may increase your suspicion for MCT disruption and may necessitate CT scans of the NOE region.

CONTROVERSIES

25. What are the indications, contraindications, and time frame for surgical repair of orbital blowout fractures?

The *indication for immediate exploration* of an orbital blowout fracture is the **rapid onset of serious intraorbital hemorrhage with decreased visual acuity.** The *indications for surgical repair* of a blowout fracture include **enophthalmos and extraocular muscle entrapment.** *Contraindications* to exploration and surgical repair of a blowout fracture include soft tissue injuries to the eye, such as hyphema, retinal tears, and globe penetration, as these injuries may be exacerbated by exploration. In addition, blowout fractures should not be repaired in the patient's only seeing eye.

The *time frame* for repair must be carefully considered, as early surgical repair is difficult when the anatomical planes and landmarks are obscured with edema and bleeding. However, waiting to long may allow the bones to heal in an abnormal position and excessive scar tissue to form, which may hamper the repair. In general, surgery should be performed 7–10 days from the date of the injury.

26. Should a lacrimal collection system injury be repaired at the same time as an MCT repair?

Except in the most severe NOE fractures, lacrimal collection system injury is an uncommon complication of NOE fracture. If a lacrimal duct injury is suspected or diagnosed at the time of the initial NOE fracture reduction and internal fixation, **repair of the duct should be delayed until after the primary surgery.** Simultaneous lacrimal system and MCT repair may produce an inadequate MCT repair and may cause injury to the canaliculi. Secondary MCT repairs are more difficult and less successful than primary MCT repairs, while secondary lacrimal collecting system repairs are usually quite successful. Therefore, the lacrimal system repair is delayed to maximize the MCT result. Lacrimal obstruction requiring dacryocystorhinostomy after NOE fracture repair ranges from 5–10%.

BIBLIOGRAPHY

1. Anonymous. Management of maxillofacial trauma. Fac Plast Surg 14:1–129, 1998.1–129, 1998.
2. Life-threatening complications and irreversible damage following maxillofacial trauma. Injury 29:253–6, 1998.
3. Facial trauma. In: Rosen P, Barkin R, Danzl F, et al (eds): Emergency Medicine: Concepts and Clinical Practice, 4th ed. St. Louis, Mosby- Year Book, Inc., 1998, pp 448–462.
4. Maxillofacial trauma in the elderly. J Oral Maxillofac Surg 57:777–782; discussion 782–783, 1999.
5. Maxillofacial Trauma: Textbook of Trauma Anesthesia and Critical Care. St. Louis, Gotta AW, Mosby Year-Book Inc., 1993, pp 529–539
6. Selecting the appropriate setting for management of maxillofacial trauma. J Oral Maxillofac Surg 57:983–989, 1999.
7. Addressing the myths of cervical spine injury management. Am J Emerg Med 15: 591–5, 1997.
8. Trauma: Management of the Acutely Injured Patient. In Sabiston DC, Lyerly HK (eds.): Textbook of Surgery: The Biological Basis of Modern Surgical Practice, 15th ed. Philadelphia, WB Saunders Co., 1997, pp 304–305.
9. Interdisciplinary treatment of severe maxillofacial trauma: A clinical report. J Prosth Dent 84:133–5, 2000.
10. Pigadas N, Avery CM: Precautions against cross-infection during operations for maxillofacial trauma. Br J Oral Maxillofac Surg 38:110–3, 2000.
11. Rhea JT, Rao PM, Novelline RA: Advances in Emergency Radiology I—Helical CT and three-dimensional CT of facial and orbital injury. Radiol Clin North Am 37: 489–513, 1999.
12. Sadrian R, Rappaport NH: An overview of maxillofacial trauma for nurses. Plast Surg Nurs 18:177–181, 1998.
13. Stanley RB: Maxillofacial trauma. In Cummings CW, et al (eds): Otolaryngology–Head and Neck Surgery, 3rd ed. St Louis, Mosby, 1998.
14. Zachariades N: Blindness after facial trauma. Oral Surg Oral Med Oral Path Oral Radiol Endo 81:34–37, 1996.

66. TEMPORAL BONE TRAUMA

Bruce W. Jafek, M.D., FACS, FRSM and Kent E. Gardner, M.D.

1. What are the most common causes of temporal bone trauma?
Temporal bone trauma can be classified into *penetrating* and *blunt*. Penetrating trauma is almost exclusively due to gunshot wounds. Blunt trauma is most commonly the result of motor vehicle accidents, but may include physical assault, falls, and bicycle accidents.

2. What are the important elements of the initial emergency history of temporal bone trauma?
Important aspects of the history include the mechanism of injury, time of onset of symptoms, and presence or absence of hearing loss, vertigo, and facial weakness. In facial nerve trauma, the prognosis and approach to treatment depend partially on whether the onset of symptoms was immediate or delayed. Often, patients with severe head trauma resulting in temporal bone trauma are unconscious. In these cases, the history must be obtained from family, paramedics, and emergency department (ED) personnel.

3. How are penetrating and blunt temporal bone trauma different?
Over 6% of temporal bone trauma is due to penetrating trauma. Penetrating temporal bone trauma is generally more destructive than blunt trauma. The amount of destruction done by a gunshot wound is related to the kinetic energy of its missile, with high-velocity weapons causing more damage than low-velocity weapons. Vascular and other intracranial injuries are more common in penetrating trauma. Facial nerve trauma is present approximately half of the time and tends to be severe. Frequently, the nerve is transected, and large segments of the nerve may be missing or damaged.

4. How are temporal bone fractures classified?

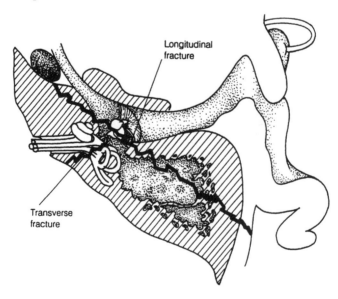

Temporal bone fractures. (From Pender DJ: Practical Otology. Philadelphia, J.B. Lippincott , 1992, p 160, with permission.)

Temporal bone fractures are classified as longitudinal fractures or transverse fractures. **Longitudinal fractures** are the most common, occurring in 70–90% of temporal bone fractures. They result from lateral blunt trauma to the temporoparietal region of the skull. This type of fracture typically begins in the thin, squamous portion of the temporal bone. The fracture line then runs across the superior external auditory canal, through the middle ear, and along the long axis of the petrous pyramid. Longitudinal fractures may involve the Eustachian tube, foramen lacerum, or foramen ovale. They also may extend into the sphenoid bone or across the midline. Longitudinal fractures cross the midline or are bilateral 30% of the time.

Transverse fractures result from a severe occipital or frontal blow. These fractures usually begin at the foramen magnum and run across the temporal bone perpendicular to the long axis of the petrous pyramid. Transverse fractures may involve the jugular foramen and almost always cause disruption of the otic capsule.

5. What should I look for when examining a patient with suspected temporal bone trauma?
- Facial nerve weakness—one of the most important physical findings to note. It is usually classified according to the House-Brackman classification.
- Hearing loss—may be *conductive or sensorineural*. Tuning forks can help distinguish between the two in the ED if the patient is conscious.
- Hemotympanum—more common with a *transverse* fracture
- Tympanic membrane perforation—more commonly seen in *longitudinal* fractures
- External auditory canal laceration with bloody otorrhea—seen in *longitudinal* fractures
- CSF otorrhea—occurs with longitudinal fractures
- CSF rhinorrhea—occurs with *transverse* fractures. Rhinorrhea results from the intact tympanic membrane directing CSF down through the Eustachian tube. CSF rhinorrhea worsens as the patient leans forward, and the patient may complain of a salty taste in the mouth.
- Nystagmus—implies damage to the vestibular system. Severe vertigo associated with nystagmus and sensorineural hearing loss implies otic capsule disruption.
- Battle's sign (see Question 6)
- Raccoon sign (see Question 6)

6. What is Battle's sign? A "raccoon" sign?
Battle's sign is postauricular ecchymosis that occurs due to fracture through the mastoid cortex. The raccoon sign is periorbital ecchymosis. Either of these signs seen in association with a history of head trauma is sufficient to make the diagnosis of probable temporal bone fracture.

7. Most temporal bone fractures are not emergencies and do not require immediate otolaryngologic consultation. What sign may necessitate early surgical intervention?
Facial nerve paralysis. A patient with the immediate onset of facial nerve paralysis, especially in association with CT findings suggesting impingement or transection, may benefit from exploration. Surgical exploration is performed as soon as the patient's condition allows.

8. Are facial nerve injuries more commonly due to transverse or longitudinal fractures?
This is a trick question. A given transverse fracture is more commonly complicated by facial nerve injury than a given longitudinal fracture: 10–20% of longitudinal and 40–50% of transverse temporal bone fractures are associated with facial nerve injury. However, the overwhelming majority of temporal bone fractures are longitudinal. Therefore, because of the greater number of longitudinal fractures vs. transverse fractures, facial nerve injuries are more commonly associated with *longitudinal fractures*.

9. What is the most commonly injured facial nerve site in *blunt* temporal bone trauma?
In *longitudinal fractures*, the **perigeniculate ganglion region** is involved in 80–93% of facial nerve injuries. The next most common site is just distal to the pyramidal eminence. In *transverse*

fractures, the **distal labyrinthine segment** is most commonly injured. Transverse temporal bone fractures are generally associated with more severe injury to the facial nerve, including transection. Longitudinal fractures are more often associated with facial nerve injuries caused by edema and hematoma.

10. In *penetrating* temporal bone trauma, what is the most commonly injured facial nerve site?

Penetrating temporal bone trauma is synonymous with gunshot wounds. Bullets tend to enter the lateral or inferior temporal bone, and tissue injury is due to dissipation of kinetic energy from the bullet. The portions of the nerve closest to the entry site and tract receive most of the energy. Therefore, the most commonly injured sites include the extratemporal nerve, the stylomastoid foramen portion of the nerve, and the vertical segment of the nerve. Transection is common with penetrating trauma and commonly requires primary repair or grafting.

11. Is CT or MRI more informative in temporal bone trauma?

A fine-cut temporal bone CT scan (1.0- to 1.5-mm cuts) with both coronal and axial views is the radiologic study of choice. This scan is extremely sensitive in evaluating the presence and extent of a temporal bone fracture. CT is also helpful in evaluating the presence of ossicular discontinuity and facial nerve lesions. MRI is less sensitive than CT in picking up fractures, ossicular discontinuity, and facial nerve trauma because bone does not show up well on MRI. Fractures are seen only because blood fills the fracture line. However, MRI is superior to CT in evaluating intracranial complications associated with temporal bone trauma. Therefore, MRI and CT can be complementary in some cases of temporal bone trauma.

12. When is an angiogram indicated in the management of penetrating temporal bone trauma?

Unless it can be determined by exam or radiologic study that the course of a bullet is lateral to the middle ear, an angiogram is *always* indicated in penetrating trauma of the temporal bone. Both the carotid and vertebral arteries should be studied. If an injury to the external carotid is noted, it is best treated with embolization at the time of angiography. Treatment of injuries to the internal carotid artery is controversial. Options include embolization, surgical revascularization, and ligation. For injuries in the petrous or intracranial portion of the internal carotid artery, which are associated with life-threatening hemorrhage, immediate embolization should be attempted.

13. How common is a CSF leak after a temporal bone fracture?

Approximately 11–27% of temporal bone fractures are complicated by a CSF leak. In longitudinal temporal bone fractures, this presents as CSF otorrhea. The diagnosis is sometimes difficult to establish due to the presence of bloody otorrhea. One way to identify a CSF leak is to check the glucose content of the otorrhea to see if it is consistent with CSF. Another way is to drip some of the bloody otorrhea on a piece of gauze or paper. If CSF is present, it will diffuse more rapidly than the blood, and a "target" or "halo" sign will be present. In transverse fractures, a CSF leak presents as clear rhinorrhea.

14. What are the common complications associated with temporal bone fracture?

Facial nerve injury, CSF leak, hearing loss, and vertigo are the most commonly recognized complications of temporal bone trauma. Cholesteatoma, vascular injuries, facial hypesthesia, diplopia, and other cranial nerve injuries may also occur. Cholesteatoma develops long after temporal bone trauma and occurs because of seeding of the mastoid cavity with squamous epithelium due to fracture of the external canal. Trauma patients are generally healthy and have well-pneumatized mastoid cavities, which are conducive to rapid cholesteatoma growth. Facial hypesthesia occurs because of damage to the Gasserian ganglion (CN V) at its location on the surface of the petrous bone. Diplopia can occur because of damage to the abducens nerve (CN VI) as it courses through Dorello's canal.

15. How do you manage a patient with a CSF leak?

Most CSF leaks stop after a few days with only conservative therapy. Conservative treatment consists of bed rest, head elevation, and avoidance of activities that increase intracranial pressure (i.e., straining, lifting, or bending over). Some advocate fluid restriction and diuretics. The use of antibiotics is controversial. If the leak persists for several days (usually 3–5), then a lumbar drain may be added to conservative therapy. If leakage persists despite lumbar drainage, then consideration is given to surgery. Indications for surgery include persistent leak despite adequate conservative therapy, recurrent meningitis, and persistent pneumocephalus. In the rare case when surgery is necessary, localization of the leak can be aided by contrast-enhanced CT, radioisotope studies, and intrathecal dye instillation.

16. What is post-concussive syndrome? How is it treated?

Most patients experience some degree of balance disturbance after temporal bone trauma. Post-concussive syndrome is a constellation of symptoms including nonspecific dizziness, headache, inability to concentrate, and fatigue. These patients tend to have normal electronystagmographic (ENG) testing and a normal audiogram. After ruling out more serious injury, these patients are treated conservatively with gradual resumption of activity, nonsteroidal analgesics, and reassurance.

17. What are the causes of vertigo when it is associated with temporal bone trauma? How should vertigo be worked up?

Causes of post-traumatic vertigo include post-concussive syndrome, concussive injury to the membranous labyrinth, cupulolithiasis, massive and disruptive injury to the labyrinth, traumatic perilymph fistula, and trauma-induced endolymphatic hydrops. Patients with post-traumatic vertigo should undergo evaluation with an ENG and audiogram, and possibly posturography.

18. How are the different types of post-traumatic vertigo differentiated and treated?

Concussive injury to the membranous labyrinth is the most common form of post-traumatic vertigo. These patients have positional vertigo and usually have a normal ENG. Concussive injury to the labyrinth is almost always self-limited and requires only symptomatic treatment.

Cupulolithiasis is a more severe form of concussive injury. The onset of positional vertigo is usually delayed. ENG generally is normal except for a positive Dix-Hallpike provocative test. Treatment usually involves the Epley maneuver or Cawthorne exercises.

Massive injury to the vestibular labyrinth occurs as the result of an otic capsule-disrupting fracture. These patients have immediate, severe vertigo, with nausea and emesis. They also tend to have a horizontal nystagmus with the fast component away from the involved ear. Initial treatment consists of vestibular suppressants and antiemetics. Physical therapy is also helpful during vestibular rehabilitation. The symptoms of an otic capsule-disrupting fracture subside over days to weeks as the CNS begins to compensate.

A **perilymphatic fistula** is characterized by vertigo and a fluctuating or progressive sensorineural hearing loss. Initial treatment consists of bed rest with expectant management. If symptoms persist, consider surgical exploration.

Trauma-induced endolymphatic hydrops usually develops months or years after head trauma. Symptoms include fluctuant hearing loss, tinnitus, and aural fullness with vertigo. The possibility of perilymphatic fistula must be considered. Treatment is consistent with that used for other forms of endolymphatic hydrops.

19. What type of hearing loss is more common in patients after temporal bone trauma?

Patients with temporal bone trauma may suffer from either **conductive hearing loss** (CHL) or **sensorineural hearing loss** (SNHL), with CHL being the more common type. CHL is usually temporary and is caused by blood in the middle ear, edema, or tympanic membrane perforation. Sometimes CHL is more permanent. Persistent CHL is due to more severe injury to the middle ear structures. SNHL is less common and is usually the result of fracture of the otic capsule.

20. What is the most common reason for persistent CHL associated with temporal bone trauma?

The most common cause is *ossicular damage*. The most common form of ossicular injury is **incudostapedial joint separation.** The incudostapedial joint is prone to injury because the long process of the incus and the stapes superstructure are at right angles to each other. When a severe blow strikes the temporal bone, the resultant torsional forces on the stapes superstructure and long process of the incus are in opposite directions. The small surface area of the stapes cannot withstand these forces, and separation occurs. Other common ossicular injuries include massive dislocation of the incus, fracture of the stapedial arch, fracture of the malleus, and epitympanic fixation of the ossicular chain.

21. How does blunt trauma cause sensorineural hearing loss?
- Disruption of the bony and membranous labyrinths from a fracture of the capsule
- Concussion injury to the inner ear without evidence of labyrinthine fracture
- Blast with noise-induced hearing loss
- Perilymph fistula
- Injury to the auditory CNS

22. What is the significance of a remote history of head trauma in a patient with recurrent meningitis?

Fractures of the otic capsule do not heal like long-bone fractures, and incomplete healing is not uncommon. Incomplete healing of a fracture line can allow ingrowth of respiratory mucosa and lead to a microscopic fistula. The fistula then can act as a highway for infection and lead to meningitis. In patients with recurrent meningitis and a past history of head trauma, a fistula should be suspected. Localization of the fistula is accomplished by CT scans, radioisotope studies, or intrathecal dye injections. Treatment of the fistula is generally with a labyrinthectomy and obliteration of the pneumatized spaces and the Eustachian tube.

23. When should patients with a CHL after temporal bone trauma be operated on?

Surgical intervention with exploration of the middle ear should be considered 3–6 months after temporal bone trauma. Some 75% of patients with CHL after trauma return to normal within this 3- to 6-month waiting period. The rest have an unhealed tympanic membrane perforation or ossicular injuries. Seventy-eight percent of patients with ossicular discontinuity can have the air-bone gap closed to within 10 dB by using ossicular reconstruction techniques.

CONTROVERSIES

24. What are the indications for post-traumatic facial nerve exploration after intratemporal facial nerve injury?

There are no universally accepted indications for facial nerve exploration after temporal bone trauma. The spectrum of facial nerve injuries resulting from temporal bone trauma is broad. At one end of the spectrum is mild facial nerve paresis. These injuries are often delayed in onset and are usually secondary to nerve edema. At the opposite end of the spectrum is complete, immediate paralysis due to transection of the nerve. Indicators of severe injury and possible benefits from surgical intervention include immediate onset of paralysis, poor prognosis by electrical testing, and evidence of nerve transection or impingement by CT scan.

Patients with only a **paresis** of the facial nerve always have good return of function and do not require surgical intervention. Patients with **delayed paralysis** of the nerve also tend to have good return of function without surgical intervention. However, some authors advocate decompression of the facial nerve in patients with delayed onset of facial nerve paralysis if electrical testing indicates a poor prognosis. **Immediate-onset paralysis** with evidence of transection or impingement of the facial nerve by CT scan, or in the setting of penetrating trauma, is also indication for surgical exploration and repair of the nerve. The indications for exploration in cases of immediate paralysis *without* evidence of nerve transection or impingement by CT scan are controversial. Electrical testing can be helpful in predicting which patients have a poor prognosis and therefore may benefit from surgical exploration.

25. How is a perilymphatic fistula diagnosed and treated?
There are two approaches to handling a suspected perilymphatic fistula: early surgical exploration and noninvasive testing and observation.

Early surgical exploration: All noninvasive test batteries are ineffective in accurately diagnosing a perilymphatic fistula. By exploring an acutely dizzy patient early, the surgeon can make the diagnosis and adequately treat the patient in a timely fashion. Delay may result in permanent labyrinthine dysfunction and deafness. Therefore, do not delay surgical exploration, especially in the patient with sudden hearing loss.

Noninvasive testing and observation: The diagnosis of perilymphatic fistula is difficult, even during surgery, and the incidence of fistulae due to indirect trauma is extremely low. Conservative therapy usually involves 1–2 weeks of bed rest with the head elevated. Many existing fistulae heal spontaneously. Patients whose symptoms worsen should have surgery. A conservative approach saves many patients from an operation and the risks of complications.

26. Should patients with a CSF leak due to temporal bone fracture receive antibiotics?
Yes: Prophylactic antibiotics may prevent the development of meningitis in the patient with a CSF leak. Antibiotics are usually harmless. Moreover, the incidence of meningitis in head trauma patients with a CSF leak is as high as 20%.

No: Most patients with temporal bone fractures and an associated CSF leak do not develop meningitis. Most leaks heal spontaneously in 4–5 days without surgical intervention. Prophylactic antibiotics have not been clearly shown to prevent meningitis, and they are typically prescribed in doses that are too small to treat most infections. Furthermore, if clinically obvious meningitis develops in the presence of antibiotics, accurate diagnosis and identification of the organism may be difficult or impossible.

LOW VELOCITY MISSILE INJURIES TO THE TEMPORAL BONE

Sabin, et al, found that the initial presentation of low-velocity missile injuries to the temporal bone included otorrhoea (69%), facial nerve injury (27%), hearing loss (65%), intracranial injuries (50%), and cranial neuropathies (58%). Vascular injury was found in 5 of 9 patients who underwent angiography. Four patients died. They concluded that low-velocity gunshot injuries can be devastating and may result in functional sequelae. Low-velocity missiles crush and lacerate surrounding structures, while high-velocity missiles cause extensive wound cavity formation and a cone of injury. Early aggressive management for intracranial, vascular, and facial nerve injury can improve the outcome.

~*Sabin, J Laryngol Otol 112:929, 1998.*

BIBLIOGRAPHY
1. Alvi A, Bereliani A: Acute intracranial complications of temporal bone trauma. Otolaryngol Head Neck Surg 119:609–613, 1998.

2. Alvi A: Battle's sign in temporal bone trauma. Otolaryngol Head Neck 118:908, 1998.
3. Chang CY, Cass SP: Management of facial nerve injury due to temporal bone trauma. Am J Otol 20:96–114, 1999.
4. Dahiya R, Keller JD, Litofsky NS, et al: Temporal bone fractures: Otic capsule sparing versus otic capsule violating clinical and radiographic considerations. J Trauma Inj Inf Crit Care 47:1079–83, 1999.
5. Goksu N, Bayazit AY, Beder L, et al: Facial reanimation after temporal bone fracture. Rev Laryng Otol Rhinol 119:313–316, 1998.
6. Hansen MC, et al: Temporal bone fractures. Am J Emerg Med 13:211–214, 1995.
7. Jones RM, Rothman MI, Gray WC, et al: Temporal lobe injury in temporal bone fractures. Arch Otolaryngol Head Neck Surg 126:131–135, 2000.
8. Kelly KE, Tami TA: Temporal bone and skull base trauma. In Jackler RK, Brackman DE (eds): Neurotology. St. Louis, Mosby, 1994.
9. Kinney SE: Trauma to the middle ear and temporal bone. In Cummings CW, et al (eds): Otolaryngology–Head and Neck Surgery, 3rd ed. St. Louis, Mosby, 1998.
10. Lancaster JL, Alderson DJ, Curley JW: Otological complications following basal skull fractures. J Roy Coll Surg Edinburgh 44:87–90, 1999.
11. Lee D, Honrado C, Har-El G, et al: Pediatric temporal bone fractures. Laryngoscope 108:816–21, 1998.
12. Lyos AT, Marsh MA, Jenkins HA, et al: Progressive hearing loss after transverse temporal bone fracture. Arch Otolaryngol Head Neck Surg 121:795–799, 1995.
13. Sabin SL, Lee D, Har-el G: Low velocity gunshot injuries to the temporal bone. J Laryngol Otol 112:929–933, 1998.
14. Shindo ML, et al: Gunshot wounds of the temporal bone: A rational approach to evaluation and management. Otolaryngol Head Neck Surg 112:533–539, 1995.
15. Wall C III, Rauch SD: Perilymph fistula pathophysiology. Otolaryngol Head Neck Surg 112:145–153, 1995.
16. Yanagihara N, Murakami S, Nishihara S: Temporal bone fractures inducing facial nerve paralysis: A new classification and its clinical significance [see comments]. ENT J 76:79–80, 83–86, 1997.
17. Yeakley JW: Temporal bone fractures. Curr Prob Diag Radiol 28:65–98, 1999.

IX. Pediatric Otolaryngology

67. THE PEDIATRIC AIRWAY

Jeffrey R. Gagliano, M.S. III and Bruce W. Jafek, M.D., FACS, FRSM

1. How does an infant's airway differ anatomically from an adult's? Are these differences important for airway management?

Several important anatomic differences exist between the infant and adult airway. The infant has narrow nares, a relatively large tongue, an elevated position of the larynx, a narrow cricoid ring, and a large occiput. Intubation of the child can be complicated by several factors, including the tongue obstructing the pharynx and difficulty with head positioning. Other considerations include the infantile larynx that, unlike the adult's, is funnel-shaped, with the narrowest region at the cricoid ring—a difference that lasts up through 8 years of age. An endotracheal tube or other foreign body that easily passes through the glottis (space between the vocal cords) may not pass through the subglottic lumen of the cricoid.

2. What unique physiology and mechanical properties of the pediatric airway increase the risk of respiratory compromise in infants vs. adults?

- *The smaller and less rigid airway* is more easily obstructed in response to infection, inflammation, or foreign body.
- *Poor collateral circulation* can complicate this obstruction.
- *Greater chest wall compliance* allows for collapse or labored breathing and a lower functional residual capacity with obstruction.
- *Horizontal rib position* (rather than angulated) yields less intercostal excursion.
- *Easily fatigable respiratory muscles* are less able to compensate for stress placed on the respiratory system.
- *Greater susceptibility to upper respiratory infections (URI)* causes edema and increased secretions that compromise ventilation.
- *Unique anatomy and physiology* yields a deceptively well-appearing child in the face of impending respiratory or circulatory collapse.

3. What percentage of infants are obligate nasal breathers?

Obligate nasal breathing is often seen in infants. The inability to tolerate nasal occlusion and mouth breathing is thought to be due to immature coordination of oral and respiratory function. Nasal breathing, combined with the high position of the larynx in the neck, allows infants to feed, swallow, and breathe simultaneously. About 92% of infants at 30–32 weeks postconceptual age and 22% of term infants are obligate nasal breathers. Nearly all infants are able to coordinate oral and respiratory function by the age of 5 months.

4. What is stridor? What are its causes?

Stridor is a symptom term for noisy breathing. The noise is created by turbulent airflow or vibration of tissues in a structural or functional narrowing somewhere between the oral cavity and distal bronchi during respiration. The key to localizing the source of stridor is characterizing the occurrence of the sound with inspiratory and/or expiratory phases of respiration.

Inspiratory stridor reflects airflow impairment above or at the level of the vocal cords. It is generally high-pitched when occurring at the vocal cords and may be low-pitched when obstruction is above the vocal cords (pharynx or supraglottic larynx).

Expiratory stridor is usually produced from airflow limitation in the distal tracheobronchial (intrathoracic) tree and gives rise to a more prolonged, sonorous sound. This may be confused with wheezing, such as in asthma.

Stridor that is both inspiratory and expiratory (**biphasic**) is usually due to obstruction immediately below the vocal cords or in the proximal (extrathoracic) trachea.

About 60% of stridor in children is localized to the larynx, 15% to the trachea, and 5% to the bronchi; 5% have an infectious cause.

5. How do you evaluate a child with stridor?

Stridor may occur in a setting of acute respiratory distress, or it may be a chronic condition. It may be due to one or more of a panoply of etiologies: congenital, inflammatory, traumatic, iatrogenic, and neoplastic.

History: the major component of the evaluation, identifying the airway abnormality in up to 80% of cases. Onset and duration of symptoms as well as initiating and possible alleviating factors are ascertained. Symptoms include dyspnea, fever, cough, voice changes, sore throat, dysphagia, apnea, and association of stridor with positioning, feeding, or crying.

Physical examination: documents the quality of stridor and its relation to phase of respiration. Signs include general appearance, vocal changes, airway sounds, drooling, subcutaneous emphysema, and respiratory effort (i.e., tachypnea, tachycardia, suprasternal or intercostal retractions) Respiratory obstruction causes hypoventilation (πPO_2 and νPCO_2), yielding signs of confusion, restlessness, and altered level of consciousness.

Radiologic evaluation: a noninvasive tool to assess the etiology of stridor. Studies include AP and lateral neck/chest radiography, AP neck barium swallow, and airway fluoroscopy. Plain films of the neck and chest during inspiration and expiration may document supraglotttic swelling, subglottic or tracheal narrowing, and shifts of the trachea and mediastinum. Barium swallow can delineate obstruction from a vascular ring causing extrinsic tracheal compression.

Definitive diagnosis of stridor generally requires **endoscopy** of the upper aerodigestive tract. Flexible fiberoptic laryngoscopy is well-tolerated in infants and young children, and confirms the cause of stridor in most cases. Fiberoptic bronchoscopy identifies abnormalities of the distal airway. Rigid endoscopy is performed under general anesthesia and is used for diagnostic as well as therapeutic purposes (e.g., laser, foreign-body removal).

6. What is the differential diagnosis of stridor and airway obstruction?

Nose and Pharynx
Congenital

Choanal atresia or stenosis	Cysts (dermoid, thyroglossal)
Nasal aperture stenosis	Macroglossia
Lingual thyroid	Encephalocele/glioma
Craniofacial anomalies	

Inflammatory

Nasal polyps	Peritonsillar abscess
Adenotonsillar hypertrophy	Retropharyngeal abscess

Neoplastic

Benign	Malignant

Foreign Body
Neuromuscular Lesions

Larynx
Congenital

Laryngomalacia	Subglottic stenosis
Webs, cysts, laryngoceles	Laryngeal atresia or clefts

Inflammatory

Laryngotracheobronchitis (croup)	Epi/Supraglottitis
Angioneurotic edema	Diptheria
Fungal infection	Tuberculosis
Sarcoidosis	

Vocal Cord Paralysis

Trauma

Intubation	Neck trauma

Foreign Body

Neoplasm

Benign: subglottic hemangioma, laryngeal papilloma, lymphangioma	Malignant

Laryngospasm

Trachea and Bronchi

Congenital

Vascular rings and slings	Webs, cysts
Subglottic (tracheal) stenosis	Tracheoesophageal fistula
Tracheomalacia	

Inflammatory

Bacterial tracheitis	Bronchitis
Bronchgenic cysts	

Foreign Body

Esophageal	Tracheal or bronchial

Neoplasm

Tracheal: subglottic hemangioma	Extraluminal: thyroid, esophagus, thymus

Trauma

Vocal cord paralysis	

Immunologic/Asthma

The most frequent causes of *congenital* airway obstruction are laryngeal anomalies, with laryngomalacia accounting for about 60%. The most frequent cause of *infectious/inflammatory obstruction* is the croup syndrome, which comprises acute inflammatory diseases of the larynx including viral croup (laryngotracheobronchitis), epiglottitis (supraglottitis), and bacterial tracheitis.

7. What is the most common cause of childhood airway obstruction?

Acute laryngotracheobronchitis, or **croup,** is the most common cause of *acute stridor* in children. Patients are usually < 2 years old, ranging from 6 months to 5 years. It is often associated with upper respiratory tract infection, primarily parainfluenza virus, as well as respiratory syncytial virus, influenza, rubeola and adenoviruses, and *Mycoplasma pneumoniae*. Croup is characterized by a barking cough with inspiratory or biphasic stridor. The stridor is usually due to edema of the subglottic space, as a result of viral infection.

Most cases are alleviated by simple home methods, such as humidification, clear liquid intake, or walks in the cool night air. Only the most severe cases cause acute airway obstruction, and their therapy includes humidification, supplemental oxygen, fluids, and nebulized racemic epinephrine. The use of oral and/or IM glucocorticoids such as dexamethasone to treat obstruction is now widely accepted as efficacious, avoiding many hospitalizations. Complications of croup include pulmonary edema, pneumonia, cardiac failure, and subsequent airway hyperreactivity.

Laryngotracheomalacia is the most common cause of *chronic stridor* in infants. It is a benign congenital disorder in which underdevelopment of the supraglottic cartilaginous structure yields a floppy airway, usually in the first 6 weeks of life. Stridor is reported most often with supine positioning, increased physical activity, and upper respiratory infections, and during feeding. Diagnosis is made with direct laryngoscopy, which shows inspiratory collapse of the epiglottis. This condition usually improves with age and resolves by age 2 without any treatment. In some cases, severe airway obstruction related to feeding, failure to thrive, obstructive sleep apnea, or severe dyspnea requires surgical epiglottoplasty.

8. What additional inflammatory conditions cause childhood airway obstruction?

Acute epiglottitis occurs much less commonly than croup in children. Prior to introduction of the HIB vaccine, *Haemophilus influenzae* type B was the most common inciting pathogen, but now, other bacterial organisms frequently cause acute epiglottitis, including nontypable *H. influenzae*, *Streptococcus pneumoniae,* groups A and C *Streptococcus pyogenes,* and *Neisseria meningitidis.* It is most frequent in patients aged 2–6 years. Signs and symptoms include rapidly developing sore throat, high fever, leukocytosis, restlessness, lethargy, and inability to control saliva. The patient's respiratory pattern is characterized by an excessively high rate with marked inspiratory stridor and retractions.

Epiglottitis is a medical emergency, since the resulting inflammation and swelling supraglottic structures (epiglottis and arytenoids) may develop rapidly and lead to complete upper airway obstruction. Intervention includes quick intubation by a skilled and experienced clinician, who is prepared to perform tracheotomy, if necessary. Direct laryngoscopy to obtain swab cultures from the epiglottis, followed by appropriate intravenous antibiotic therapy, is required. The epiglottis usually returns to normal size after 48 hours.

Bacterial tracheitis (pseudomembranous croup) is a severe form of croup that may occur at any age and most likely represents bacterial superinfection in a child with pre-existing viral croup. *Staphylococcus aureus* is the most common inciting pathogen; however, *H. influenzae,* group A *S. pyogenes,* Neisseria species, and *Moraxella catarrhalis* also may be cultured from tracheal secretions. Localized bacterial invasion of the tracheal mucosa results in edema, purulent secretions, and pseudomembranes, but negative blood cultures. The initial clinical presentation is similar to viral croup, but patients subsequently develop high fever, toxicity, pneumonia (up to 60%), and progressive upper airway obstruction that is unresponsive to conventional croup treatment. Lateral x-rays show a normal epiglottis, but confirm subglottic and tracheal narrowing, as well as large crusts within the airway. The diagnosis is made by endoscopic examination of the airway that reveals copious purulent secretions and crusts.

Management of bacterial tracheitis includes airway protection with an endotracheal tube, frequent suctioning, and repeated endoscopies due to recurrent plugging and crusting. IV antibiotics should follow culture results and sensitivities, but should initially cover *S. aureus.* Other inflammatory conditions leading to airway obstruction include spasmodic laryngitis, head and neck abscesses, inflammatory nasal obstruction, and oropharyngeal obstruction.

9. How are croup, epiglottitis, and bacterial tracheitis differentiated pathologically and clinically?

Distinguishing and Classic Characteristics of Croup,
Bacterial Tracheitis, and Epiglottitis

FEATURE	CROUP	BACTERIAL TRACHEITIS	EPIGLOTTITIS
Age	< 2 years	Any age	3–5 years
Organism	RSV, parainfluenza	*Staphylococcus aureus*	*Haemophilus influenzae*
Site of involvement	Subglottic	Trachea	Supraglottic
Stridor	Biphasic	Expiratory	Inspiratory
Voice	Barking cough	Hoarseness	Unaffected
Position forward	Not characteristic	Not characteristic	Erect, chin jutting
Swallowing	Unaffected	Unaffected	
Treatment	Humidity, inhaled steroids, racemic epinephrine, antibiotics	Bronchoscopy, suctioning, IV antibiotics, intensive care	Artificial airway, humidity, IV monitoring

From Cummings CW, et al (eds): Current Therapy in Otolaryngology – Head and Neck Surgery, 6th ed. St. Louis, Mosby, 1998, p 424; with permission.

10. **Which *iatrogenic* disorders can lead to airway obstruction in the child?**

The most common causes of iatrogenic stridor are from laryngeal obstruction and include intubation, instrumentation, and surgery. **Recurrent laryngeal nerve paralysis** may be secondary to surgical trauma or pressure-induced ischemia following routine intubation. Paralysis of this nerve due to surgery is most commonly unilateral, although bilateral paralysis has also been reported. Paralysis due to pressure-induced ischemia is usually self-limited. **Endotracheal intubation** may result in airway obstruction or nerve ischemia after removal, due to the mechanical trauma and irritation of the tube. **Acquired subglottic stenosis** may be seen in neonates or older children subjected to long-term intubation. There are several causes of iatrogenic **nasal obstruction,** including scar tissue formation following tonsil or adenoid surgery, prolonged administration of topical nasal decongestants, and many systemically administered medications that cause nasal stuffiness as a side effect. **Birth trauma** due to difficult delivery, neck torsion and abnormal cervical traction due to unusual intrauterine positioning have all been implicated, as well.

11. **Which *traumatic* disorders cause childhood airway obstruction?**

Foreign bodies can precipitate airway obstruction by lodging in virtually any region of the upper aerodigestive tract. Nasal foreign bodies often cause unilateral, and less commonly cause bilateral, purulent and malodorous rhinorrhea. Foreign bodies in the larynx or hypopharynx often present with inspiratory stridor. In the trachea, they may mimic croup.

Radiographic imaging is often inadequate for identification and localization of the object, because many foreign bodies are radiolucent. However, forced expiratory (obtained by manually compressing the abdomen during expiration) and inspiratory chest x-rays do offer additional insight and should be obtained. Forced expiratory studies may show mediastinal deviation away from the affected side as well as hyperinflation on the affected side as the foreign body impedes expiratory airflow. Inspiratory films may show localized hyperinflation, since the aspirated object often traps air distally by the ball-valve effect. If the airway is completely obstructed, characteristic radiographic findings include atelectasis and related volume loss. Endoscopy often serves as the ultimate tool necessary for identification and removal of the inciting foreign body.

Many **other types of trauma** can cause airway obstruction, including mandibular fractures causing retrodisplacement of the tongue, blunt or penetrating cervical trauma, dislocation of the arytenoid cartilages, laryngeal fracture, and compression of the airway lumen secondary to hematoma. Traumatic injury to the nose can precipitate airway obstruction. Exposure to hot air, smoke, or steam (thermal trauma) or inhalation/ingestion of caustic chemicals may lead to airway obstruction from massive mucosal edema.

12. **Which *neoplastic* disorders most commonly cause airway obstruction in the child?**

Hemangioma is the most common head and neck neoplasm in children. It may appear anywhere in the upper aerodigestive tract. Hemangiomas of the larynx may cause inspiratory or biphasic stridor due to their subglottic location.

Juvenile nasopharyngeal angiofibroma is the most common vascular mass found in the nasal cavity. The condition is seen almost exclusively in males aged 7–21 years. Most present with nasal obstruction and recurrent epistaxis. The tumor is locally invasive and can lead to gross facial deformity or direct intracranial extension.

A **teratoma** is a neoplasm with tissue elements from all three germinal layers. The nasopharynx is a common location for such tumors, and the patient with a teratoma may present with varying degrees of nasal obstruction. Cervical teratomas may also cause airway obstruction due to extrinsic pressure, and surgical resection is necessary.

Lymphangiomas are soft, compressible masses representing areas of regional lymphatic dilation. Approximately 90% of these lesions present before age 3. Airway compromise may occur from intraoral or laryngeal extension.

Recurrent respiratory papillomatosis can be seen in any portion of the upper aerodigestive tract and is the most common benign neoplasm of the larynx in children. The lesions, generally caused by the human papillomavirus (HPV 6, 11, and 16), commonly present with respiratory obstruction, hoarseness, croupy cough, stridor, and even aphonia.

13. Are radiographic studies helpful in evaluating upper airway obstruction? Which ones?

An accurate diagnosis of the etiology of upper airway obstruction can usually be obtained from history, physical examination, and endoscopy. However, many lesions can be identified non-invasively with radiography. A lateral view, **plain-film** x-ray with the neck extended helps to identify adenotonsillar hypertrophy, epiglottitis, or retropharyngeal abscess. The anteroposterior view may show tracheal deviation, asymmetry or narrowing of the subglottis, and vocal cord paralysis when obtained during phonation and deep respiration. All views are helpful when evaluating radiopaque foreign bodies, although most of these foreign bodies are radiolucent. Chest x-rays help in diagnosing pneumonia, areas of hyperaeration, or atelectasis. **Upper gastrointestinal studies** identify tracheoesophageal fistulas, vascular rings, and gastroesophageal reflux. **Fluoroscopy** can identify dynamic obstructions, such as laryngomalacia, tracheomalacia, vocal cord paralysis, and foreign bodies, and it localizes the obstruction site in obstructive sleep apnea. **CT and MRI** help to identify and characterize pathology located within soft tissue structures. Anomalies of the great vessels are best visualized with noncontrast MRI.

14. What are the indications for endotracheal intubation and tracheostomy in children?

In general, prolonged endotracheal intubation is well tolerated and managed more effectively than tracheostomy in infants from birth to 6 months of age. In the presence of severe inflammatory glottic or tracheal disease, edema in the area of the cricoid may cause pressure against the tube, and endotracheal intubation should be maintained only long enough for tracheostomy to be performed. To avoid subglottic injury, tracheostomy should be considered in a child over 6 months of age when intubation is required for > 10–14 days.

15. What surgical options are available when managing subglottic stenosis?

Mild to moderate laryngeal stenosis in infants and children can be managed with the **anterior cricoid split procedure.** It is performed only when the child has failed extubation and has discrete, mild to moderate subglottic narrowing. The procedure is through an external neck incision and involves dividing the cricoid cartilage, upper tracheal ring, and lower portion of the thyroid cartilage anteriorly. The patient is intubated with a nasotracheal tube that serves as a stent. The stent is usually removed after 5–10 days.

Endoscopic treatment of subglottic stenosis with laser and dilation has the advantage of avoiding a tracheotomy, but is generally successful only in treating stenosis of < 50%. When stenosis of the lumen is > 70%, *open reconstruction* is generally recommended. Several operative approaches are used. With anterior subglottic stenosis, an anterior *autogenous costal cartilage graft* is appropriate. With more circumferential stenosis, the cricoid may be divided anteriorly, posteriorly, and possibly laterally, with placement of a stent and additional grafts.

16. What is gastroesophageal reflux disease (GERD)? How does it affect children?

Reflux of gastric contents into the esophagus is a normal phenomenon surrounding the inherent patency of the gastroesophageal pseudo-sphincter. When systemic gastrointestinal or respiratory symptoms are the result of such reflux, GERD is the diagnosis. Failure to thrive and recurrent pulmonary symptoms are the most common complications of GERD in children. It is uncommon to see the pediatric patient with the hallmark adult symptoms of heartburn, vomiting, or dysphagia, a factor often contributing to misdiagnosis. GERD has been implicated in the pathogenesis of a variety of respiratory disorders, including aspiration pneumonia, chronic cough, wheezing, reactive airway exacerbation, sinusitis, laryngitis, and apnea. Symptoms seem to be mediated through mucosal inflammation, edema, and protective airway reflexes resulting from abnormal gastric acid exposure. There is an increased incidence of GERD in premature infants with respiratory distress syndrome, in neurologically impaired children, and in children with congenital esophageal anomalies.

17. How is pediatric GERD diagnosed? What is the treatment?

Diagnosis is usually accomplished clinically in thriving infants age < 6 months. The gold standard for diagnosis is mucosal biopsy with a prolonged or 24-hour esophageal dual-pH study.

Reflux is diagnosed if the pH $<$ 4 for $>$ 5–10% of the time at the lower probe and $>$ 4% of the time at the upper probe, during the period that the probe is in the esophagus.

GERD associated with respiratory symptoms usually responds to conventional medical anti-reflux therapy. Reflux can often be limited with lifestyle modifications, including small and frequent feedings, formula thickened with rice cereal, post-prandial uprightness for at least 1 hour, and no eating for 3 hours prior to bedtime. Use of an H_2-blocker like ranitidine (Zantac), proton pump inhibitor like omeprazole (Prilosec), and/or an agent that promotes gastric emptying like cisapride (Propulsid) is an effective pharmacologic regimen. Rarely, if the child's GERD causes (1) persistent vomiting with failure to thrive, (2) severe esophagitis or esophageal stricture, or (3) apneic spells or chronic pulmonary disease that is unresponsive to medical therapy, then surgical fundoplication is indicated.

CONTROVERSIES

18. Describe obstructive sleep apnea. How is it manifested in the pediatric airway?

Parents will say, "He always breathes through his mouth"; "She snores like a truck driver"; or "At night, she sounds like a power saw!" Sleep apnea and upper airway obstruction may not always be accompanied by such florid descriptions. This relatively newly classified phenomenon has yielded increasing surgical interest over the past 15 years. Obstructive sleep apnea (OSA) describes the syndrome in which airway obstruction results in temporary apnea while sleeping. It is defined as air flow obstruction for 6–10 seconds that is associated with respiratory effort, brady-cardia, oxygen desaturation, and/or termination with gasping and agitated arousal. OSA's incidence in 4- to 5-year-old children, the population with the most abundant lymphoid tissue, is reported as high as 2%. The number of sites, severity, and location of obstruction are extremely variable. Factors contributing to pediatric apnea include: adenotonsillar hypertrophy, cleft palate and posterior pharyngeal flap, craniofacial disorders, familial factors, nasal obstruction, laryngeal and tracheobronchial lesions, neurologic impairment, and obesity.

19. List some side effects of pediatric OSA.

OSA is associated with an array of adverse effects. Some children develop failure to thrive, a condition thought to be a result of obligate mouth breathing, slow eating, anosmia due to nasal obstruction, and growth hormone deficiency due to diminished REM sleep. The most frequent cardiac effect is bradycardia. Alterations in blood pressure during apnea can decrease systolic blood flow, which may compromise cerebral perfusion, causing a condition known as cerebral anoxia in susceptible infants. Apnea has been implicated in the pathophysiology of SIDS. Infants at higher risk for SIDS have been shown to have higher rates of apnea. Daytime behavioral changes include hypersomnolence and poor school performance, presumably due to chronic sleep deprivation. The development of frank cor pulmonale and other signs of right heart failure are extremely rare.

20. Discuss the diagnosis and treatment of pediatric OSA.

Diagnosis of OSA is made by polysomnography in a certified sleep lab that can objectively assess sleep efficiency, obstructive events per hour, blood oxygen desaturation, associated cardiac arrhythmias, and sleep architecture. The otolaryngologist's evaluation of the upper aero-digestive tract is essential to reveal evidence of discrete obstruction and subsequent therapeutic intervention.

Be cautious when considering surgery, because of significant possible complications involving anesthesia, respiratory distress, and sudden death in OSA patients. Nonsurgical options, including weight loss (if obesity exists), constant positive airway pressure (CPAP) or bilevel positive airway pressure (BiPAP), nasal strips, artifical airway, oral devices, treatment of allergies and GERD, and drug therapy, should be tried prior to surgery. CPAP/BiPAP is effective in 75–80% of patients; however, compliance is low, and only 40% of patients consistently use the facemask for 4 or more hours per night. Current surgical treatment options include tonsillectomy +/- adenoidectomy, nasal surgery (e.g., septoplasty), craniofacial surgery (mandibular advancement), revision of posterior pharyngeal flap, tracheotomy, uvulopalatopharyngoplasty, and laser-assisted uvulopalatoplasty.

Multiple studies have shown improvement with tonsillectomy and adenoidectomy in OSA patients. Note, however, that one study reported a 15–65% weight gain in 75% of 41 patients undergoing this surgery.

BIBLIOGRAPHY

1. Chung CJ, Fordham LA, Mukherji SK: The pediatric airway: A review of differential diagnosis by anatomy and physiology. Neuroimaging Clin North Am 10:161–180, 2000.
2. Cotton RT: Management of subglottic stenosis. Otol Clin North Am 33:111–130, 2000.
3. Cotton RT: Subglottic stenosis in children, and Holinger LD: Foreign bodies of the airway and esophagus. In Gates GA (ed): Current Therapy in Otolaryngology – Head and Neck Surgery. St. Louis, Mosby, 1998, pp 465–473.
4. Drake AF: Controversies in upper airway obstruction. In Bailey BJ (ed): Head and Neck Surgery– Otolaryngology. Philadelphia, Lippincott-Raven, 1998, pp 885–896.
5. Friedman EM: Tracheobronchial foreign bodies. Otol Clin North Am 33:179–186, 2000.
6. de Jong AL, Kuppersmith RB, Sulek M, Friedman EM: Vocal cord paralysis in infants and children. Otol Clin North Am 33: 131–150, 2000.
7. Larsen GL, Accurso FJ, Deterding RR, et al: Respiratory tract & mediastinum. In Hay Jr WW, et al. (eds): Current Pediatric Diagnosis and Treatment, 15th ed. New York, Lange/McGraw-Hill, 2001, pp 428–475.
8. Myer CM, Cotton RT: Pediatric airway and laryngeal problems. In Lee KJ (ed): Essential Otolaryngology–Head and Neck Surgery, 6th ed. Norwalk, CT, Appleton & Lange, 1995, pp 889–904.
9. Orenstein SR: Management of supraesophageal complications of gastroesophageal reflux disease in infants and children. Am J Med suppl 4a:139s–143s, 2000.
10. Patterson R, Harris KE: Idiopathic anaphylaxis. Allerg Asthma Proc 20(5):311–315, 1999.
11. Rencken I, Patton WL, Brasch RC: Airway obstruction in pediatric patients. From croup to BOOP. Radiol Clin North Am 36(1):175–187, 1998.
12. Silva AB: Airway manifestations of pediatric gastroesophageal reflux disease. In Wetmore, et al. (eds): Pediatric Otolaryngology. New York, Thieme, 2000, pp 619–634.
13. Sommer D, Forte V: Advances in the management of major airway collapse: The use of airway stents. Otol Clin North Am 33:163–178, 2000.
14. Wiet GJ, Long FR, Shiels II WE, Rudman DT: Advances in pediatric airway radiology. Otol Clin North Am 33:15–28, 2000.
15. Zalzal GH, Tran LP: Pediatric gastroesophageal reflux and laryngpharyngeal reflux. Otol Clin North Am 33:151–162, 2000.

68. TONSILS AND ADENOIDS

Gresham Richter, M.D. and Bruce W. Murrow M.D., Ph.D.

1. Where is Waldeyer's ring?

Waldeyer's ring is the lymphoid tissue located in the nasopharynx and oropharynx at the entrance to the aerodigestive tract. The structures composing this ring are the faucial (palatine) tonsils, pharyngeal tonsils (adenoids), lateral "bands" on the lateral wall of the oropharynx, and the lingual tonsil at the base of the tongue.

2. Where are the adenoids and tonsils located?

The adenoids are located midline along the posterior aspect of the nasopharynx at the level of the posterior chonae and extend laterally to the eustachian tube orifices. When enlarged, the adenoids can contribute to both mechanical and functional obstruction of the nose and eustachian tube. The palatine tonsils lie along the lateral wall of the oropharynx between the anterior and posterior pillars and extend from the soft palate to the tongue base. At their base, they can appear to blend into the lingual tonsil.

3. The palatine tonsils lie in a fossa produced by what three muscles?

The *palatoglossus* muscle forms the anterior pillar, and the *palatopharyngeus* muscle forms the posterior pillar. The tonsil is bound laterally by the *superior constrictor* muscle.

4. Which blood vessels supply the palatine tonsils?

The tonsils are supplied by several branches of the external carotid artery. These branches include the tonsillar (main supply) and ascending palatine branches of the facial artery, the ascending pharyngeal artery, the dorsal lingual branch of the lingual artery, and the palatine branch of the maxillary artery.

5. What is the function of the tonsils and adenoids?

The tonsils and adenoids are lymphoid structures and likely play a role in immunity. Their position is appropriate for exposure to both inhaled and ingested antigens. They are composed of B lymphocytes, primarily, and T lymphocytes. Antigen exposure can produce secretory antibodies and lymphokines. Hyperplasia is thought to result from B cell proliferation during high doses of antigen exposure. It is generally felt that removal of tonsil and adenoid tissue does not produce significant problems immunologically.

6. Can tonsils and adenoids grow back after adenotonsillectomy?

Yes. If all lymphoid tissue is not removed during surgery, the residual tissue may hypertrophy and again cause symptoms.

7. How is tonsillar hypertrophy graded?

Tonsil size is graded according to the percentage projection from the anterior tonsillar pillar toward the midline. A 1+ tonsil projects 0–25% from the anterior tonsillar pillar toward the midline; 2+ projects 25–50%; 3+ projects 50–75%; and 4+ projects 75–100% ("**kissing tonsils**").

8. At what age is adenotonsillar disease most prevalent?

Adenotonsillar disease is often considered a disease of childhood. In fact, tonsillectomies are the most common major surgical procedures performed in children. The tonsils and adenoids are most active between the ages of 4 and 10 years in response to a variety of antigenic challenges, and it is during this time that adenotonsillar disease most often occurs. Although involution begins after puberty, tonsillar disease frequently occurs in adults as well.

9. Name the most common infectious etiologic agents involved in adenotonsillar disease.

Common bacterial pathogens include group A β-hemolytic streptococci (GABHS), non-GABHS bacteria, and β-lactamase-producing organisms such as *Bacteroides,* nontypable *Haemophilus, Staphylococcus aureus,* and *Moraxella catarrhalis.* Common viral pathogens include adenovirus, coxsackievirus, parainfluenza, enteroviruses, Epstein-Barr virus, herpes simplex virus, and respiratory syncytial virus.

10. What are the symptoms and signs of tonsillitis?

Sore throat, dysphagia, enlarged erythematous tonsils with exudate, fever, halitosis, and tender cervical nodes are classic symptoms and signs of acute tonsillitis. Chronically enlarged tonsils can obstruct the oropharynx and cause snoring, obstructive sleep apnea, nocturnal coughing or choking, and voice changes. Sufficiently enlarged adenoids can obstruct the nasal choanae and eustachian tube, leading to nasal obstruction with rhinorrhea, and middle ear problems including a plugged feeling and otitis media.

11. Mononucleosis can produce exudative, swollen tonsils that appear indistinguishable from bacterial infections. What can help in the etablishment of a diagnosis?

Mononucleosis is caused by the Epstein Barr virus. A history of recent exposure and, on physical exam, generalized lymphadenopathy along with splenomegaly is consistent with mononucleosis. Useful laboratory results include increased lymphocytosis and atypical lymphocytes on the blood smear differential as well as a positive monospot and heterophil antibody titres.

12. Describe the nonsurgical treatment of adenotonsillar disease.

It is often difficult to distinguish viral from bacterial tonsillitis/pharyngitis. Most viral infections are self-limiting and require only palliative care. In fact, treatment of mononucleosis with amoxacillin can cause a rash. Still, throat cultures should be performed but, in reality, often are not. Penicillin is the initial drug of choice for culture-positive streptococcal infections.

13. When should a patient with bacterial tonsillitis be considered for surgery?
- 7 infections in 1 year
- 5 infections/year for 2 consecutive years
- 3 infections/year for 3 consecutive years
- >2 weeks missed from school or work in any 1 year

14. What are the absolute indications for tonsillectomy?
- Obstructive sleep apnea or cor pulmonale
- Malignancy or suspected malignancy
- Tonsillitis resulting in febrile convulsions
- Persistent or recurrent tonsillar hemorrhage

15. What are some relative indications for an elective tonsillectomy?
- Recurrent acute or chronic tonsillitis
- Peritonsillar abscess
- Eating or swallowing disorders
- Tonsillolithiasis
- Halitosis
- Orofacial and dental abnormalities

16. When is a tonsillectomy and adenoidectomy contraindicated?
- Blood dyscrasias (leukemias, purpuras, hemophilia, etc.)
- Uncontrolled systemic diseases (diabetes, heart disease, etc.)
- Cleft palate
- Acute infections

17. What is the most common reason for tonsillectomy?

Obstructive tonsillar hyperplasia (usually +3 and +4 lesions).

18. What surgical techniques are available for removing tonsils?

The original "**cold steel**" tonsillectomy has mostly given way to the **electrocautery (hot)** technique. In the former, a serated blade is used to "scrape" the tonsil downward, and a snare is employed to amputate the inferior pole, usually leaving significantly bleeding vessels that are then controlled. Electrocautery allows more careful coagulation of the blood vessels to the tonsil, as they are exposed during the dissection. Although hot dissection is thought to reduce perioperative blood loss, it remains controversial whether this is at the expense of prolonged postoperative pain and recovery time when compared to the cold blade technique. More recently *radiofrequency ablation* and *laser tonsillectomies* have been employed with some success in reduction of post-operative pain and bleeding. However, these techniques are still being debated.

Regardless of the tools, the basic tonsillectomy involves entry into the normally loosely ad-herant plane between the tonsillar capsule and the lateral superior constrictor muscle (peritonsi-lar space) and extricating the tonsil along this plane. Deviation from this plane into the tonsil or underlying muscle can create bothersome intraoperative bleeding. Multiple infections can ob-scure this plane and make dissection more difficult. Care is also taken to leave the anterior and posterior pillar tissue. Also, the palatine tonsils often can blend into the lingual tonsil inferiorly, and care must be taken not to "chase" the tonsillar tissue into the lingual tonsil, with potential dis-section into the vascular tongue base, which can increase the risk of postoperative bleeding.

19. Describe the symptoms and signs of adenoiditis.

The symptoms of adenoiditis are difficult to differentiate from bacterial or viral upper respi-ratory tract infections. Fever, purulent rhinorrhea, nasal obstruction, and otalgia are common. Postnasal drip, congestion, chronic cough, and halitosis can also occur during chronic infections. Moreover, patients often present with snoring, mouth breathing, "adenoidal facies," and symp-toms of otitis media or sinusitis during chronic infections with secondary nasopharyngeal ob-struction.

20. What is the appearance of the classic "adenoidal facies"?

Adenoidal facies are characterized by an open mouth, nasal-mental elongation, flattened mid-face, and dark circles under the eyes.

21. What treatment is available for adenoiditis or adenoid hypertrophy?

Medical treatment of infectious adenitis is the same as for tonsillitis. **Nasal steroids** can be used to treat adenoid hypertrophy that causes nasal obstruction. Adenoiditis that is not appropri-ately responsive to medical treatment can be treated surgically with **adenoidectomy.** Under gen-eral anesthesia and indirect visualization with a mirror, an adenoid curette is placed intraorally and seated superorily to the adenoid pad An inferior movement of the curette "cuts" the adenoids free. Care is taken to stay mostly midline and avoid injury to the lateral torus tubaris (opening to the eustachian tube). Residual adenoid tissue can by removed with an adenoid punch, also under indirect observation with a mirror. Hemostasis is undertaken via a combination of pressure from "tonsil packs" placed in the nasopharynx and electrocautery. Alternatively, electrocautery using a suction bovie can be used alone to remove or shrink the adenoid tissue. Regardless of the method, the goal is to remove adenoidal obstruction of the posterior choanae.

22. What are some proposed indications for adenoidectomy?

- Recurrent or chronic middle ear disease
- Obstructive adenoid hypertrophy
- Obligate mouth breathing or snoring
- Recurrent acute or chronic adenoiditis
- Sleep apnea

23. What does the postoperative management of adenotonsillectomy involve?

The patient and parents of children should be told to expect pain, postoperative bleeding, tem-porary weight loss, and halitosis. Pain is always an issue, and good pain control is a necessity to promote oral intake and minimize dehydration. In addition, oral antibiotics have been shown to decrease postoperative pain in children. If bleeding occurs, it should be brought to the attention of the physician; if significant, it will require an office or emergency department (ED) visit with evaluation by an ENT physician. A soft-food diet is recommended. Patients should not participate in heavy activity for 2 weeks after the procedure. Although tonsillectomies and adenoidectomies are commonly performed as outpatient surgeries, it is wise to admit patients with complicated cases, especially if the procedure is done for obstructive sleep apnea.

24. What are the complications of tonsillectomy and adenoidectomy?

- Bleeding (up to 2 weeks after procedure)
- Airway obstruction
- Dehydration and weight loss
- Velopharyngeal insufficiency
- Pulmonary edema (especially after relief of obstruction)
- Death

25. What is the incidence of postoperative tonsillectomy bleeding and mortality associated with tonsillectomy?

Postoperative bleeding ranges from 0.1% to 8%, depending on severity. Mortality is usually reported around .002% and is mostly due to anesthetic complications and postoperative hemorrage, usually within the first 24 hours after surgery.

26. How is postoperative bleeding managed?

Postoperative bleeding generally occurs either soon after the procedure, while the patient is still in the hospital, or within the first 2 weeks after the procedure. Carefully examine the tonsillar fossae (including the most inferior aspect adjacent to the tongue), looking for active bleeding sites or evidence of clot. About 5 days after the surgery, when the eschar sloughs off from the tonsillar fossae, a small number of **blood streaks** may be found in the spit; if only temporary, they may be managed with observation. With more **significant bleeding that has currently stopped,** particularly if a child (lower blood volume than adult), the patient can be admitted overnight to the hospital with observation and preparedness (NPO status) to take the patient to the operating room (OR) in case of abrupt re-bleeding. If **active bleeding** is encountered, it should be stopped. Some cases can be adequately handled with some type of cauterization in the office or ED if the bleeding point is easily identifiable and the patient is cooperative (rarely a child). Otherwise, the patient should be taken to the OR for control of the bleeding, which may include electrical cauterization and/ or suturing. Note that when a patient comes to the ED with a post-tonsilliectomy bleed, he or she should be examined by an otolaryngologist, not just the ED doctors.

27. Why can velopharyngeal insufficiency occur after adenoidectomy?

Velopharyngeal insufficiency (VPI) occurs when there is incomplete closure of the soft palate against the posterior pharyngeal wall. This is manifest by hypernasal speech and nasopharyngeal regurgitation. In children, adenoid tissue significantly adds to the bulk of the posterior pharyngeal wall. The soft palate abuts against this wall during speech and swallowing. An adenoidectomy reduces this bulk and can lead to incomplete closure, resulting in VPI.

28. What is the frequency of post-surgical VPI?

Different studies show the incidence of VPI after adenoidectomy to range from 1/1500 to 1/10,000 in normal patients. The incidence of VPI in patients with palatal disorders, such as submucous cleft, is much higher.

29. On examination, you see a bifid uvula. Is it safe to proceed with adenotonsillectomy?

The presence of a bifid uvula has been associated with various disorders of the soft palate. *Submucous cleft* is the most common of these disorders. Adenotonsillectomy with a submucous cleft leads to a higher incidence of *velopharyngeal insufficiency.* Carefully evaluate the palate prior to tonsillectomy and adenoidectomy in *any* patient, but pay special attention to patients with a bifid uvula. If a submucous cleft is encountered, some feel that a "superior" adenoidectomy can be performed. This adaptation leaves some bulk in the posterior pharyngeal wall, allowing adequate velopharyngeal closure after surgery.

30. In patients with extensive adenotonsillar tissue obstructing the airway, what pulmonary problem may occur after adenotonsillectomy?

Pulmonary edema may develop. The long-term obstruction by adenotonsillar tissue produces a state of increased PEEP (positive end-expiratory pressure). After removal of the obstructing tissue, the excess PEEP is relieved suddenly, and fluid can move into the interstitual and alveolar spaces, resulting in a picture of pulmonary edema with decreased blood oxygen saturation. This can occur intraoperatively or a few hours later. Treatment involves diruesis for mild cases, or intubation with re-establishment of increased PEEP in more severe cases.

31. What is a peritonsillar abscess?

A peritonsillar abscess is a collection of pus in the potential space that surrounds the tonsil, between the tonsillar capsule and the superior constrictor muscle of the lateral pharyngeal wall. This process develops as an infection in a peripheral tonsillar crypt that penetrates through the tonsillar capsule and enters the peritonsillar space. Over half of patients who present with peritonsillar abscess have a history of previous tonsillar infections. The bacterial makeup of these infections is mixed aerobic and anerobic pathogens.

32. What are the typical signs and symptoms of a peritonsillar abscess?

Patients with peritonsillar abscess usually have a history of a sore throat for at least 3–4 days, with fever, dysphagia, odynophagia, and a "hot potato" or muffled voice, as well as trismus (decreased ability to open mouth) and drooling. Airway obstruction is uncommon. Examination reveals an inflamed oropharynx with infected, swollen tonsils. The peritonsillar area, usually unilaterally, is also inflamed and swollen, with a bulge in the soft palate superior to the tonsil and displacement of the uvula toward the contralateral side, away from the midline. Occasionally, fluctuance is demonstrated on palpation.

33. How is a peritonsillar abscess managed?

Needle aspiration with recovery of pus can be diagnostic and therapeutic, but incision with drainage is usually the definitive approach. Care must be taken to avoid injury to the closely positioned carotid artery, especially with distorted anatomy from the swelling. These procedures are performed in the office or ED. After drainage, broad-spectrum antibiotics with strong anerobic coverage, such as clindamycin, are recommended. Some recommend that if the patient has had a prior peritonsillar abscess, a tonsillectomy should be considered after complete resolution of the infection.

CONTROVERSIES

34. Is it safe to perform an adenotonsillectomy as an outpatient procedure for uncomplicated patients?

Those who advocate that this procedure be performed on an outpatient basis feel that it is more cost-effective. They also cite a low incidence of major postoperative complications. In opposition, others argue that an adenotonsillectomy is a major surgery fraught with serious postoperative complications; these complications are best handled in the inpatient setting. Criteria for overnight stay include children who are vomiting or experiencing postoperative bleeding, have poor oral intake, live $> 30–45$ minutes from the hospital, come from neglected environments, have other medical problems, or are < 3 years old.

35. How old should the patient be before undergoing adenotonsillectomy?

There is no set age, but several studies show an increased incidence of complications with children < 3 years of age. When indicated, tonsillectomy and adenoidectomy (T&A) are viable options for this age group, but both parents and physicians need to be aware of the increased complication rate. Patients in this age group are probably not candidates for routine outpatient surgery.

36. What is the role of antibiotic and steroid administration following T&A?

Several studies show earlier recovery, less postoperative pain, and fewer complications with the use of antibiotics and steroids following T&A. Other studies show no significant difference. Advocates of their use cite minimal adverse effects in the face of potential benefits. Opponents cite unnecessary costs, development of resistant bacterial strains, and potential complications.

37. What is the relationship between *prions* and tonsils? How does this affect the ENT surgeon?

Prions are proteinaceous, infectious agents capable of invading the CNS and leading eventually to progressive dementia (i.e., Cruetzfedt-Jacob Disease; vCJD). These agents have recently been described to also accumulate within lymphoreticular tissue. Tonsillar biopsy specimens of patients with vCJD also show extensive prion invasion. Instrument-to-patient transmission has been described, and prions contaminating surgical instruments have proven to be resistant to standard sterilization techniques. Because the incidence of vCJD is unknown, and considering the number of tonsillectomies performed each year, tonsillectomy instruments may pose a substantial risk to patients *and* surgeons for acquiring vCJD. Disposable tonsillectomy trays have been proposed, but remain a debated issue. Nonetheless, ENT surgeons asked to perform tonsil biopsies on potential vCJD patients should exercise extreme caution and sterile technique with disposable instruments.

PEDIATRIC PULMONARY EDEMA
POST TONSILLECTOMY AND ADENOIDECTOMY

Negative-pressure pulmonary edema (NPPE) continues to be reported as a complication of prolonged upper airway obstruction seen by anesthesia providers during induction or emergence from T&A. The majority of patients reported to have experienced NPPE have been healthy, without underlying pulmonary or cardiac disease. Factors associated with the occurrence of NPPE include young, male patients and patients with long periods of airway obstruction (e.g., markedly hypertrophic tonsils and adenoids). Overzealous intraoperative fluid administration and preexisting heart and lung disease also have been implicated as predisposing factors. NPPE is the result of a marked decrease in intrathoracic pressure caused by ventilatory efforts against an upper airway obstruction in a disruption of the normal intravascular Starling mechanism, ultimately leading to the transudation of intravascular proteins and fluid into the pulmonary interstitium. The onset of NPPE is usually rapid, and without prompt recognition and intervention, the outcome can be fatal.

~Thomas, AANA Journal 67:425, 1999

BIBLIOGRAPHY

1. Bhaskar K: Diet following tonsillectomy. Pediatr Nurs 10:25–7, 1998.
2. Brodsky L: Tonsillitis, tonsillectomy, and adenoidectomy. In Bailey B, Calhoun K (eds): Head and Neck Surgery–Otolaryngology, 2nd ed. Philadelphia, Lippincott-Raven Publishers, 1998, pp 441–454.
3. Burton MJ, Towler B, Glasziou P: Tonsillectomy versus non-surgical treatment for chronic / recurrent

acute tonsillitis. Cochrane Database of Systematic Reviews [computer file]. (2):CD001802, 2000.

4. Casselbrant ML: What is wrong in chronic adenoiditis/tonsilitis anatomical consideration. Int J Ped ORL 49 (supp 1): S133-S135, 1999.
5. Frosh A: Prions and the ENT surgeon. J Laryngol Otol 113:1064–1067, 1999
6. Hatton RC: Bismuth subgallate-epinephrine paste in adenotonsillectomies. Ann Pharmacother 34:522–5, 2000.
7. Hellier WP, Knight J, Hern J, et al: Day case paediatric tonsillectomy: A review of three years experience in a dedicated day case unit. Clin Otolaryngol Allied Sci 24:208–12, 1999.
8. Hollis LJ, Burton MJ, Millar JM: Perioperative local anaesthesia for reducing pain following tonsillectomy. Cochrane Database of Systematic Reviews [computer file]. (2):CD001874, 2000.
9. Hultcrantz E, Linder A, Markstrom A, : Tonsillectomy or tonsillotomy? A randomized study comparing postoperative pain and long-term effects. Int J Ped ORL 51:171–76, 1999.
10. Marshall T: A review of tonsillectomy for recurrent throat infection [see comments]. Br J Gen Pract 48:1331–5, 1998.
11. Maw R: Re-evaluating the ENT procedures. Practitioner 244:608, 612–4, 617, 2000.
12. Nelson LM: Radiofrequency treatment of obstructive tonsillar hypertrophy. Arch Otolaryngol Head Neck Surg 126:736–740, 2000.
13. Nicklaus PJ, Herzon FS, Steinle EW: Short stay outpatient tonsillectomy. Arch Otolaryngol Head Neck Surg 121:521, 1995.
14. Nunez DA, Provan J, Crawford M: Postoperative tonsillectomy pain in pediatric patients. Arch Otolaryng Head Neck Surg 126:837–41, 2000.
15. Peeters A, Van Rompaey D, Schmelzer B, et al: Tonsillectomy and adenotomy as a one day procedure? Acta ORL Belgica 53:91–7, 1999.
16. Randall DA and Hoffer ME. Complications of thonsillectomy and adenoidectomy. Otolaryngol Head Neck Surg 118: 61–68, 1998.
17. Richardson MA: Sore throat, tonsillitis, and adenoiditis. Med Clin North Am 83:75–83, 1999.
18. Strachan DP, Cook DG: Health effects of passive smoking. 4. Parental smoking, middle ear disease and adenotonsillectomy in children. Thorax 53:50–56, 1998.

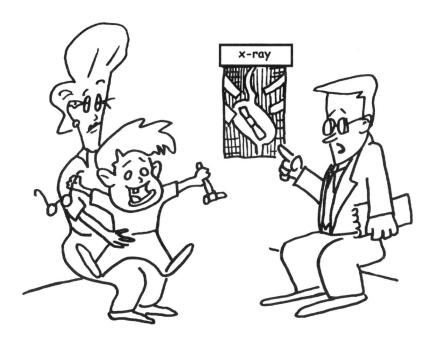

**"The good news is that we can retrieve the lipstick.
The bad news is that your plan doesn't cover cosmetic surgery."**

Jim Gough

69. CONGENITAL MALFORMATIONS

Michelle Stanford, M.D. and Kenny H. Chan, M.D.

1. How does the differential diagnosis of a congenital neck mass differ with its location?

Common congenital neck lesions that are centrally located include thyrogolossal duct and dermoid cysts. Laterally located congenital neck masses include branchial anomalies and lymphangiomas.

2. How does a branchial fistula form? A branchial cyst? A branchial sinus?

The branchial apparatus consists of five mesodermal arches, of which the first three are clinically significant. On the external wall, these arches are lined with ectodermal grooves or clefts; on the internal wall, they are lined with endoderm pouches. Each arch contains a cartilaginous portion, an artery, nerve, and musculature that begins to develop in the fourth week. As the structures within each arch proliferate, a cervical sinus forms. The cervical sinus eventually is obliterated by the growth of the surrounding structures.

Of all of the branchial arches, the second arch is the most commonly malformed. A **branchial sinus** is open into the skin or lumen of the foregut and ends blindly in the deep tissues of the neck. A **branchial fistula** is caused by the persistence of an internal and external opening. A **branchial cyst** occurs when the cervical sinus remains patent and the external opening is obliterated; this malformation is more commonly seen in adults.

3. What are the possible complications of a lymphangioma?

Cervical lymphangiomas, also known as **cystic hygromas,** do not usually produce symptoms, although the cosmetic deformity is often of concern. Large lymphangiomas in the anterior neck can cause **airway** or pharyngeal **compression.** These cystic spaces can also become infected, forming an **abscess. Hemorrhage** into the cyst may also occur. A lymphangioma often presents when it becomes associated with infection or hemorrhage.

4. Why does a thyroglossal duct cyst move on swallowing?

A thyroglossal duct cyst is a remnant of the thyroid gland's descent from the foramen cecum, at the base of the tongue, to the pretracheal space. Because of the close proximity to the hyoid bone superiorly and the attachment to the thyroid gland inferiorly, the lesion moves during swallowing. Thyroglossal duct cysts are the most common anterior midline neck masses in children. These masses must be removed because they have the potential for neoplastic transformation.

5. Compare a teratoma and a dermoid cyst.

Both are anomalies involving pluripotential embryonal cells. Teratomas are composed of all three germ layers and are much larger than dermoid cysts. Dermoid cysts are composed of ectoderm and mesoderm and tend to occur along the lines of embryonic fusion (midline). Dermoid cysts characteristically have an adipose matrix that appears "cheesy." Dermoid cysts do not exclusively occur in the neck.

6. Name the six types of tracheoesophageal fistulas.

- Isolated esophageal atresia without fistula (6–7%)
- Esophageal atresia with proximal tracheoesophageal fistula (1%)
- Esophageal atresia with distal tracheoesophageal fistula (86%)
- Esophageal atresia with proximal and distal tracheoesophageal fistula (1–5%)
- Tracheoesophageal fistula without atresia (5%), also called H-type
- Esophageal stenosis without fistula (1%)

In cases of atresia, the presentation is usually the inability to swallow, excess salivation, and

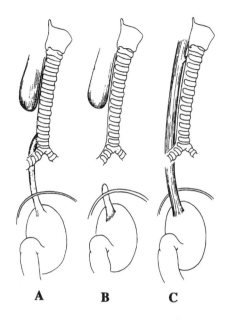

Esophageal atresia. *A,* The most common form of esophageal atresia (85%) consists of a dilated proximal esophageal pouch and a connection of the distal esophagus to he carina of the trachea. *B,* Pure esophageal atresia. *C,* Fistula of the H-type without atresia. (From Coran AG (ed): Surgery of the Neonate. Boston, Little, Brown, 1978, p 46, with permission.)

A   B   C

episodes of coughing and cyanosis in the first few days of life. The presentation depends on the severity of the atresia. The H-type often presents later, with recurrent problems with pneumonia, coughing when fed, or abdominal distention.

7. Which is the most common malformation associated with the supraglottis?

Of the structures in the upper aerodigestive tract, the larynx is the most commonly affected with anomalies. Affecting the supraglottis, laryngomalacia is a congenital flaccid larynx that is diagnosed by high-pitched stridor. The problem is usually self-limited, and treatment is unnecessary.

8. What are the most common malformations of the glottis?

The glottis may be affected by **unilateral vocal cord paralysis,** usually a self-limited condition. When **bilateral vocal cord paralysis** occurs, a thorough work-up should be performed to rule out other concurrent malformations (i.e., Arnold-Chiari syndrome). **Webs** usually affect the anterior part of the glottis and cause aphonia. **Posterior clefts** are rare, but occur because the tracheoesophageal septum fails to develop.

9. What are the two most common malformations of the subglottis?

Congenital stenosis of the subglottis is generally secondary to a deformed cricoid cartilage. Stenosis is defined by an anteroposterior diameter of < 4 mm in the newborn. A **hemangioma** of the subglottic area usually presents in the third or fourth week of life. Spontaneous regression of these lesions can occur. When the lesion is obstructing the airway, treatment includes systemic corticosteriod, tracheotomy, and surgical removal.

10. What are the two groups of tracheal malformations? What causes them?

Intrinsic malformations are caused by maldevelopment of the trachea. Some examples of intrinsic malformations include tracheal agenesis, stenosis (hypoplasia), tracheomalacia, tracheomegaly, and tracheal diverticula.

Extrinsic malformations are secondary to compression of the airway from the structures that surround it. Causes include vascular (i.e., innominate artery compression or other aberrant malformations, such as a double aortic arch or aberrant right subclavian artery), masses in the neck and mediastinum, and an enlarged thyroid.

11. Describe the common congenital malformations of the auricle.

The most common malformations of the auricle are microtia, preauricular cysts, and canal atresia. **Microtia** is hypoplasia of the external ear. It can be associated with or without **atresia** of the external auditory canal. It may be present as an isolated deformity or may be accompanied by hemifacial or bilateral facial microsomia. There are three types of microtia. In *grade I,* the auricle is misshapen, but the landmarks are recognizable. In *grade II,* the auricle is hook-shaped or looks like a question mark. In *grade III,* only one or two protuberances mark the position of the lobule. Current therapy for microtia is reconstructive surgery using an autologous rib graft for the framework in a multistage operation. With the advent of bone-anchored hearing devices to correct conductive hearing loss secondary to canal atresia, alternative treatment consists of implanting additional osseous-integrating posts for the attachment of a prosthesis.

A **preauricular pit/cyst** is a remnant of the first branchial or pharyngeal groove. Surgical excision is required when chronic drainage or infections occur.

12. Explain the anomalies of the first branchial groove.

The first branchial groove gives rise to the external auditory canal (EAC). Anomalies are divided into aplasia, atresia, stenosis, and duplication of the EAC. **Aplasia** occurs when the first branchial groove does not develop. The groove usually persists as a tract. **Atresia** anomalies occur when the EAC is present, but the lumen is not. The lumen is blocked by bone, fibrous tissue, or both. **Stenosis** occurs when the lumen is narrowed, which occurs in varying degrees of severity. **Duplication** occurs when the EAC develops normally, but the tract persists from the canal to the skin of the neck.

13. What are the common congenital malformations of the nose?
- Choanal atresia
- Dermoid cysts
- Nasal gliomas and encephaloceles

14. How do gliomas and encephaloceles differ?

Both gliomas and encephaloceles comprise ectodermal neural tissue of the brain that has remained in the nasal cavity or nasopharynx following embryologic development. Encephaloceles are herniated glial tissue that always maintain the communication with the CSF. They are differentiated from gliomas by the presence of a defect in the cranium that allows for the herniation to occur. Unlike encephaloceles, gliomas are not always connected to the CSF.

15. What anomalies commonly occur with choanol atresia?

Choanal atresia is the most common nasal anomaly. Atresia of the nares can be unilateral or bilateral, bony or membranous, and complete or incomplete. Bilateral atresia is a serious and life-threatening airway emergency. Most choanal atresia occurs along with other anomalies; hence the CHARGE mnemonic:

    C Coloboma
    H Heart disease
    A Atresia, choanal
    R Retarded development of the CNS
    G Genital hypoplasia
    E Ear anomalies or deafness

16. How do cup ear deformities and prominent ear deformities differ?

A **cup ear deformity** is a congenital malformation of the auricle in which the upper and middle portions are abnormal and the lower portion is normal. The upper portion is bent forward and downward. The middle portion is generally large and at a 90° angle from the skull. It can be present in various degrees of severity. In a **prominent ear deformity,** the child has protruding ears. Measured from the mastoid to the ear, an angle of $> 40°$ or a distance of > 20 mm characteristically exists. Both cup ear and prominent ear deformities can be improved with reconstructive surgery.

CONTROVERSIES

17. Is preoperative imaging required before removing a midline anterior neck mass?

An ectopic thyroid can be the only functioning thyroid tissue present in a patient. It can also mimic a thyroglossal duct cyst. Injudicious removal of an ectopic thyroid may result in permanent thyroid replacement therapy for a patient. Therefore, ongoing controversy revolves around obtaining a preoperative radionuclide scan and/or a sonogram of the neck before operative intervention.

18. Explain the two theories of congenital cholesteatoma formation.

Theory 1—The more commonly approved theory states that an ectodermal cell rest remains behind the tympanic membrane in the postnatal period. Proliferation of these cell rests results in the formation of a cholesteatoma (cyst-like mass that is filled with desquamating debris).

Theory 2—Most children with cholesteatoma have had otitis media with an effusion. This theory states that the cholesteatoma is the result of metaplasia secondary to middle ear inflammation.

BIBLIOGRAPHY

1. Brown Rl, Azizkhan Rg: Pediatric Head And Neck Lesions. Pediatr Clin North Am 45:889–905, 1998.
2. Coppit GL III, Perkins JA, Manning SC: Nasopharyngeal teratomas and dermoids: A review of the literature and case series. Int J Ped ORL 52:219–27, 2000.
3. Drolet BA, Esterly NB, Frieden IJ: Hemangiomas in children [see comments]. New Engl J Med 341:173–81, 1999.
4. Dubois J, Garel L: Imaging and therapeutic approach of hemangiomas and vascular malformations in the pediatric age group. Ped Radiol 29:879–93, 1999.
5. Gallagher PG, Mahoney MJ, Gosche JR: Cystic hygroma in the fetus and newborn. Semin Perinatol 23:341–56, 1999.
6. Ghaneim A, Atkins P: The management of thyroglossal duct cysts. Int J Clin Pract 51:512–3, 1997.
7. Josephson GD, Spencer WR, Josephson JS: Thyroglossal duct cyst: The New York Eye and Ear Infirmary experience and a literature review. ENT J 77:642–4, 646–7, 651, 1998.
8. Organ GM, Organ CH Jr: Thyroid gland and surgery of the thyroglossal duct: exercise in applied embryology. Wrld J Surg 24:886–90, 2000.
9. Paczona R, Jori J, Czigner J: Pharyngeal localizations of branchial cysts. Eur Arch ORL 255:379–81, 1998.
10. Rohrich RJ, Lowe JB, Schwartz MR: The role of open rhinoplasty in the management of nasal dermoid cysts. Plast Reconst Surg 104:1459–66; quiz 1467; discussion 1468, 1999.
11. Sie KC, Tampakopoulou DA; Hemangiomas and vascular malformations of the airway. Otol Clin North Am 33:209–20, 2000.
12. Wagner RB: The history of mediastinal teratoma. Chest Surg Clin North Am 10:213–22, xi, 2000.
13. Woodruff WW, Kennedy TL: Non-nodal neck masses. Semin Ultrasound CT MR 18:182–204, 1997.

70. GENETIC ISSUES IN OTOLARYNGOLOGY

Anne L. Matthews, R.N., Ph.D. and Nathaniel H. Robin, M.D.

1. What are the major inheritance patterns for single gene disorders?

Autosomal dominant (AD): Only a single copy of the mutated gene is needed for expression of the phenotype. "Autosomal" means the abnormal gene is carried on one of the non-sex-linked chromosomes, numbers 1 through 22. Often, the disease is present in many generations of a family. When one parent has the disease, the risk for passing on the mutant gene is 50% in each pregnancy.

Autosomal recessive: Two copies of the mutated gene are needed for expression of the phenotype. In such cases, both parents are always carriers, and therefore have a 25% risk that each future pregnancy will result in a child with the same disease. Usually there is no family history of the disease in multiple generations, but it may be seen among siblings.

X-linked: The abnormal gene is carried on the X chromosome. Most X-linked disorders are **recessive,** implying that a female who carries the mutant X-linked gene is normal because she has a second normal gene on her other X chromosome. However, a carrier female has a 50% chance of having an affected son, and a 50% chance of having a carrier daughter. Men with X-linked recessive disorders have carrier daughters and normal sons.

Some X-linked genetic traits manifest problems in both men and women who carry the mutant gene. These are called X-linked **dominant** disorders because the abnormal X-linked gene's effect is dominant over the corresponding normal gene on the other X chromosome. Males are usually more severely affected than females, and in some cases the disease is lethal in males, so only females may be observed with the particular disease. Both daughters and sons of women with X-linked dominant traits have a 50% chance of inheriting the abnormal gene. Affected men can only pass the trait to their daughters, and in every case, the daughter is affected.

2. For AD diseases, why is it so hard to identify which family members are affected?

Expressivity and **penetrance**. Ideally, the same phenotype or condition would be evident in all affected members in a classic dominant family history. In reality, however, dominant diseases vary in how they manifest. This is called **variable expressivity**. Another important concept is penetrance. **Reduced penetrance** means that a carrier of a dominant gene may not have any detectable phenotypic expression.

Lastly, many AD diseases are the result of **new mutations.** In these cases, the mutation in the affected individual is thought to have occurred in the egg or sperm that formed him or her, with both parents being normal. Clinically, a person may be affected with a dominant disorder and have a documented negative family history. With each pregnancy, the individual who is affected by the mutation has a 50% risk of transmitting the abnormal gene to each offspring, but the risk to the parents is below 1% in most cases.

3. Multifactorial genetic inheritance is supposed to be the most common cause for most isolated congenital malformations, such as isolated cleft lip and/or palate. What does this mean?

Many common disorders run in families, but they are not associated with single-gene, chromosomal, or teratogenic factors. Because these traits are caused by many factors, both genetic and environmental, they are called multifactorial. Multifactorial disorders recur within families at a rate above what would be expected by chance alone, but below that for a single gene trait. A geneticist can estimate the approximate heritability, or the importance of genetic factors in a given trait, and recurrence risks. The empiric risk to first-degree relatives, as determined by family studies, is approximately the square root of the population risk. As expected, the recurrence risk is greater when > 1 family member is affected. Similarly, the more severe the malformation, the greater the recurrence risk. In many multifactorial traits, one sex is more frequently affected for reasons that are not always understood. For example, cleft lip is more common in males than females. Therefore, a female with a cleft lip has a greater chance than a male with a cleft lip of having a child with a cleft lip.

4. What are the indications for obtaining chromosome studies?

Reasonable criteria for obtaining cytogenetic studies are the presence of two major malformations, or a single major malformation with two or more minor malformations. A major malformation is an anomaly that has a significant effect on an individual's health, while a minor anomaly refers to a medically insignificant departure from normal development. The likelihood of finding a cytogenetically detectable abnormality is approximately 1–3% in a child with one major and two or more minor anomalies.

Note that chromosome analysis with fragile X testing should be considered in every child with developmental delay and/or mental retardation, even in the absence of other abnormalities.

Minor Anomalies	Major Malformations
High-arched palate	Growth retardation
Cleft uvula	Mental retardation/developmental delay
Wide-set eyes	Sensorineural hearing impairment
Abnormal slant of palpebral fissures	Congenital heart defects
Micrognathia	Spina bifida
Short/abnormally shaped fingers	Genitourinary malformations
Hernia	Cleft lip with/without cleft palate
Pectus excavatum/carinatum	Cleft palate alone
Large auricles	Microcephaly
Short neck	Absent or hypoplastic ears
Synophrys	Renal anomalies/absent kidney
Abnormal fingerprints and hand creases	Eye anomalies/blindness

5. Is cleft lip with or without a cleft palate really a different anomaly than cleft palate alone?

Yes. While affecting related structures, these are distinct entities based on developmental, genetic, and clinical data. First, cleft lip with or without a cleft palate (CLP) and cleft palate alone (CPA) arise from distinct defects at different embryologic ages. CLP is caused by a failure of fusion of the fronotnasal prominence with the lateral prominences at approximately 6 weeks, while CPA is caused by a failure of fusion of the lateral palatine ridges at approximately 9 weeks gestation. Furthermore, a parent with a CLP has an elevated chance of having a child with a CLP, but not CPA. For CLP, the recurrence risk ranges from 1–7%, depending on the sex of the affected parent and the severity of CLP (unilateral cleft lip, for example, has a lower recurrence risk than bilateral cleft lip and palate).

6. What are the syndromes I should be concerned about in a child with a cleft lip and or palate?

When a child with a cleft is encountered, conduct a genetic evaluation. It is important to ensure that the defect is isolated and not part of a syndrome. Approximately 10–25% of CLP is associated with a genetic syndrome. In contrast, 25–40% of cleft palates without cleft lips are associated with genetic syndromes.

There are numerous genetic syndromes that have CLP and CPA as one finding. Below are some that are important to keep in mind because they are relatively common:

Cleft Lip With/Without Cleft Palate	Cleft Palate Alone
Trisomy 13	Velocardiofacial syndrome
Wolff-Hirschhorn syndrome (4p-)	Stickler syndrome
Opitz G syndrome	Apert syndrome
Oral-facial-digital syndrome	Treacher Collins syndrome
Van der Woude syndrome	Van der Woude syndrome

7. What is Pierre Robin sequence? How is it different from cleft palate alone?

Pierre Robin sequence occurs in about 1 in 30,000 births and affects both males and females equally. Although its inheritance is most likely multifactorial, it can occur as part of a syndrome. The initiating defect of Pierre Robin sequence may be hypoplasia of the mandibular area prior to 9 weeks gestation. This hypoplasia restrains the tongue posteriorly, thus impairing closure of the posterior palatal shelves at the midline. Cardinal features of this sequence include striking micrognathia, glossoptosis, and cleft palate. Newborns with Pierre Robin are at risk of apnea due to an obstructed airway. It is important to recognize that approximately half of Pierre Robin sequence is part of a genetic syndrome. The most common syndromes are Stickler syndrome (50%; see Question 19) and velocardiofacial syndrome (25%; see Question 9).

8. What is van der Woude syndrome, and why is it on both lists?

Van der Woude syndrome (VDWS) is an AD disorder that is characterized by CLP, CPA, and lip pits. This is an extremely variable disorder. Within a family, there may be affected individuals with only lower lip pits (these are actually accessory salivary glands), and others with CLP or CPA. The occurence of **mixed clefting type** (CLP and CPA in the same family) sets VDWS apart from nearly all other syndromes with clefting. Other conditions that feature mixed clefting type include Rapp-Hodgkin, Hay-Wells, and ectodermal dysplasia-ectrodactyly-clefting syndromes.

9. What is velocardiofacial syndrome (VCFS)?

VCF is an AD disorder that is characterized by velopharyngeal insufficiency or cleft palate, hypernasal speech, behavioral or psychiatric problems, learning disabilities, conotruncal heart defects, and characteristic facial appearance. It is caused by a deletion in chromosome 22q11 (del22q11). While in approximately one-third of cases this deletion is visible on routine chromosome analysis, for two-thirds it is detectable only through specialized testing, called FISH (fluorescence in-situ hybridization). VCFS is really one representation of the spectrum of conditions caused by this chromosome deletion. When accompanied by hypocalcemia and thymic hypoplasia, it is called **DiGeorge syndrome.** It has an incidence of 1 in 2–4000, making it the most common microdeletion syndrome.

10. What is choanal atresia?

Embryologically, the bucconasal membrane ruptures at the seventh week of gestation. If this rupture fails to occur, the primitive nasal cavity does not communicate with the pharynx, resulting in choanal atresia. The incidence of this malformation is 1 in 5000 live births. Choanal atresia affects females to males in a 2:1 ratio. In 90% of cases, the defect is a bony atresia, with the remaining 10% being membranous. Although this disorder is usually unilateral and diagnosed later in life, bilateral atresia is usually recognized in the neonatal period. Because newborns are obligate nose breathers, those affected by a bilateral atresia exhibit cyanosis.

11. How does lop or cup ear occur?

Lop or cup ear defect represents one of the most common malformations of the external ear. It can be seen as an isolated trait, or as one finding in a child with a genetic syndrome. As an isolated entity, lop/cup ear has an incidence of 1 in 1000 births, and it is inherited as an AD trait. In this disorder, hypoplasia of the superior one-third of the auricle causes a downward folding and deficiency of the superior aspect of the helix. Most of the auricle originates from the second branchial arch. The tragus and a small part of the helix arise from the first branchial arch. If the antihelix fails to unfold between the 12th and 16th weeks of development, a protruding helix persists, resulting in lop or cup ear.

The mildest form of this defect may be the result of intrauterine constraint and will resolve in the first year of life. Otherwise, the lop/cup ear can be surgically corrected in severe cases. Among these cases have been a few reports of nonsyndromic lop/cup ear defects that are seen as an AD trait in families. Rarely, the lop or cup ear is associated with a genetic syndrome.

12. What is the significance of auricular tags?

Auricular appendages or tags are common, minor anomalies that are usually located just anterior to the auricle near the tragus. When multiple, auricular tags often follow a line of predilection where the first and second branchial arches join. In most cases, auricular tags are as an isolated finding, but they can be seen as part of many genetic syndromes, such as oculo-auriculo-vertebral spectrum (Goldenhar syndrome), which usually includes auricular tags. One study reported that approximately 2% of individuals with auricular tags have some associated syndrome. Another report found that among neonates who had an isolated ear tag, 13% had some degree of sensorineural hearing impairment. Therefore, it is reasonable to do hearing screens in all children with this finding.

13. What are the most common causes of congenital hearing impairment? Perinatal hearing loss? Postnatal hearing loss?

A common **prenatal** (intrauterine) cause of hearing loss is intrauterine infection. Low birthweight and microcephaly are often associated with such infections. In these cases, an ophthalmologic evaluation may reveal chorioretinitis. **Perinatal** (caused at the time of birth) causes of hearing impairment may be due to hypoxia, hyperbilirubinemia, infection, and ototoxic drugs. A sloping high-frequency hearing loss is suggestive of a perinatal etiology. The major **postnatal** cause of severe to profound sensorineural deafness is bacterial meningitis.

14. What does "Capital D Deaf" mean?

The term "deaf" implies a severe to profound hearing inability. "Capital D Deaf" refers to a group of individuals who are hard of hearing or deaf and who do not consider their deafness a disease or a handicap. Members of the Deaf community embrace their hearing inability as part of their identity, shared history, and social customs. Many members of the Deaf community have a negative attitude toward medicine because they believe that medicine's primary goal is to "fix" their auditory inability. To the Deaf, this perceived attitude is inappropriate and paternalistic, and they view medicine as a threat to their community. These negative attitudes extend to cochlear implants, genetic testing, and genetic research.

"Hearing loss" implies that an individual had hearing at some point, so the term "hearing impairment" is used by health professionals as a general term to denote any level of hearing inability. Individuals with a diminished hearing ability prefer the term "hard of hearing."

15. How much of hearing impairment is due to genetic factors?

To answer this question, we must first divide hearing impairment by the age of onset. **Prelingual hearing impairment** is that which occurs before language acquisition, or age 3 years. This has an incidence of 1/1000 babies, and is divided into syndromic and nonsyndromic forms. Approximately one-third of pediatric hearing impairment is part of a genetic syndrome. Of nonsyndromic hearing impairment, recent studies estimate that 60–80% is due to genetic factors, with the remainder due to environmental causes, most commonly unidentified congenital infections. Autosomal recessive is most common, accounting for approximately 85%, with autosomal dominant making up most of the rest.

The percentage of **progressive and adult-onset hearing loss** that is genetic is less well characterized, but autosomal dominant is most common, and the amount of mitochondrially inherited deafness is probably underrecognized.

Note that 90–95% of hearing impairment occurs without a family history, and that the lack of a family history does *not* exclude a genetic basis for the hearing impairment.

16. What is the most common genetic cause of pediatric nonsyndromic hearing loss?

Mutations in *GJB2*, the gene for Connexin 26 (CX26), cause approximately 30% of cases of sporadic hearing impairment, and over 50% of cases in which there is an affected sibling. Studies have shown that approximately 1 in 31 American Caucasians carry a Cx26 mutation, with Ashkenazi Jews having an even higher carrier rate. One particular Cx26 mutation, called 35delG, accounts for two-thirds of all mutations in non-Ashkenazi Jewish individuals, while 4% of Ashkenazi Jews carry another mutation, 167delT. A dozen or so other genes are known to cause pediatric deafness, but Cx26 is the only one for which testing is clinically available.

17. How many deafness genes are there?
As many as 100+ genes may be involved in nonsyndromic hearing impairment. Currently, approximately 60 loci (the chromosomal location of a gene) are known, and the actual gene has been identified for about 24. All but a few select genes are very rare. Loci of deafness genes are denoted by DFNA, for autosomal dominant deafness genes; DFNB, for autosomal recessive deafness genes; and DFN for X-linked deafness genes. These figures are changing constantly. The most up-to-date information is available at http://dnalab-www.uia.ac.be/dnalab/hhh/.

18. Sensorineural hearing loss may be associated with inner ear anomalies. Describe the most common autosomal inner ear dysmorphologies.
Scheibe aplasia is the most common of the inherited inner ear anomalies. It is usually inherited in an autosomal recessive pattern and may also be seen in association with Usher syndrome. Although the bony labyrinth, utricles, and semicircular canals are normal, a membranous cochlea-saccular aplasia is characteristic.
Michael aplasia is inherited in an AD manner. Although this aplasia has a wide phenotypic spectrum, it is usually characterized by complete developmental failure of the inner ear. Typically, Michael aplasia is associated with a normally developed middle ear and external auditory canal.
Mondini aplasia is characterized by incomplete development of the bony or membranous labyrinth. The cochlea may be represented by a single curve, and the vestibule and semicircular canals may be abnormally wide or completely absent. Hearing may be unaffected, or complete hearing loss may be present. Mondini aplasia may be inherited as an AD trait, but is also found as part of the autosomal recessive Pendred syndrome (see Question 19). In fact, up to 20% of deaf children with Mondini aplasia have mutations in the Pendred syndrome gene, even without the thyroid findings.
Alexander aplasia is associated with an abnormal cochlear duct. The basal coil and its adjacent ganglion cells are the most affected. Patients with an Alexander aplasia have a high-frequency hearing loss.

19.   What are the most common genetic syndromes that feature hearing impairment?
Usher syndrome is an autosomal recessive disorder characterized by sensorineural hearing loss and retinitis pigmentosa. This is genetically heterogeneous, with a number of different genes causing the same phenotype.
Pendred syndrome is another autosomal recessive condition. It is characterized by prelingual deafness and goiter. Individuals demonstrate a partial failure of iodine organification. About half of these individuals are euthyroid; the remainder are hypothyroid. Pendred syndrome accounts for about 5% of congenital deafness. Genetic testing for the Pendred syndrome gene *pendrin* is available only on a research basis.
Waardenburg syndrome is one of the more readily recognizable and better known hearing impairment syndromes. Diagnostic criteria include partial albinism (white hair patch, different color eyes), telecanthus, some degree of hearing impairment, hair turning gray at an early age, and an affected first-degree family member.
There are four types of Waardenburg syndrome. Telecanthus is present in type 1, absent in type 2. Type 3 features craniofacial findings plus multiple other anomalies. Type 4 is associated with Hirschsprung disease. Hearing impairment occurs in 50% of type II patients, compared to only 20% of those with type I. The gene for Waardenburg syndrome 1 is PAX3 on chromosome 2; Waardenburg syndrome 2 is MITF; Waardenburg syndrome 3 is homozygosity for Pax3 mutations; and type 4 is EDNRB.
Stickler syndrome, also called hereditary arthro-ophthalmopathy, is an AD disorder characterized by high myopia, flat midface, early adult arthritis, micrognathia, and cleft palate either alone or associated with the Pierre Robin sequence. Progressive, sensorineural, high-frequency

hearing loss is seen in many cases. Stickler syndrome is caused by mutations in either COL2A1, COL11A1, or COL11A2. Individuals with COL11A2 mutations are distinguished by their lack of eye involvement. Also, mutations in COL11A2 can cause nonsyndromic hearing impairment.

Branchio-oto-renal (BOR) syndrome involves abnormalities of the branchial arch, including ear pits and tags, cervical fistulae, and hearing impairment. In addition, about two-thirds of patients have renal involvement, ranging from clinically insignificant differences to major renal anomalies. Hearing loss may be sensorineural, conductive, or mixed. BOR syndrome is an AD disorder caused by mutations in the gene EYA1 on chromosome 8.

Treacher Collins syndrome, or mandibulofacial dysostosis, is an AD craniofacial disorder. Manifestations include microtia, aural meatal atresia, and conductive hearing loss. Sensorineural hearing loss and vestibular dysfunction may also be present. Facial manifestations include malar hypoplasia with underdevelopment of zygomatic arches resulting in down-turned palpebral fissures, coloboma of lower lids, and a hypoplastic mandible. The gene for Treacher Collins is called *treacle,* on chromosome 5.

Neurofibromatosis (NF) is a neurocutaneous disorder. Bilateral acoustic neuromas are found in 95% of patients with NF type II. NF type I is associated with cutaneous findings, including café-au-lait spots and cutaneous and plexiform neurofibromas; rarely, it is associated with unilateral acoustic neuromas. However, patients with both types of NF should receive audiologic evaluation.

20. If a child of two hearing patients has a sporadic hearing loss, what is the recurrence risk for later children?

This is the most common scenario, as 90–95% of deaf children are born to hearing parents. The recurrence risk for these parents is 10–16%, but this can be modified with Cx26 testing.

21. If two hearing parents have two deaf children, what is the recurrence risk? What if one deaf parent has one deaf child?

In the first scenario, it is assumed that the deafness is autosomal recessive; and therefore there is a 25% recurrence risk for each subsequent pregnancy. Over 50% of such cases are caused by Cx26 gene mutations.

For the second scenario, the most likely explanation is that the deafness is due to an AD gene, and the recurrence risk is then 50% for each subsequent pregnancy.

22. What testing should be offered to families to provide appropriate genetic counseling and recurrence risks?

Families should be offered genetic testing for Cx26 gene mutations if the deafness appears to be nonsyndromic, i.e., no other malformations are present or etiology is identified. Families should receive genetic counseling prior to and after testing so that the limitations of the genetic test, as well as issues regarding recurrence risks, are understood.

23. Which factor complicates a family pedigree of otosclerosis?

Otosclerosis, the most common genetic cause of adult-onset hearing loss, is an AD disorder. However, because of decreased penetrance, only 40% of gene carriers actually demonstrate otosclerosis. Thus it is difficult to determine specific recurrence risks.

24. What otolaryngologic problems exist for individuals with craniosynostosis syndromes?

Individuals with a craniosynostosis syndrome, such as Apert, Crouzon, Pfeiffer, Saethre-Chotzen, or Jackson-Weiss syndrome, often have highly arched palates, middle ear disease, and conductive hearing loss. Furthermore, some of these children have upper airway abnormalities, such as choanal atresia and tracheal rings.

25. Which particular chromosomal defects have otolaryngologic considerations?

Trisomy 21, trisomy 13, cri du chat (5p–), Wolf-Hirschhorn (4p–), and deletion of the long arm of chromosome 18 (18q–). Trisomy 13 and Wolf-Hirschhorn are associated with cleft lips with or without cleft palates. The typical, mewing cry described in infants with cri du chat syndrome is ascribed to abnormal laryngeal development. In patients with 4p deletion, the endolarynx is narrow and diamond-shaped, with a persistent interarythroid cleft. Individuals with 18q– are at risk for narrow or atretic ear canals, contributing to frequent otitis media and deafness.

26. Are there otolaryngologic considerations in evaluating a child with Down syndrome?
Children with Down syndrome are at increased risk for upper respiratory tract infections. They are susceptible to frequent otitis media due to eustachian tube dysfunction. They also are predisposed to mixed hearing losses, because they often have significant middle ear anomalies. Assessment of audiologic function is essential because significant hearing losses in young children affect all aspects of development. Children with Down syndrome are susceptible to upper airway obstruction because of their narrow nasopharynx, narrow oropharyngeal airway, and macroglossia. Over 50% of Down syndrome patients have obstructive sleep apnea.

27. Why is an otolaryngologist likely to evaluate a patient with cystic fibrosis?
The children often have severe and chronic pansinusitis. Ten percent develop obstructive nasal polyposis, which is usually refractory to medical or surgical management. Lastly, as many as 40% of individuals with CF develop sensorineural hearing loss. While some have speculated that this hearing loss is caused by the potentially ototoxic antibiotics these patients receive (e.g. aminoglycosides), there is no evidence to support this.

CONTROVERSIES

28. In offering genetic counseling for a congenital deformity in a child, the mother of the child asks *you*, "What would be the possibility of a second child having the same congenital malformation?" Believing that the deformity could have been caused by one abnormal gene from each parent, you have obtained blood from the mother, father, and child. In carrying out the genetic testing, it is incidentally determined that the "father" is *not* this child's biological father. With whom should you discuss this information?
Obviously you can omit the child—he is too young, now. That's the simple part of this Brave New World–type question. Ethicists will have the opportunity to debate this one for a long time: some experts estimate that false paternity occurs in as many as 10% of genetic testing cases. But you may find yourself on the "front line" and, if so, will have to provide a single answer to this question—and actually act upon it.

This question was considered at length in Johns Hopkins News (Winter, 2001, p. 54) and the consensus of a panel of "experts" was that the mother should be informed that the malformation would not recur with offspring of "this (potential) father," since this father was not the father of this child. How the mother chose to share the information would be up to her, but it was concluded that she should be encouraged to share the information with her husband, the potential father of additional offspring. The husband could be informed that he would not father "additional children with the same congenital abnormality," omitting the exact reason *unless he asked the basis for the opinion*. Alternatively, neither the father nor the mother might be informed about the false paternity, and the question could be answered, "Subsequent children born of this marriage would not inherit the deformity." The difficulty would come, of course, if the parents asked further questions that required a broader explanation. At that point, you would have to decide whether to tell the truth, or to *lie* to one or both of them—and act upon this decision.

In view of the unexpectedly high incidence of false paternity, this situation will become a greater issue as additional DNA testing occurs. There is one way of avoiding these dilemmas. Parents can be routinely presented with a **written statement** before genetic testing takes place in which they are informed that difficult social issues, such as the discovery of mistaken paternity, could arise from information obtained from blood samples. They then can be asked to **sign an agreement** stating that the clinician should exercise discretion in divulging that information; this, of course, puts this ethical dilemma squarely on your back.

The issue of the sensitivity and specificity of the testing in this area introduces a whole new set of ethical questions and is far beyond the scope of this chapter, but presents a real issue. This is not a recent dilemma. An archeology study by Brigham Young University of preserved Egyptian mummies over 4000 years old determined that one of the "children" of a pharaoh, mummified with his "parents," was not, in fact, the child of that father, although his DNA did match his mother's. Thus, new technology uncovered a very old indiscretion. And Native Americans (Navahos) identify children according to the clan of the mother (maternal lineage), since the identity of the mother is always known with certainty.

BIBLIOGRAPHY

1. Brookhauser PE: Genetic hearing loss. In Bailey BJ (ed): Head and Neck Surgery–Otolaryngology, 2nd ed., Philadelphia, J.B. Lippincott, 1998.
2. Cohen MM, Gorlin RJ, Fraser FC: Craniofacial Disorders. In Rimoin DL, Conner JM, Pyeritz RE (eds): Emery and Riomoin's Principles and Practice of Medical Genetics, 3rd ed. New York, Churchill Livingstone, 1996.
3. Cohn ES, Kelley PM: Clinical phenotype and mutations in connexin 26 (DFNB1/GJB2), the most common cause of childhood hearing loss. Am J Med Genetics 89:130–6, 1999.
4. Cohn ES, Kelley PM, Fowler TW, et al: Clinical studies of families with hearing loss attributable to mutations in the connexin 26 gene. Pediatrics 103:546–550, 1999.
5. Crockett DM, Seibert RW, Brumstead RM: Cleft lip and palate: The primary deformity. In Bailey BJ (ed): Head and Neck Surgery–Otolaryngology, 2nd ed., Philadelphia, J.B. Lippincott, 1998.
6. Kimberling WJ, Orten D, Pieke-Dahl S: Genetic heterogeneity of Usher syndrome. Adv ORL 56:11–8, 2000.
7. Krutovskikh V, Yamasaki H: Connexin gene mutations in human genetic diseases. Mutation Res 462:197–207, 2000.
8. Lewin B: Genes VII. London, Oxford Univ Press, 1999.
9. McGuirt WT, Lesperance MM, Wilcox ER, et al: Characterization of autosomal dominant nonsyndromic hearing loss loci: DFNA 4, 6, 10 and 13. Adv ORL 56:84–96, 2000.
10. Morris DP, Saeed SR: The common causes of hearing loss in adults. Practitioner 244:70–4, 76–7, 79–80 passim, 2000.
11. Morrison, AW, Balantyne J, Martin MC, Martin A (eds): Hereditary deafness. In Deafness. London, Whurrn Publishers, 1993.
12. Pfister M, Lalwani AK: DFN4: Nonsyndromic autosomal dominant X-linked sensorineural hearing impairment. Adv ORL 56:196–199, 2000.
13. Rehm HL, Morton CC: A new age in the genetics of deafness. Gene Med 1(6):295–302, 1999.
14. Scriver CR, Childs B, Beaudet A, et al: Metabolic and Molecular Basis of Inherited Disease. Philadelphia, McGraw-Hill Professional Publishing, 2000.
15. Usami S, Abe S, Akita J, et al: Sensorineural hearing loss associated with the mitochondrial mutations. Adv ORL 56:203–211, 2000.
16. Van Laer L, McGuirt WT, Yang T, et al: Autosomal dominant nonsyndromic hearing impairment. Am J Med Genetics 89:167–174, 1999.
17. Willems PJ: Genetic causes of hearing loss, N Engl J Med 342:1101–1108, 2000.

71. CLEFT LIP AND PALATE

David A. Hendrick, M.D.

1. Who treats clefts?

Clefts are surgically repaired by otolaryngologists and plastic surgeons trained in pediatric facial plastic surgery. However, the treatment is not purely surgical, and children with clefts should be treated by a team that includes reconstructive surgeons, dentists, pediatricians, otologists, speech pathologists, audiologists, psychologists/psychiatrists, nutritionists, and geneticists.

2. Do race or sex predilections exist in the incidence of cleft lip or palate?

Asians and Native Americans have the highest rate. African-Americans have the lowest rate. Males have more cleft lips and cleft lips with cleft palates. Females have more isolated cleft palates.

3. Do clefts demonstrate any inheritance patterns?

Clefts may be related to a known teratogenic insult or part of a recognized malformation syndrome. Others are transmitted with incomplete penetrance in a multifactorial nonmendelian pattern. Therefore, genetic counseling for families with nonsyndromic clefts can be complex. Cleft recurrence in a family ranges from 2–17%, depending on the number of affected parents and siblings.

4. Embryologically, when do cleft lips and/or palates develop?

The upper lip, nose, and palate form in two phases. Anterior to the incisive foramen, the upper lip, nose, and premaxilla develop during the second month of gestation. Posterior to the incisive foramen, the palate develops during the third month. Disruptions during these critical periods predispose to clefts.

5. What is the primary palate? The secondary palate?

The primary and secondary palates are separated by the incisive foramen. The **primary palate** consists of the lip, alveolar arch, and palate anterior to the incisive foramen (the premaxilla). The **secondary palate** consists of the soft palate and hard palate posterior to the incisive foramen.

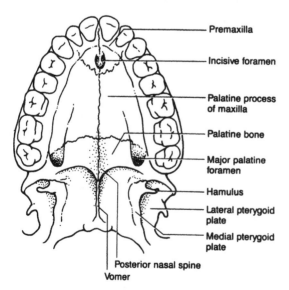

Premaxilla

Incisive foramen

Palatine process of maxilla

Palatine bone

Major palatine foramen

Hamulus

Lateral pterygoid plate

Medial pterygoid plate

Posterior nasal spine

Vomer

Basic anatomy and divisions of the palate. (From Randall P. LaRossa D: Cleft palate. In McCarthy JG (ed): Plastic surgery. Philadelphia, W.B. Saunders, 1990, p 2726, with permission.)

6. What is a complete cleft lip? An incomplete cleft lip?

A complete cleft lip includes a cleft of the entire lip and the underlying premaxilla, or alveolar arch. An incomplete cleft lip only involves the lip.

7. What is a Simonart's band?

In the case of a severe, incomplete cleft lip, a thin remnant of tissue, or "band," in the floor of the nasal vestibule bridges the medial and lateral lip elements across the cleft.

8. What is a submucous cleft?

In a child with a submucous cleft, the musculature of the palate is deficient. However, the palate looks intact because the overlying oral and nasal mucosa are present. A **zona pellucida,** or bluish midline streak on the soft palate, is the result of the muscular diastasis. A submucous cleft is characterized by a bifid uvula and loss of the posterior nasal spine. A notch may be present in the posterior hard palate. A child with a submucous cleft may have difficulties with speech because the soft palate does not function normally.

9. Describe the initial priorities for managing a newborn with a cleft.

The initial priorities are **feeding assistance** for the infant and **counseling** for the family. Infants must develop adequate suction around a nipple and need frequent rests and burping as they often swallow much air ("aerophagia"). Special nipples, such as the "Habberman Feeder," can bypass or occlude the cleft; bulb syringes can eliminate the need for suckling; and a palatal prostheses can occlude an extremely wide cleft palate.

10. What kinds of problems can an otolaryngologist expect to encounter in the cleft palate patient?

Aside from the feeding problems and the cleft repairs, the otolaryngologist can expect to deal with eustachian tube dysfunction and velopharyngeal dysfunction.

Eustachian tube dysfunction is secondary to the hypoplastic levator and tensor veli palatini muscles, which control the eustachian tube. Eustachian tube dysfunction can lead to chronic otitis media, possible formation of cholesteatomas later in life (in 7% of patients with cleft palate), conductive hearing deficits, and associated speech delays. With increasing age, eustachian tube function usually normalizes.

Velopharyngeal dysfunction is due to deficiencies in the palatal and pharyngeal musculature and/or inadequate palatal length. Velopharyngeal dysfunction can lead to speech articulation difficulties and potential **velopharyngeal insufficiency** (VPI). VPI is characterized by hypernasal speech and nasal regurgitation of food and liquids. Note that these problems are inherent to cleft palate and are *not* associated with isolated cleft lips.

11. Aside from cleft repair, what interventions should the otolaryngologist consider?

- Pressure equalization tube placement
- Otitis media management
- Cholesteatoma management
- Audiologic monitoring
- Speech therapy coordination
- VPI surgery

12. What is the "Rule of 10's"?

The "Rule of 10's" is a guideline for when it is reasonable and safe to repair a cleft lip in an infant. When an infant is >10 weeks old, >10 lbs in weight, and has a serum hemoglobin of >10 g/dl, general anesthesia for surgical repair of the cleft lip can be performed. Repair of cleft palates is delayed until later.

13. When should cleft palates be repaired?

The "board answer" to this question is *after* the first anterior molars erupt and *before* the posterior molars erupt, which typically occurs between 18 and 24 months of age. The idea here is to minimize adverse effects of the developing palate and occlusal relationships. However, some centers prefer to repair cleft palates between 10 and 18 months of age, when articulate speech skills are being developed.

14. Name the muscular deficiencies associated with cleft lip and palate.

In a cleft lip, the orbicularis oris muscle is deficient at the cleft. Muscle fibers tend to follow the cleft up into the base of the nose and must be dissected out to be reapproximated across the cleft. In a cleft palate, the (1) levator veli palatini muscle, (2) tensor veli palatini, (3) uvular muscle, (4) palatopharyngeus muscle, and (5) palatoglossus muscle normally have midline raphes and are therefore all deficient at the palate's cleft. Muscle fibers normally form a muscular "sling" across the soft palate, but in clefts they tend to have abnormal insertions into the posterior margin of the hard palate. Reconstruction of this muscular sling is critical to functional success after palatoplasty.

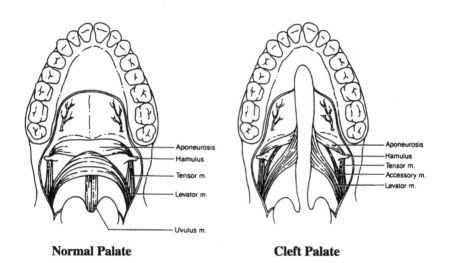

Normal Palate   **Cleft Palate**

Musculature of the normal and cleft soft palate. Not illustrated are the palatopharyngeus muscle (comprises the posterior tonsillar pillar) and the palatoglossus muscle (comprises the anterior tonsillar pillar). (From Randall P, LaRossa D: Cleft palate. In McCarthy JG (ed): Plastic surgery. Philadelphia, W.B. Saunders, 1990, p 2726, with permission.)

15. Describe the Millard repair.

The Millard repair is the most popular method of cleft lip repair and involves a **rotation advancement technique.** The philtrum of the lip is rotated downward as a flap, and the lateral lip segment is advanced across the cleft and into the space left behind by the central lip segment. Unlike other methods, the final suture line of the Millard repair closely recreates the philtrum of the lip.

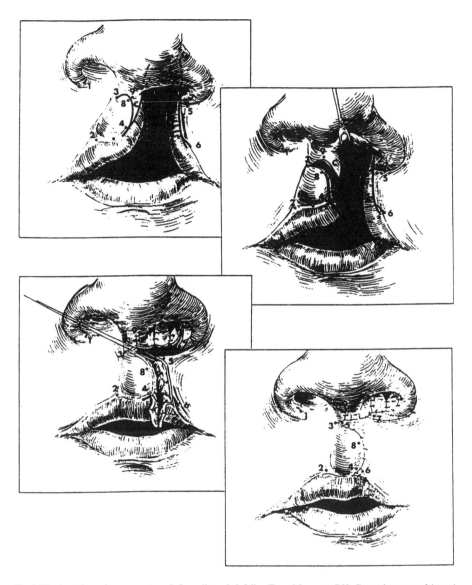

The Millard rotation-advancement repair for unilateral cleft lip. (From Musgrave RH: General aspects of the unilateral cleft lip repair. In Grabb WC, Rosenstein SW, Bzoch KR (eds): Cleft Lip and Palate: Surgical, Dental, and Speech Aspects. Boston, Little, Brown, 1971, pp 197-200, with permission.)

16. What are some other methods of cleft lip repair?
- Lip adhesion (Randall-Graham)—less commonly performed today
- Straight-line repair (Rose-Thompson)—very limited applications
- Rectangular flap repair (LeMesurier)—not as aesthetic as Z-plasty flap methods
- Triangular flap repairs (including Skoog, Bardach, and Tennison-Randall repairs)—all variations on Z-plasty techniques; best for wide cleft lip defects.

17. List the critical elements or goals of successful cleft lip repairs.
- Correct alignment of cupid's bow
- Correct approximation of the orbicularis oris muscle
- Symmetric reconstruction of the lip vermilion
- Creation of a nasal floor and vestibular sill
- Symmetric placement of the nasal alar bases and columella

18. What are the methods of cleft palate repair?

The **V–Y pushback** (Oxford method) and **two-flap palatoplasties** are the most commonly used techniques for repairing incomplete and complete clefts of the palate, respectively. The essential difference between these two methods is whether or not the anterior premaxilla mucoperiosteum is included with the posterior-based pedicled flaps. Of these two methods, only the V–Y pushback provides additional palate length, and only the two-flap technique provides adequate closure of the cleft alveolus, thereby defining their favored roles. Other methods of palatoplasty include:

Four-flap palatoplasty—essentially converts a more complete cleft palate into a shorter, incomplete cleft case to take advantage of the V–Y pushback technique for palatal lengthening. The mucoperiosteum of the anterior hard palate is raised as two anteriorly based flaps, which are then reapproximated across the anterior cleft. A standard V–Y pushback is then performed using the two remaining posterior-based flaps.

Von Langenbeck palatoplasty—basically a precursor to the two-flap technique, in which the flaps are bipedicled both posteriorly and anteriorly. Rarely used except perhaps for clefts of the soft palate only.

Schweckendiek's primary veloplasty—a less extensive version of the Von Langenbeck technique designed to close only the soft palate as part of a staged approach. Rarely used now.

Furlow palatoplasty—an "opposing Z-plasty" technique for closing and elongating the soft palate. Oppositely oriented Z-plasties are employed to close the nasal and oral mucosal surfaces. The muscle sling can be reconstructed by retaining and reorienting the muscle fibers with the appropriate flaps of the Z-plasties.

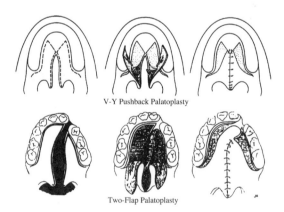

V-Y Pushback Palatoplasty

Two-Flap Palatoplasty

The V-Y pushback and two-flap palatoplasties. (From Randall P, LaRossa D: Cleft palate. In McCarthy JG (ed): Plastic surgery. Philadelphia, W.B. Saunders, 1990, p 2744, with permission; and from Bumsted RM: The Management of Cleft Lip and Palate. Rochester, MN, American Academy of Otolaryngology, 1980, pp 34, 37, with permission.)

19. List the goals and critical elements of successful cleft palate repairs.
- Separation of the nasal and oral cavities through closure of both mucosal surfaces
- Construction of a water-tight, air-tight velopharyngeal valve

- Preservation of facial growth
- Good development of aesthetic dentition and functional occlusion

In addition to the above basic goals, most surgeons believe that reconstruction of the muscular sling of the soft palate is essential for good functional results of the repair.

20. What are the most common postoperative complications of cleft palate repair?

Hypernasal speech is the most common complication following cleft palate repair, occurring in up to 30% of patients. **Oral-nasal fistulas** are the second most common complication and occur in 10–21% of cleft palate repairs. These fistulas typically occur at either end of the hard palate (i.e., at the anterior alveolus or at the junction of the soft and hard palate).

21. Which secondary procedures are associated with cleft lip and palate surgery?

Secondary procedures are those following the initial repairs of the cleft lip and palate. Besides revisions of the lip and palate, procedures are often necessary to address velopharyngeal insufficiency, alveolar clefts, and nasal deformities.

22. How is velopharyngeal incompetence (VPI) managed?

The deficiency should be assessed with various diagnostic tools, including speech articulation tests, cinefluoroscopy, lateral neck x-rays, manometry, and nasopharyngoscopy. **Speech therapy** should begin with parental counseling when the child is 6 months old, and individual child therapy should begin when the child is about 4 years of age. **Dental prosthesis** may improve palatal lift. About 20–25% of VPI cases may need **surgery.** Methods include secondary palatal lengthening (e.g., Furlow palatoplasty), pharyngeal augmentation (narrow the anteroposterior diameter of the nasopharynx using soft tissue or implants), and pharyngeal flaps (convert the incompetent nasopharynx into two lateral "ports"). Pharyngeal flaps require good lateral pharyngeal wall motion for functional success.

23. What are the rhinoplasty concerns in the surgical management of the cleft lip patient?

Most patients have a nasal deformity that becomes more apparent and severe with age. Classically, the cleft nose deformity involves:

- Shortened columella with its base angled to the noncleft side
- Nasal spine deviation to the noncleft side, with a similar deflection of the caudal septum toward the noncleft side and a compensatory hypertrophy of the cleft side inferior turbinate
- Medial crura of lower lateral cartilage collapsed inferomedially on the cleft side
- Lateral crura of lower lateral cartilage collapsed and buckled on the cleft side. Generally it will be weaker and longer than the noncleft lower lateral cartilage.
- Deflection of the nasal tip toward the cleft side due to the above deficiencies
- Relative stenosis of the nasal valve on the cleft side

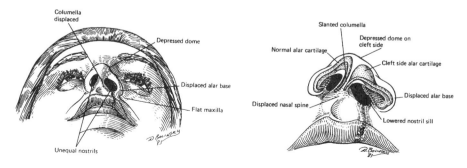

The cleft nose. (From Smith HW: The Atlas of Cleft LIp and Cleft Palate Surgery. New York, Grune & Stratton, 1983, pp 290, 293, with permission.)

- Hypoplastic maxilla on the cleft side, causing lateralization of the alar base and widening of the nare
- Possible deviation of the bony nasal pyramids toward the cleft side
- Broad nasal dorsum
- Thick skin over the nasal tip

CONTROVERSIES

24. How is the cleft alveolus surgically managed?

Ultimately, the cleft alveolus must be reconstructed to provide for alveolar arch integrity and for tooth eruption or support at the cleft. Traditionally, this requires placement of bone grafts harvested from the iliac crest, rib, or cranium. Cancellous bone from the iliac crest has been favored by most surgeons; others prefer cortical or corticocancellous onlay grafts from the rib or cranium.

The timing of repair is controversial, with most centers performing "secondary" grafting prior to canine eruption during the stage of mixed dentition (9–12 years of age). Some centers continue to perform "primary" grafting in early childhood at the time of cleft lip repair.

25. In a child with a cleft, when should the nasal tip deformities be repaired?

Partial correction of the nasal deformities is accomplished at the time of primary lip repair by reconstructing the nasal sill, straightening or lengthening the columella, and placing the alar base in a more symmetric position. The timing for nasal tip rhinoplasty is controversial, with some surgeons attempting repairs at the time of primary lip repair and others waiting until 6–10 years of age. More complete rhinoplasty is deferred until facial growth is nearly complete, at approximately 14–18 years of age.

BIBLIOGRAPHY

1. Bender PL: Genetics of cleft lip and palate. J Pediatr Nurs 15:242–249, 2000.
2. Crocket DM, Seibert RW, Bumsted RM: Cleft lip and palate. In Bailey B (ed): Head and Neck Surgery–Otolaryngology, 2nd ed. Philadelphia, J.B. Lippincott, 1998, pp 816–831.
3. Cockell A, Lees M: Prenatal diagnosis and management of orofacial clefts. Prenat Diag 20:149–151, 2000.
4. Kobayashi J, Kimijima Y, Yamada S, et al: 4p- syndrome and 9p tetrasomy mosaicism with cleft lip and palate. J Craniomaxillofac Surg 28:165–70, 2000.
5. Lambrecht JT, Kreusch T, Schulz L: Position, shape, and dimension of the maxilla in unoperated cleft lip and palate patients: Review of the literature. Clin Anat 13:121–33, 2000.
6. Lorenz HP, Hedrick MH, Chang J, et al: The impact of biomolecular medicine and tissue engineering on plastic surgery in the 21st century. Plast Reconstr Surg 105:2467–2481, 2000.
7. Mills JL: Folate and oral clefts: Where do we go from here? New directions in oral clefts research. Teratol 60:251–252, 1999.
8. Madorsky SJ, Wang TD: Unilateral cleft rhinoplasty: A review. Otol Clin North Am 32:669–82, 1999.
9. Molsted K: Treatment outcome in cleft lip and palate: Issues and perspectives. Crit Rev Oral Biol Med 10:225–239, 1999.
10. Rivkin CJ, Keith O, Crawford PJ, et al: Dental care for the patient with a cleft lip and palate. Part 1: From birth to the mixed dentition stage. Br Dent J 188:78–83, 2000.
11. Schutte BC, Murray JC: The many faces and factors of orofacial clefts. Human Molec Genetics 8:1853–1859, 1999.
12. Seibert RW, Bumsted RM: Cleft lip and palate. In Cummings CW, et al (eds): Otolaryngology–Head and Neck Surgery, 2nd ed. St. Louis, Mosby, 1998, pp 1128–1164.
13. Steinberg B, Padwa BL, Boyne P, et al: State of the art in oral and maxillofacial surgery: treatment of maxillary hypoplasia and anterior palatal and alveolar clefts. Cleft Palate Craniofac J 36:283–291, 1999.
14. Strauss RP: The organization and delivery of craniofacial health services: the state of the art. Cleft Palate Craniofac J 36:189–195, 1999.

X. Related Specialties

---

72. TASTE AND SMELL

Miriam R. Linschoten, Ph.D. and Bruce W. Murrow, M.D., Ph.D.

---

1. What are papillae?

Papillae are specialized structures that are involved in taste. Three of the four types of papillae contain taste buds.

- The **fungiform papillae** are located on the anterior two-thirds of the tongue. Each fungiform papilla contains 0–18 taste buds. Fungiform taste buds contribute about 750 taste buds to the oral cavity.
- Several **foliate papillae** are located on the posterior lateral surface of the tongue. These papillae consist of a series of clefts containing as many as 1300 taste buds.
- The **circumvallate papillae** are located on the posterior dorsal tongue. Humans have 8–12 circumvallate papillae arranged in an inverted V-form. The total number of circumvallate taste buds is about 2400, which is roughly half the total number of buds in the oral cavity.
- The **filiform papillae** are distributed over the entire dorsal surface of the tongue. These structures contain no taste buds, but help in sustaining tastants on the surface of the tongue.

The soft palate, larynx, pharynx, and epiglottis contain extrapapillar taste buds situated within the epithelium.

2. Describe the topographic map of taste

Many textbooks describe specific locations on the tongue where each of the four basic tastes—sweet, salty, sour, and bitter—are exclusively detected. Unfortunately, this so-called topographic map does not exist: each of the basic tastes can be perceived on all loci in the mouth containing taste buds. There are, however, differences with respect to how strong a certain concentration is perceived at different loci; for instance, the same bitter stimulus will taste stronger at the back of the tongue than at the tip, but it will taste bitter at both places.

3. How are taste buds innervated?

The lingual taste buds are innervated by three cranial nerves (CN). The chorda tympani branch of the facial nerve (CN VII) supplies the taste buds in all the fungiform papillae and some buds in the foliate papillae. The remaining foliate taste buds receive innervation from the lingual branch of the glossopharyngeal nerve (CN IX). This last branch also provides innervation to the circumvallate papillae. The vagus nerve (CN X) innervates buds in the epiglottis and larynx. CN VII carries taste information from the anterior two-thirds of the tongue, while CN IX is responsible for taste from the posterior one-third of the tongue.

4. What is the role of the trigeminal nerve in taste and smell disorders?

While the trigeminal nerve (CN V) provides most of the sensory innervation of the face, the trigeminal nerve fibers of the nose, oral cavity, and eye are sensitive to chemical stimuli in addition to mechanical, proprioceptive, and nociceptive stimuli. This sensitivity is considered part of the **common chemical sense** and serves as a protective mechanism to warn of the presence of potentially dangerous chemicals. Trigeminal chemoreception is not a simple sensory system. Stimulation of trigeminal chemoreceptors modulates perception of subsequent or concurrent chemical stimuli. It is important to verify the function of this protective sense, especially in patients with other chemosensory dysfunction. Vicks VapoRub is often used to test whether the nasal trigeminal function is intact.

5. Where is the olfactory epithelium located?

To date, the *exact* boundaries of the olfactory epithelium (OE) are still unclear. It is located in the superior aspect of the nasal vault. Historically, the OE in humans has been described around the cribiform plate in the olfactory cleft and measuring 0.1 to 2 cm^2. Recent evidence indicates that the OE can include locations more anteriorly and inferiorly than previously thought, such as around the anterior insertion of the middle turbinate.

6. Which cells make up the olfactory epithelium?

The OE is made up of four cell types:

The **olfactory receptor cell** (ORC) is responsible for transducing the odorants into electrical signals. These cells have an elongated cell body with a dendritic process and terminal bulb that reaches the epithelial surface, and a basal axonal process that projects to the olfactory bulb. The dendritic bulb has cilia, which contain the olfactory receptors for odorant molecules.

Sustenticular cells are elongated cells that have microvilli protruding from their apical surface and provide a supporting role to the ORCs that they surround.

Microvillar cells are flask-shaped cells with a tuft of microvilli at their apical surface. The function of these cells is still not understood, though some have proposed a possible receptor role for them.

Basal cells, which by their very name describes their position in the olfactory epithelium, are thought to be progenitor cells that replenish the above cell types in the regenerative epithelium.

7. Describe how an olfactory receptor cell responds to an odorant.

The odorant binds to a receptor on the cilia of an olfactory receptor cell and starts a cascade of biochemical changes that ultimately results in the production of an action potential. In particular, the odorant binds to a G-protein–coupled receptor that activates adenylate cyclase and produces cAMP, which in turn opens a nonselective cation channel. An influx of Ca$^+$ then activates Ca-sensitive chloride channels that allow the efflux of Cl$^-$ from the cell and causes the cell to depolarize. This generator current produces an action potential in the cell body that propagates along the axon to the olfactory bulb.

Another potential pathway involves odorant binding to a different G-protein–coupled receptor that results in production of IP$_3$. The IP$_3$ opens a nonselective Ca$^+$ channel and leads to depolarization of the cell.

The relative contribution to olfaction of each of these pathways continues to be studied. While more research has been done in animals than in humans, the overall principles of stimulation as described above appear to occur in human ORCs.

8. What percentage of the human genome is related to olfactory receptor genes?

Over 1% of the human genome. However, many of these may encode for pseudogenes that are not expressed.

9. What is the difference between smell, taste, and flavor?

Most patients presenting with a smell disorder complain that they are unable to taste. This phenomenon is mainly a question of language and definition. There is an overlap between taste, smell, and flavor. **Taste** refers to the sensations (sweet, sour, salty, bitter) arising from the taste receptors. **Smell** refers to the sensations arising from the olfactory receptors. There are many different smell qualities for which no satisfactory classification exists. **Flavor** is the combined sensation of taste, smell, temperature, texture, and pungency.

A patient with nasal obstruction has have a decreased sense of smell, and therefore the flavor of foods changes. Questions to help make the distinction are: are you able to taste the sweetness of sugar, the saltiness of pretzels, the sourness of a lemon, the bitterness of black coffee? Some confusion between sour and bitter is common and does not indicate a taste problem. Perfumes, Vicks VapoRub, and cleaning agents (such as ammonia and bleach) have a trigeminal component, and the ability to "smell" these does not imply a normal functioning sense of smell.

10. What percentage of flavor is due to smell?

Flavor is the combined perception of taste, smell, texture, temperature, and pungency. Of these, smell has the largest input. It is estimated that about 80% of flavor comes from smell.

11. What is the "jelly bean" test?

In the jelly bean test, the nose is held closed while a flavored jelly bean is placed in the mouth and chewed. Under these conditions the jelly bean "tastes" sweet, or sour, but the specific flavor (e.g., grape, strawberry) can only be identified when the air is allowed to flow freely through the nose, so that smell contributes to the sensation. While jelly beans have not been used extensively in clinical practice, this paradigm does effectively demonstrate the interaction of taste and smell to produce flavor, and the importance of intact smell to flavor perception.

12. What happens to olfaction with age?

Olfactory function decreases with age. This is likely due to a combination of anatomical and physiologic changes. With increasing age, the intact olfactory epithelium at birth becomes patchy, as if the regenerative powers of the olfactory epithelium are unable to keep up with the accumulation of insults. At the ORC level, recent research indicates that ORCs from older patients appear to become less selective to odorants. Psychophysical tests demonstrate diminished olfactory sensitivity in subjects from whom isolated ORCs show diminished selectivity.

13. Define the terms hypogeusia, ageusia, dysgeusia, and gustatory agnosia.

These terms refer to different types of **gustatory dysfunction.** *Hypogeusia* is the diminished sensitivity to one or more tastants. *Ageusia* is an inability to detect any or all qualitative gustatory sensations. *Dysgeusia* (or parageusia) is a distortion or perversion in the perception of a tastant (such as a sweet food being perceived as bitter) or the perception of a taste that occurs in the absence of an external stimulus (a phantom taste). *Gustatory agnosia* refers to the inability to classify or identify a tastant verbally, even though the ability to distinguish between tastants may be normal. Hypogeusia, ageusia, dysgeusia, and gustatory agnosia may be partial, complete, or selective.

14. Define anosmia and hyposmia.

These terms describe different types of **olfactory dysfunction.** Anosmia is the inability to qualitatively detect an olfactory sensation. Total anosmia is the complete inability to detect olfactory sensation, while partial anosmia is the inability to detect some, but not all, odorants. Along the same lines, total hyposmia is a decreased sensitivity to all odorants, while partial hyposmia is a decreased sensitivity to some odorants.

15. What is dysosmia? Olfactory agnosia?

Dysosmia may be either a distortion in the perception of an odor (**parosmia**) or the perception of an odor when no olfactory stimulus is present (**phantosmia**). *Olfactory agnosia* is the inability to classify or identify an odorant verbally even though the patient may find it recognizable.

16. How do you categorize the loss of olfactory and gustatory sensitivity?

Anatomic categories for losses include transport losses, sensory losses, and neural losses.
- **Transport losses** result from conditions which interfere with the accessibility of the receptor cells. For olfaction, this may involve swollen nasal mucosa or structural obstructions, such as neoplasms, polyps, or a deviated septum. In gustation, transport losses are caused by bacterial colonization of the taste pores, oral inflammation, or xerostomia.

- **Sensory losses** are the result of injuries to the receptor cells. Olfactory sensory loss may occur with viral infections, exposure to toxic chemicals or antiproliferative drugs, and radiation to the head and neck. Gustatory sensory loss is caused by drugs that affect cell turnover, radiation therapy, viral infections, and endocrine disorders.
- **Neural losses** are caused by damaged peripheral and central pathways. In olfaction, neural losses occur with neoplasms of the anterior cranial fossa, head trauma, neurosurgical procedures, and neurotoxic substances. Kallmann's syndrome also leads to neural olfactory loss. Neural gustatory losses stem from neoplasms, head trauma, and damage to the afferent nerves with dental and otologic procedures.

17. In your evaluation of a patient, what are the key questions to ask?
- Questions that differentiate between taste and smell disorders (Are you able to taste salty, sweet, sour, and bitter substances? Can you smell flowers or cooking odors?)
- Questions that address the duration and onset (gradual or sudden) of the disorder as well as events concurring with the disorder.
- Questions about current and past history of diseases, trauma, surgeries, and medications.

18. What should you look for on physical exam of a patient with a taste or smell problem?
A patient with taste or smell problems should undergo a complete head and neck physical exam. However, the nose, oral cavity, and pharynx take on greater importance. Examine the nose for obstruction (e.g., polyps, tissue mass) and infection (e.g., erythematous swollen mucosa, purulent drainage). Likewise, examine the nasopharynx and oropharynx for obstruction and infection (adenoids). Investigate the oral cavity for infection (thrush), loss of tongue papillae, mass, trauma, postsurgical changes, and xerostomia. When examining the ears, keep in mind potential pathologic involvement of the facial nerve and its chorda tympani branch. In the cranial nerve exam, pay particular attention to CNs I (identification of coffee in the office setting), V, VII, and IX.

19. How do you proceed with the work-up?
You may wish to refer the patient to a Taste and Smell Center for psychophysical testing. The most common clinical tests examine the ability to detect and identify odorants and tastants. Testing should be unilateral as well as bilateral. For taste testing, differences in the sensitivity or suprathreshold sensation might exist between the two halves of the tongue. Differences may also exist between the anterior and posterior parts on one side of the tongue. To evaluate dysgeusia, topical anesthesia can be helpful in determining the site of origin. Blood tests could help determine whether the disorder is the result of hyponatremia, liver disease, or kidney disease. If you suspect that the patient's symptoms are the result of chronic sinus infections, a sinus CT is indicated. If the patient has other neural symptoms, an MRI may be necessary to evaluate for brain lesions.

20. What is the UPSIT?
UPSIT is an acronym for University of Pennsylvania Smell Identification Test, which aids in the objective evaluation of a loss of smell. It is a 40-item smell identification test; the patient scratches and sniffs an odorant and picks the corresponding label from four possible answers. The test has been standardized for age and gender. For instance, for a 50-year-old, a normal score ranges from 35 to 40 for women and from 36 to 40 for men.

21. What are the major causes of taste disorders?
Pure taste disorders are not as well documented as smell disorders. However, viral infections and head trauma have been reported to result in dysgeusias. Many medications have been associated with taste dysfunction.

22. Which diseases are associated with taste disorders?
Loss or distortion of taste is less prevalent than loss of smell. However, taste disorders may be debilitating. Taste pathways may be interrupted by lesions such as acoustic neuromas. Bell's

palsy may also lead to taste dysfunction. Taste alteration during radiation therapy and chemotherapy have been well-documented. Epilepsy, psychiatric disorders, hypothyroidism, and diabetes are also reported to have secondary taste symptoms.

23. What is burning mouth syndrome (BMS)?

BMS is an intra-oral pain disorder that occurs despite a clinically normal appearance of the oral mucosa. The tongue tip, anterior hard palate, and oral lower lip are most frequently affected. For most patients, the burning pain starts midmorning or early afternoon and is followed by dry mouth, dysgeusia, and thirst. Most patients diagnosed with BMS are postmenopausal women. The etiology is still unclear. The dysgeusia involves either a persistent taste or an alteration in taste perception. The persistent taste is most commonly described as bitter and/or metallic in quality. Complaints of altered tastes include all taste qualities—sour and bitter taste stronger than normal, sweet tastes weaker, and salt tastes either stronger or weaker.

Some patients find relief with clonazepam, a benzodiazepine, which is often used as an anticonvulsant. Treatment starts at 0.25 mg of clonazepam at bedtime for 1 week. The daily dose can be increased by 0.25 mg each week, up to a total dosage of 3 mg.

24. Can a mouthwash cause a taste disorder?

Yes. Antibacterial mouth-rinses containing chlorhexidine or hexetidine might induce disorders ranging from persistent taste loss to transient selective losses for one or two qualities. Both agents are also associated with dysgeusia.

25. What are the major causes of smell disorders?

- **Nasal and paranasal sinus disease** often is accompanied by diminished olfactory acuity for several likely reasons. Obstruction of the nasal passages results in restriction of airflow to the olfactory epithelium, presumably altering the ability to smell. In many cases, excess mucus and infectious byproducts convey an obnoxious odor, which is detected only by the patient and distorts and covers everyday odors.
- **Upper respiratory tract infections** should be considered if the anosmia or hyposmia is sudden in onset.
- **Head trauma,** with or without loss of consciousness, can result in anosmia. It is often bilateral and permanent, although some variations have been reported.
- **Inhalation of volatile chemicals** has been implicated in anosmia and hyposmia. Presumably, these toxic fumes cause direct damage to the olfactory receptor cells.

26. Both sinus disease and upper respiratory infections may lead to taste and smell complaints. How are the etiologies differentiated?

The primary distinction revolves around the time of onset. Although patients with sinus disease may detect occasional "whiffs" of odor, overall they report a slowly deteriorating sense of smell. In contrast, a post-viral loss is often very sudden in onset; most patients know the exact day when their sense of smell became impaired.

27. What are other causes of smell disorders?

Congenital, aging, postsurgical (neurosurgery, nasal), neurodegenerative-associated, systemic disease, idiopathic.

28. What treatments are available for olfactory loss?

Some olfactory losses, depending on etiology, are amenable to treatment. Cases that are due to obstruction of the olfactory cleft may respond to treatment. In particular, if sinus disease or nasal polyposis is present, medical treatment or functional endoscopic sinus surgery can alleviate the obstruction and relieve the olfactory loss. Patients that are found to have steroid-dependent olfactory deficits obtain relief of their olfactory loss, albeit often only temporary, with oral steroids as a therapeutic effect in addition to the diagnostic benefit.

Surgery may also be beneficial for patients with dysosmia. Some surgeons have reported removing the olfactory epithelium with some success in outcome. However, this is a difficult surgery at the base of the brain (cribiform plate) that can lead to CSF leaks and intracranial entry; it should only be attempted by surgeons with extensive experience doing the procedure.

Olfactory pathology related to toxic and chemical exposure can be limited or improved with removal of the offending agent. Nasal topical steroids may have benefits for recovery in addition to addressing inflammatory/obstructive effects. Some have tried supplemental therapy such as zinc and Gingkoba for treatment of some olfactory deficits; however, the efficacy of these agents has not been proven by experimental study.

Unfortunately for most post-traumatic and post-viral losses, no specific treatment is available, and only time will determine the degree of recovery.

29. Which diseases are associated with smell disorders?

Neurologic Diseases	Systemic Diseases
Alzheimer's disease	Diabetes mellitus
Parkinson's disease	Graves' disease
Myotrophic lateral sclerosis	Other thyroid disease
Familial dysautonomia	Arthritis and related autoimmune diseases
Multiple sclerosis	Psychiatric disorders
Myasthenia gravis	Inherited disorders (e.g., Kallmann's
Temporal lobe epilepsy	syndrome)

30. What is Kallmann's syndrome?

Kallmann's syndrome, transmitted in an autosomal dominant pattern with variable penetrance, consists of congenital hypogonadotropic eunuchoidism and anosmia. This syndrome illustrates the probable association of smell and sexual development. Some of these patients have shown agenesis of the olfactory bulbs and stalks, incomplete development of the hypothalamus, or no olfactory epithelium in the olfactory cleft. Patients with Kallmann's syndrome also have a high incidence of renal abnormalities, cryptorchidism, deafness, diabetes, and midline facial deformities.

31. How often do patients who suffer head trauma subsequently have a taste or smell disorder?

Review of the literature reveals numerous case reports detailing loss of smell following head trauma. In summary, 5% of all head trauma victims suffer from anosmia. Dysgeusia in head trauma is rare, but well-documented reports indicate that it occurs in 0.4% of all cases.

32. What is the mechanism for loss of smell in head trauma?

Head trauma often produces a coup counter-coup situation where the brain initially slides in one direction and then in the reverse in relation to the skull. This causes sheering of the olfactory neural fibers (fila) as they transverse the small perforations in the cribiform plate. Often, patients suffer a permanent olfactory loss. Even though the olfactory fila are, in principle, capable of regeneration, scarring at the cribiform plate is thought to seal off the holes that the olfactory fila use to normally traverse the cribiform plate. However, several reports describe approximately a third of trauma-related patients recovering olfactory function. Perhaps in these patients a traction type of injury allows recovery. In general, recovery can take up to 1 year or more, but if there is no sign of recovery by 6 months, the chances are much less.

33. Describe the taste and smell effects of cardiovascular drugs.

Angiotensin-converting enzyme inhibitors, especially **captopril** and **enalapril,** have been reported to affect both taste and smell function. Although estimates vary, as many as 20% of patients using captopril develop a loss of taste or smell. Captopril may also lead to sweet, salty, and metallic phantogeusias. These side effects often resolve when captopril is discontinued, although a persistent taste change may linger for over a year.

Calcium channel blockers can produce taste and smell disorders. Nine percent of patients taking nifedipine report hyposmia, while others report a sweet, salty, or metallic phantogeusia. Diuretics (e.g., acetazolamide, amiloride, and hydrochlorothiazide), antiarrhythmics, and antihyperlipidaemics have all been associated with taste or smell problems.

34. Do other drugs commonly affect taste and smell?

Acetazolamide, used to treat glaucoma and mountain sickness, almost always causes a mild bitter taste when patients drink carbonated beverages. This effect resolves within 48 hours after the drug is discontinued. Although rare, many antibiotics are capable of causing taste or smell dysfunction. Some of these might persist after discontinuing the drug. **Gentamicin** can cause persistent hyposmia, and **doxyxycline** can cause persistent dysosmia or anosmia. Antiprotozoals commonly affect taste and smell. Specifically, **metronidazole and pentamidine,** both parenteral and inhaled forms, induce hypogeusia and metallic phantogeusia. About one-third of patients taking the antirheumatic drug **penicillamine** develop hypogeusia or dysgeusia. Over 10% of patients treated with **gold** for rheumatoid arthritis develop a dysgeusia that may precede stomatitis. Several antithyroid drugs have been associated with taste and smell disorders, especially **carbimazole, thiamazole,** and **methimazole**. Anxiolytics and antidepressants are mainly implicated in taste disorders. **Bromocriptine,** an antiparkinsonian drug, may cause phantosmias in 9% of patients, and **levodopa** may cause dysosmia, bitter phantosmia, or hypogeusia in 20–40% of patients. **Felbanate,** an anticonvulsant, causes dysgeusia in 6% of patients.

35. Does the psyche play any role in taste and smell disorders?

Yes. Depressed persons may exhibit chemosensory dysfunction. When compared with normal controls, depressed patients often exhibit hypogeusia. In contrast, depression does not lead to hyposmia. A recent study found that patients with chemosensory distortions or hallucinations (dysgeusia and dysosmia) had significantly higher scores on the Beck Depression Inventory. The same study found a close relationship between dysgeusia and antidepressant use. However, you must distinguish between the effects of the medication and the effects of the underlying condition. Burning mouth syndrome may also be related to affective disorders such as depression; however, be cautious in interpreting these complaints as purely psychogenic.

Conversely, a patient who suffers from a taste or smell disorder may become depressed. Because taste and smell play an important role in one's sense of safety and pleasure, distortions often affect general well being.

36. What are the consequences of smell and taste loss?

The most concerning effect of a loss of smell is related to safety. Fire, natural gas, and spoiled food are all identified mainly by smell. Patients with significant smell loss should be advised of this problem and should take protective measures, such as fire/smoke alarms, natural gas detectors, and strict adherence to marked dates on foods. In addition, smell and taste play an important role in the hedonic pleasures of life (e.g., dining, enjoyment of wine, perfumes). Hence, quality of life can be greatly affected by smell and taste pathology. Weight gain, weight loss, and depression are all common in patients with taste and smell disorders.

CONTROVERSIES

37. What is the vomeronasal organ? What role may it play in adult chemosensation?

The vomeronasal organ (VNO) contains chemosensory cells that respond to pheromones and is important to animals in mating and other social interactions. The existence of this structure and, if present, its functionality in adult humans is controversial. The VNO has clearly been demonstrated in fetal tissue, and in adults there often is an unmistakable pit on the anterior-inferior septum. External electrode recordings from this structure (ElectroVomeroGram) have been obtained with substances that are thought to be candidates for human pheromones. However, the actual significance of the VNO to humans is not clearly elucidated.

38. Can tonsillectomy cause the loss of taste?

There are numerous reports of taste loss and taste distortions after tonsillectomy. Taste dysfunction after tonsillectomy is most likely the result of either mechanical damage to the glossopharyngeal nerve (pressure of blade or clamp) or of accidental cutting of the glossopharyngeal nerve. This nerve reportedly sometimes runs rather superficially.

It is thought that the glossopharyngeal and the chorda tympani nerves mutually inhibit each other. When either of the four nerves is damaged or cut, a release of inhibition takes effect. This results in the intact nerves trying to compensate for the loss. The patient complains of diminished taste sensations and/or distorted taste. A spatial taste test should be performed to localize the origin of the problem.

39. What is the role of zinc in taste and smell disorders?

Zinc is commonly prescribed in the treatment of taste and smell disorders. There is, however, no evidence that it is helpful. A double-blind study demonstrated that it was no more effective than a placebo in the treatment of taste and smell dysfunction. Zinc appears to be helpful only when the patient is zinc-deficient to begin with.

BIBLIOGRAPHY

1. Doty RL: Handbook of Olfaction and Gustation. New York, Marcel Dekker, 1995.
2. Henkin RI: Drug-induced taste and smell disorders. Drug Safety, 11:318–377, 1994.
3. Jafek BW, Gordon, ASD, Moran DT, Eller PM: Congenital anosmia. Ear Nose Throat Journal 69: 331–337, 1990.
4. Jafek BW, Eller PM, Esses BA, Moran DT: Post-traumatic anosmia: Ultrastructural correlates. Arch Neurol 46:300–304, 1989.
5. Leopold DA: Physiology of olfaction. In Cummings CW, et al (eds): Otolaryngology–Head and Neck Surgery, 3rd ed. St. Louis, Mosby, 1998.
6. Leopold DA: et al: Anterior distribution of human olfactory epithelium. Laryngoscope 110:417–421, 2000.
7. Rawson NE: Human olfaction. In Finger TE, Silver WL, Restrepo D (eds): Neurobiology of Taste and Smell. New York, John Wiley, 2000.
8. Norgren R: Gustatory system. In Paxinos G (ed): The Human Nervous System. New York, Academic Press, 1990, pp 845–861.
9. Seiden AM: Taste and Smell Disorders. New York, Thieme, 1997.
10. Monti-Bloch L, et al: The human vomeronasal system. A review. Ann NY Acad Sci 855:373–89, 1998.
11. T. V. Getchell LM, et al (eds): Smell and Taste in Health and Disease. New York, Raven Press, 1991.
12. Doty RL (ed): Handbook of Olfaction and Gustation. New York, Marcel Dekker, Inc., 1994.
13. Doty RL, et al. University of Pennsylvania Smell Identification Test: A rapid quantitative olfactory function test for the clinic. Laryngoscope 94:176–178, 1984.

73. ALLERGY & IMMUNOLOGY

Betty Luce, R.N., Kay Rhew, M.D., and William H. Wilson, M.D.

1. What is the primary function of the immune system?
The human immune system is a highly complex system of cells, cell products, and enzymes. The immune system differentiates self from non-self, and seeks to eliminate elements that are foreign to the body. Most immune functions are under fundamental *genetic* control.

2. How does the immune system function in the allergic condition?
Allergy is a hypersensitive state acquired through exposure to a particular allergen (foreign protein). Re-exposure to the antigen reveals an increased capacity on the part of the individual to react. This altered capacity is a function of both *genetic predisposition* and *repeated exposure* to the allergen. All cells in the immune system are derived from stem cells in the bone marrow. The lymphocyte plays a major role in both humoral immunity (B cells) and cell-mediated immunity (T cells).

3. Describe humoral immunity.
In humoral immunity, B lymphocytes produce the five classes of immunoglobulins: IgA, IgM, IgG, IgD, and IgE. With the stimulus of a specific antigen, B lymphocytes in association with T-helper lymphocytes produce antibodies specific to the antigen, which results in an immune response. Antibodies produce reactions specific to their type. For example, IgE attaches to antigen on the surface of a mast cell, causing mediator (e.g., histamine) release.

4. Describe cell-mediated immunity.
The T lymphocytes are involved in cell-mediated immunity. Subtypes of the T lymphocytes, T-helper and T-suppressor cells, produce soluble factors called *lymphokines* to enhance or suppress an immunologic response. The T-helper cell amplifies an antibody response by increasing B cell production, thus increasing the number of antibodies to a particular antigen, while a T-suppressor cell decreases antibody production to an antigen. Immunotherapy is designed to activate the function of T-suppressor cells.

5. What are natural killer cells?
Natural killer cells (NK) are non-T and non-B cells that may be of monocyte lineage, although recent research suggests most are derived from lymphocytes. NK cells can bind IgG to receptors on their cell surfaces. It has been shown that certain antibodies can mediate lysis of virus-infected cells by this mechanism in vitro. There is evidence suggesting such activity plays a role in host defense against viruses and tumors.

6. What are the functions of the five classes of immunoglobulins?
IgE normally makes up less than 1% of serum immunoglobulins, and can be detected in cord blood at birth. It is involved in *immediate (type I) hypersensitivity* (see Question 13), and may also be elevated in other disease states such as parasitic disease. IgE molecules attached to a mast cell must be bridged by an antigen to incite an allergic reaction.

IgG is a single immunoglobulin molecule, making up about 75% of all serum immunoglobulin. There are four subclasses of IgG, three of which are capable of binding complement. IgG4 is the source of *blocking antibodies* stimulated by immunotherapy injections. IgG receptors are present on neutrophils and killer cells. Recurrent severe sinopulmonary infections may be manifestations of a depressed immune response secondary to IgG deficiency. Maternal IgG levels are carried over for about 6 months after birth, longer if the infant is breast fed. This gives adequate time for the infant's IgG to develop.

IgA makes up about 15% of serum immunoglobulins, and is found in all secretory and mucosal tissue in the respiratory, gastrointestinal, and genitourinary tracts, as well as in secretions such as breast milk and saliva. Two IgA molecules (*dimer*) joined with epithelial secretions form an immunocompetent S-IgA molecule. This molecule provides *surface protection to the mucous membranes* against antigens. Secretory IgA (S-IgA) constitutes greater than 80% of all antibodies produced in mucosa-associated lymphoid tissues in humans. IgA levels rise slowly in the first year of life.

IgM is a large immunoglobulin made up of five monomer units, and represents about 8% of serum immunoglobulins. It is the body's *earliest defense* against bacteria. It is the first rise in response to initial exposure to antigen or bacteria, and is later supplanted by the reaction of IgG in subsequent exposures. IgM rises rapidly in the first year of life.

IgD is a monomer similar to IgG, making up less than 1% of serum immunoglobulins. Its function is unknown at this time.

7. What is the role of histamine in the allergic response?

Histamine is present in the mast cell and basophil. Two types of histamine receptors are found on cell surfaces: H_1 receptors are found on smooth muscle of vessels, bronchi, and gastrointestinal mucosa, while H_2 receptors are found on suppressor T cells, basophils, mast cells, neutrophils, and gastric cells. Histamine causes increased vascular permeability, edema, and vasodilation. It is the mediator of the skin test (whealing) response; the primary mediator of a type I (IgE) allergic response; and possibly a factor in late-phase allergic response. Certain foods such as chocolate and red wine are known to stimulate production of histamine, even in the absence of a hypersensitivity response.

8. Is heparin also a mediator?

Yes. Heparin may assist in suppressing histamine production. It assists in production of phagocytes, and may block tissue damage associated with an allergic response.

9. What are prostaglandins?

Prostaglandins are formed from arachidonic acid, and are of several different types. The prostaglandin active in an immediate hypersensitivity response is PGD2, which is spasmogenic and vasoactive, and inhibits platelet aggregation. The overproduction of PGD2 can be moderated by dietary change, which can increase production of PGD1 and PGD3, helpful in mediating an inflammatory response. (Increasing consumption of monounsaturates such as olive oil, avocado, nuts, and flax seed while reducing consumption of saturated fat [animal] is a common therapeutic recommendation.)

10. Describe the functions of leukotrienes, platelet-activating factor, and interleukins.

Leukotrienes, also formed from arachidonic acid, are the vasopermeability factors responsible for delayed or prolonged anaphylactic reactions, particularly to aspirin.

Platelet-activating factor stimulates platelets to release histamine.

Interleukins are produced by the action of a macrophage acting as an antigen-presenting cell to T lymphocytes. There are at least 10 different types of interleukins known at this time. Among the actions of the different types are:

- Stimulus for the production of inflammatory reactants
- Activation of NK cells
- Growth factor for mast cell differentiation from precursor cells to mature cells
- Increases synthesis of IgG and IgE and growth of mast cells
- Growth and differentiation of eosinophils
- Maturation of B cells into immunoglobulin-secreting cells.

11. What is complement?

Complement is a group of plasma proteins that act through enzymatic activity to cause cell lysis. Complement is particularly significant in type II and type III hypersensitivity (see Question 13). The *complement cascade* is activated by an antigen-antibody complex, and is active on the cell surface. When the sequence is complete, the complex penetrates the cell surface, allowing water into the cell and electrolytes out, resulting in cellular swelling and lysis.

12. Define hypersensitivity.

Immune response to antigens or immune complexes can result in tissue damage. These reactions are called hypersensitivity reactions.

13. What is the Gell and Coombs classification of the mechanisms of hypersensitivity?

Gell and Coombs defined four classes of hypersensitivity:

Type I hypersensitivity occurs in atopic immediate hypersensitivity diseases. Chemical mediators are released that cause vasodilation, increased vascular permeability, bronchospasm, and edema. Bronchial asthma, urticaria, analphylaxis, and allergic rhinitis are examples of type I reactions.

Type II hypersensitivity involves cytotoxic reactions, with either IgG or IgM, in which the immunoglobulin reacts on the cell surface with the cell-bound antigen, resulting in lysis of the cell. Hemolytic anemias, transfusion reaction, and myasthenia gravis are examples of Type II reaction.

Type III hypersensitivity involves immune-complex diseases. The antigen-antibody binding activates complement in the circulation, initiating a characteristic neutrophil inflammatory response. Commonly affected are serosal surfaces such as peritoneum, pleura, joints, kidney, and skin. Systemic lupus erythematosus, rheumatoid arthritis, serum sickness, and glomerulonephritis are examples of type III reaction

Type IV hypersensitivity is characterized by delayed reactions, and is cell-mediated. Macrophages also function as antigen-presenting cells, releasing interleukin-1, which promotes the proliferation of helper T cells; these in turn regulate delayed hypersensitivity reactions. Dendritic cells and Langerhan's cells are recognized as extremely efficient antigen-presenting cells, as well. Contact dermatitis, tuberculin hypersensitivity, and granulomatous hypersensitivity are examples of Type IV reaction. Clinically, Type IV reactions are seen on skin tests of yeast and molds, indicating chronic exposure to fungal antigens produced by mucocutaneous infections.

14. Define anaphylactic shock.

Anaphylactic shock is an acute IgE-mediated allergic reaction in a sensitized person. Clinical manifestations may be immediate or delayed, and include pruritis, urticaria, angioedema, hypotension, respiratory distress secondary to laryngeal edema, laryngospasm or bronchospasm, abdominal pain, and shock. Fatal anaphylaxis is due to airway obstruction.

15. What is the proper management of an acute anaphylactic reaction?

Airway management is the first priority. Intubation is indicated, and ventilation should begin with 100% oxygen. If laryngeal edema is unresponsive to epinephrine, surgical airway management may be indicated. Hypotension should be treated with epinephrine, glucagons, volume expansion with crystalloid or colloid, followed by titration to blood pressure and urine output. Resistant bronchospasm should be treated with inhaled β-agonists, such as albuterol or metaproterenol.

16. What is atopy?

Atopy is a term used clinically to describe allergic symptoms. Atopy specifically implies:
- Genetic predisposition
- The antibody produced (*atopic reagin*) is deposited in cutaneous tissue.
- The primary reaction produced is edema.

Principal atopic manifestations are bronchial asthma, vasomotor rhinitis, atopic dermatitis, and chronic urticaria.

17. What are the indications that allergy may be an etiologic factor in pediatric otolaryngic disease?

The history might include a positive family history for allergy, colic in infancy, numerous formula changes secondary to intolerance, a fussy baby who sleeps poorly, eczema, and reported intermittent erythema of the external ear following exposure to certain foods.

Physical exam characteristics may include chronic middle ear effusion, a transverse supratip crease (commonly associated with the "allergic salute," a habit of wiping the itchy nose in an upward fashion), "allergic shiners" (dark circles under the eyes due to venous stasis), Dennie's lines (allergic eye creases just under the lower lid), massive enlargement of tonsils and adenoids, hypertrophic lymphoid follicles on the posterior wall of the pharynx (cobblestone appearance), lateral pharyngeal lymphoid bands, bruxism, malocclusion, and mouth breathing.

18. Is a positive skin test necessary to identify allergic disease?

No. A positive whealing response identifies type I (IgE-mediated) allergy, which accounts for only atopic patients. Non-atopic allergies (headache, arthus reactions, delayed hypersensitivity) are typically type II, III or IV reactions, and do not display a whealing response to skin testing. Skin tests should be inspected after 48 hours for a type IV response. Type IV responses are most commonly seen in response to yeast and mold testing Clinically, type IV reactions are occasionally seen to food and pollen antigen skin tests.

19. What are the contraindications to skin testing?

Patients who are taking β-adrenergic blockers, tricyclic antidepressants, and monoamine oxidase (MAO) inhibitors should not be skin tested, as these drugs may complicate treatment of anaphylaxis. Patients who take antihistamines need to be forewarned to discontinue their use before the scheduled appointment, as residual effects may interfere with accurate SET results (see Questions 46 and 47). Short-acting antihistamines (diphenhydramine, fexofenadine) should be discontinued for 24 hours; long-acting antihistamines (loratadine, certirizine) will interfere with skin testing results for up to 3 weeks. Patients taking systemic corticosteroids should be advised to delay skin testing until 2 weeks following discontinuation, as the anti-inflammatory effects of the steroid may preclude satisfactory SET results.

20. How is allergic diathesis identified in the absence of a positive skin test?

A comprehensive history and physical assessment will identify the allergic patient. A questionnare is often employed to ensure that complete information is obtained.

In addition to the **chief complaint,** the patient should be questioned specifically regarding *symptoms of pollen, dust, mold, contact, and food allergies.*

The **system review** addresses other symptoms that the patient may not have associated with allergy, such as fatigue, sleep disorder, sore mouth or tongue, nausea, bloating, edema, headache, dizziness, fluctuating hearing loss, tinnitus, chronic external otitis, muscle and joint pain, frequent urination, menopausal or PMS symptoms, dry or cracking skin, and skin rash, particularly in the antecubital fossae.

A review of **previous illnesses** may reveal chronic sinus disease, recurrent tonsillitis or ear infections, bronchitis, asthma, migraine, and hives. Previous surgeries may include nasal polypectomy or sinus surgery, tonsillectomy, or myringotomy.

Medication history may reveal that antihistamines, aminophylline, steroid or bronchodilator inhalers, beta blockers, diuretics, and steroids are frequently prescribed.

The **family history** should investigate the incidence of autoimmune disease, diabetes, alcohol and drug abuse, as well as allergic disease.

The patient's **health habits** and **dietary history** should be assessed, particularly eliciting information regarding the use of tobacco, recreational drugs, alcohol, soft drinks, chocolate, and excessive amounts of sugar. Frequency of consumption of the common food offenders (cow's milk, corn, wheat, soy, fungal derivatives, and nightshade family—tomato, pepper, potato) should be noted, along with known food intolerances.

The patient's home and work **environment** should be investigated. Particularly, questions should be asked about water damage or excessive mold in the environment. Pet ownership or frequent **exposure** to birds and animals should be ascertained.

Social history is important to assess the effects of **stress** on the allergic patient. Job-related stress, divorce, and financial or family problems may exacerbate allergic symptoms.

21. Is allergic fungal sinusitis a true allergy or an infection?

A 1999 study from the Mayo Clinic reevaluated the current criteria for diagnosing allergic fungal sinusitis (AFS) and determined the incidence of AFS in patients with chronic rhinosinusitis (CRS). Fungal cultures of nasal secretions were positive in 96% of 210 consecutive CRS patients, with AFS diagnosed in 93% of consecutive surgical cases based on histopathologic findings and culture results. IgE-mediated hypersensitivity to fungal allergens was not evident in the majority of AFS patients. The study concluded that a more accurate terminology for AFS would be **eosinophilic fungal sinusitis.**

Manning studied patients using fungal-specific antigen, skin testing specific IgE and IgG antibodies and inhibition RAST (see Question 48). He also analyzed sinus mucosa from 14 patients by immunohistocytochemistry for eosinophilic inflammatory mediators, neurotoxin, and neutrophil mediators. The results of these two studies suggested that allergic fungal sinusitis is an antigen-triggered IgE and IgG mediator hypersensitivity response with a late-phase inflammatory reaction involving release of eosinophilic mediators.

According to Mabry et al., the differential diagnosis for AFS includes allergic mucin sinusitis (no fungi demonstrable), mycetoma (fungal forms filling one sinus without allergic mucin), or saprophytic fungal growth within a diseased sinus (positive culture without other features). The authors describe characteristic features of AFS: chronic pansinusitis with polyposis, tenaceous allergic mucin with a light green or grey color, and "peanut butter" texture. Histologically, this material contained numerous eosinophils and Charcot-Leyden crystals. Fungal stains showed the presence of noninvasive hyphae.

22. List some dietary sources of fungal derivatives.

Dietary sources of fungal derivatives are yeasts; products of fermentation such as vinegar and alcoholic beverages; aged and/or moldy cheese (e.g., brie, cheddar); mold-containing foods such as raisins, prunes, and black tea; foods potentially containing aflatoxins (peanuts in the shell); foods contaminated by mold during processing (fruit juice concentrates); and foods of fungal origin (e.g., mushrooms). Malt is derived from fermented barley. Yeast is added to many manufactured foods to improve the flavor or aroma.

23. What is the therapeutic regime for allergic fungal sinusitis?

Dietary and environmental avoidance of molds and dust, combined with immunotherapy, have proven effective in reducing the recurrence of sinus disease. To be effective, **dietary elimination** of fungal derivative antigens must be as complete as possible. Note that mold is ubiquitous in foodstuffs, and *total* elimination is not possible. Patients are advised to read labels carefully before purchasing processed food. **Environmental control** of obvious mold contamination is equally important, as mold spores are an ordinary component of all exterior and interior environments, making 100% avoidance impossible.

Immunotherapy is based on both type I and type IV reactions, as indicated by skin testing. Type IV reactions are treated at a dilution 5-fold weaker than the end point as indicated by the T-cell response observed 48 hours post-testing. A typical pattern of sensitivity includes a mixture of type I and type IV reactions to inhalant and ingested molds.

Marple and Mabry report excellent treatment results of AFS with a regime of: (1) careful preoperative evaluation and medical preparation, (2) meticulous exenterative surgery, (3) closely supervised immunotherapy with relevant fungal and non-fungal antigens, (4) medical management, including topical and systemic corticosteroids as needed, (5) irrigation and self-cleansing by the patient, and (6) close clinical follow-up, with endoscopically-guided debridement when necessary. They report that this combination has greatly reduced the need for steroid therapy, eliminated the need for maintenance systemic steroids, and reduced the rate of revision surgery to virtually zero.

24. What species of mold are implicated in allergic disease?

The main hazardous species belong to the families Aspergillus, Penicillium, Cladosporium, Mucor, Stachybotrys, Absidia, Alternatia, Fusarium, and Cryptostroma. The greatest risks are associated with aspergillus and penicillium, which have been implicated as causative agents in asthma, hypersensitivity pneumonitis, pulmonary mycosis, and fungal sinusitis. Mold spores commonly produce an allergic response (rhinitis, dermatitis, sinusitis). Mold may also produce mycotoxins (see Question 25), and may pose a health threat to farmers and workers in food industries. In particular, stachybotrys mycotoxin is prevalent in buildings with indoor air problems.

25. What are the effects of chronic exposure to mold spores and/or mycotoxins?

Mycotoxins may cause a variety of short-term as well as long-term adverse health effects, ranging from immediate toxic response and immunosuppression to a potential long-term carcinogenic effect. Symptoms include dermatitis, recurring cold and flu-like symptoms, burning sore throat, headaches and excessive fatigue, diarrhea, mental confusion, and depression. In addition to mycotoxins, volatile organic compounds (musty odors) released from actively growing fungi have been associated with trigeminal nerve irritation. The "common chemical sense" responds to pungency, not odor, by initiating avoidance reactions such as breath holding, paresthesias, itching, burning, swelling of mucous membranes, and dilation of surface blood vessels. Decreased attention, disorientation, diminished reflex time, and dizziness can result from such exposure.

26. How does host resistance and immune response to fungal infections differ from other infectious agents?

Jones describes studies demonstrating that clearing of dermatophyte infection depends on a cell-mediated response. Those subjects who mounted decisive delayed-type hypersensitivity reactions more often effectively cleared the fungal infection. Those who had absent or defective cellular immunity were predisposed to chronic or recurrent dermatophyte infection. The presence of an acute, inflammatory infection was correlated with a type IV reaction to a trichophyton skin test, while chronic infection was associated with a high IgE-mediated response and a low T-cell-mediated response. Other studies have shown that the therapeutic efficacy of systemic antifungals is differentially potentiated by cytokines or cytokine antagonists, and is influenced by host immune reactivity.

27. What is an Id reaction?

The Id reaction or autoeczematization is a cutaneous response to an infection in a remote location. The cause is unknown, but it is hypothesized that increased stimulation of normal T cells by altered skin constituents with lowering of the irritation threshold may be responsible. Dereberry reported that an Id reaction from fungal infection may be responsible for some cases of chronic otitis external. Successful treatment consisted of a yeast elimination diet and immunotherapy with dermatophyte extracts (trichophyton, oidiomycetes, and epidermophyton).

28. Is chronic serous otitis media (OM) an allergic disease?

Shambaugh suspected allergy as an etiology of chronic draining mastoid cavities or middle ears of patients with OM, and recommended that "surgical mastoidectomy is not indicated. With competent allergic diagnosis and management, preferably by the otologist trained in allergic methods, the otorrhea is . . . bought under control."

Hurst reports that the middle ear is unusual in that it contains no lymphoid tissue, and normally has a very weak response to antigen challenge. However, a previously sensitized middle ear does present a vigorous immune response when presented with antigen. In subjects who have primed eosinophils and neutrophils circulating in their blood, mediators present in the middle ear will attract and activate those cells, with the resultant chronic release of *eosinophil cationic protein* (ECP).

Studies of patients with OME have shown that effusion ECP and tryptase are elevated only in atopic patients, and that total serum IgE is not definitively different from a control group. Allergic reactions, infectious inflammation, and local immunologic response associated with persistent bacterial pathogens or viruses have been considered to be factors responsible for eustachian tube dysfunction leading to otitis media. Allergy has been shown to be almost as potent as bacterial infection in producing an inflammatory response in the middle ear. This may explain why the allergic patient is particularly unable to clear the resultant fluid spontaneously. In a child who is "otitis prone," bacterial or viral OM will proceed to the development of refractory effusion.

Stenfors reported that immunoglobulin activity is specific in combating bacterial pathogens invading the middle ear. IgA prevents bacteria from attaching to the epithelium, has no pro-inflammatory effect, and does not activate complement. IgG antibodies have a phygocytoxic effect on bacteria, and prevent bacteria from penetrating the epithelium. IgG is pro-inflammatory and can activate a complement cascade.

Other research examined the different mediators of inflammation contained in sticky, glue-like effusion in the middle ear. Results suggested a strong complement activation and consequent inflammation in children with chronic OME. Complement damage to the epithelial lining is prevented by a strong expression of regulators *membrane cofactor protein* (MCP) and *protectin* (CD59).

29. Which allergens are commonly implicated in chronic otitis media?

Chronic middle ear effusion in children is most commonly associated with allergy to a food. Patients typically have an atopic history with an incidence of 43% allergic rhinitis, 40% asthma, and 21% atopic eczema. There is a high incidence of adverse reactions to cow's milk (7.5% of infants), and of this group, many are allergic to eggs (58%), soy (47%), oranges (35%), and peanuts (35%). Prolonged breast feeding and dietary control are preferred methods of management. Cow's milk allergy is not transitory; only 28% of children reach clinical tolerance by age 2, 56% by age 4, and 78% by age 6. Even if a child appears to become milk-tolerant, subsequent atopic disorders frequently develop.

30. What role does allergy play in Meniere's disease?

Wilson theorized that initial hypersensitization of the patient to penicillin might be responsible for the eventual antigenic excitation of a perverse labyrinthine response by commonly ingested fungal derivatives or exposure to mold spores. He achieved a 26% success rate in treating patients with complete elimination of all known allergic offenders and hyposensitization for proven inhalant allergens. At the time of the study (1974), Wilson reported that attempts to hyposensitize to ingested yeasts and products of fermentation were unsuccessful.

Dereberry reported evidence that allergy and immunologic factors play a role in some Meniere's patients. Meniere's disease is thought to be related to function of the endolymphatic sac (ELS). The ELS has a highly vascular subepithelial space containing numerous fenestrated blood vessels that are peripheral and "leaky." At least three mechanisms by which allergy may play a role in causing dysfunction of the the ELS are: the ELS itself may be a "target organ" of mediator released from systemic inhalant or food reactions; deposition of circulating immune complex may produce inflammation and interfere with the sac's filtering capability; and a predisposing viral infection may produce a mild impairment of ELS function, which may interact with allergies, causing the sac to decompensate. The endolymphatic sac is the seat of immune reactivity in the inner ear. Repeated inflammatory reactions can produce dysfunction and eventual Meniere's disease.

31. What is the etiology of nasal polyps? How can recurrence be prevented after removal?

Nasal polyps are caused by allergy and infectious process. Polyps are commonly seen in triad with aspirin allergy and asthma. Steroids and decongestants can be used on a temporary basis to offer relief of obstruction. Polyps that obstruct the airway and sinus ostia may be a contributing cause of chronic sinus infection and require surgical removal. Recent research has shown that nasal polyp-infiltrating plasma cells are mainly IgA-secreting cells, a part of the mucosal immune system. The IgA production is partly dependent on IL-10 and TNF-α. The absence of IgE-secreting cells suggested that a type I sensitivity is not necessary for the development of nasal polyps.

Recurrence can often be prevented by control of the allergic condition—dietary and environmental controls with immunotherapy, if needed.

32. What is the etiology of chronic thrush?

Clinically, chronic thrush has been associated with a poor immune response to mucocutaneous fungal infections. Dietary and environmental control of fungal sources, and immunotherapy may improve the response to topical oral antifungal medications.

Research has shown that decreased salivary flow, decreased secretion of antimicrobial proteins in saliva, and reduced effect of polymorphonuclear leukocytes in the saliva of the aged and immunocompromised patient increase the risk factor for oral candidiasis. Other studies have shown that candidiasis with hyposalivation may induce pain in the tongue without manifestation of objective abnormalities.

33. What is the initial recommendation for the control of allergies?

The first and most important strategy is avoidance of the allergen(s). This may involve:

1. **Control dust and mold in the home and work environments.** Clean-up and repair of water leaks and other moisture damage; the use of mold inhibitors and ozone to kill mold spores remaining after decontamination; regular cleaning of furnace ducts; use of electrostatic or HEPA filters and dehumidifiers; and proper ventilation for bathrooms, clothes dryers, and kitchen appliances will reduce ambient mold in interior air. Swamp coolers should be avoided because the water-soaked filter pads accumulate moldy growth, carried by the cool air to seed the interior with mold spores. Avoidance of carpets, drapes, excessive plants, stuffed animals, and other décor reduces dust exposure. Attention to drainage problems outside the house can be helpful: excessive watering of lawns, moisture and mold growth in crawl spaces, shrubs planted too close to the foundation, and improper channeling of drain spouts away from the foundation creates soil saturation, causing elevated humidity which contributes to interior growth of mold.

2. **Limit exposure to pollens.** Avoid the use of attic fans, which pull in mold spores and pollens from outside air. Keep windows closed at night, and use air conditioners during pollen season.

3. **Limit exposure to birds and animals.** At the very least, exclude pets from sleeping spaces. The sleeping area must be thoroughly cleaned and sanitized to remove all vestiges of fur, feathers, or saliva. Ideally, an allergic patient should not own pets.

4. **Eliminate exposure to allergenic foods.** Food allergens that have been identified by history and/or skin testing should be totally eliminated. This involves not only ingested food choices, but the presence of the food as an additive (corn and soy are ubiquitous in the American diet), as a filler or excipient in medications (corn starch or dextrose in IV fluids), or as an ingredient in toothpaste or mouthwash.

5. **Control stress.** Stress reduction may involve counseling, lifestyle change, or other factors generally outside the venue of the ENT physician. A regular program of exercise and meditation are excellent recommendations known to be effective in controlling excess production of cortisol.

34. What is the allergic threshold response?

Many individuals are genetically predisposed to allergy but never experience allergic symptoms. This avoidance is possible because their exposure to allergens has never reached the concentration or *threshold* that precipitates symptoms. The threshold may be reached by an overwhelming exposure to one allergen, or it may be the cumulative effect of exposure to several. It is possible to control allergic symptoms by controlling exposure to the most obvious or frequently encountered allergens. This limits the total number of circulating antibodies at any given time.

Infection increases the likelihood or severity of an allergic response. Deficiencies of IgA or

IgG may increase the susceptibility to infection, due to compromised immunocompetence of mucosal surfaces. Mobilization of the immune system to fight infection results in disruption of the homeostasis which may have been attained by dietary and environmental controls and immunotherapy.

Stress lowers the allergic threshold by increasing cortisol output in the "fight or flight" mode, reducing the availability of the body's normal physiologic cortisol to deal with inflammation. Recent evidence demonstrates that physiologic amounts of cortisol are needed to develop and maintain normal immunity, and that there is a feedback relationship between the immune system and the hypothalamic-pituitary-adrenal axis.

35. Are all food allergies mediated by the immune system?

No. Non-immunologic food reactions include:

Chemical hypersensitivity

- Caffeine may cause headache, anxiety, palpitations.
- Histamine release from foods such as alcohol, chocolate, strawberries, tomatoes may cause headaches, tachycardia, urticaria.
- Tyramine hypersensitivity may cause headache and urticaria; tyramine is found in aged cheese, red wines, liver, brewers yeast. Monoamine oxidase inhibitors interfere with metabolism and clearance of tyramine; foods containing tyramine should be avoided by those taking this medication.
- Vasoactive amines include phenyethylamine and dopamine found in chocolate, serotonin in cheeses.

Enzyme intolerance abnormalities

- Lactase deficiency occurs in approximately 5–20% of North Caucasian individuals, and 60–90% in other races and areas of the world.
- Phenylketonuria—avoidance of foods containing phenylalanine, especially aspartame is necessary.

Idiosyncratic reactions to foods (mechanism of action not always well understood)

- Asthma can be induced by ingestion of sulfites or FD&C Yellow No. 5.
- Hyperkinetic behavior is observed in children following the ingestion of food-coloring agents or excessive sugar.
- "Chinese Restaurant Syndrome" can result from consumption of excessive amounts of monosodium glutamate.
- Migraine headaches may follow consumption of chocolate or aspartame.

36. What are the classifications of immunologic food reactions?

In the U.S., "food allergy" has been identified with immediate or type I hypersensitivity to a food which occurs within 1 hour of ingestion, is IgE mediated, and results in the classic symptoms of angioedema and urticaria. European literature uses the term "allergy" to include all types of Gell and Coombs immune hyperreactions, I, II, III, and IV.

Within this context, food reactions may be classified as "immediate" (about 5% of food allergy reactions), or "delayed" (about 95% of food allergy reactions). The type III response appears to be most prominent in·delayed food reactions.

Based on clinical observations, Rinkel, Randolph, and Zeller proposed two categories of food allergy—fixed and cyclic.

37. How do "fixed" and "cyclic" food allergies differ?

A *fixed* food allergy is usually present from a very early age in an atopic individual. The amount of food that must be eaten to become sensitized is unknown. Atopic infants have reportedly become sensitized to minute quantities of food allergens present in the mother's breast milk. A fixed food allergy always produces an *immediate* reaction. Allergies to peanuts, shellfish, nuts, and food dyes are typical fixed allergies, with potentially fatal consequences of ingestion. Tolerance is never developed.

Cyclic food allergies are nonanaphylactic and are developed in response to frequency of exposure to the food. As noted above, most *delayed* responses are thought to be type III. Frequent consumption results in the formation of antigen excess, forming soluble immune complexes which cause low-grade chronic symptoms. On dietary exclusion, antigen concentration falls, precipitable immune complexes are formed, and "acute serum sickness" results (withdrawal symptoms). Prolonged elimination of the antigen results in any immune complexes being in antibody excess, and soluble again, thus clearing symptoms.

While the "serum sickness immune complex" model explains multiple manifestations of food allergy reaction, the reason for occurrence in a particular shock organ (ear, nose, skin) remains unexplained.

38. What are the stages of a cyclic food reaction?

Cyclic food allergy is a function of frequency of exposure. The pioneering work of Herbert Rinkel led to classification of the stages of food allergy:

Masking stage (commonly seen in the office)
- Patient is not born with allergy to the food.
- Sensitization is caused by frequent ingestion.
- Clinical symptoms develop slowly.
- Initial food ingestion causes temporary stimulation.
- When stimulation wears off, symptoms develop.
- Patient craves food to continue stimulation.
- **Immunologic—antigen is in excess, with pseudotolerance.**

Withdrawal stage (may or may not occur, depending on severity of food addiction)
- Eliminating food leads to withdrawal symptoms, often severe.
- Stage lasts up to 4 days.
- **Immunologic—antigen clears, leaving high levels of antibody; may be in a complex with tissue that is antigenically similar to the food, such as the synovium or GI tract in a type II reaction.**

Hyperacute stage (lasts 4–12 days)
- Remission of symptoms, cytotoxic reactions have ceased.
- Oral challenge leads to a marked reaction.
- **Immunologic—ingested antigen combines with available amount of immune complexes.**

Active sensitization state (length is a function of severity of allergy)
- Remission of symptoms as long as avoidance is continued
- Little or no tolerance of more than one exposure to the food

Latent sensitization state
- Ingestion of food causes intermittent and mild symptoms.
- Continued elimination will lead to tolerance; without antigenic stimulation, antibodies will decrease

Tolerance (3 months to 2 years)
- Food ingestion no longer produces symptoms.
- Food must be rotated every 4 days.
- **Immunologic—little or no antibody present, but memory cells "remember" food.**

Full cycle (if food is again ingested frequently)
- Tolerance stage may last 2–4 weeks.
- Latent sensitization develops (mild symptoms).
- Active sensitization develops (symptoms each time).
- Masking stage occurs.
- **Immunologic—increasing antigen exposure leads to the formation of immune complexes and increased symptoms.**

A delayed food reaction can take place up to 72 hours after the ingestion of the food. Aberrant cytokine production has been associated with atopic disease. Recent research studied the effect of oral food allergen challenges on serum cytokine production. Results showed that patients with late-onset reactions were found to have lower levels of IL-10 concentration than did their immediate-reacting counterparts. These patients are likely to show a negative skin test.

39. What is the oral challenge feeding test?

Herbert Rinkel developed the concept of the oral challenge feeding test, which consists of total removal of the suspected food allergen from the diet for 4 days. On the 5th day, the food is fed in a pure form, unaccompanied by other foods, twice in the morning. After elimination during the day, the food is fed with the evening meal, accompanied by other foods. If reaction is noted after the initial feeding, other feedings are suspended. The patient is watched for symptoms up to 72 hours following the feeding.

Food challenges are most effective diagnostically when a single allergenic food is suspected, or when other offenders have previously been eliminated.

40. Does the oral challenge test work if multiple food allergies are mediated by different immune mechanisms, or if there are multiple shock organs?

It may be necessary to repeat challenge feedings of different foods, if confusing results are obtained with the first challenge. In practice, patients may discover that certain symptoms are specific to one food, while another food causes other symptoms. In the period following elimination of the known offender, they may report adverse reactions to previously unsuspected food offenders.

41. Are foods ever cross-reactive with pollen allergy?

Many allergic individuals react both to pollens and foods, and some report a potentiating effect between specific combinations. Research has identified a family of proteins called *profilin*, present in plant families, that are capable of acting as pan-allergens causing cross-reactivity. For example, a cross-reactivity has been documented between the summer squash family (cantaloupe, zucchini) and ragweed; and between grass and the lily family (onions, garlic). In practice, it is possible to reduce symptoms of pollinosis during season by avoiding the cross-reactive food.

42. What is latex allergy? Do foods ever cross-react with latex?

Latex is an emulsion of rubber globules derived from the sap of plants of the Euphorbiacea family. Within the last 15 years, it has become a cause of serious allergic reactions. The major allergen appears to be a protein fragment known as rubber elongation factor; it causes contact dermatitis, pruritus, urticaria, conjunctivitis, rhinitis, and asthma. In recent years, a number of cases of anaphylaxis have been reported, particularly among those frequently exposed such as healthcare workers, latex industry workers, and patients who undergo frequent operative procedures. Latex sensitivity is so exquisite in sensitized individuals that they must avoid even the environments where latex is used. Aerosolized latex from the powder in gloves of coworkers has been known to cause reaction. Cross-reactions with avocado, bananas, chestnuts, and fruits have been reported.

43. What is seasonal allergic rhinitis? What is the standard medical treatment for this condition?

Tree, grass, and weed pollens in their seasons may cause symptoms of allergic rhinitis in susceptible individuals. Symptomatic relief may be afforded by prescription antihistamines (Allegra, Claritin), natural antihistamines (Quercitin with vitamin C), freeze-dried Stinging Nettles), natural homeopathic remedies (Zicam for allergy), mast-cell inhibitors (Nasochrom), and nasal steroids (Beconase). Saline nasal irrigation may facilitate ciliary action to wash away secretions, but has the disadvantage of washing away secretory IgA in the process. Immunotherapy may offer relief to those whose symptoms are not adequately controlled by medication or local measures.

44. What is the relationship of pollinosis to food allergy in aggravating chronic allergic symptoms?

Uncontrolled seasonal pollen allergies may exacerbate perennial symptoms caused by food allergy. This is explained by the concept of the **total load** and/or the allergic threshold (see Question 34). Total load refers to the sum effect of all uncontrolled allergens on the atopic individual.

45. What is perennial allergic rhinitis? What is the standard medical treatment for this condition?

Perennial symptoms may be caused by allergy to foods, ingested and inhalant molds, dust, pets, and chemicals. Treatment should be based on avoidance and immunotherapy rather than medication to suppress symptoms. Recent animal research has shown that preservatives commonly used in nasal sprays and drops (benzalkonium chloride and potassium sorbate) can lead to nasal lesions, including intraepithelial glandular formation, inflammatory cell infiltration, vascular hyperplasia, and edematous change. Prolonged use is not recommended.

46. What is immunotherapy?

Immunotherapy is the attenuation of the atopic individual's allergic response by hyposensitization to specific allergens. Using either the skin endpoint titration (SET) or RAST method of determination, the relieving dose of an antigen is established to the specific tolerance of the patient. Symptomatic relief is safely, rapidly, and efficiently obtainable with these techniques, which are both quantitative and qualitative.

47. What is SET?

Quantitative Skin Endpoint Titration was introduced by Herbert Rinkel in the 1940s. The technique consists of:

- Intradermal application of 0.01–0.02 cc of antigen to produce a 4-mm wheal at a presumed nonreacting level of the antigen (usually N-5 strength).
- Progressively stronger 5-fold dilutions are applied until the first 2 mm or greater increment in whealing is observed.
- Continue applying progressively stronger dilutions through two dilutions beyond the dilution where progression begins.
- The endpoint is determined to be at the level of a 7-mm wheal. Progressive whealing response must be noted to determine a valid endpoint.
- Immunotherapy is commenced with a dose of 0.1 cc of the antigen at the endpoint determined by the testing.

Advantages of this technique are:
- Both quantitative and qualitative
- Highly reproducible
- Very sensitive
- Safe to begin immunotherapy at a therapeutic dose
- Objective
- Identifies type IV reactions as well as type I reactions

Disadvantages are the time needed to test and the volume of supplies needed.

48. What is RAST?

RAST stands for radioallergosorbent test, which is an *in vitro* measure of specific IgE determination. Allergens are chemically linked to solid-phase supports (usually paper discs) that are incubated with a droplet of serum from the patient. If specific IgE antibodies are present in the serum, they will bind with the allergen to form a complex. In a second step, the discs are incubated with radio-labeled IgE antibodies from another species, usually rabbit. After incubation, all free-labeled anti-IgE is washed away, leaving the specific IgE with a radioactive tag to be counted. The Modified RAST (MR) Scoring System has shown a 95% accuracy in response to properly performed nasal or conjunctival provocation test with the antigen.

In RAST-based immunotherapy, the recommended initial doses are administered in inverse proportion to the individual MR score. In other words, a high specific antibody score indicates the need for a very dilute allergen concentration. Once initial doses are successfully administered, the dose is doubled at each subsequent visit until customary maximal levels are reached. (This is dependent on clinical response.)

Recommended practice suggests that prior to starting immunotherapy, an intradermal skin test of the specific antigen mixture is placed. If a wheal of 15 mm or less is produced, the initial dose is administered subcutaneously.

RAST testing may be preferred to SET in atopic patients who show dermatographia or have extensive skin involvement. RAST is not effective in the diagnosis and treatment of non-atopic hypersensitivity.

CONTROVERSY

49. How did SET become the treatment of choice for ENT physicians?
Actually, this is not really controversial. Otolaryngic allergy is indebted for its present metholodogy to a physician who was not an otolaryngologist. Herbert Rinkel introduced quantitative skin endpoint titration, based on the pioneering work of Hansel, in the 1940s while concurrently developing a regime to identify and treat food allergies by elimination. Rinkel worked extensively with Theron Randolph (the father of clinical ecology) and ENT allergy pioneers, Dor Brown, Russell Williams, William Wilson, and James Willoughby to develop a system of allergy treatment more effective for their ENT patients than the scratch or prick methods of skin testing, which were in prevalent use at that time. For a number of years, courses to train otolaryngologists were taught yearly in Cheyenne and Jackson Hole, Wyoming by this group. Dr. Brown was a founder of the Pan American Allergy Society, which continues to offer a yearly training course based on Rinkel's techniques. The first instructional course program at the ASOOA (predecessor of AAOA) in 1971 was organized by Dr. Hugh Powers, and 32 instructional courses were given. By 1985, membership in the AAOA had passed the 1000 mark necessary for membership in the American Medical Association. Today, the AAOA is the largest subspecialty group of the American Academy of Otolaryngology.

BIBLIOGRAPHY

1. Ammann HM: Is Indoor Mold Contamination a Threat to Health? http://www.doh.wa.gov/ehp/oehas/mold.html
2. Corey JP: Allergic Fungal Sinusitis: Role of Immunotherapy, Antifungals and other Adjunctive Therapies http://www.invitroallergy.org/99mtng/abstracts/Corey.htm
3. Corthesy B, Spertini F: Secretory immunoglobulin A: From mucosal protection to vaccine development. Biological Chemistry 380(11):1251–62, 1999.
4. Dereberry, MJ: Allergic and immunologic aspects of Meniere's Disease. J Otolaryngol Head Neck Surg 114(3):360–365, 1996.
5. Dereberry MJ: Fixed vs. Cyclic Food Allergies. Notes presented at AAOA July 24, 1996.
6. Dereberry MJ, Berliner KI: Foot and Ear Disease—The dermatophid reaction. Laryngoscope 106:181–186, 1996.
7. Gray Environmental, Inc: Common Toxigenic Fungi Found Indoors. http://www.grayenvironmental.com/mold.htm
8. Hurst DS: Literature Review of Middle Ear Disease in *Kid's Ear Disease, Fluid & Allergy, http://home.earthlink.net/~meear/Review.html*
9. Hurst DS: The Middle Ear: A Possible Target Organ for Allergy in Children with Otitis Media with Effusion. Presented at AAOA, September 2000.
10. Cho J-H, et al: Long-Term Use of Preservatives on Rat Nasal Respiratory Mucosa: Effects of Benzalkonium Chloride and Potassium Sorbate. Laryngoscope 110:312–317, 2000.
11. Jones HE: Immune response and host resistance of humans to dermatophyte infections. J Am Acad Dermatol 28(5 Pt 1):S12-S18, 1993.
12. Mabry RL, Manning SC, Mabry CS: Immunotherapy in the treatment of allergic fungal sinusitis. J Otolaryngol Head Neck Surg 116:31–35, 1997.
13. Manning S: Further Evidence for Allergic Pathophysiology in Allergic Fungal Sinusitis. Otoscope 2(2), April 1997. http://depts.washington/edu/otoweb/OtoScope6.html
14. Marei MA, al-Hamshary AM, Abdalla KF, Abdel-Maaboud AI: A study on secretory IgA in malnourished children with chronic diarrhea associated with parasitic infections. J Egyptian Soc Parasitol 28(3):907–13, 1998.
15. Mencacci A, Cenci E, Bacci A, Bistoni F, Romani L: Host immune reactivity determines the efficacy of

combination immunotherapy and antifungal chemotherapy in candidiasis. J Infect Dis 181(2):686–94, 2000.

16. Nalebuff DJ: Use of RAST Screening in Clinical Allergy: A Cost-Effective Approach to Patient Care. Ear Nose Throat J 107–121, 1985.

17. Narkio-Makela M, Jero J, Meri S: Complement activation and expression of membrane regulators in the middle ear mucosa in otitis media with effusion. Clin Exp Immunol 116(3):401–9, 1999.

18. Osaki T, Yoneda K, Yamamoto T, Ueta E, Kimura T: Candidiasis may induce glossodynia without objective manifestation. Am J Med Sci 319(2):100–105, 2000.

19. Pediatric Database: Dietary Protein Intolerance. http://www.icondata.com/health/pedbase/files/DIETARYP.HTM

20. Ponikau JE, Sherris DA, Kern EB, et al: The Diagnosis and Incidence of Allergic Fungal Sinusitis. Mayo Clin Proc. 74:877–884, 1999.

21. Sanchez-Segura A, Brieva JA, Rodriguez C: Regulation of immunoglobulin secretion by plasma cells infiltrating nasal polyps. Laryngoscope 110(7):1183–1188, 2000.

22 Snyder OP, Poland DM: Adverse Reactions to Food, Food Allergy and Sensitivity. Hospitality Institute of Technology and Management, June 1997, St. Paul, MN. http://www.hi-tm.com/Documents/Allergy.html

23. Sutas Y, Kekki OM, Isolauri E: Late-onset reactions to oral food challenge are linked to low serum interleukin-10 concentrations in patients with atopic dermatitis and food allergy, Clin Exp Allergy 30(8):1121–8, 2000.

24. Trotsky M: Immunology for the Otolaryngic Allergist. Otolaryngol Clin North Am 25(1):151–162, 1992.

25. Ueta E, Tanida T, Doi S, Osaki T: Regulation of *Candida albicans* growth and adhesion by saliva. J Lab Clin Med 136(1):66–73, 2000.

26. University of Texas Southwestern Medical Center at Dallas: Clinics and Services Information: Allergic Fungal Sinusitis. http://www2.swmed.edu/oto/clin/afs.htm

27. Vanderbilt Medical Center: Chronic Fungal Sinusitis. http://www.mc.vanderbilt.edu/peds/pidl/infect/fungsinu/htm

28. Wilson L: Focus On . . . The Etiology of Allergy. Medical Sciences Bulletin http://pharminfo.com/pubs/msb/allergy_et.html

74. RADIOLOGY OF THE HEAD AND NECK

Caroline L. Hollingsworth, M.D., David Rubinstein, M.D.,
and B. Burton Putegnat, M.D.

1. What are the major advantages and disadvantages of MRI in head and neck imaging?

Advantages

- Multiple pulse sequences to characterize lesions
- Multiplanar imaging without reconstructing images
- Demonstration of arteries and veins without contrast
- No use of ionizing radiation
- Direct imaging of bone marrow

Disadvantages

- MRI takes significantly more time than CT; claustrophobia may interfere with exam
- More sensitive to patient motion (e.g., swallowing) than CT
- Contraindicated in patients with pacemakers, some aneurysm clips, cochlear implants, neurostimulators, and other metallic foreign bodies
- Does not delineate cortical and trabecular bone detail as well as CT
- Higher cost than CT

2. What structures are located in the parapharyngeal space? Why is this space important radiographically?

The parapharyngeal space runs from the skull base to the hyoid bone and is just deep to the pharyngeal mucosa and superficial to the carotid sheath. Inferiorly, it communicates openly with the submandibular space. The parapharyngeal space contains relatively few structures: fat, the mandibular branch of the facial nerve, the pterygoid venous plexus, and branches of the ascending pharyngeal artery.

Although a rare source of primary pathology, this space is extremely important as a radiographic landmark because the fat makes it readily visible on MR and CT images of the suprahyoid neck. Due to its central anatomic position, the origin of pathologic processes within the deep fascial spaces of the neck can be identified by the specific displacement pattern of the parapharyngeal space. The parapharyngeal space may provide a path for pathology to extend superiorly to the skull base. (See figures.)

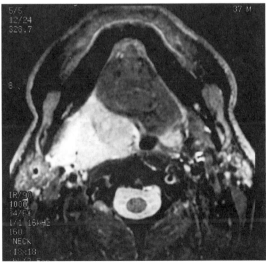

T2-weighted MRI of the suprahyoid neck depicts a homogeneously hyperintense mass with its center in the parapharyngeal space. The right carotid sheath is displaced posterolaterally. (Courtesy of Gregory Chaljub, M.D., Department of Radiology, University of Texas Medical Branch at Galveston.)

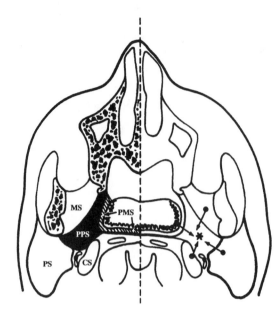

Axial view of the midnasopharynx illustrates the parapharyngeal space, carotid space, masticator space, pharyngeal mucosal space, and parotid space as well as the displacement pattern typical of a mass located in one of these spaces. (From Harnsberger HRic: Handbook of Head and Neck Imaging, 2nd ed. St. Louis, Mosby, 1995, p 18, with permission).

3. What is the most common benign tumor of the parapharyngeal space?

Pleomorphic adenomas of ectopic salivary gland tissue are the most frequently encountered benign tumors of the parapharyngeal space. It is important to determine whether the tumor actually originates from the deep lobe of the parotid gland, because the surgical approaches differ. A tumor that originates in the deep lobe may be accessible with a transparotid approach, which presents less risk to the facial nerve than an oral or submandibular approach. (See figure.)

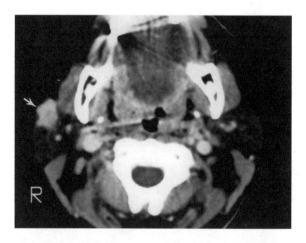

Axial CT of a pleomorphic adenoma (*white arrow*) located in the superficial lobe of the right parotid gland. (Courtesy of Gregory Chaljub, M.D., Department of Radiology, University of Texas Medical Branch at Galveston)

4. Describe the location, contents, and anatomic relations of the masticator space.

The masticator space runs anterolateral to the parapharyngeal space from the temporal fossa to the mandible. Important structures contained within this space include the muscles of mastication (masseter, temporalis, and medial and lateral pterygoid) as well as the third portion of the fifth cranial nerve. The majority of masses in the masticator space originate from an infection secondary to dental caries or dental extraction. Neoplasm or infection may spread to the skull base by tracking along the mandibular division of the trigeminal nerve or temporalis muscle. (See figures.)

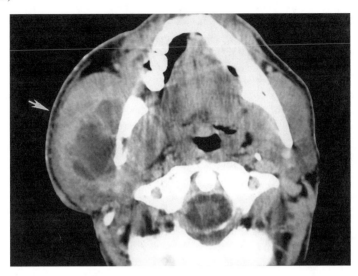

Axial CT image of an abscess (*white arrow*) located in the masticator space. (Courtesy of Faustino Guinto, M.D., Department of Radiology, University of Texas Medical Branch at Galveston)

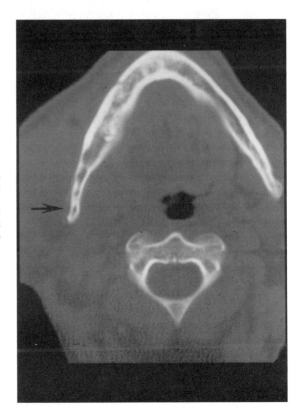

Axial CT image with bone widows shows bone destruction associated with osteomyelitis (*black arrow*) of the mandible secondary to an abscess. (Courtesy of Faustino Guinto, M.D., Department of Radiology, University of Texas Medical Branch at Galveston.)

5. When a lesion is localized to the carotid space, what are the most common entities in the differential diagnosis?

The borders of the carotid space are the jugular and carotid foramina superiorly, the deep lobe of the parotid laterally, the retropharyngeal space medially, and the aortic arch inferiorly. This space is surrounded by a tough fascia formed from the three layers of the deep cervical fascia. Since this space communicates intracranially via the jugular foramen, it provides the opportunity for intracranial and extracranial spread of disease. You must know the contents of the space to formulate a differential diagnosis. The contents include important vascular (common carotid artery and internal jugular vein), neural (cranial nerves IX–XII and sympathetic plexus), and lymphatic structures (deep cervical chain, including the jugulodigastric or sentinel node). **Paraganglioma, schwannoma, and nodal metastasis** from a squamous cell carcinoma are the most common lesions found within the carotid space. (See figure.)

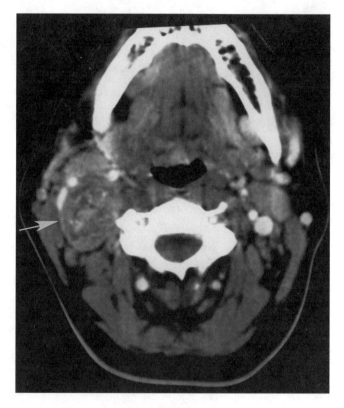

Right carotid space schwannoma (*white arrow*) on axial contrast-enhanced CT. (Courtesy of Faustino Guinto, M.D., Department of Radiology, University of Texas Medical Branch at Galveston)

6. Describe the characteristic appearance of a paraganglioma on CT and MRI.

MRI of a paraganglioma reveals a heterogeneous, tubular mass in the carotid space, jugular foramen, or middle ear, characterized by multiple areas of low intensity that represent flow voids. On CT, a paraganglioma characteristically appears as an intensely enhancing mass. Paragangliomas produce irregular, permeative bony changes around the jugular foramen, whereas schwannomas, another lesion found in the jugular foramen, produce regular, smooth, scalloped changes. Carotid body tumors separate the internal and external carotid arteries. (See figures.)

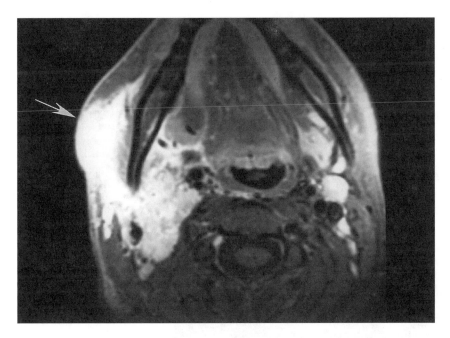

Enhanced fat-saturated T1-weighted MRI depicts a paraganglioma (*white arrow*) on the right involving the parapharyngeal and masticator spaces inferiorly. (Courtesy of Gregory Chaljub, M.D., Department of Radiology, University of Texas Medical Branch at Galveston)

Magnetic resonance angiogram (MRA) shows marked widening of the carotid sheath on the right secondary to the presence of a paraganglioma located at the carotid bifurcation. (Courtesy of Gregory Chaljub, M.D., Department of Radiology, University of Texas Medical Branch at Galveston)

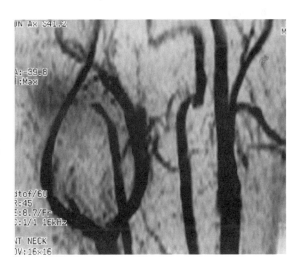

7. What is the most appropriate imaging technique for evaluating a suspected abscess of the head and neck?

Both MRI and CT can be used to evaluate an abscess for the presence of osteomyelitis. CT has the advantages of being faster and more economical. On CT, an abscess usually appears to have a thick wall surrounded by inflammatory changes. These changes are usually characterized by enhanced soft tissue with or without septations. (See figure.)

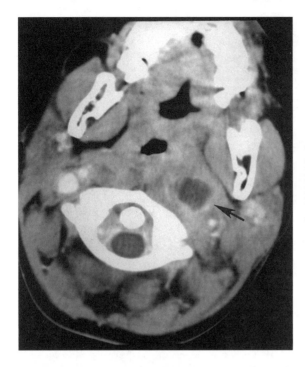

Contrast-enhanced axial CT demonstrating an abscess (*black arrow*) with a
hypodense center and peripheral enhancement. (Courtesy of Susan John,
M.D., Department of Radiology, The
University of Texas Medical Branch at
Galveston)

**8. Which clinical conditions may mimic a retropharyngeal space abscess on radiologic
evaluation?**

Fluid that has collected in the retropharyngeal space, for whatever reason, often appears radiologically identical to a retropharyngeal abscess. Such a collection may be due to various
causes, including surgery or venous obstruction from superior vena cava syndrome. In addition,
internal jugular thrombosis causing transudation of fluid into the retropharyngeal space, or distal
lymphatic obstruction that impairs drainage from the retropharyngeal space, may also mimic an
abscess on radiologic evaluation.

9. Describe the clinical presentation and radiologic appearance of branchial cleft cysts.

Ninety-five percent of branchial cleft abnormalities are derived from the second branchial
cleft. In children, the usual presentation is a submandibular mass that may be associated with a
sinus tract opening just above the clavicle. In young adults, the appearance of a submandibular

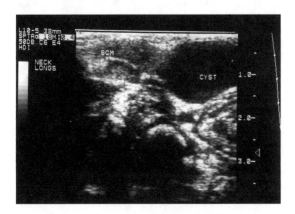

Ultrasound of a second branchial cleft
cyst at the anterior border of the sternocleidomastoid (SCM). (Courtesy of Susan John, M.D., Department of Radiology, The University of Texas Medical
Branch at Galveston)

mass is often preceded by viral infection or trauma. Ultrasound, often performed in pediatric cases, typically shows a well-circumscribed, hypoechoic lesion. Sectional imaging often shows a simple cystic mass at the angle of the mandible along the anterior margin of the sternocleido-mastoid muscle. The cyst characteristically displaces the carotid space posteromedially, the ster-nocleidomastoid muscle posterolaterally, and the submandibular gland anteromedially. It is important to image a suspected branchial cleft cyst to differentiate it from jugulodigastric node adenopathy, which may present similarly. (See figures.)

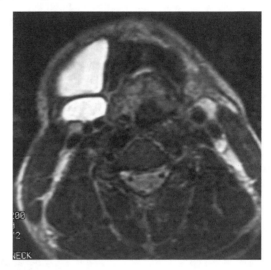

T2-weighted axial MRI of a second brachial cleft cyst at the anterior margin of the right sternocleidomastoid. (Courtesy of Gregory Chaljub, M.D., Department of Radiology, University of Texas Medical Branch at Galveston)

10. What are the usual locations of thyroglossal duct cysts?

Thyroglossal duct cysts may be found anywhere along the course of the duct. The duct arises from the foramen cecum in the posterior tongue and extends inferiorly through the muscle of the tongue and the mylohyoid muscle at the floor of the mouth, into the anterior neck to the normal position of the thyroid gland, posterior to the strap muscles. Most cysts occur below the level of the hyoid bone and in the midline. The cysts may be imbedded in the strap muscles. They rarely contain carcinomas, but may become infected.

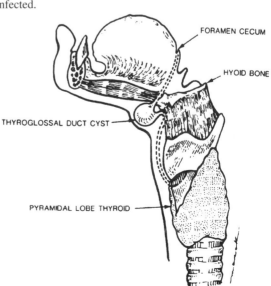

Sagittal view of the migration tract of a thyroglossal duct cyst. Harnsberger HRic: Handbook of Head and Neck Imaging, 2nd ed. St. Louis, Mosby, 1995, p 206, with permission).

11. Discuss the application of CT and MRI in the evaluation of a neck mass that is suspected to be malignant.

Although a thorough clinical examination is fundamental in the evaluation of a neck mass, radiologic imaging is often essential for diagnosis. CT or MRI can determine precise anatomic relationships, presence of an occult primary that has led to cervical metastases, and the solid or cystic nature of the mass. MRI is most helpful in defining the extent of neoplastic infiltration. Discrete lesions are well demonstrated by both modalities. CT is faster and more helpful with patients who have trouble holding still or controling their secretions. The MRI or CT should be performed before biopsy to avoid confusion due to changes created by the biopsy.

12. What characteristics of a lymph node on CT or MRI suggest malignancy?

The characteristics of a lymph node that suggest malignancy include the presence of central necrosis, ill-defined margins indicating extracapsular spread to adjacent tissues, and size. Nodes in the parotid or retropharyngeal chains are classified as malignant if their maximum diameter is > 1.0 cm. There is less consensus in the case of nodes in the spinal accessory, deep cervical, or submandibular groups. Many authorities believe that in these chains, only nodes > 1.5 cm should be called malignant. Others maintain that the increase in specificity is not worth the decrease in sensitivity, and that all nodes > 1.0 cm should be considered malignant.

In the presence of a known malignancy, nodes with central necrosis (with central low attenuation by enhanced CT or central low intensity by T1-weighted, contrast-enhanced MRI) are considered to be malignant regardless of their size. Similarly, nodes with ill-defined margins are considered malignant with extranodal spread of neoplasm. (See figure.)

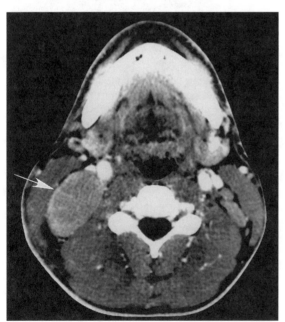

Axial CT of an enlarged lymph node (*white arrow*) present in the right jugular chain. (Courtesy of Faustino Guinto, M.D., Department of Radiology, University of Texas Medical Branch at Galveston)

13. Can neoplastic invasion of the carotid artery be accurately determined radiologically?

No imaging modality can determine neoplastic invasion of the carotid artery with 100% accuracy. Demonstration of fat between the artery and neoplasm by any modality indicates that the artery is not involved. The likelihood of involvement of the artery increases with increased circumferential contact of the neoplasm with the artery. The wall of the carotid artery can be seen only with ultrasound, but even this modality is not 100% accurate in determining invasion of the artery by an adjacent neoplasm. The wall may appear affected when it is not. MRI and CT demonstrate the lumen of the artery and adjacent structures, but not the arterial wall. Consequently, both modalities only estimate the likelihood of invasion by the degree of circumferential contact. Angiography can demonstrate only the lumen of the artery and is the least sensitive method for determining invasion of the wall.

14. Why are both CT and MRI indicated in the evaluation of suspected rhabdomyosarcoma?

Rhabdomyosarcoma is the most common soft tissue sarcoma and the second most common solid tumor in children. Both CT and MRI are important in the evaluation because treatment decisions are made based on bone involvement and exact extent of soft tissue spread. **Bone destruction,** a common feature of rhabdomyosarcomas, is best demonstrated by CT. The **margins of the neoplasm,** including intracranial spread, are best demonstrated by MRI. (See figures.)

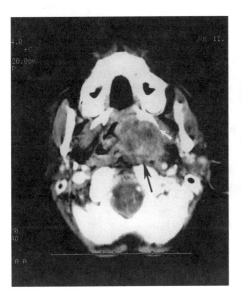

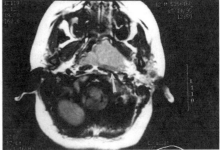

Rhabdomyosarcoma (*white arrow*) demonstrated on MRI. (Courtesy of Susan John, M.D., Department of Radiology, University of Texas Medical Branch at Galveston)

Rhabdomyosarcoma (*black arrow*) with bone destruction (*white arrow*) demonstrated on CT. (Courtesy of Susan John, M.D., Department of Radiology, University of Texas Medical Branch at Galveston)

15. What are the important radiologic findings in evaluating a cholesteatoma before surgery?

The radiologist must make several important observations when assisting in the preoperative evaluation of a cholesteatoma. The relationship of a cholesteatoma to the facial nerve must be established to determine the risk of injury to this structure. Extension of the lesion into the sinus tympani should be evaluated radiographically because it is an area that cannot be visualized during surgery (mastoid approach). The status of the tegmen tympani (intact or not) helps to predict complications involving the temporal lobe. The relationship of the lesion to the membranous labyrinth helps to establish the risk of fistula formation postoperatively. The location of the lesion relative to the ossicles also helps with surgical planning.

16. How are congenital anomalies of the ear best defined?

Because the middle and external ear arise from different structures than the inner ear, congenital anomalies affect either the external ear (with possible involvement of the middle ear) or the inner ear. The structures of the external and middle ear consist mainly of bone and air-filled spaces. Air and bone are well differentiated from each other by CT, but both appear black on MRI.

As a result, CT is the best modality to demonstrate stenosis or atresia of the external canal, possible involvement of the middle ear cavity and the ossicles, and the location of the descending portion of the facial nerve in its bony canal. The membranous labyrinth of the inner ear is filled with fluid and can be imaged by MRI. The membranous labyrinth is surrounded by the bony labyrinth, which can be imaged by CT. Because CT allows better spatial resolution than MRI, the structures of the inner ear are better defined by CT.

The resolution of MRI is improving, however, and new techniques allow sections ≤ 1 mm. MRI may provide better or complementary data in the future.

17. How are vascular anomalies that cause pulsatile tinnitus best evaluated?
Although angiography and MRI can demonstrate the course of the internal carotid artery and the jugular vein, CT best demonstrates the relationship of these vessels to the middle ear. CT determines whether the lateral margin of the carotid canal is intact and demonstrates the aberrant carotid artery in the middle ear. Similarly, CT determines whether the bony covering of the jugular bulb is intact and demonstrates any portion of the jugular vein in the middle ear. Correct identification of these anomalies is important to prevent a disastrous biopsy of misplaced but otherwise normal vessels.

18. What is the most common location of neoplasms in the posterior fossa?
In the posterior fossa, the cerebellopontine angle is the most common location of neoplasms. Although approximately 90% of primary neoplasms in the cerebellopontine angle are acoustic neuromas, other lesions must be considered. Meningiomas, epidermoid tumors, and facial nerve schwannomas account for approximately 5% of the remaining primary tumors. Other primary tumors are rare in this location. (See figure.)

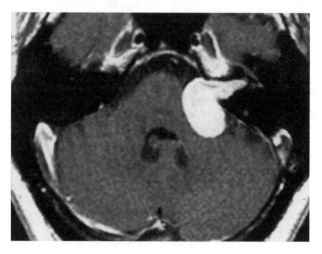

T2-weighted axial MRI of an acoustic neuroma located in the left cerebellopontine angle with extension into the internal auditory canal. (Courtesy of Gregory Chaljub, M.D., Department of Radiology, University of Texas Medical Branch at Galveston)

19. What is the appropriate radiologic evaluation of a patient with a history of trauma to the temporal bone?
Once the patient's circulatory and respiratory status is stable, radiologic studies should include a high-resolution CT to evaluate the skull base for fractures. When evaluation of the vasculature is clinically indicated, angiography best demonstrates the luminal anatomy, but MRI and MRA may be sufficient to characterize vascular injuries.

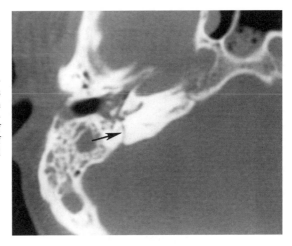

Unenhanced axial CT with bone windows shows a longitudinal right petrous fracture (*black arrow*) extending from the posterior portion of the petrous pyramid to the bony labyrinth. (Courtesy of Gregory Chaljub, M.D., Department of Radiology, University of Texas Medical Branch at Galveston)

20. Describe the appropriate radiologic evaluation of a patient with cerebrospinal fluid (CSF) rhinorrhea.

CT or MRI of the skull base should be performed. If the initial study does not show an abnormality that could cause a CSF leak, but demonstrates possible CSF in the paranasal sinus or mastoid air cells, a **CT cisternogram** may be helpful. For this study, contrast is injected intrathecally by a lumbar puncture. The patient's head is lowered below the level of the lumbar spine to move the contrast into the head. The presence of contrast in air cells indicates a CSF leak. CT best demonstrates fractures, but MRI best demonstrates skull-base anomalies such as encephaloceles. (See figure.)

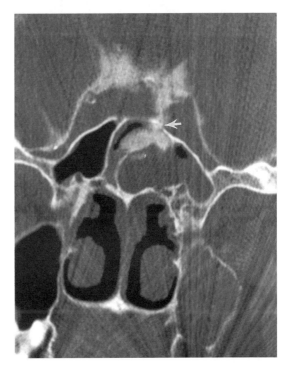

CT cysternogram with a CSF lead into the posterior ethmoid and sphenoid sinuses secondary to a fracture (*white arrow*) through the right planum sphenoidale and left carotid sulcus. (Courtesy of Gregory Chaljub, M.D., Department of Radiology, University of Texas Medical Branch at Galveston)

21. Discuss radiologic imaging of the paranasal sinuses.

Although the sinuses have traditionally been evaluated with plain films, CT offers superior imaging and is now the gold standard. The presence of air-fluid levels without history of recent trauma or lavage is evidence of an acute inflammatory condition. Mucoperiosteal thickening in the absence of air-fluid levels may indicate either acute or chronic disease. Severe unilateral sinusitis may result from a bacterial or fungal process. It may also represent sinuses obstructed by inverted papilloma, polyp, or another lesion. Fungal causes, most commonly *Aspergillus,* should be considered when a hyperdense area (thought to represent calcium, iron, and manganese) is seen in the context of chronic sinusitis.

22. What is the significance of incidental ethmoid or sphenoid sinusitis in a patient who has had a CT for an unrelated condition?

The majority of patients with incidental ethmoid sinus abnormalities have localized disease involving only a few of the air cells. The demonstrated mucosal thickening may indicate the presence of granulation tissue, acutely or chronically edematous mucosa, or a clinically silent ethmoid sinusitis. In most patients, particularly adults, this finding has little clinical significance. Approximately 10% of patients undergoing CT of the head for other reasons are found to have ethmoid sinus disease. However, incidentally discovered sphenoid sinusitis is much less common. Because of the anatomic location and proximity to neurovascular structures, neurologic and optic complications are found in up to 25% of patients with severe sphenoid sinusitis.

23. Which imaging modality is best for evaluating a nontraumatic brachial plexopathy?

MRI is the modality of choice because of its ability to acquire images in multiple planes. Coronal and parasagittal images best demonstrate the anatomy of the brachial plexus and the surrounding structures. CT demonstrates the area only in axial images. In addition, intravenous contrast is necessary to delineate blood vessels with CT, but not with MRI. CT images obtained at or below the level of the shoulders may be degraded by beam-hardening artifact.

24. What radiographic findings confirm the diagnosis of epiglottitis?

In an equivocal presentation of epiglottitis, lateral neck radiographs are a useful diagnostic tool. The patient must be accompanied by a physician who is capable of securing the airway in the event of rapid respiratory decompensation. Important signs of epiglottitis include a swollen epiglottis, arytenoid prominence, and aryepiglottic folds. This constellation creates the **classic "thumb-print" sign.** Air trapping secondary to airway obstruction may lead to dilatation of the hypopharynx.

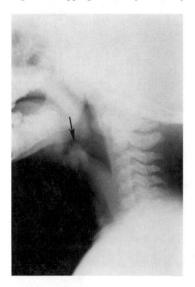

Lateral neck radiograph of a patient with a swollen epiglottis creating the classic "thumb print sign" indicative of epiglottitis. (Courtesy of Susan John, M.D., Department of Radiology, University of Texas Medical Branch at Galveston)

CONTROVERSIES

25. What is the role of radiology in the diagnosis and treatment of juvenile angiofibromas?
    Both CT and MRI can demonstrate the nasopharyngeal mass, which may indent the posterior margin of the maxillary sinus, involve the infratemporal fossa, or extend into the nasal cavity. CT best demonstrates bone destruction if the skull base is involved, but MRI best shows the involvement of the cavernous sinus or other intracranial structures. Angiography also demonstrates the extent of this benign but invasive vascular neoplasm, but does not define its exact relationship to surrounding structures. Angiography provides a road map of the feeding vessels for preoperative intra-arterial embolization of the neoplasm. Even the radiotherapist may be involved in the treatment of extensive angiofibromas.

ACKNOWLEDGMENT

    Special thanks to members of the Department of Radiology at the University of Texas Medical Branch at Galveston for their support and guidance.

BIBLIOGRAPHY

1. Caldemeyer KS, Mathews VP, Righi PD, et al: Imaging features and clinical significance of perineural spread or extension of head and neck tumors. Radiographics 18:97–110; quiz 147, 1998.
2. Davis JP, Maisey MN, Chevretton EB: Positron emission tomography—A useful imaging technique for otolaryngology, head and neck surgery? [editorial]. J Laryngol Otol 112:125–127, 1998.
3. Dillon WP: Head and neck imaging. Am J Neuroradiol 21:25–28, 2000.
4. Fischbein N, Anzai Y, Mukherji SK: Application of new imaging techniques for the evaluation of squamous cell carcinoma of the head and neck. Semin Ultrasound CT MR 20:187–212, 1999.
5. Fordham LA, Chung CJ, Donnelly LF: Imaging of congenital vascular and lymphatic anomalies of the head and neck. Neuroimag Clin North Am 10:117–136, 2000.
6. Ginsberg LE: Imaging of perineural tumor spread in head and neck cancer. Semin Ultrasound CT MR 20:175–86, 1999.
7. Koch BL: Imaging extracranial masses of the pediatric head and neck. Neuroimag Clin North Am 10:193–214, 2000.
8. Mack MG, Vogl TJ: MR imaging of the head and neck. Eur Radiol 9:1247–1251, 1999.
9. Salvolini L, Bichi Secchi E, Costarelli L, et al: Clinical applications of 2D and 3D CT imaging of the airways—A review. Eur J Radiol 34:9–25, 2000.
10. Zeifer A: Sinus imaging. In Bailey BF, et al (eds): Head and Neck Surgery–Otolaryngology, 2nd ed. Philadelphia, J.B. Lippincott, 1998.

75. ANESTHESIA IN OTOLARYNGOLOGY

Matthew Flaherty, M.D.

1. What premedications are appropriate for the otolaryngology patient?

Anxiolytics such as benzodiazepines provide sedation and relief of anxiety preoperatively. Some anxiolytics, such as Versed, can produce amnestic benefits. Opioids can be given to provide analgesia. Undesirable reflexes, such as salivation or increase in vagal tone, can be prevented with anticholinergics. Postoperative nausea and vomiting can be better controlled with the use of preoperative antiemetics (droperidol and ondansetron) and by providing gastric emptying with metoclopramide or intraoperative gastric suction.

2. Why is malignant hyperthermia (MH) important to the otolaryngologist?

Malignant hyperthermia only occurs after exposure to the potent inhalational anesthetics (halothane, isoflurane, etc.) or the muscle relaxant succinylcholine. These are the "triggering anesthetics" and are among the most common anesthetics used today. It is essential to prevent this exposure by delivering non-triggering anesthetics, such as propofol and nitrous oxide. The otolaryngologist and anesthesiologist must recognize patients that are susceptible. Patients may not experience MH with every prior anesthetic exposure, since prior anesthetics may have been the non-triggering type.

The overall incidence is generally about 1 in 40,000 anesthetics in adults and 1 in 10,000–15,000 in children. It is rarely reported in children under 3 years of age. All those with a family history of MH and those with a history of a questionable reaction to anesthesia must be considered potential MH patients, and preoperative preparations should be made. Since the otolaryngologist often sees a high percentage of children—patients often receiving their first general anesthetic—he or she should be especially aware of the possibility of and treatment for this dread condition.

3. What causes malignant hyperthermia?

Malignant hyperthermia is an inherited membrane defect that occurs primarily in skeletal muscle. When these patients are exposed to triggering drugs (e.g., potent inhalation anesthetics and succinylcholine), calcium is released at an enhanced rate from the sarcoplasmic reticulum. The excess calcium overwhelms the ATPase pump responsible for returning calcium from the mycoplasm to the sarcoplasmic reticulum, and a hypermetabolic state results. This decreases the amount of ATP available to the cell. Without ATP, the actin-myosin crossbridge cannot detach, and muscle remains contracted, resulting in rigidity.

MH is inherited in an autosomal dominant fashion and has a highly variable clinical presentation. Patients with *any* family history of MH, "fevers" associated with anesthesia, or unexplained death during surgery must be referred to the anesthesiologist for preoperative planning. Current research is focusing on chromosomal analysis and DNA linkages. Mortality due to MH is currently 5–20% after a patient receives a triggering anesthetic.

4. How does malignant hyperthermia present?

MH is primarily a clinical diagnosis. Signs and symptoms are related to the hypermetabolism of skeletal muscle and generally include tachycardia, trismus, muscle rigidity, hyperventilation, cyanosis, sweating, unstable blood pressure, and increased temperature. Laboratory tests commonly show hypercarbia, hyperkalemia, respiratory and metabolic acidosis, hypoxia, myoglobinuria, and an increased creatine kinase (often > 20,000 IU).

5. Describe local anesthetics.

Local anesthetics block sodium channels, which results in an inability of the cell to achieve threshold potential. A propagated action potential fails to develop, and therefore conduction is blocked. Structurally, local anesthetics consist of an aromatic moiety with a substituted amine. The linkage between the two is either an ester or an amine. The linkage tends to create a number of clinical similarities; therefore, local anesthetics are grouped into either the **ester** or **amide** group. Amides are often metabolized in the liver, and esters in the plasma (by pseudo-cholinesterase). Ester local anesthetics may cause allergic reactions because they are metabolized to para-aminobenzoic acid (PABA). Amide local anesthetics rarely cause allergic reactions.

Helpful memory aid: Amide local anesthetics have two i's in their names: lidocaine, bupivacaine, mepivacaine, etidocaine, and prilocaine. Ester local anesthetics have one i: tetracaine, cocaine, chloroprocaine, and procaine.

6. Which local anesthetic is unique (almost) to otolaryngology?

Cocaine is one of the local anesthetics used almost exclusively in otolaryngology. Its unique advantage is vasoconstriction, which other local anesthetics lack. In fact, lidocaine is a vasodilator and is often prepared with epinephrine. Cocaine is used topically on mucosal surfaces, providing anesthesia and vasoconstriction to provide a bloodless surgical field.

7. What are the toxic doses of the common local anesthetics?

Lidocaine 5 mg/kg without epinephrine, 7 mg/kg with epinephrine. Bupivicaine 2–3 mg/kg. Cocaine 4 mg/kg (although idiosyncratic reactions may occur at lower doses, and higher doses may be well tolerated by some patients).

8. Describe common side effects related to topical cocaine anesthesia.

Cocaine was the first known drug to have local anesthetic action and is still used routinely by many otolaryngologists for topical anesthesia to facilitate nasal surgery. Systemic absorption is unpredictable by the nasal route. Cocaine can sensitize the myocardium to arrhythmias, especially in association with epinephrine and halothane. It may also cause hypertension.

9. How much epinephrine is contained in each milliliter of 1:200,000 solution?

Epinephrine 1:200,000 is frequently added to local anesthetic solutions and contains 5 μg/ml. At a concentration of 2 μg/kg, patients receiving halothane anesthesia have increased ventricular ectopy.

10. How is the airway best secured during an ENT procedure in the mouth?

If the procedure is in the mouth, oral endotracheal tubes may be used. The surgeon may need to move the tube from side to side, and the anesthesiologist should be notified each time it is moved. Specialized endotracheal tubes called RAE tubes are formed with a sharp bend to angle the tube past the chin and face, or nose. RAE tubes are often used for tonsillectomies. Occasionally, the oral endotracheal tube will obstruct the surgical field, or the jaws will be wired shut during the case, and in these cases, the endotracheal tube is passed via the nostril to the nasopharynx and then into the trachea. Extensive trauma or radical resection sometimes requires tracheotomy.

11. Why must nitrous oxide be used carefully when performing surgery in the middle ear?

Nitrous oxide is 34 times more soluble than nitrogen and therefore will enter an air-filled cavity rapidly, resulting in increased pressure. This situation can be problematic in the case of ear surgery, where pathology may limit normal venting of the middle ear via the eustachian tube. To avoid complications, nitrous oxide is not commonly used during middle ear surgery. However, if it is used, it should be discontinued 15 minutes or more before surgical closure of the middle ear cavity.

12. Discuss the unique anesthetic considerations during laser surgery.

It is important for the patient to be protected from inadvertent laser exposure, and laser-related fires must be prevented. The operative site should be draped with wet towels. All personnel in the operating room, as well as the patient, should wear protective eyewear. Avoid nitrous oxide because it supports combustion, and the inspired oxygen concentration is lowered to the lowest acceptable oxygen saturation, usually guided by the pulse oximeter.

Laser surgery in the airway is often in close proximity to the endotracheal (ET) tube; the possibility of airway fire exists. Specialized ET tubes for laser surgery are designed to resist laser ignition, although even these tubes are occasionally ignited. The smoke of a burning ET tube contains a variety of toxic chemicals. When a tube is ignited, regardless of the type, it must be removed immediately. If tracheal tissue continues to burn, it should be irrigated with saline solution. Reintubation should follow quickly, since the airway may rapidly become edematous in response to thermal and chemical injury. The ET tube cuff is the thinnest and most easily ignited part of the tube. The cuff is often filled with saline or water when laser surgery is planned, and when laser energy strikes the cuff, it may puncture the cuff, and the subsequent leak of fluid may extinguish a potential fire. Methylene blue dye also may be used to color the fluid, alerting the surgeon to a punctured cuff if blue dye is seen leaking into the surgical field.

Airway fires may be avoided by performing surgery without an ET tube. For example, laser surgery is often accomplished via a ventilating bronchoscope, which has no flammable components.

13. What are the special anesthesia considerations during direct laryngoscopy or endoscopy?

During direct laryngoscopy or endoscopy, access to the patient's airway must be shared between the otolaryngologist and anesthesiologist. This must be done in a way that oxygenation and ventilation are adequately maintained. Inhaled anesthetics may have significant leak since no cuff is present on the direct laryngoscope. Intravenous anesthetics are preferred. If using an ET tube, it helps to use the smallest size that can still allow adequate ventilation. The ET tube may be displaced during various surgical maneuvers, and both surgeon and anesthesiologist must be alert to maintain its position. Alternative methods of oxygenation may be used, such as a ventilating bronchoscope or laryngoscope. Topical anesthetics may facilitate these procedures, as will the use of anticholinergics to control secretions.

It is important to remember that patients undergoing these procedures may have significant airway pathology, and attention to airway maintenance is the priority.

14. What are the special considerations in patients with malignancies of the head and neck?

A high degree of suspicion must be maintained for a difficult airway. Approximately 50% of the tracheal lumen may be obstructed before a patient experiences any symptoms. However, once a patient is under general anesthesia, a mass in or around the trachea may become more apparent. Often, when muscle relaxants are administered, the muscles of the airway lose tone and a tumor may suddenly obstruct the airway. Alternative methods of airway management, such as an awake tracheotomy or awake fiberoptic intubation, may be indicated. Tobacco and ethanol abuse is associated head and neck cancer. Patients may have hepatic damage from extensive alcohol abuse. Coagulopathy associated with liver disease may contribute to extensive airway bleeding. Some patients may have had radiation therapy, leading to epiglottic fibrosis or laryngeal edema. Smoking is associated with increased secretions, increased airway irritability, and chronic obstructive pulmonary disease.

15. What are the unique anesthetic considerations in thyroid surgery?

Elective patients should be rendered euthyroid and continue their medications through the morning of surgery. Tracheomalacia may develop in response to encroachment of an enlarged thyroid. Careful preoperative examination of the airway should seek to identify potential airway difficulties.

16. What are the more common acid-base disorders seen in the postoperative period?

Respiratory acidosis is most common secondary to residual anesthetics and neuromuscular blocking agents causing hyperventilation. Metabolic acidosis may occur when surgical blood loss or third-space losses are underappreciated and volume resuscitation is inadequate. Respiratory alkalosis is also common due to pain or anxiety and consequent hyperventilation.

17. How can endotracheal tube placement be confirmed?

The continuing presence of carbon dioxide in exhaled gas is the single best confirmation. Any other method of confirmation, as follows, is more subjective: Direct visualization of the tube in glottic opening. Symmetric bilateral chest movement with manual ventilation. Presence of bilateral breath sounds with auscultation. Absence of air movement during epigastric auscultation. Maintenance of arterial oxygen saturation. Condensation of water vapor in the tube lumen during exhalation.

18. How can a difficult airway be recognized prior to surgery?

The **Mallampati classification** evaluates the patient according to the relative size and position of the tongue to the palate. Class I and II airways (good to moderate visualization of the posterior pharynx when the mouth is fully open with tongue extended) are usually manageable with conventional laryngoscopy. Class III and IV airways (poor to no posterior pharynx visualized) predict higher incidences of difficulty when intubating by conventional laryngoscopy. Inability to extend the head, a small mouth, limited mouth opening, prominent upper incisors, and any distorting airway pathology can all lead to a difficult airway, and require special attention and planning.

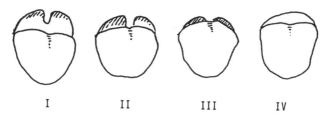

I   II   III   IV

The Mallampati classification of posterior pharyngeal visualization. In class I and II airways, the uvula is completely or partially seen, respectively. In class III and IV airways, the base of the uvula or soft palate only may be seen, respectively.

19. A patient with Down syndrome is scheduled for tonsillectomy. Are there special concerns regarding the airway?

Down syndrome is associated with macroglossia and atlantoaxial instability. Preoperative assessment should always include airway examination. Patients may have no preoperative cervical spine symptoms and still suffer intraoperative cervical spine and spinal cord damage if the neck is flexed or extended beyond its normal range of motion. Radiologic exam prior to surgery is occasionally indicated depending on the degree of head extension and flexion planned intraoperatively.

20. You premedicated a patient with topical phenylephrine; intraoperatively, the blood pressure begins to rise. The anesthesiologist wants to give a beta blocker to lower it. Do you agree?

No! This scenario has caused a number of fatalities, primarily in children. Phenylephrine (an alpha-1 agonist) causes vasoconstriction. The systemic vascular resistance would be very high if you measured it. Cardiac output is probably already lowered. The addition of the beta blocker at this time reduces the heart rate and contractility; cardiac output may fall to dangerous levels. The preferred antihypertensive is a direct vasodilator such as hydralazine or sodium nitroprusside.

21. The anesthesiologist tells you that the patient is becoming tachycardic. What are the potential causes of intraoperative tachycardia?
Tachycardia during general anesthesia may be secondary to hypoxia, and this is always checked first. Next are cardiac arrhythmias, ventricular tachycardias, and supraventricular tachycardias. Secondary causes include hypercarbia, pain, fever, sepsis, malignant hyperthermia, and thyrotoxicosis. Drugs such as atropine, glucopyrrolate, catecholamines, isoflurane, pancuronium, and cocaine all can cause tachycardia.

CONTROVERSIES

22. Should a child with a minor upper respiratory infection (URI) undergo general anesthesia?
In support of surgery: Although URIs can increase the risk of perioperative respiratory complications, in the absence of fever and productive cough, most children will experience minimal intraoperative and postoperative difficulties. Procedures such as typanostomy and tubes may alleviate infections and improve patient comfort. It is difficult to define when the upper respiratory irritation associated with an infection has subsided, but the mucosa usually returns to normal within 6–8 weeks. Many children will have a new URI within this time period, further extending the delay in surgery.

In support of postponement: URIs increase the irritability of the airway and lead to increased bronchospasm, laryngospasm, and desaturation. Pulmonary aspiration, negative pressure pulmonary edema, and aggravated postoperative respiratory infection can arise from these airway reflexes and their treatment. Prolonged hospitalization and morbidity may result from anesthesia during acute infection and recovery.

23. Masseter muscle rigidity occurs in a child during anesthetic induction for elective surgery. Do you proceed with surgery or stop and reschedule?
In support of stopping: Masseter muscle rigidity (MMR) is an early sign of malignant hyperthermia (MH). If the triggering anesthetic is stopped, the patient may recover without further symptoms. Continuing the inhaled anesthetic may lead to MH. Instead of continuing with surgery, time is better spent preparing for the treatment of MH. The child can return for elective surgery with a nontriggering anesthetic.

In support of continuing: MMR is common in children, and as many as 1 in 100 children receiving halothane and succinylcholine will have MMR to some degree, lasting 2–3 minutes. MMR is usually easily overcome after that time. MH is rare (1 in 10,000–15,000 anesthetics in children). It is unlikely then that the MMR will develop into MH. The anesthetic could be changed to a nontriggering type at this time, and the surgery could proceed.

ANESTHETIC AGENTS AND THE PREGNANT HEALTH WORKER

The relationship between exposure to trace concentrations of waste anesthetic gases in the operating room and the possible development of adverse health effects has concerned healthcare professionals for numerous years. Results of studies have been conflicting. In the late 1960s and early 1970s, some U.S. and European epidemiologic studies of operating room personnel showed an increase in the incidence of adverse health effects, including spontaneous abortion and development of congenital abnormalities in offspring. However, subsequent analysis of these studies by two independent groups showed that the apparent increase in adverse health effects was most likely due to flaws in study methods and data collection. A later prospective study showed *no causal relationship* between exposure to trace concentrations of waste anesthetic gases and adverse health effects. Each institution should have a waste anesthetic gas management program that includes scavenging of waste anesthetic gases, work practices to reduce contamination, documented maintenance and regular checking of all equipment, and education of all personnel on this subject. A mechanism for reporting work-related health problems should be in place in each institution.

~McGregor, Mayo Clin Proc 75:273, 2000

BIBLIOGRAPHY

1. Aranda M, Hanson CW 3rd: Anesthetics, sedatives, and paralytics. Understanding their use in the intensive care unit. Surg Clin NA 80:933–947, 2000.
2. Brown A: Anesthesia. In Cummings CW, et al (eds): Otolaryngology–Head and Neck Surgery, 2nd ed. St. Louis, Mosby, 1998.
3. Butler MG, Hayes BG, Hathaway MM, et al: Specific genetic diseases at risk for sedation/anesthesia complications. Anesth Analges 91:837–855, 2000.
4. Denborough M: Malignant hyperthermia [see comments]. Lancet 352:1131–1136, 1998.
5. Griffis CA: Human immunodeficiency virus/acquired immune deficiency syndrome-related drug therapy: anesthetic implications. CRNA 10:107–116, 1999.
6. Groudine SB, et al: New York State guidelines on the topical use of phenylephrine in the operating room. The phenylephrine advisory committee. Anesthesiology 92(3):859–864, 2000.
7. Hollmann MW, Durieux ME: Local anesthetics and the inflammatory response: A new therapeutic indication? Anesth 93:858–875, 2000.
8. Hopkins PM: Malignant hyperthermia: Advances in clinical management and diagnosis. Br J Anaesth 85:118–128, 2000.
9. McAuliffe MS, Hartshorn EA: Anesthetic drug interactions. Quarterly update. CRNA 10:184–190, 1999.
10. McCarthy TV, Quane KA, Lynch PJ: Ryanodine receptor mutations in malignant hyperthermia and central core disease. Human Mutation 15:410–417, 2000.
11. McGregor DG: Occupational exposure to trace concentrations of waste anesthetic gases. Mayo Clin Proc 75:273–277, 2000.
12. O'Keeffe NJ, Healy TE: The role of new anesthetic agents. Pharm Ther 84:233–248, 1999.
13. Shafer SL: The pharmacology of anesthetic drugs in elderly patients. Anesth Clin NA 18:1–29, 2000.
14. Stolworthy C, Haas RE: Malignant hyperthermia: A potentially fatal complication of anesthesia. Semin Periop Nurs 7:58–66, 1998.
15. Tetzlaff JE: The pharmacology of local anesthetics. Anesth Clin North Am 18:217–33, 2000.
16. Vervloet D, Magnan A, Birnbaum J, et al: Allergic emergencies seen in surgical suites. Clin Rev Allergy Immunol 17:459–467, 1999.
17. Warner DO: Preventing postoperative pulmonary complications: The role of the anesthesiologist. Anesth 92:1467–1472, 2000.

76. THE EYE AND ORBIT

David M. Kleinman, M.D., David W. Johnson, M.D., and Jon M. Braverman, M.D.

1. What is an afferent pupillary deficit?

An afferent pupillary deficit is a condition due to disease along the afferent (incoming light signal) pathway, in which the pupillary response to direct light stimulation in the abnormal eye is sluggish as compared to the uninvolved eye. This phenomenon is also called a **relative afferent pupillary deficit** (RAPD) because the pupillary responses are being compared. It can be graded from mild (1+) to severe (4+). Another frequently used term to describe this condition is the **Marcus Gunn pupil.**

2. What are the causes of an RAPD?

An RAPD can be caused by optic nerve disease (ischemia, trauma, infection, inflammation, tumor, glaucoma) and severe retinal problems (large retinal detachments, infections, central retinal artery or vein occlusions). Media opacities such as a cataract or a corneal scar will not cause an RAPD.

3. How do you test for an RAPD in the setting of injury to the iris constrictor mechanism?

The iris sphincter or its innervation can be damaged during blunt or penetrating ocular trauma, and this problem can interfere with the direct pupillary light response in the injured eye. In this situation, careful attention must be applied to the consensual pupillary response when light is presented to the injured eye during the swinging flashlight test. In low ambient light, a bright test light is passed back and forth between both eyes as the direct and consensual reflexes are noted and compared. If an RAPD is present in the affected eye, the consensual pupillary response in the healthy eye is diminished as compared to its response to direct light stimulation. Thus, the status of the retina and optic nerve can be established in the setting where one eye has a pupil that does not react due to trauma.

4. Name the four basic ocular emergencies, and describe their immediate treatments.

Chemical burn: Following chemical exposure, the eye must be irrigated with normal saline administered in large quantities as soon as possible.

Acute glaucoma: Symptoms include eye pain, blurred vision, seeing halos around objects, headache, and nausea or vomiting. On examination, the eye is red, the pupil is generally partially dilated, and corneal haze is seen. Initial management involves topical β-blockers, topical β-agonists, and oral carbonic anhydrase inhibitor (i.e., acetazolamide, 500 mg po). Intravenous acetazolamide or osmotic agents (i.e., mannitol) are used in severe cases.

Central retinal artery occlusion: This condition is diagnosed in the setting of acute unilateral painless loss of vision. An RAPD is present, and on funduscopic examination, the retina appears pale, except for a cherry red spot in the center of the macula (posterior retina). Ocular massage can be administered in an attempt to dislodge the central retinal artery emboli and facilitate their transfer downstream in the retinal circulation. Anterior chamber paracentesis, oral carbonic anhydrase inhibitors, and/or inspired carbogen (95% O_2/5% CO_2, to dilate the retinal arterioles) may be used to treat this condition as well.

Ruptured globe: This is suspected in the setting of periocular trauma (especially penetrating) with subconjunctival hemorrhage, decreased vision, and a shallowed or deepened anterior chamber; sometimes, obvious scleral or corneal lacerations are seen. An eye shield should be placed to protect the eye, and broad-spectrum intravenous antibiotics (i.e., a cephalosporin and aminoglycoside) are administered. Additional emergent care includes tetanus toxoid, if applicable, and antiemetics, if needed.

Note: emergent ophthalmologic consultation is indicated in all of these situations.

5. Can a ruptured globe present with normal intraocular pressure?

Yes. When the integrity of the eye is violated, the uvea can plug the rupture site and allow the eye to maintain pressure. This is especially true for posterior ruptures and for patients with ruptures where there is a delay in the attainment of medical attention. These wounds generally require surgical management; the diagnosis of a ruptured globe should not only be made when there is an extremely low intraocular pressure in the setting of blunt or penetrating trauma.

6. What is a hyphema, and how can this condition cause permanent visual loss?

A hyphema is defined as blood in the anterior chamber of the eye. Trauma is the most frequent cause, and the blood arises from tears in iris vessels. When blood is inside the eye, it can block the outflow of aqueous into the trabecular meshwork, thus causing acute rises in intraocular pressure. If the intraocular pressure remains at high levels for an extended period of time, permanent damage to the optic nerve can result. Additionally, the cornea can become blood stained when the intraocular pressure rises in a blood filled eye. Corneal blood staining can take years to resolve. The management of a hyphema is somewhat controversial, but close ophthalmologic follow up is an important facet of care.

7. Is there any blood test that should be obtained when an African-American patient presents with a hyphema?

A sickle cell screen needs to be ordered when individuals in this sub-group of the population develop a hyphema because under the low oxygen tensions in the anterior chamber red blood cells can sickle. Sickled red cells can cause rapid and severe rises in intraocular pressure. Patients carrying a gene for hemoglobin S or C need closer evaluation, as pressure control or an anterior chamber washout may often be required.

8. What conditions should be suspected in the evaluation of blunt (as opposed to penetrating) ocular and orbital trauma?

Blunt trauma can cause contusive injury to the globe and optic nerve directly or indirectly by force transmission along the orbital bones towards the orbital apex. This explains why some patients suffer from symptomatic visual loss due to traumatic optic neuropathy absent signs of direct globe injury. With direct globe trauma one needs to consider multiple levels of potential trauma pathology including: traumatic iritis, iris root tears with or without associated hyphema, traumatic cataract with or without subluxation, vitreous hemorrhage, retinal tears or detachment, globe rupture, orbital blow-out fractures.

9. What is traumatic optic neuropathy?

Traumatic optic neuropathy (TON) is the result of indirect traumatic injury to the optic nerve. Direct penetrating injuries of the optic nerve are excluded, but compression from edema or orbital bone fragments is included in the definition of this condition. Visual loss and an RAPD are necessary to make this diagnosis, and other ocular injuries should not be sufficient to account for the findings. The mechanisms that cause TON are multiple and not mutually exclusive. They include tears or shear injuries of the optic nerve, bone fractures of the optic canal injuring the nerve, and vascular compromise, inflammation, and/or hematomas involving the optic nerve. The condition is either instantaneous or delayed (primary or secondary TON), and secondary injury has a better prognosis as its effects may be somewhat reversible.

10. What are the cardinal diagnostic signs of an orbital blow-out fracture?

Blunt globe trauma typically produces an inferior and/or medial wall blow-out fracture. Common to both configurations is the propensity for orbital soft-tissue entrapment, which can produce a dysmotility syndrome reflective of the direction and amount of orbital tissue tethered in the fracture ostium. The so-called *restrictive* myopathy can present variably as an inability to look up or down, and sometimes there are medial and lateral deficits as well. If the orbit floor fractures

The Eye and Orbit

through the infraorbital canal, there may be a deficit in sensation along the distribution of the infraorbital nerve. Orbital volume expansion (blow-*out*) can also produce diplopia and ptosis secondarily, but this tends to be a later finding. CT imaging with direct coronal views provides the best detail of the orbital wall anatomy.

11. What are the possible complications of surgical repair of an orbital blowout fracture?
Orbital cellulitis
Persistent or late enophthalmos
Extrusion of the implant
Optic nerve injury with vision loss
Injury to the neurovascular bundle along the orbital floor causing infraorbital hypesthesia
Retrobulbar hemorrhage
Oculomotor nerve palsy
Ectropion or skin traction from the incision
Extraocular muscle injury

12. What is dacryocystitis, and how is it diagnosed and treated?
Dacryocystitis is an infection in the lacrimal sac, which is located in the lacrimal fossa above each bony nasolacrimal canal. Predisposing factors include obstruction of the nasolacrimal system due to prior infection, trauma, or tumor (rare). A history of epiphora (spontaneous tearing) is not uncommon in patients with obstruction of the nasolacrimal system. Acute infection of the lacrimal sac presents as a tender red nodule on the lateral upper aspect of the nose. There may be mucopurulent retrograde discharge into the ipsilateral eye or crusting of the eyelid on the affected side. Patients may be febrile and have other constitutional signs such as anorexia or nausea.

Treatment consists of parenteral antibiotics (topical eyedrops usually ineffective due to the obstruction). (Incision and drainage are contraindicated due to the propensity for chronic fistula formation.)

13. What are the indications for an emergent lateral canthotomy?
A lateral canthotomy and lateral tendon cantholysis must be performed in the setting of a retrobulbar hemorrhage with sustained high intraocular pressure, or when this elevated pressure is associated with an afferent pupillary deficit. A retrobulbar hemorrhage generally is secondary to trauma. Awake patients present with symptoms of pain and decreased vision; however, severe head injury is not an uncommon comorbidity. Proptosis, resistance to retropulsion, subconjunctival hemorrhage extending posteriorly, elevated intraocular pressure, afferent pupillary deficit, and restriction of extraocular motility can be found in varying degrees on examination. Intraocular pressure and pupil reactivity should be monitored closely. Orbital cellulitis, globe rupture, and carotid cavernous fistula should be considered in the differential diagnosis.

14. What clinical findings differentiate preseptal from postseptal (or orbital) cellulitis? When should imaging be obtained?
In the setting of eyelid edema and erythema, chemosis (conjunctival edema), decreased visual acuity, restriction of extraocular movements, and proptosis all point toward orbital involvement and are indications for intravenous antibiotics and CT imaging. Thin cut coronal and axial views are most helpful. MRI is indicated when CNS manifestations are present.

15. How is orbital cellulitis staged?
Stage 1 Preseptal (periorbital) cellulitis: Inflammation anterior to the orbital septum, with edema, erythema, warmth, and tenderness; one or both eyelids may be involved.
Stage 2 Subperiosteal abscess: Preseptal cellulitis present, as well as an abscess between the bony wall of the orbit and the periorbita; clinically, chemosis, asymmetric proptosis, extraocular muscle restriction, and decreased vision may be present.

Stage 3 Orbital cellulitis: Inflammation within the retrobulbar contents of the orbit, but enclosed by the periorbita; clinical findings include marked preseptal cellulitis, chemosis, proptosis (generally axial), ophthalmoplegia, and decreased vision.

Stage 4 Orbital abscess: Orbital cellulitis and abscess in the retrobulbar tissue; the findings are those of orbital cellulitis, but with more severe proptosis and visual loss.

Stage 5 Cavernous sinus thrombosis: Inflammation within the cavernous sinus in addition to the findings of orbital cellulitis; this condition may become bilateral; CN III, IV, and VI palsies are present, episcleral venous dilation occurs; meningitis may be present.

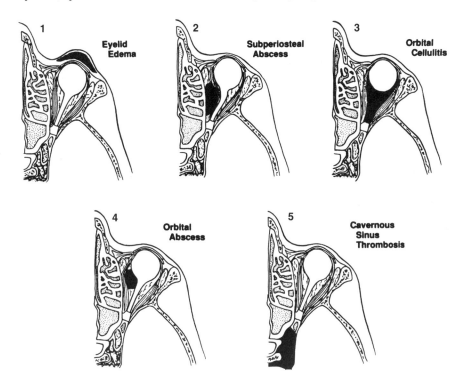

Stages of orbital cellulitis. (From Stankiewicz JA, Newell DJ, Park AH: Complications of inflammatory diseases of the sinuses. Otolaryngol Clin North Am 26:641, 1993; with permission.)

16. How are periorbital and orbital cellulitis treated?

The patient with **periorbital cellulitis** can generally be treated on an outpatient basis with oral antibiotics and warm compresses to the inflamed area three times daily. Conjunctivitis is treated if present. Patients who appear noncompliant, toxic, fail to respond, or are < 5 years of age will need hospitalization and IV antibiotics. The patient is followed daily until improvement is noted.

The patient with **orbital cellulitis** is hospitalized. Broad-spectrum intravenous antibiotics are initiated, nasal decongestant spray is administered as needed, and antibiotic ointment is applied three times daily if corneal exposure from proptosis is present. The patient is re-evaluated frequently. Surgical drainage of the sinuses is indicated urgently if visual acuity decreases, if the patient's condition deteriorates over 24 hours, or if it fails to improve over 48–72 hours. Repeat imaging may be necessary. Exploration and drainage of subperiosteal or orbital abscesses are indicated.

17. What are the etiologies of orbital cellulitis?

Sinusitis is the cause of orbital cellulitis 70–80% of the time. The ethmoids are most commonly involved. Other causes include cutaneous infections (from lacerations, abrasions, or impetigo), penetrating trauma, lacrimal infection, odontogenic sources, or dental or mid-facial surgery.

18. Why is orbital cellulitis in a diabetic concerning?
Infection with mucormycosis should be considered in any diabetic with orbital cellulitis. Rhinocerebral mucormycosis is a fungal disease that spreads rapidly from the paranasal sinuses and orbit to the brain; untreated, it is fatal. This infection is most likely to be seen in a patient with diabetic ketoacidosis. The diagnosis should also be considered in immunocompromised patients, in patients receiving steroid or antibiotic therapy, and in patients with severe burns or malignancies who demonstrate orbital or periorbital inflammation. Appropriate treatment includes correcting the underlying disorder, antifungal therapy, and debridement.

19. What are the possible complications of orbital cellulitis?

Retrobulbar abscess	Elevated intraocular pressure
Cavernous sinus thrombosis	Central retinal artery or vein occlusion
Ophthalmoplegia	Optic neuritis
Orbital apex syndrome	Endophthalmitis
Permanent cranial nerve dysfunction	Meningitis
Variable degrees of visual loss	Death

20. How does the anatomy of the orbit predispose to the spread of infection from the sinuses?
The thin walls of the orbit and their close proximity to the sinuses facilitate spread in complicated sinusitis. The lamina papyracea is exceptionally thin and fragile; it forms the lateral wall of the ethmoid labyrinth and a significant portion of the medial wall of the orbit. Additionally, the venous system of the orbit predisposes to hematogenous spread of infection to the orbit. The veins around and within the orbit, including the superior and inferior ophthalmic veins, form a diffuse network of interconnected valveless branches, and the direction of blood flow depends on local pressure gradients. Thus, communication between the nose, ethmoids, face, orbit and cavernous sinus exists.

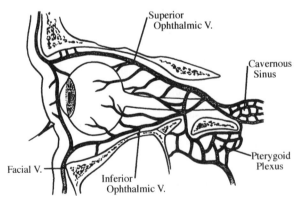

The venous network around the face, orbit, and cavernous sinus. (From Stankiewicz JA, Newell DJ, Park AH: Complications of inflammatory diseases of the sinuses. Otolaryngol Clin North Am 26:640, 1993; with permission.)

21. What is the orbital septum?
The orbital septum is a thin fibrous membrane that arises from the periorbita of the orbital rim and extends into the eyelids. It lies between the orbicularis muscle and the tarsus of the lids. The superior orbital septum blends at the superior tarsus with the levator palpebrae superioris aponeurosis. The inferior orbital septum blends with the inferior tarsal plate. Laterally and medially, the orbital septum forms the lateral and medial palpebral ligaments, respectively. This membrane acts as a barrier between the eyelids and orbit.

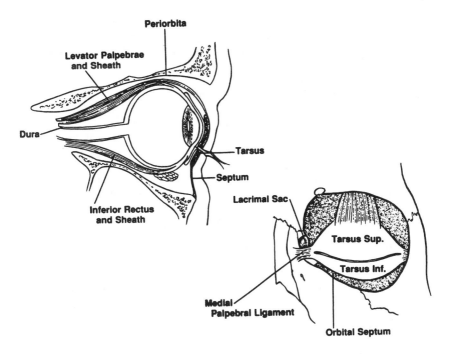

Anatomy of the orbital septum. (From Stankiewicz JA, Newell DJ, Park AH: Complications of inflammatory diseases of the sinuses. Otolaryngol Clin North Am 26:642, 1993; with permission.)

22. How is a retinal detachment different from a posterior vitreous separation?

A retinal detachment occurs when the neurosensory retina separates from the posterior inner lining of the globe (retinal pigment epithelium, Bruch's membrane, and choroid). This condition causes temporary and possibly permanent visual loss. A posterior vitreous separation is when the posterior cortical vitreous moves forward, breaking free from its attachment to the optic nerve and macula. A posterior vitreous separation is a normal part of aging; generally no treatment is required, but occasionally a retinal tear can be identified. Both conditions can present with photopsia (flashes of light) and a sudden onset of new floaters. A central or peripheral scotoma (blind area in the visual field) is more likely to be noted in patients with retinal detachments. These clinical signs may be seen with a retinal detachment but not a posterior vitreous separation: an afferent pupillary deficit and a decreased red reflex. Retinal detachments are not always seen with the direct ophthalmoscope, and referral to an ophthalmologist is indicated.

23. Name the three different types of retinal detachments.

Rhegmatogenous retinal detachments are caused by small or large holes in the retina which allow fluid to enter the subretinal space and dissect the retina anteriorly from its normal anatomic position. A *tractional retinal detachment* is caused by the contraction of fibrovascular proliferative membranes thereby detaching the retina. *Exudative retinal detachments* are caused by the leakage of fluid from the retinal vessels or a site posterior to the retina. Tumors or inflammatory diseases are the most common causes of exudative retinal detachments.

24. What are the special concerns in the evaluation of eyelid lacerations?

The location of the laceration with respect to critical structures such as the lacrimal drainage system, the canthal tendons, or the levator palpebrae superioris dictates the surgical repair strategy. One must differentiate skin-muscle lacerations from marginal lid lacerations (that which involves the underlying tarsal plate, which is the "endoskeleton" of the eyelids). Separate closure of the tarsal plate is indicated in these full-thickness lid lacerations. Attention should be paid to the orientation of the laceration as it relates to the propensity for secondary lid malposition due to contractile wound scarring. Careful probing of the lacrimal canaliculi is indicated when lid lacerations could potentially involve these structures.

25. What is amblyopia, and how can it be prevented?

Amblyopia is diminished vision in an eye that is secondary to problems in visual system maturation taking place from birth to age seven or eight. The eye can be functionally and anatomically normal with decreased vision being the only finding. Ambyopia can also be present along with ocular abnormalities. Its effects can be minimized by identifying predisposing conditions such as certain types of strabismus (misalignment of the eyes), media opacities (i.e. cataract), or large imbalances in refractive error between the two eyes, and correcting them as is best possible. The better seeing eye can be patched for a period of time to allow the amblyopic eye to learn to see better. This management is typically performed under the close supervision of a pediatric ophthalmologist and should be carried out at as early an age as possible to be maximally effective.

26. What is the most common cause of blindness occurring in patients between the ages of 20 and 64?

Diabetic retinopathy. Much of the severe visual loss encountered in diabetics, however, is preventable. Good blood glucose control, treatment of hypertension, and regular eye exams are important aspects to maintaining useful vision in these patients. Retinal laser treatments are generally preventative, and are best administered before visual loss occurs.

27. When is a third nerve palsy worrisome? Why?

A third nerve palsy is concerning when the pupil is involved because a posterior communicating artery aneurysm is a common etiology. Emergent CT or MRI/MRA is indicated, and cerebral angiography is frequently necessary as well. Pupil-sparing third nerve palsies generally have a microvascular etiology (i.e., diabetes), but imaging is necessary in certain subsets of patients.

28. What is the differential diagnosis for a red eye?

Conjunctivitis	Corneal abrasion
Blepharitis	Iritis
Episcleritis	Acute angle closure glaucoma
Scleritis	Subconjunctival hemorrhage
Inflamed pinguecula or pterygium	Dry eye syndrome
Corneal or conjunctival foreign body	

29. Which findings point toward a malignancy in an eyelid lesion?

Lid lesions that grow rapidly, destroy the lash line, interfere with the meibomian orifices, ulcerate, cause inflammation, or recur after excision are more likely to be malignant. Benign and malignant tumors of the eyelids can have similar appearances, and biopsy is generally necessary to establish a diagnosis.

30. Discuss the treatments for the ocular complications of facial nerve palsy.

Exposure keratitis, which can be very severe, is the main concern in patients with a facial nerve palsy, as this cranial nerve innervates muscles that close the eye. Treatment for mild exposure problems entails the frequent use of artificial tears. If the artificial tears are being used more frequently than four times daily, preservative-free solutions should be used. Lubricating ointment should be applied at night, but the eye also may be taped shut at night. For cases not responding to these measures where regeneration of the nerve is expected, a moisture chamber can be worn around the eye, temporary plugging of the puncta can be performed, or temporary external eyelid weights can be used. In more severe or permanent cases, a gold weight or eyelid spring can be placed in the upper lid to help it close, or a tarsorrhaphy (lid suturing procedure) can be performed. Artificial tears are utilized adjunctively with the latter procedures.

31. What are the risks of contact lens wear?

Whether worn for refractive correction or cosmetic enhancement, a soft or rigid contact lens potentially can cause trauma and secondary infection to the cornea and conjunctiva. Conditions that predispose the eye to dryness or chronic inflammation (Sjögren syndrome, allergic conjunctivitis) increase the chances of having contact lens–related complications. Perhaps the single most common underlying reason for contact lens–related complications is intentional overwear. Patients should be advised to always remove the lenses and resort to spectacle wear if redness or irritation develops.

32. What is one of the most important pieces of medical advice to give to a monocular patient?

Monocular patients should be told to wear eye protection whenever they are in a situation that may result in accidental injury to the eye, i.e., working, outdoor activities, sports activities, etc. Patients with one eye are at a statistically higher risk for suffering an injury in their only seeing eye. They should be counseled to avoid activities where eye injuries are common (i.e., contact sports). Additionally, these patients should probably avoid both contact lens wear and refractive surgery—although complications are relatively infrequent and the risk of a visually devastating problem should not be assumed.

CONTROVERSIES

33. How is traumatic optic neuropathy (TON) managed?

When inflammation and edema of the nerve itself are the most likely etiologies, management of this condition becomes controversial. Although spontaneous improvement in patients with TON is well documented, most ophthalmologists will treat these injuries with intravenous corticosteroids. The doses vary, however, from conventional doses of dexamethasone or methylprednisolone to megadoses of methylprednisolone at spinal cord injury levels. Optic canal decompression has been utilized for the treatment of this condition as well. The timing of surgery is also controversial, but patients are usually started first on IV corticosteroids, and if the condition worsens or does not improve within a few days, then decompression surgery may be recommended. Surgical decompression of the optic canal is not performed at all medical centers in the United States. There are no randomized controlled studies comparing the various therapies.

34. Is the presence of an orbital floor fracture sufficient indication for surgical repair?

Different specialties consider different constellations of surgical indicators. It is probably an oversimplification to equate the presence of a floor fracture with the need for surgical intervention. Ophthalmologists consider the size and displacement of the fracture along with an estimation of the increase in orbital volume, which is a risk factor for late enophthalmos. The presence of a restrictive dysmotility is also an indication for surgical dissection to release entrapped orbital soft tissue. It is sometimes difficult to differentiate a restrictive myopathy (entrapment) from a paretic motility problem (which is not a surgical indicator) with direct observation alone. Given that there are potentially significant complications from an orbital floor dissection, the decision to operate should be carefully contemplated.

BIBLIOGRAPHY

1. Berestka JS, Rizzo JF: Controversy in the management of traumatic optic neuropathy. Int Ophth Clin 34:87, 1994.
2. Busch T, Sirbu H, Aleksic I, et al: Anterior ischemic optic neuropathy: a complication after extracorporal circulation. Ann Thor CV Surg 4:354–358, 1998.
3. Dickersin K, Manheimer E: Surgery for nonarteritic anterior ischemic optic neuropathy. Cochrane Database Syst Revs [computer file]. (2):CD001538, 2000.
4. Li KK, Teknos TN, Lauretano A, et al: Traumatic optic neuropathy complicating facial fracture repair. J Craniofac Surg 8:352–355; discussion 356–359, 1997.

5. Moseley I, Gass A: Magnetic resonance imaging in optic neuropathy. Clin Neurosci 4:302–319, 1997.
6. Osguthorpe JD, Hochman M: Inflammatory sinus disease affecting the orbit. Otolaryngol Clin North Am 26:657, 1993.
7. Pomeranz HD, Rizzo JF, Lessell S: Treatment of traumatic optic neuropathy. Int Ophth Clin 39:185–194, 1999.
8. Potarazu SV: Ischemic optic neuropathy: Models for mechanism of disease. Clin Neurosci 4:264–269, 1997.
9. Rhee DJ, Pyfer MF, Friedberg MA, Rapuano CJ: The Wills Eye Manual: Office and Emergency Room Diagnosis and Treatment of Eye Disease, 3rd ed. Philadelphia, Lippincott Williams and Wilkins, 1999.
10. Retina and Vitreous. Basic and Clinical Science Course. San Francisco, American Academy of Ophthalmology, 1999.
11. Strome SE, Hill JS, Burnstine MA, et al: Anterior ischemic optic neuropathy following neck dissection. Head Neck 19:148–152, 1997.
12. Vaughan DG, Asbury T, Riordan-Eva P: General Ophthalmology, 15th ed. Stamford, CT, Appleton & Lange, 1999.

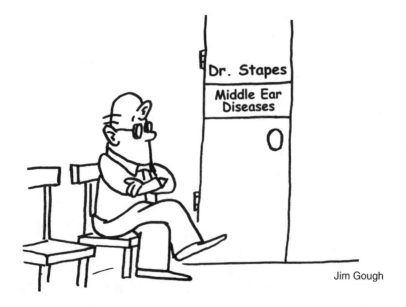

Jim Gough

77. COST-EFFECTIVE OTOLARYNGOLOGY

Bruce W. Jafek, M.D., FACS, FRSM and Arlen D. Meyers, M.D., M.B.A.

1. What does cost-effective otolaryngology mean?
Practicing cost-effective otolaryngology means using as few resources as possible to achieve a desired outcome or to get maximum benefit from an expenditure of resources.

2. How are healthcare costs defined?
Healthcare costs can be divided into direct and indirect components. **Direct costs** are the values of goods and services used to detect, treat, and rehabilitate individuals with a disease or impairment. **Indirect costs** include those used to administer the healthcare system (e.g. administration, insurance transactions). There are several other ways to measure costs, including average costs, marginal costs, fixed costs, and variable costs. Accounting for the true "cost" of a given treatment or service can be extremely difficult.

3. So what is "health"?
Defining health is a challenge. Definitions range from a narrow statistical definition (e.g., length of life) to a broad philosophical definition. To most of us, the definition is simply the presence or absence of disease. More broadly, the World Health Organization (1978) defined health as "complete physical, mental, and social well-being, and not merely the absence of disease or injury." Expanding on this concept, Evans and Stoddart included function, well-being, and prosperity, as a result of the interactions of medical care, the environment, socioeconomic status, genetic endowment, and individual behavior. Kindig concluded, "If an optimal allocation of societal resources for improving health outcomes is desired, we not only have to understand the interactions, but the relative costs with each, so that health output can be maximized for the resources available." Therefore, if resources were unlimited, we would not have to deal with the cost-effectiveness question and could just blindly increase the investments in all areas, until perfect health was achieved. However, society cannot afford all of the technology that medicine can devise, nor meet all of the needs of the consumer. Therefore, some sort of allocation ("rationing," to use an unpopular word) must take place. And cost-effectiveness will continue to be an etherial "buzz-word" until an optimal investment strategy is devised for the utilizaiton of our limited resources in an attempt to improve and maintain health, however that is ultimately defined.

4. What country spends the greatest percent of its gross domestic product (GDP) on health care?
The United States, followed by Canada, Germany, Japan, and Great Britain. Richard Scott, former CEO of Columbia/Hospital Corporation of America observed, "Health care consumes 13.7% of our GDP. A fairer system would make better use of the money we now spend, and it would allow us to provide compassionate care to all Americans."

5. What about the quality and performance of the U.S. healthcare system?
Ideally, our high level of expenditures would result in a population that is healthier than in other countries that spend less. While it is true that our technology and specialized care are probably the best in the world, it is not appropriate to automatically conclude that our population has better health or that further increases in healthcare expenditures will make us healthier. Kindig observed that our current efforts focus on the process (e.g., procedure rates and patient satisfaction) and not on outcome measures, leaving public and private purchasers of health care without adequate guidance on healthcare investment decisions. If the system is to be improved, explicit financial incentives must be developed to insure progress in the improvement of the health status of populations. Such a focus would turn attention to outcomes, rather than structure or process, and

unleash forces that would capture the attention of health providers, health institutions, and other health-enhancing sectors of society that are currently not held accountable for such outcomes.

6. How are benefits defined?

The outcome of a given treatment can be measured in several ways. **Cost minimization** assumes a given outcome and seeks methods for achieving this outcome at lesser costs. **Cost-effectiveness** analysis expresses the outcome in units that can be measured objectively, such as measures of disability or 5-year survival. **Cost-benefit** analysis converts the costs and benefits into dollars. **Cost-utility** analysis expresses the denominator as the worth of a change in health status. The most commonly used unit for this measurement is **quality-adjusted life-years,** an arbitrarily defined measure of the quality of life times the number of years that this is maintained. A more recently devised measure is **health adjusted life expectancy,** a combination of life, disease, and disability.

4. What features of otolaryngology affect cost-effective practice?

Several features of otolaryngology have important implications for cost-effective practice:
- Otolaryngologists represent only 1.5% of all physicians in the U.S.
- Many other specialists care for patients with otolaryngology complaints.
- Otolaryngology concentrates on the pediatric and geriatric age groups, with the care of the geriatric patient being three times as costly as that of the younger patient.
- Otolaryngology is primarily an office- and ambulatory-based specialty.
- Medications constitute an important part of patient management in otolaryngology.
- Approximately 1 in 30 patients seen by otolaryngologists requires an operation.

5. Where is there potential to save money in otolaryngology?

The 20 most common otolaryngology procedures account for 87% of all otolaryngology operations performed in the U.S. These are relatively low-cost, high-volume procedures. Unfortunately, the precise indications for several of these operations are unclear (e.g., tonsillectomy, sinus surgery, septoplasty, and bilateral myringotomy with tubes). Managed care and capitation have forced a reevaluation of the necessity for many of these procedures, with an emphasis on refining indications, documenting outcome, and reducing costs.

6. How can otolaryngologists use fewer resources to achieve a given result?

Altering certain practice patterns offers the most potential for optimizing the use of resources.
- Eliminating unnecessary tests and office visits
- Determining appropriate place of care
- Prescribing appropriate medications, particularly antibiotics
- Using appropriate prehospitalization and postdischarge ancillary services to minimize length of stay
- Basing therapeutic decisions on data, rather than anecdote.

7. How can the costs of ambulatory surgery be reduced?

Surgeons should not routinely order unnecessary preoperative lab tests. Frequently, ASA class I patients only need a preoperative hematocrit. Routine studies to screen for clotting disorders, EKGs in patients < 50 years old, chest x-rays, routine pregnancy tests, and routine preoperative urinalyses are not cost-effective.

The use of perioperative medications should be strictly monitored and limited to those with proven effectiveness.

Quality improvement programs should be in place to identify adverse trends, such as postoperative infections, hospital readmission following ambulatory surgery, and drug reactions.

8. When should prophylactic antibiotics be used in otolaryngologic surgery?

Prophylactic antibiotics are indicated in patients undergoing **clean-contaminated** (e.g. surgery from the skin [clean] through into the mouth [contaminated, but not infected]) head and neck surgery. Patients having clean salivary gland surgery, thyroid surgery, most ear surgery, trauma surgery, and cosmetic procedures do not benefit from prophylactic antibiotics. When prophylactic antibiotics are administered, they should be given preoperatively and for 24–48 hours postoperatively at the appropriate dose.

9. When should you order sinus x-rays in patients with nasal and sinus complaints?

Routine x-rays of the paranasal sinuses have limited sensitivity and specificity when compared to CT scans. They are of some value in monitoring the progress of an air-fluid level of the maxillary sinus during treatment. In general, however, a limited coronal CT scan of the sinuses without contrast administration is the image of choice for evaluating sinusitis.

10. When should you take a culture of the ear, nose, or throat?

Cultures of the ear canal, nasal cavity, and nasopharynx are usually not helpful in managing infections of those regions. Situations in which sinus aspiration or tympanocentesis may be helpful include:

- Failure of the patient to respond to medical management
- Outright or impending infectious complication
- Suspicion of a resistant organism causing infection.

11. Which antibiotic should be used to treat acute otitis and sinusitis?

Amoxicillin is still the initial drug of choice. Clinicians should be aware, however, of emerging resistant strains of *Haemophilus* and *Pneumococcus;* antibiotics may require adjustment according to the clinical response of the patient.

12. Do all patients with squamous cell cancer of the head and neck need staging panendoscopy?

Probably not. Although there are not enough data to say for sure yet, patients with lesions of the anterior floor of the mouth can probably be staged adequately with fiberoptic laryngoscopy in the office and an MRI. The MRI is used to look for second primaries and metastatic lymph nodes.

13. When should a patient with ENT problems be referred to an otolaryngologist?

The American Academy of Otolaryngology–Head and Neck Surgery has published referral guidelines for primary care practitioners covering the most common ENT ambulatory problems. Request a copy at One Prince Street, Alexandria, VA 22314, or fax (703) 683-5100, or contact them by email at webmaster@entnet.org.

CONTROVERSY

14. Can primary care practitioners take care of ambulatory otolaryngologic problems more cost-effectively than specialists and still maintain quality of care?

The data are insufficient to say. Studies in the past have looked at specific diseases in an attempt to determine if primary care or specialty care is more cost-effective in these situations. However, until we get a better handle on how to measure general health quality, account for comorbidity, and define the outcomes, we will not have an accurate answer.

ACCESS TO ADEQUATE HEALTH CARE

While access to adequate health care is the stated goal of societies, poverty not only excludes people from the benefits of healthcare systems but also restricts them from participating in decisions that affect their health. The resulting health inequalities are well documented, and the search for greater equity attracts many concerned players and initiatives. Fundamental to the success of these efforts, however, is the need for people to be able to negotiate their own inclusion into health systems and demand adequate health care. This calls for a restatement of the centrality of people in public health and its practice. New forms of communication and cooperation are required at all levels of society, nationally and internationally, to ensure equitable exchange of views and knowledge to formulate appropriate action to redress inequalities and improve people's health and well-being.

~Macfarlane, Lancet 356:787, 2000

BIBLIOGRAPHY

1. Alsarraf R, Alsarraf NW, Kato BM, et al: Meta-analysis in otolaryngology. Arch Otol-HNS 126:711–716, 2000.
2. Bergmo TS: An economic analysis of teleconsultation in otorhinolaryngology. J Telemed Telecare 3:194–199, 1997.
3. Brown D, Kresevic D, Nosan P: Head and neck patients. An innovative, cost-effective approach. Nurs Mgt (Chicago) 29:27–29, 1998.
4. Casiano RR, Numawa JR: Efficacy of computed tomographic image—guided endoscopic sinus surgery in residency training programs. Laryngoscope. 110:1277–1282, 2000.
5. Derkay CS: Pediatric otolaryngology procedures in the united states: 1977–1987. Int J Ped ORL 25:1–12, 1993.
6. Dohar JE, Bonilla JA: Processing of adenoid and tonsil specimens in children: a national survey of standard practices and a five-year review of the experience at the Children's Hospital of Pittsburgh. Otol-HNS 115:94–7, 1996.
7. Dranove D: The Economic Evolution of American Healthcare. Princeton, NJ, Princeton Univ Press, 2000.
8. Fuchs VA: Who Shall Live? New York, Basic Books, 1974.
9. Gates GA: Cost-effectiveness considerations in otitis media treatment. Otol-HNS 114:525–30, 1996.
10. Hadley JA: Overview of otolaryngic allergy management. an eclectic and cost-effective approach. Otol Clin NA 31:69–82, 1998.
11. Hogikyan ND, Pynnonen M: Indirect laryngeal surgery in the clinical voice laboratory: the renewal of a lost art. ENT J 79:350, 354, 357–8, 2000.
12. Kim JY, Lee CH: Clinical study on the efficacy of tonsilloadenoidectomy. Acta Oto-Laryng (Supp) 454:265–272, 1988.
13. Kindig DA: Purchasing Population Health. Ann Arbor, Univ Mich Press, 1997.
14. Macfarlane S, Racelis M, Muli-Musiime F: Public health in developing countries. Lancet 356:787–788; 841–6, 2000.
15. Meyers A, Eiseman B: Cost-Effective Otolaryngology. Philadelphia, B.C. Decker, 1990.
16. Rosbe KW, Jones D, Jalisi S, et al: Efficacy of postoperative follow-up telephone calls for patients who underwent adenotonsillectomy. Arch Otol-HNS 126:718–21, 1998.
17. Strauss M, Bellian K: Otolaryngology care unit: A safe and cost-reducing way to deliver quality care. Laryngoscope 109:1428–1432, 1999.

XI. Critical Care Issues

78. FLUID AND ELECTROLYTE MANAGEMENT

J. Honey Onstad, M.S. IV and Bruce Murrow, M.D., Ph.D.

1. Water composes what percentage of the human body?

Total body water (TBW) ranges from 50–70%. Women tend to possess a higher relative adipose content and less TBW. A kilogram of water is approximately equivalent to 1 liter. Therefore, a 70-kg man is composed of about 42 L of water.

2. How is this water distributed?

Total body water is distributed into three functional compartments—the intracellular, extracellular, and interstitial spaces. The intracellular compartment is the largest, accounting for 30–40% of total body weight. The intravascular and plasma compartments combine to form the extracellular fraction, contributing 5%. The interstitial compartment contributes the remaining 15%.

3. What three factors should be considered when estimating fluid needs?

Therapy should be directed toward maintaining or correcting three facets of fluid needs. Maintenance therapy replaces sensible and insensible fluid losses that occur with normal body functioning. Replacement therapy is aimed at correcting previous deficits such as losses associated with trauma. Finally, replacement therapy is estimated for ongoing losses associated with the underlying disease process.

4. How do you calculate maintenance fluids?

The following formula, which calculates maintenance need in ml/day, can be used in adults or children and is based on weight. This formula

$$0–10 \text{ kg} = 100 \text{ ml/kg}$$
$$11–20 \text{ kg} = 1000 \text{ ml} + (50 \text{ ml/kg for every kg over 10})$$
$$> 20 \text{ kg} = 1500 \text{ ml} + (20 \text{ ml/kg for every kg over 20})$$

For example, a 12-kg child would need a maintenance of 1000 ml + (50 ml $\times$ 2 kg) =1100 ml/day.

Applying the **4, 2, 1 rule** is perhaps an easier way to calculate fluid requirements. This formula calculates maintenance need in ml/hr.

$$0–10 \text{ kg} = 4 \text{ ml/kg}$$
$$11–20 \text{ kg} = 40 \text{ ml} + (2 \text{ ml/kg for every kg over 10})$$
$$> 20 \text{ kg} = 60 \text{ ml} + (1 \text{ ml/kg for every kg over 20})$$

For example, a 70-kg man needs a maintenance of 60 ml + (1 ml $\times$ [70–20] kg) = 110 ml/hr.

In general, use D_5W 1/2 NS with 20 KCl for adults. Children have decreased ability to concentrate urine, therefore D_5W 1/4 NS with 20 KCl is preferred.

To maintain obligatory **sodium** losses from urine, feces, and sweat, healthy adults need 1–2 mEq Na/kg/day and children need 1 mEq Na/kg/day. To maintain obligatory **potassium** losses, a healthy adult also needs 0.5–1.0 mEq K/kg/day. An appropriate maintenance regimen in a healthy adult would be 2500 ml of 0.45% NaCl with 5% dextrose and 20 mEq KCl/L. A previously healthy patient may need calcium, magnesium, phosphorus, vitamin, and protein replacement after 1 week of parenteral therapy.

5. What are the electrolyte compositions of commonly used IV fluids?

FLUID	Na^+ mEq/L	K^+ mEq/L	Cl^- mEq/L	HCO_3^- mEq/L	Ca^{2+} mEq/L	Kcal/L	GLUCOSE g/L
1/2 NS	77	0	77	0	0	0	0
NS	154	0	154	0	0	0	0
D_5W	0	0	0	0	0	170	50
$D_{10}W$	0	0	0	0	0	340	100
LR	130	4	109	28	3	9	0

NS = normal saline, D_5W = detrose 5% in water, LR = lactated Ringer's

6. What are the electrolyte compositions of bodily fluids?

	Na^+	K^+	Cl^-	HCO_3^-	VOLUME (ml/DAY)
Bile	145	5	100	35	50–800
Diarrheal	60	35	40	30	Variable
Gastric	60	10	130	0	100–4000
Pancreatic	140	5	75	115	100–800
Saliva	60	20	15	50	500–2000
Sweat	50	5	40	0	100–4000
Urine	60	30	40	0	1000–1600

7. How do you calculate plasma osmolality?
Plasma Osm = $(2 \times Na)$ + glucose/18 + BUN/2.8

8. How can you best assess daily fluctuations in fluid status?
Changes in fluid status are best assessed through diligent input, output, and daily weight records.

9. What is the minimum acceptable urinary output in a postoperative adult patient? In a child?
Minimal urine output for an adult is 30 ml/hr (0.5 ml/kg/hr), and for children is 1–2 ml/kg/hr. Lower flows suggest hypovolemia or a decrease in intravascular volume.

10. What are the most reliable clinical indicators of hypovolemia?
Tachycardia, orthostasis, decreased pulse pressure, and decreased urine output are the most sensitive and reliable clinical indicators of hypovolemia. Systolic blood pressure is a late and insensitive indicator, usually remaining stable until 20–30% of blood volume is lost.

11. How do you administer albumin?
Albumin is usually administered in a 25% solution. For every 100 ml of 25% albumin solution, the plasma volume will expand approximately 500 ml.

12. Name four sources of ongoing fluid loss.
Loss of body fluid is one of the most common sources of ongoing volume deficit. Nasogastric suctioning is best replaced with D_5W 1/2 NS with 20 mEq KCl/L. The potassium concentration may need to be increased if the deficit persists. Fluid deficits caused by diarrhea are replaced with Ringer's lactate with the possible addition of 10 mEq KCl/L. **Fever** significantly contributes to insensible fluid loss, causing 2–2.5 ml/kg/day loss for each degree above 37°C. Excessive fever replacement is best accomplished with D_5W 1/2 NS with 5 mEq KCl/L. Other potential sources of ongoing fluid losses are **third spacing** and burns.

13. Describe "third spacing."

Third spacing refers to a situation in which fluid is drawn from the vascular space and accumulates in tissues and hollow visceral spaces. This sequestered fluid becomes nonfunctional, unable to participate in transport processes. Third spacing leads to a functional volume depletion. Attempts to restore the intracellular and extracellular fluid deficits only lead to further "third space" fluid accumulation. This situation is seen in surgical patients with hemorrhagic shock, ischemic injury, postoperative wounds, bowel obstruction, infection, trauma, burns, and peritonitis.

14. What is the relationship between blood glucose and serum sodium?

For each 100 mg/dl that the blood glucose level is above 100 mg/dl, the serum sodium is reduced by 1.6 mEq/L. This is a condition known as **pseudohyponatremia.**

15. What are the symptoms of severe hyponatremia? What happens if the hyponatremia is corrected too quickly?

Hyponatremia usually does not produce symptoms until the concentrations drop to 120–125 mEq/L. These levels may produce neurologic symptoms, such as confusion, lethargy, nausea, vomiting, seizures, and coma.

Overly vigorous correction of hyponatremia may lead to a situation in which the brain is surrounded by a hypertonic plasma, dehydrating surrounding tissue. This condition is known as **osmotic demyelination syndrome** or **central pontine myelinosis.** A symptomatic sodium deficit therefore should be corrected no faster than 2 mEq/L/hr and should not exceed 12 mEq/L/day. The correction maneuvers should cease if the patient becomes asymptomatic or if the serum levels reach 120–125 mEq/L.

16. What are the two most common causes of hypernatremia in the critical care setting?

In the ICU, hypernatremia is usually caused by the iatrogenic administration of salts with insufficient water. Diabetes insipidus may also lead to hypernatremia.

17. You believe that your patient has developed a hypovolemic hypernatremia. How should you correct this disturbance?

First, correct the volume status with lactated Ringer's or isotonic saline, and then correct any remaining sodium abnormality with 0.2% saline or 5% dextrose in water. You can calculate the patient's water deficit with the following formula.

Water deficit (liters) = 0.6 × weight (kg) × [serum Na − 140] / serum Na

18. Describe the EKG changes associated with hyperkalemia and hypokalemia.

The heart is the first organ to reflect changes in potassium concentration. EKGs are therefore important tools in guiding therapy. Increasing serum potassium levels will lead to **peaked T waves** followed by a prolonged PR interval, absent P waves, prolonged QRS-T, and finally, sine waves. Decreasing potassium levels lead to **flattened T waves,** followed by the appearance of U waves and, finally, depressed ST segments with flat or inverted T waves and prominent U waves.

19. What is the appropriate treatment of hyperkalemia?

Plasma potassium levels greater than 6.5 mEq/L can seriously derange organ function, and levels above 10 mEq/L can cause fibrillation and death. Therefore, the treatment must be expedient. If potassium is greater than 6.0 mEq/L, perform an EKG. If EKG changes are present, immediate treatment is required.

First, stop all potassium intake and discontinue potassium-sparing diuretics, ACE inhibitors, and mineralocorticoids . Then protect the heart (reversible depolarization) with immediate calcium chloride infusion (500 mg slow IV push). Next, the goal is to shift potassium into the cell and to remove potassium from the body. To shift potassium into cells, use 50 ml D5 with 10–15 units regular insulin, IV push. Beta-2 agonists (e.g., Albuterol) can also be used. To remove potassium from the body, use Kayexelate, diuretics, or hemodialysis. Kayexalate can be given orally, 20–60 g with 100–200 ml of sorbitol, or as an enema, 40 g with 40 g sorbitol in 100 ml of water.

20. How does catabolism in the postoperative period affect potassium?

In the postoperative period, catabolism often leads to an increase in the serum potassium levels. For this reason, it is important to monitor the potassium concentration carefully, ensuring that it is not iatrogenically overcorrected when calculating maintenance requirements.

CONTROVERSIES

21. What are colloids? When are they indicated?

Albumin and synthetic colloids (hetastarch or "Hespan" and dextran) are two commonly used colloids, also referred to as **volume expanders.** They are often used to treat previous fluid deficits. These substances have a high molecular weight (> 8000 kD) and are unable to rapidly pass capillary membranes. They are, theoretically, confined to the vascular space, where they exert a high osmotic force. This pressure retains fluid in the blood vessels. Blood products can also be used as efficient colloids.

Keeping in mind that all colloids are extremely expensive, they should be used only in situations where intravascular replenishment is critical. Crystalloids have lower molecular weight (< 8000 kD), yet can also effectively increase the intravascular volume. However, crystalloids cannot maintain the high intravascular osmotic pressure. Therefore, crystalloids require as much as four times the volume of colloids to achieve equivalent hemodynamic effects.

BIBLIOGRAPHY

1. Anonymous: Part 8: Advanced challenges in resuscitation. Section 1: Life-threatening electrolyte abnormalities. Resuscitation 46:253–259, 2000.
2. Antonelli Incalzi R, Gemma A, Capparella O, et al: Postoperative electrolyte imbalance: Implications for elderly. J Nutr Health Aging 2:34–38, 1998.
3. Beck LH: Fluid and electrolyte balance in the elderly. Ger Nephr Urol 9:11–14, 1999.
4. Boldt J: Volume replacement in the surgical patient—does the type of solution make a difference? Br J Anaesth 84:783–793, 2000.
5. Bohn D: Problems associated with intravenous fluid administration in children: Do we have the right solutions? Curr Opin Peds 12:217–221, 2000.
6. Bridges EW: Fluids and electrolytes in surgical patients. In Bailey BJ (ed): Head and Neck Surgery– Otolaryngology. Philadelphia, J.B. Lippincott, 1998, pp. 2373–2385.
7. Gomella LG: Clinician's Pocket Reference. Stanford,CT, Appleton & Lange, 1997, pp 169–170.
8. Hewitt-Taylor J: Children in intensive care: Physiological considerations. Nurs Crit Care 4:40–45, 1999.
9. Holliday MA, Friedman AL, Wassner SJ: Extracellular fluid restoration in dehydration: A critique of rapid versus slow. Ped Neph 13:292–297, 1999.
10. Jauniaux E, Gulbis B: Fluid compartments of the embryonic environment. Human Repro Update 6:268–278, 2000.
11. Leelanukrom R, Cunliffe M: Intraoperative fluid and glucose management in children. Paed Anaesth 10:353–359, 2000.
12. Nolan J: Fluid replacement. Br Med Bull 55:821–843, 1999.
13. Okuda T, Kurokawa K, Papadakis MA: Fluid and electrolyte disorders. In Tierney LM, McPhee SJ, Papadakis MA (eds): Current Medical Diagnosis and Treatment. New York, McGraw-Hill Companies, 2000, pp 860–870.
14. Rosenthal MH: Intraoperative fluid management—what and how much? Chest. 115(5 Suppl):106S–112S, 1999.
15. Vincent JL: Strategies in body fluid replacement. Minerva Anest 66:278–284, 2000.
16. Welk TA: Clinical and ethical considerations of fluid and electrolyte management in the terminally ill client. J IV Nurs 22:43–47, 1999.
17. Woods I: Perioperative optimisation of fluid management improves outcome. Minerva Anest 66:285–287, 2000.

79. ACID-BASE DISTURBANCES

Brennan T. Dodson, M.S. IV

1. What are the normal arterial blood gas (ABG) values for pH, PCO2, and [HCO₃⁻]?

	LOW	NORMAL	HIGH
pH	< 7.37 (acidemia)	7.40	> 7.43 (alkalemia)
PCO2	< 35 (hypocapnia)	40	> 45 (hypercapnia)
[HCO₃⁻]	< 20	24	> 28

2. What are the normal compensatory responses to the primary acid-base disorders?

DISORDER	PRIMARY CHANGE	COMPENSATORY RESPONSE AND PH CHANGES
Respiratory acidosis	Increased PCO_2	
Acute		Every 10 mmHg increase in PCO_2 = 1 mEq/L increase in [HCO_3^-], 0.08 decrease in blood pH
Chronic (after 3–5 days)		Every 10 mmHg increase in PCO_2 = 3–4 mEq/L increase in [HCO_3^-], 0.03 decrease in blood pH
Respiratory alkalosis	Decreased PCO_2	
Acute		Every 10 mmHg decrease in PCO_2 = 2 mEq/L decrease in [HCO_3^-], 0.08 increase in blood pH
Chronic		Every 10 mmHg decrease in PCO_2 = 4–5 mEq/L decrease in [HCO_3^-], 0.03 increase in blood pH
Metabolic acidosis	Decreased [HCO_3^-]	Every 1 mEq/L decrease in [HCO_3^-] = 1–1.3 mmHg decrease in PCO_2
Metabolic alkalosis	Increased [HCO_3^-]	Every 1 mEq/L increase in [HCO_3^-] = 0.6–0.7 mmHg increase in PCO_2

3. What is respiratory acidosis? How is it diagnosed?

Respiratory acidosis is characterized by increased blood PCO_2 or **hypercapnia** (from alveolar hypoventilation) with a decreased blood pH or **acidemia** (pH < 7.37). It is diagnosed with an **ABG** and **basic chemistry panel.**

4. What are the differences between acute and chronic respiratory acidosis?

In *acute* respiratory acidosis, each 10 mmHg increase in alveolar CO_2 results in a large change in arterial pH, with a minimal change in the concentration of plasma bicarbonate ([HCO_3^-]) (see Question 2). During the acute phase, there is minimal change in plasma HCO_3^- because renal compensation does not fully mature until 3–5 days of hypercapnia. **Renal compensation** occurs via proximal tubule secretion of hydrogen ions and distal tubule increases in HCO_3^- production and retention. After acute hypoventilation has been present for 3–5 days and renal compensation has matured, this acute condition is now called chronic respiratory acidosis.

Chronic respiratory acidosis is distinguished from acute respiratory acidosis by the presence of elevated plasma HCO_3^-, a normal or near-normal pH (secondary to renal compensation), and persistent, stable hypercapnia. As a result, each 10 mmHg increase in PCO_2 results in a large increase (up to 3–4 mEq/L) in plasma HCO_3^-, with smaller changes in blood pH (See Question #2).

5. An obese, 63-year-old patient with documented obstructive sleep apnea (OSA) presents to the ED complaining of somnolent episodes. He is probably experiencing what acid-base disorder?

Respiratory acidosis, due to upper airway obstruction and obesity. This patient's upper airway obstruction and obesity prevents adequate alveolar ventilation; therefore, he retains more metabolically produced CO_2, leading to a chronic respiratory acidosis.

6. What are some other causes of respiratory acidosis?

Any disease process that limits alveolar ventilation can cause respiratory acidosis. In addition to **airway obstruction** by OSA and bronchial or bronchiolar obstruction, **medullary respiratory center inhibition** (e.g., drug overdose, central sleep apnea, primary CNS disease), **neuromuscular disorders** that decrease respiratory muscle activity (e.g., myasthenia gravis, Guillain-Barré syndrome, myopathy), **pulmonary disease** (e.g., chronic obstructive pulmonary disease, asthma, pneumothorax, pneumonia, pulmonary edema), **chest wall abnormalities** (e.g., kyphoscoliosis, obesity, rib fractures), and **mechanical hypoventilation** (e.g., inadequate ventilator settings) can cause hypercapnia and acidemia.

7. What are the clinical features of acute respiratory acidosis?

Most commonly, acute respiratory acidosis is due to acute hypoventilation and is accompanied by **hypoxemia** or low arterial oxygen tension (PaO_2 < 60 mmHg). Untreated hypoxemia results in rapid deterioration of organ function—seen first in the most oxygen-sensitive organ system, the CNS, causing **lethargy, confusion, stupor, and coma.** Because renal compensation is slow, a greater degree of blood acidemia is seen in acute respiratory acidosis. The cardiovascular system is particularly sensitive to acidemia, as arterial pH declines below 7.20 and peripheral arterial tone and myocardial contractility diminish, **reducing blood pressure. Ventricular and atrial arrhythmias** can develop as acidemia increases sympathetic input to the heart and lowers fibrillation thresholds. In the CNS, acidemia results in **vasodilation and increased CSF pressure,** contributing further to CNS depression. In the pulmonary system, acidemia results in **pulmonary hypertension,** further increasing cardiac stress.

8. How do you treat acute respiratory acidosis?

Treatment involves identifying the underlying cause, **securing an airway,** and ventilating to **restore PO_2** levels. Hypoxemia, if present, causes greater morbidity/mortality than hypercapnia. The patient may require surgical and/or medical management to treat the cause of the hypoventilation, or simple ventilation until drug levels diminish to acceptable levels (e.g., depressant overdose). **Intubation and assisted ventilation** may be indicated when respiratory failure is eminent. You will never be faulted for securing an airway and ventilating a patient early on in respiratory failure, as the patient is more likely to be weaned from the ventilator than resuscitated from cardiac arrest.

9. What must you be careful of when treating an episode of acute respiratory acidosis in a patient with chronic respiratory acidosis from COPD?

Posthypercapnic alkalosis. Though a patient's PCO_2 may be returned to normal levels, serum HCO_3^- remains elevated, as renal excretion of HCO_3^- is slow to develop. Electrolyte and volume deficits must be corrected, as excretion of HCO_3^- is slowed with low potassium, low chloride, and hypovolemia. In chronic respiratory acidosis, the patient's **respiratory drive becomes hypercapnia-dependent,** making ventilator weaning difficult with a "normal" PCO_2. The patient's PCO_2 levels should be returned to levels consistent with the patient's chronic respiratory acidosis.

10. What is respiratory alkalosis? How do you distinguish acute from chronic respiratory alkalosis?

Respiratory alkalosis, characterized by decreased blood PCO_2 (**hypocapnia**) with increased blood pH (**alkalemia**), results from any disease process that causes hyperventilation through direct or indirect stimulation of the CNS respiratory center.

In *acute* respiratory alkalosis, for each 10-mmHg decrease in blood PCO_2, the plasma bicarbonate level decreases by 2 mEq/L, while the blood pH increases by 0.08. After a few hours of acute hypocapnia, renal compensation begins via a proximal decrease hydrogen ion secretion and distal decrease in the reabsorption of bicarbonate. After 8–12 hours, a measurable decrease in plasma HCO_3^- is seen.

Chronic respiratory alkalosis is marked by hypocapnia with maximally decreased plasma HCO_3^-. In chronic respiratory alkalosis, for each 10-mmHg decrease in blood PCO_2, the plasma bicarbonate level decreases by 5–6 mEq/L, while the blood pH increases by only 0.02. After 36–72 hours, plasma HCO_3^- should be maximally lowered, usually to 16–18 mEq/L, and should remain stable despite persistent or worsening hypocapnia.

11. What are the clinical features of a respiratory alkalosis?

Acute respiratory alkalosis is a relatively benign, self-limited condition; however, morbidity can be significant and is often more associated with the etiologic pathology than with the alkalemia itself. Acute hypocapnia results in a **reduction in cerebral blood flow** (up to 20%) causing symptoms of **light-headedness and confusion,** and even transient convulsions, obtundation, and syncope. Cardiovascular changes, **decreased cardiac output and decreased arterial blood pressure,** occur with hyperventilation and hypocapnia in anesthetized patients. In patients with significant cardiac disease, respiratory alkalosis can result in **atrial or ventricular arrhythmias;** patients receiving glucose or insulin infusions can develop **decreased blood phosphate levels.**

12. What are the common causes of a respiratory alkalosis?

Among outpatients, **anxiety** and **pregnancy** (with associated hyperventilation) are common causes of respiratory alkalosis; **liver failure** and **gram-negative sepsis** are more common in the critically ill. The major etiologies of respiratory alkalosis include **hypoxemic drive** (pulmonary disease with an A-a gradient, cardiac disease with a right-to-left shunt, cardiac disease with pulmonary edema, severe anemia, high altitude), **acute and chronic pulmonary disease** (pulmonary embolism, emphysema), **over-stimulation of medullary respiratory center** (psychogenic or neurologic disorders, liver failure with encephalopathy, sepsis, salicylate ingestion, pregnancy), and **mechanical overventilation.**

13. A 55-year-old man, status-post treatment for esophageal carcinoma, presents with a 3-month history of progressive dysphagia and an inability to eat anything by mouth for the last 3 weeks. On exam, he appears mild to moderately cachetic. What acid-base disturbance will this man probably demonstrate?

Metabolic acidosis with an increased anion gap, secondary to starvation ketosis. A severe tumor obstruction of the upper digestive tract is preventing this patient from obtaining adequate nutrition, while the patient's catabolic breakdown of muscle and fat for his daily caloric needs leads to a state of metabolic ketoacidosis (causing an increased anion gap).

14. What is metabolic *acidosis?* How do you predict the PCO_2 and assess the adequacy of the respiratory compensation?

Metabolic acidosis is an acid-base disorder characterized by **acidemia with decreased plasma HCO_3^-;** the compensatory response is through increased ventilation, inducing hypocapnia. This condition may be due to a loss of plasma HCO_3^- or a gain in H+ (that lowers pH and depletes plasma HCO_3^-). The compensated PCO_2 can be predicted by multiplying the last two digits of the pH by 100. If the PCO_2 is higher than your calculation, the respiratory compensatory response is inadequate, and the patient has a metabolic acidosis *and* a respiratory acidosis.

Example: if pH = 7.25,   predicted PCO2 = 0.25 × 100 = 25 mmHg

15. What is the anion gap? How is it calculated?

The anion gap (AG; also known as the plasma unmeasured anion gap) represents unmeasured blood anions that are necessary for maintaining electroneutrality; it is calculated by subtracting the measured plasma anions from the measured plasma cations. The unmeasured anions of the anion gap are made up of (50–60%) albumin, phosphates/sulfates (40%; from tissue metabolism), and lactic/keto acids (from incomplete combustion of carbohydrates and fatty acids). The AG is useful in the differential diagnosis and classification of metabolic acidosis, as the etiology and treatment is different in **high gap** metabolic acidosis vs. **normal gap** metabolic acidosis. Basically, a high gap signifies the presence of organic acids in the blood that deplete the plasma HCO_3^- and, therefore, elevate the AG. This is clearly seen by the equation,

$$\text{Anion gap} = [Na+] - ([Cl^-] + [HCO_3^-]) \qquad \text{Normal anion gap} = 12\ (\pm 2)\ mEq/L$$

A high AG usually indicates renal failure (increased sulfate, phosphate, organic anions) or the overproduction/decreased utilization of organic acids (ketoacids, lactic acid).

16. What causes a low anion gap?

A low AG (<12 mEq/L) may indicate a **loss in unmeasured anions** (e.g., hypoalbuminemia), a **gain in Cl- or HCO_3^-** with no change in Na+, a **gain in cations** with no change in serum osmolality (IgG cationic paraprotein multiple myeloma), **bromide intoxication** (Br- ions are incorrectly counted as Cl- ions), and **severe hyperlipidemia.**

17. What are the clinical features of metabolic acidosis?

While most clinical features are attributable to the etiologic disease, severe metabolic acidosis (pH < 7.2) can cause **deteriorating cardiac function** and **hypotension,** as acidemia causes resistance to catecholamines in the peripheral vasculature. This peripheral resistance can limit the vasocontrictive effects of endogenous/exogenous epinephrine, causing a **blunted homeostatic pressor response** and **less success in resuscitating** the acidotic patient. **Kussmaul respiration** (deep rapid respiration) develops as the respiratory system attempts to compensate for blood acidemia by expelling CO_2, lowering arterial PCO_2.

18. List the causes of normal gap metabolic acidosis.

A simple **loss of HCO_3^- or a gain of H+** (without a detectable accompanying plasma anion) causes normal gap metabolic acidosis in the absence of a cause for a low AG.

19. How does a normal gap metabolic acidosis differ from a high gap metabolic acidosis?

A normal gap acidosis is usually caused by **loss of bicarbonate or addition of H+** to the extracellular fluid, while a high gap acidosis results from the **accumulation or ingestion of organic acids.** In normal gap acidosis, HCO_3^- is lost through diarrheic stool or in urine; in high gap acidosis, organic acids accumulate after they are overproduced, ingested, or not excreted by the kidneys.

20. List the most common causes of normal gap metabolic acidosis. How can they be remembered?

Drugs (acetazolamide, spironolactone, beta-blockers, triamterine)
Renal tubular acidosis

Bicarbonate loss through intestine (diarrhea, pancreatic fistula)
Ostomies (ureterosigmoidostomy or ileostomy)
Dilution of plasma bicarbonate (via rapid infusion of normal saline)
Ingestion of exogenous acids (ammonium chloride, methionine, cystine, calcium chloride)

Remember who cares for the patient? **DR. BODI**

21. What are the most common causes of high gap metabolic acidosis? How can they be remembered?

Methanol ingestion
Uremia

Diabetic ketoacidosis
Paraldehyde
Ingestion of toxins
Lactic acidosis
Ethylene glycol ingestion
Salicylate overdose

Remember **MUDPILES.**

22. How is metabolic acidosis treated?

Identify and correct the underlying disorder. If asymptomatic with mild to moderate acidemia, no treatment is necessary. If pH < 7.25 or HCO_3^- < 15, **HCO_3^- replacement** is necessary. **Calculate the HCO_3^- deficit,**

HCO_3^- deficit = 0.4 × patient wt (kg) × (25 − measured HCO_3^-)

(1 "amp" or ampule of bicarbonate = 50 mEq $NaHCO_3$)

Infuse 50% of deficit over first 12 hours, and recheck ABG and chem 7 (see Question 27) after 4 hours of infusion; continue infusion to correct bicarbonate to only about 15–16 mEq/L. This method of conservative replacement will avoid an **"overshoot" central alkalosis,** a complication of excessive HCO_3^- administration. Conservative therapy is indicated in renal failure or heart failure patients, as excessive sodium bicarbonate administration can cause volume overload, hypernatremia, and a hyperosmolar state.

23. Define metabolic *alkalosis.* What are the two types of metabolic alkalosis?

Metabolic alkalosis is an acid-base disorder characterized by **alkalemia** with **increased plasma HCO_3^-**; the compensatory response is through decreased ventilation, inducing hypercapnia. Metabolic alkalosis results from a **loss of H+ or a gain of HCO_3^-**. It is divided into two types based on urinary chloride levels, chloride-responsive metabolic alkalosis (urinary chloride level is < 10–20 mEq/L) and chloride-unresponsive metabolic alkalosis (urinary chloride level is > 10–20 mEq/L). Hypokalemia and hypovolemia often exacerbate metabolic alkalosis.

24. What causes each type of metabolic alkalosis?

Chloride-responsive metabolic alkalosis is caused by contraction alkalosis, excessive use of diuretics, prolonged vomiting or NG suction, excessive bicarbonate infusion, and villous adenoma. *Chloride-unresponsive* metabolic alkalosis is caused by severe potassium depletion and mineralocorticoid excess.

25. Which is the most common primary acid-base disorder seen in surgical patients? What three factors usually lead to this disorder?

Metabolic alkalosis. The three factors which produce this disorder in surgical patients are (1) **volume depletion** (third-spacing, prolonged NPO), (2) **potassium depletion,** and (3) **loss of gastric secretions** through excessive NG suction.

26. How is a metabolic alkalosis treated?

Correct underlying disease, **correct hypovolemia** with normal saline (or other isotonic solution containing chloride), and **correct hypokalemia** (after confirming adequate renal function) with IV fluids containing KCl or KCl elixir/tabs given PO or NG.

CONTROVERSIES

27. Can an ABG be used to diagnose an acid-base disorder?

No, not by itself. While an ABG gives an accurate assessment of arterial pH, PCO_2, and PO_2, the [HCO_3^-] is a calculated value and can be incorrect. A basic chemistry panel or "chem 7" (containing sodium, potassium, chloride, bicarbonate, BUN, creatinine, and glucose) is required to accurately measure the plasma HCO_3^-. Additionally, the chem 7 can be used to identify any comorbid electrolyte or renal abnormalities.

ACID-BASE BALANCE IN POTENTIAL ORGAN DONORS

An abnormal blood pH may cause the loss of donor organs through harmful physiological consequences. The organ procurement coordinator must correctly analyze the acid-base abnormality and treat its cause while normalizing the blood pH. The mechanical ventilation parameters are changed to correct acidemia or alkalemia by altering the $PaCO_2$. Thereafter, hydrochloric acid or sodium bicarbonate may be administered to correct the calculated metabolic acid-base deficit. The types of acidosis or alkalosis, dead space effect during mechanical ventilation, base excess, base deficit, and the appropriate evaluation of blood lactate are also discussed as related to the correction of the acid-base status throughout donor care.

~Powner, Progress Transplant 10:98, 2000

BIBLIOGRAPHY

1. Bartholow C, Whittier FC, Rutecki GW: Hypokalemia and metabolic alkalosis: Algorithms for combined clinical problem solving. Comp Therapy 26:114–120, 2000.
2. Bryan-Brown CW, Gutierrez G: Pulmonary gas exchange, transport, and delivery. In Ayres SM, Grenvik A, Holbrook PR, Shoemaker WC (eds.): Textbook of Critical Care, 3rd ed. Philadelphia, WB Saunders Co, 1995, pp 776–784.
3. Eddy VA, Morris JA Jr, Cullinane DC: Hypothermia, coagulopathy, and acidosis. Surg Clin North Am 80:845–854, 2000.
4. Fall PJ: A stepwise approach to acid-base disorders. Practical patient evaluation for metabolic acidosis and other conditions. Postgrad Med 107:249–250, 253–254, 257–258 passim, 2000.
5. Heering P, Ivens K, Thumer O, et al: Acid-base balance and substitution fluid during continuous hemofiltration. Kidney Int 56 Suppl 72:S37–40, 1999.
6. Kollef MH: Critical care. In Carey CF, Lee HH, Woeltje KF (eds): The Washington Manual of Therapeutics, 29th ed. Philadelphia, Lippincott-Raven, 1998, pp 170–189.
7. Mahnensmith RL: Electrolyte and acid-base disorders. In Bone RC, Dantzker DR, George RB, et al (eds): Pulmonary & Critical Care Medicine. New York, Mosby-Yearbook Inc., 1998, pp 34–55.
8. Marik PE: Acid base disturbances. In Marik PE (ed): The ICU Therapeutics Handbook. New York, Mosby, 1996, pp 140–149.
9. O'Brien WJ: Fluids and electrolytes. In Berry SM, Bass RC, Heaton KM, et al (eds): The Mont Reid Surgical Handbook, 4th ed. St. Louis, Mosby-Year Book, 1997, pp 27–31.
10. Powers F: The role of chloride in acid-base balance. J IV Nurs 22:286–291, 1999.
11. Schuller D: Pulmonary diseases. In Carey CF, Lee HH, Woeltje KF (eds): The Washington Manual of Therapeutics, 29th Ed. Philadelphia, Lippincott-Raven, 1998, pp 190–212.

80. NUTRITIONAL ASSESSMENT AND THERAPY

Brenda Fishman, M.S. III

1. How is nutritional status evaluated?

Nutritional status is best evaluated with an initial history, review of systems, and physical exam. Muscle atrophy (examine the temporal muscles and the interosseous muscles of the hands) and edema suggest malnutrition. Skin, hair, eyes, mouth, nails, extremities, abdomen, skeletal muscle, and fat stores are all important to evaluate. Anthropometric measurements, although imprecise, may be used to estimate nutritional loss. The skinfold thickness of the triceps estimates body fat, while the midarm muscle circumference estimates skeletal muscle mass. Indirect calorimetry is used in the critical patient to estimate caloric expenditure.

2. Is there a blood test that can correctly detect nutritional status?

Unfortunately, there is no blood test that can accurately determine nutritional status. However, measuring serum albumin, serum transferrin, and serum prealbumin cans help evaluate a patient's protein and nutritional status. These tests have limited usefulness because serum proteins levels are altered by many factors besides nutritional status (hydration, liver function, disease states, and surgery). However, they can be of some help, as follows:

Serum albumin (normal = 3.5–5.8 mg/dl): Evaluates nutritional status over previous 3 months. Bad measure of acute changes in dietary status (< 3 weeks). False increases with dehydration and decreases with liver & renal disease.

Half-life = 18–21 days   Degree of depletion: mild (2.8–3.4), moderate (2.1–2.7), severe (<2.1)

Serum transferrin (normal = 200–400 mg/dl): Evaluates nutritional intake of several weeks.

Half-life = 7–9 days   Degree of depletion: mild (150–200), moderate (100–149), severe (<100)

Serum prealbumin (normal = 16.6–43.1 mg/dl): Evaluates nutritional status of previous week. False increases with renal disease and decreases with liver disease.

Half-life = 2–3 days   Degree of depletion: mild (10–15), moderate (5–9), severe (< 5)

3. What are risk factors for malnutrition?

Poverty, chronic disease, multiple prescription medicines, inadequate nutrition education, alcoholism, poor social structure, involuntary weight loss/gain, and nonambulatory or homebound status are all risk factors for malnutrition.

4. If a patient is receiving inadequate nutrition, which tissues will show nutritional deficiencies first?

The hair, skin, and mouth are most susceptible to nutrition deficiencies because of the rapid cell turnover of epithelial tissue. Mucosal changes of the gastrointestinal tract are reflected by problems such as diarrhea and anorexia.

5. What is a quick way to estimate a patient's ideal body weight?

Males: For 5 feet, 106 lbs is considered ideal weight. For each additional inch over 5 feet, add 6 lbs.

Females: For 5 feet, 100 lbs is considered ideal weight. For each additional inch over 5 feet, add 5 lbs.

6. If weight loss is noted during an initial history, how do you determine if it is significant?

Weight loss in excess of 10% ideal body weight suggests malnutrition. Unfortunately, many critically ill patients are edematous, and the measured weight may not reflect the real body cell mass. To determine if the weight loss is significant, consider the patient's current weight and the time period of the loss. Percent weight change = [(usual weight − current weight)/ (usual weight)] × 100.

7. How is basal metabolic rate (BMR) calculated?

The BMR is the resting energy requirement (kcal/kg/day) and can be calculated with the Harris-Benedict equation. This equation, based on body surface area, calculates the daily energy expenditure. The formula is based on healthy, resting adults and must be modified depending on the severity of the patient's condition, amount of activity, and stress factors (trauma, burns). It also relies on the patient's weight, which may be affected by edema or ascites, and should be modified for patients who are over 125% of their ideal body weight.

For example, in a patient with a fever, the BMR increases 13% for each °C of temperature elevation. In general, the basal caloric need for a nonstressed person at bedrest is 25–35 kcal/kg/day. Most hospitalized patients require 35–45 kcal/kg/day. Postoperative patients and those with multiple trauma, sepsis, or extensive burns have a significantly increased metabolism, requiring 50–70 kcal/kg/day. However, it is important not to overfeed patients, because this predisposes them to liver statosis, hyperglycemia, electrolyte imbalances, macrophage dysfunction, and respiratory problems due to increased CO_2 production.

Females (kcal/day): $655 + (9.60 \times W) + (1.8 \times H) − (4.7 \times A)$

Males (kcal/day): $66 + (13.7 \times W) + (5.0 − H) − (6.8 \times A)$

where W is actual or usual weight (kg), H is height (cm), and A is age (years).

8. What is the difference in daily protein requirement between an unstressed person and a surgical patient?

An unstressed,well-nourished person needs 0.6–1.0 g/kg/day of protein. Postoperatively, a patient needs 1.5–2.0 g/kg/day, and a highly catabolic patient requires at least 2 g/kg/day of protein. These increased requirements occur with excessive gastrointestinal losses, such as diarrhea, nasogastric suction, or exudation. Skin processes such as exfoliative diseases, burns, and draining wounds may also increase protein requirements.

Nitrogen balance may be calculated with the following formula:

$$\text{Nitrogen balance (g/d)} = \frac{\text{protein intake (g/d)} − [\text{UUN (g/d)} + 4]}{6.25}$$

where UUN is urine urea nitrogen.

If a patient has a negative nitrogen balance, the patient is experiencing increased protein catabolism and could benefit from nutritional therapy. Patients with renal failure or hepatic cirrhosis may have impaired nitrogen excretion or metabolism, and protein administration should be approached carefully.

9. Define enteral nutrition.

Enteral nutrition is the administration of nutrients through the existing and functional gastrointestinal tract. This therapy may be supplemental to an oral diet, or it may fulfill all caloric, protein, and hydration requirements.

10. When is enteral nutrition indicated?

- Any patient with a functional GI tract who is unable to fulfill his or her nutritional requirements for > 4 days
- A patient who has unintentionally lost > 10% of normal body weight
- Patients suffering severe protein malnutrition (kwashiorkor) or severe protein-calorie malnutrition (marasmus)
- Some postoperative patients, malnourished cancer chemotherapy or radiation patients, trauma patients, and bone marrow transplant candidates

11. Are there potential complications to enteral nutrition?

The two main complications are **aspiration pneumonia** and **diarrhea.** To avoid aspiration, feedings may need to be changed from large-volume boluses to small-volume continuous feedings. In patients at high risk for aspiration, the feedings may be directed into the jejunum. To prevent diarrhea, hyperosmolar or bolus feedings should be avoided. Bacterial overgrowth in the solution may also lead to diarrhea.

12. A severely malnourished patient with esophageal cancer needs nutritional therapy. She is alert and cooperative. What type of therapy should you initiate?

This patient is unlikely to be capable of an oral regimen. A nasogastric tube could be placed distal to the lesion, and enteral therapy initiated. Alternatively, a percutaneous endoscopic gastrostomy tube may be placed either endoscopically or via an open approach, in anticipation of long-term enteral therapy.

13. Which disease state will appear first in an ill, hospitalized patient who is receiving only 5% dextrose?

Kwashiorkor (nonadapted protein-calorie malnutrition) can develop within 2 weeks of a patient receiving only 5% dextrose. The patient's fat reserves and muscle mass usually remain unaltered—giving a deceptive appearance of adequate nutrition. However, signs of kwashiorkor include increased hair fragility, hypopigmentation, edema, and skin breakdown or delayed wound healing. This condition compromises the muscles of the respiratory system, the heart, and the immune system.

14. What is parenteral nutrition?

Parental nutrition is the administration of all daily requirements of water, calories (dextrose, lipid, etc.), protein (amino acids), vitamins (A, B1, B3, B6, B12, Biotin, C, D, E, and folic acid), minerals (copper, selenium, manganese, chromium, iodine, and zinc), and essential fatty acids and nutrients.

15. How is total parenteral nutrition (TPN) delivered?

Central lines are superior, as they allow for the administration of a high-concentration, low-volume, 25–45% dextrose solution. Peripheral catheters only permit a 5–15% solution and therefore require a higher volume.

16. Which vitamin deficiency is most commonly seen with TPN?

Because it is omitted from the daily multivitamin preparation, patients may become vitamin K deficient.

17. A critically ill patient on mechanical ventilation is receiving a parenteral formula that is approximately 50% carbohydrate and 50% lipid emulsion. Why such a high fat content?

Fat oxidation produces one-third less CO_2 than glucose oxidation. Therefore, a patient in respiratory failure would benefit from this solution because it provides adequate calorie content without producing hypercapnia.

18. What is a respiratory quotient (RQ)? How is it measured?

RQ is the ratio of carbon dioxide production to oxygen consumption. A normal RQ is 0.8–0.9. This value may be measured in the ICU with a metabolic cart, which uses a closed-circuit, indirect calorimetric method. Caloric needs are subsequently based on this ratio. The RQ may be manipulated by changing carbohydrate and fat concentrations in the TPN formula.

19. Explain the other metabolic complications of TPN.

- Acidosis is common, and alkalosis is occasionally seen.
- Hyperglycemia and hyperosmolarity may occur within the first few days of therapy. Hyperglycemia should be treated with regular insulin IM or SC, with subsequent insulin added

directly into the TPN bottles. Insulin should be initiated at 5–10 U/L of 25% dextrose. A glucose of > 200 mg/dl can lead to diuresis and inhibition of WBC function.

- Hypoglycemia may result with the abrupt cessation of TPN, especially if insulin has been supplemented. A severe hypoglycemia can be treated with 10% D/W IV. To prevent hypoglycemia, taper TPN cessation over 48 hours.
- Electrolyte imbalances are often corrected by the addition or elimination in subsequent TPN bags.
- An elevation of blood urea nitrogen (BUN) often occurs when TPN is started. If the BUN increases to 75 mg/dl, regimen modification is indicated.
- If a malnourished patient is unable to increase his or her minute ventilation, TPN may cause hypercapnia. Because CO_2 production is greater with carbohydrate metabolism than with fat metabolism, carbohydrate administration should be reduced or substituted with fat.
- Vitamin K deficiencies are frequent, as this vitamin is not included in the standard multivitamin regimen. Deficiencies should be identified and corrected in subsequent TPN bags.
- After extensive TPN, trace minerals such as copper, manganese, iodine, molybdenum, and selenium may become deficient.
- Patients may experience a wide array of lipid reactions. Immediate reactions include dyspnea, cyanosis, cutaneous reactions, nausea, vomiting, flushing, fever, and dizziness. Delayed reactions include hepatomegaly, jaundice, splenomegaly, thrombocytopenia, and leukopenia.
- TPN administration also may cause liver dysfunction, gallbladder disease, and metabolic bone disease.

20. Name the three nonmetabolic complications of TPN.

- Placement of a central catheter may induce pneumothorax, arrhythmia, and air emboli. The subclavian, carotid, superior vena cava, and thoracic duct may be punctured with placement.
- Venous thrombosis may be a late complication of central line placement. Low-dose heparin administration to the TPN bag may reduce this risk.
- With TPN comes the risk of catheter infection.

21. You initiate TPN for a critically ill patient. What lab tests should be monitored, and how often?

Draw a full electrolyte panel—including Na^+, K^+, Cl^-, HCO_3^-, glucose, BUN, creatinine, PO4, Mg, albumin, calcium, liver function tests, and a complete blood count with a differential—on initiation of TPN administration. Monitor intake, output, and weight daily. Electrolytes and glucose should be monitored daily for 3 days until they stabilize. Then, these values may be checked every 3–4 days. Evaluate albumin and liver function tests every 10–14 days. Evaluate trigylceride levels closely if lipid emulsion is being administered.

22. What is refeeding syndrome? How can it be avoided?

Refeeding syndrome occurs in patients who are severely malnourished when they receive nutrition support that is energy rich (particularly carbohydrate rich). The high carbohydrate intake leads to increased cellular uptake of electrolytes and extremely low serum phosphorous, potassium, and/or magnesium. This large electrolyte shift can lead to lethargy, muscle weakness, cardiac dysfunction, fatigue, and, potentially, death. Refeeding syndrome can be avoided by initially only providing patients with half of their energy requirement based on current dry body weight (about 20 kcal/kg/day). In addition, phosphorous, potassium, magnesium, glucose, and fluid status must be closely monitored.

CONTROVERSIES

23. When is parenteral nutrition indicated?

Patients requiring TPN are usually critically ill patients who do not have a functional GI and/or are unable to fulfill caloric, protein, and hydration requirements. TPN is designed to maintain nutrient balance, restore depleted nutrients, and rest the GI tract. This therapy is often used when protein and calorie depletion is severe, or when the course of the illness is predicted to deplete the nutritional status of the patient. Bowel rest with parental nutrition is often indicated in Crohn's disease, inflammatory colitis, and severe pancreatitis.

When evaluating a patient for nutritional supplementation, if a patient has a functional gut, enteral nutrition is usually superior to TPN. The parental route may increase cost and morbidity. In addition, parenteral nutrition cannot provide a diet that is as complete as enteral nutrition.

NUTRITIONAL DEFICIENCIES

Most of the prevailing chronic diseases in the world have an important nutritional component that directly causes a specific disease, enhances the risk through phenomena of promotion, exerts a beneficial effect in decreasing risk, or prevents the disease. For example, regular intake of foods with saturated fats such as meat and certain dairy products raise the risk of coronary heart disease. The total mixed-fat intake is associated with a higher incidence of the nutritionally linked cancers, specifically cancer of the postmenopausal breast, distal colon, prostate, pancreas, ovary, and endometrium. International studies in geographic pathology have shown that a given disease may have vastly different incidence and mortality as a function of residence. Validation of these approaches can be the basis for public health recommendations and health-promotion activities. Nutritional lifestyles that offer the possibility of a healthy, long life can be adopted by most populations in the world.

~Weisburger, Nutrition 16:767, 2000

BIBLIOGRAPHY

1. Beyer P: Medical nutrition therapy for upper gastrointestinal tract disorders. In Mahan LK, Escott-Stump S (eds): Krause's Food, Nutrition, and Diet Therapy, 10th ed. Philadelphia, WB Saunders, 2000.
2. Bloch AS, Mueller C: Enteral and parenteral nutrition support. In Mahan LK, Escott-Stump S (eds): Krause's Food, Nutrition, and Diet Therapy, 10th ed. Philadelphia, WB Saunders, 2000.
3. Escott-Stump S. Nutrition and Diagnosis-Related Care, 4th ed. Baltimore, Williams & Wilkins, 1998.
4. Fish J, Seidner DL: Enteral nutrition support. In Morrison G, Hark L (eds): Medical Nutrition and Disease, 2nd ed. Malden, Blackwell, 1999.
5. Garrow JS, James WPT, Ralph A (eds): Human Nutrition and Dietetics, 10th ed. New York, Churchill Livingstone, 2000.
6. Grodner M, et al: Foundations and Clinical Applications of Nutrition: A Nursing Approach, 2nd ed. St. Louis, Mosby, 2000.
7. Matarese L, Steiger E: Parenteral nutrition support. In Morrison G, Hark L (eds): Medical Nutrition and Disease, 2nd ed. Malden, Blackwell, 1999.
8. Morgan SL, Weinsier RL (eds): Fundamentals of Clinical Nutrition, 2nd ed. St. Louis, Mosby, 1998.

81. BLOOD PRODUCTS AND COAGULATION

Chitra Rajagopalan, M.D.

1. Which blood components are commonly available in a hospital blood bank?
Most hospital blood banks have packed red blood cells (RBCs), fresh frozen plasma, platelets, and cryoprecipitate readily available for transfusion. Other products, such as whole blood, single donor platelets, and antithrombin III may be obtained from the local blood center.

2. Define the terms "type and screen" and "type and crossmatch."
Type and screen refers to a process of determining a patient's ABO and Rh blood type and screening the patient's serum for the presence of unexpected antibodies directed against RBC antigens. *Type and crossmatch* refers to a type and screen, a major crossmatch (compatibility testing using the patient's serum and donor unit red blood cells), and selecting compatible units.

3. How do you decide whether to request a type and screen or a type and crossmatch?
Request a type and screen for surgical procedures that have minimal blood loss intraoperatively, e.g., septoplasty. If you encounter an unexpected bleeding problem in the operating room, crossmatch compatible blood can be available within 10–20 minutes.

Request a type and crossmatch when there is a high probability of perioperative blood loss or the patient has a history of a bleeding disorder. When crossmatched blood is requested, compatible units are selected, labeled with the patient's name, and separated from the general blood bank inventory.

4. What is a maximum surgical blood order schedule (MSBOS)?
Every hospital blood bank has a list of commonly performed surgical procedures and the median numbers of units transfused for those procedures. The MSBOS is established as a collaborative document between the hospital blood bank and the surgeons, and is used routinely in determining the number of units of blood that will be required for a surgical procedure. Use the MSBOS as a guideline. Patients with a history of a bleeding disorder should be evaluated; additional units or modified blood components may be required prior to surgery.

SURGICAL PROCEDURE	UNITS
Branchial cleft cyst	T&S
Glossectomy	2
Laryngectomy	2
Radical neck dissection	4
Mandibulectomy	2
Ethmoidectomy	T&S
Mastoidectomy	T&S
Rhinoplasty/septoplasty	T&S
Maxillectomy	2
Tongue dissection	4
Vascular tumor resection (e.g., angiofibroma)	6
Myringotomy	—

T&S = type and screen, units = number of packed red cells to be requested, — = no T & S or units to be requested

5. What is autologous blood? When should you request autologous units for your patients?
When a patient donates a unit of blood for himself or herself, it is termed autologous blood. These units are reserved for the same donor/patient and are usually discarded if not used. Autologous blood is usually collected prior to an elective surgical procedure. Some patients are not suitable for autologous blood donation. For example, if the patient has a bacteremia or a metastatic

tumor, autologous blood is not collected. The MSBOS can be used to decide which patients qualify for this procedure and how many autologous units will be needed.

Autologous blood is traditionally prepared as a unit of packed RBCs. Whole blood, platelets, cryoprecipitate, or fresh frozen plasma may be ordered as special requests.

6. What is directed blood?

When a patient's family members or friends donate a unit of blood for the patient, it is termed directed blood. All directed blood units are subject to the same screening tests as homologous units. Directed blood collected from family members is irradiated to eliminate the risk of graft-versus-host disease. If the patient is not transfused with these directed units, the units can be given to another patient (unlike autologous blood units).

7. What is fibrin glue?

Fibrin glue, or fibrin adhesive, consists of two components: human fibrinogen solution and thrombin solution. This adhesive provides fixation of tissues and hemostasis. It has been applied topically in various surgical procedures, including ossicular reconstruction, securing of tympanic membrane grafts, following endoscopic sinus surgery, and during thyroidectomies. To eliminate the risk of disease transmission by this product, many surgeons request autologous cryoprecipitate.

8. Which routine screening tests (for infectious disease) are performed on homologous blood donors?

Hepatitis B surface antigen
Hepatitis B core antibody
RPR for syphilis (rapid plasma reagin test)
Hepatitis C antibody

HIV types 1 and 2 antibody
Human T-cell leukemia virus (HTLV I/II) antibody
Cytomegalovirus (CMV) antibody (special circumstances)
Nucleic acid test/PCR

These tests are performed on every unit of homologous blood collected in the United States.

9. What are the risks of transmitting HIV-1, HTLV 1, hepatitis B virus (HBV), and hepatitis C virus (HCV) to patients?

The current risks of transmission of these infections per unit of blood transfused are:

HIV 1   1 in 430,000 to 1 in 676,000
HTLV-1   1 in 50,000 to 1 in 640,000
HBV   1 in 50,000 to 1 in 250,000
HCV   1 in 10,000 to 1 in 100,000

When obtaining an informed consent for a blood transfusion, risks must be discussed with the patient. Since the introduction of the NAT test, the true incidence of post-transfusion HCV is not known. Other viruses such as CMV, Epstein-Barr virus, HAV, and parvovirus B19 can also be transmitted through a blood transfusion.

10. How is compatibility determined for various blood components?

The only blood components that require crossmatch compatibility are packed red cells and whole blood. Fresh frozen plasma and platelets are issued as ABO compatible and Rh type specific. No compatibility testing is required (including ABO and Rh) for cryoprecipitate.

11. Which is the most common type of transfusion reaction?

Fortunately, the most common type of transfusion reaction is a **febrile nonhemolytic transfusion reaction.** This reaction is most often due to antibodies directed against WBC antigens. Because fever is also an early sign of a **hemolytic** transfusion reaction, it should not be ignored. After the blood bank has confirmed the compatibility status of the unit implicated in the reaction, you can resume the transfusions. The unit in question, however, is discarded after the serologic work-up. It is recommended that patients with previous febrile nonhemolytic transfusion reactions be premedicated with antipyretics such as acetaminophen (*not* aspirin) 30 minutes prior to subsequent transfusions and be given leukopoor blood products. A serious but uncommon cause of fever may be due to bacterial contamination of the unit.

12. How do you recognize a transfusion reaction in an anesthetized patient?
Some clues to recognizing a transfusion reaction in the OR are:

Fall in blood pressure	Oozing from IV sites
Pink urine	Shock
Unexplained bleeding	

This situation is tricky, and several factors in the OR mask the detection of a transfusion reaction. Your anesthesiologist is aware of this entity and can help.

13. A patient in your outpatient clinic tells you that during a tooth extraction several years ago, he had extensive bleeding. What laboratory screening tests should you request for the initial work-up?
The following screening tests will assist you in identifying most, but not all, hemostatic defects:

CBC with platelet count	Fibrinogen level
Prothrombin time (PT)	Bleeding time*
Activated partial thromboplastin time (aPTT)	

*The usefulness of the bleeding time test has been challenged by many coagulationists due to the variables associated with performing the procedure. Therefore, several hospitals do not offer this test. The newer platelet function analyzers are quickly replacing the bleeding time test. The most useful preoperative screening test to predict bleeding is a thorough clinical history including medication history.

14. What are the *initial* screening tests for a patient with a history of a thrombotic disorder?
A careful history and examination to determine predisposing factors, such as family history of thrombosis, obesity, malignancy; prolonged immobility; or postoperative status. Laboratory tests should include: PT, aPTT, antithrombin III, proteins C and S, plasminogen, thrombin time, and lupus inhibitor assay.

15. During the operative procedure your patient bleeds excessively and oozes from all IV sites. What laboratory tests would you request to assess the bleed?
Several systemic or localized pathologic processes may lead to activation of the coagulation or fibrinolytic systems and predispose to disseminated intravascular coagulation (DIC). In such situations, the underlying cause must to identified to initiate specific therapy. Typically, laboratory evidence of DIC is characterized by a precipitous drop in platelet count; elevation of PT, aPTT, and thrombin time; and a positive D-dimer test. DIC may progress from the acute to a chronic state.

CONTROVERSIES

16. What is the usual requirement for transfusion for a patient undergoing head and neck cancer surgery? Why is this important?
Patients with a normal hemoglobin level who do not require flap reconstruction and do not have either a T3 or T4 primary stage tumor have the lowest probability (.02, according to Weber) for requiring blood transfusion. Patients at highest risk (.65) are those with a less than normal hemoglobin level, who require flap reconstruction, and have a T3 or T4 primary tumor stage. Based on a model, an algorithm was developed to serve as a guideline for preoperative transfusion plan-

ning. Weber concluded that by using the TPRA model to prepare guidelines for preoperative transfusion planning, costs could theoretically be reduced by 50% without significantly increasing the risk of exposing patients to allogeneic blood transfusion. In addition, some studies suggest that matched groups of patients who *receive transfusions* do more poorly, survival-wise, than those who do *not* receive transfusions. This difference is postulated to be related to some negative immune alteration by the transfused blood.

ANEMIA AND COAGULATION DISORDERS IN ADOLESCENTS

The transition of childhood to adulthood includes changes to nearly all parts of the body including the blood and the coagulation system. Some disorders, like iron deficiency anemia, develop as the result of rapid growth. Approximately 10% of American adolescents are anemic, and the prevalence is far greater in high-risk populations, such as urban, indigent African-American adolescents, in which 40–50% of young women are anemic. Adolescents at greater-than-average risk for developing iron deficiency anemia, such as athletes involved in lengthy, intense physical activities and pregnant adolescents, should be screened for anemia. Many blood problems are inherited, but the first manifestations may not emerge until adolescence, as in the case of an adolescent girl discovered to have von Willebrand's disease during an evaluation of excessive menstrual bleeding. Besides iron deficiency anemia and von Willebrand's disease, other common hematologic disorders seen in adolescent patients include immune thrombocytopenic purpura, hemophilia, thrombocytosis, and hypercoagulable disorders.

~Hord, Adoles Med 10:359, 1999

BIBLIOGRAPHY

1. Burnouf T, Radosevich M: Reducing the risk of infection from plasma products: Specific preventative strategies. Blood Rev 14:94–110, 2000.
2. Cattaneo M, Lecchi A, Agati B, et al: Evaluation of platelet function with the PFA-100 system in patients with congenital defects of platelet secretion. Thromb Res 96:213–217,1999.
3. Conlon B, Daly N, Temperely I, et al: ENT surgery in children with inherited bleeding disorders. J Laryngol Otol 110:947–949, 1996.
4. Davis BR, Sandor GKB. Use of fibrin glue in maxillofacial surgery. J Otolaryng 27:107–116,1998.
5. Gewirtz AS, Miller ML, Keys TF: The clinical usefulness of the preoperative bleeding time. Arch Path Lab Med 120:353–356,1996.
6. Lucas GF, Leach M. Transfusion-related acute lung injury. Transfus Med 10: 91–93, 2000.
7. Peterson P, Hayes TE, Arkin CF, et al: The preoperative bleeding time lacks clinical benefit: College of American Pathologists and American Society of Clinical Pathologists' position article. Arch Surg 133: 134–139,1998.
8. Sazama K, DeChristopher PJ, Dodd R, et al: Practice parameters for the recognition, management and prevention of adverse consequences of blood transfusion. Arch Path Lab Med 124: 61–70, 2000.
9. Schrieber GB,Busch MP, Kleinmann SH, et al: The risk of transfusion transmitted viral infections. New Engl J Med 334:1685–1690, 1996.
10. Selesnick S, al-Rawi M: Adhesives in otology and neurotology. Am J Otolaryng 18: 81–89,1997.
11. Simon TL, Alverson DC, AuBuchon J, et al: Practice parameter for the use of red blood cell transfusions. Arch Path Lab Med. 122:130–138, 1998.
12. Weber RS: A model for predicting transfusion requirements in head and neck surgery. Laryngoscope 105(8 Pt 2 Su 73):1–17, 1995.

82. WOUND HEALING AND DEHISCENCE

David C. Roska, D.O., Bruce W. Jafek, M.D., FACS, FRSM

1. Describe the physiologic phases of wound healing.

The **early phase** consists primarily of hemostasis and inflammation. Hemostasis is created by immediate, local vasoconstriction and by aggregation of platelets and fibrin due to exposed extravascular collagen. The inflammatory response involves the presence of neutrophils and macrophages. Neutrophils phagocytize damaged tissue and bacteria and predominate during the first 48–72 hours. Neutrophils are then replaced by macrophages, which are a primary source of cytokines that stimulate fibroblast proliferation, collagen production, angiogenesis, and other healing processes.

The **intermediate wound-healing phase** includes mesenchymal cell proliferation, angiogenesis, and epithelialization. These processes predominate 2–4 days after wounding, and are mediated by cytokines. Fibroblasts are the primary mesenchymal cell involved in wound healing. Incisional wounds are generally re-epithelialized completely in 24–48 hours.

The **late wound-healing phase** is predominated by collagen production and wound contraction. Fibroblast synthesizing of collagen begins 3–5 days after injury and continues for 2–4 weeks. Wound contraction begins 4–5 days after wounding and continues for 12–15 days. Myofibroblasts are found in wounds during contraction and first appear on day 3 post-wounding; they predominate until approximately day 21 after wounding.

The **terminal wound-healing phase** has scar remodeling as its hallmark. About 21 days post-wounding, net accumulation of collagen becomes stable. Old collagen is broken down, and new collagen is synthesized in a denser, more organized fashion along stress lines. Intra- and inter-molecular cross-links are the major contributors to increased wound breaking strength. Remodeling continues over a 12-month period; therefore, decisions regarding operative scar revision should not be made prematurely.

2. How much strength do wounds regain?

Skin obtains approximately 30% of its normal tensile strength by 3 weeks, and 60% by 6 weeks. At 6 months the maximum tensile strength of wounded skin is attained, which is at best only about 80% that of unwounded skin.

3. Which are the predominate types of collagen in wounds?

Normal dermis contains approximately 80% type I collagen and 20% type III collagen. At 24 hours after wounding, invading fibroblasts synthesize and secrete type I and III collagen, forming a neomatrix. Type III collagen is elevated for 3–4 days before type I collagen levels increase. However, most collagen in wounds and normal skin is type I.

4. Describe the three types of wound closure.

First intention healing (primary healing)—The edges of the wound are immediately reapproximated after injury.

Second intention healing (secondary healing)—The wound edges are left unopposed, allowing the wound to heal spontaneously through production of granulation tissue, wound contraction, and re-epithelialization.

Third intention healing (delayed primary closure)—The wound is allowed to heal spontaneously for a period of days to weeks, and is then actively closed.

5. What is granulation tissue?

Granulation tissue consists of inflammatory cells—macrophages and fibroblasts—and a gel-like matrix of collagen, hyaluronic acid, and fibronectin containing a newly formed vascular network. It is the red, granular, moist tissue that is characteristic of secondary healing.

6. How do you determine whether the wound should be closed?

All wounds contain bacteria, but several factors affect the degree of contamination of each wound, including: blood supply to the wound, amount of necrotic debris, local wound care requirements, and the use of systemic or topical antibiotics. Generally, infection exists when bacteria have proliferated to levels beyond 10^5 organisms per gram of tissue. Therefore, most wounds can be successfully closed when organisms/g of tissue are less then 10^5.

An important exception: any wound infected with Group B streptococci should *not* be closed, as this is the only bacterial species identified to cause infection at lower bacterial concentrations.

7. List the most common local factors that impair wound healing.

Infection	Radiation
Foreign bodies	Previous trauma
Ischemia/hypoxia	Venous insufficiency
Cigarette smoking	Local toxins

8. List the most common systemic factors that impair wound healing.

Malnutrition	Alcoholism
Cancer	Chemotherapeutic agents
Diabetes mellitus	Jaundice
Systemic corticosteroids	Old age
Uremia	

9. What are the clinical signs of an infected wound?

Inflammation and infection are identified by the cardinal signs of redness, heat, swelling, and pain. These are easily remembered in Latin as *rubor, calor, tumor,* and *dolor,* respectively.

10. Describe the best way to treat infected wounds.

Infected wounds should be opened and drained, and all necrotic tissue sharply debrided away. Any blood clots, debris, and foreign bodies are then removed. The wound should be maximally irrigated with a physiologic saline solution. Dressing changes can be done every 4 hours. Oral and or topical antibiotics can be used as clinically indicated.

11. When is antibiotic prophylaxis appropriate in head and neck surgical wounds?

Surgical site infections account for 14–16% of all nosocomial infections. Once the decision has been made to use prophylactic antimicrobial agents, they should be administered not more than 30–60 minutes before surgery. For example, in operations requiring incisions through oral or pharyngeal mucosa:

Likely Pathogen	Prophylactic Regimen	Adult Dosage
Staphylococcus aureus, streptococci, oropharyngeal anaerobes	Clindaycin with or without gentamicin *or*	600 mg IV for 24 hours 1.5 mg/kg IV
	cefazolin with or without metronidazole	1–2 g IV 0.5 g IV

12. What is wound dehiscence?

Wound dehiscence occurs when infection spreads throughout the layers of the wound, causing the wound to break down. This usually occurs 7–10 days postoperatively.

13. What are methods for wound closure?

Options in order of complexity are: (1) direct wound approximation; (2) skin grafts; (3) local flaps; and (4) distant flaps.

14. When should skin grafts be used?

Skin grafts may be used to cover large wounds that are covered by healthy granulation tissue. The graft is placed over the wound and becomes vascularized from the underlying tissue. The graft can be a split-thickness skin graft, which includes the epidermis and part of the dermis. Split-thickness skin grafts are more commonly used because they vascularize rapidly. A full-thickness skin graft includes all of the epidermis and dermis.

15. How do a keloid and a hypertrophic scar differ?

Both are caused by excess collagen synthesis during wound repair and are more common in darker-skinned and younger patients. *Keloids* are a firm mass of scar tissue that extends beyond the initial wound edge into tissue that was not damaged originally, and may continue to grow even after 6 months. Keloids commonly occur on the earlobes, mandible, and anterior neck. *Hypertrophic scars* are confined to the wound area and usually stabilize by 3 months.

16. List the treatment strategies available for keloids and hypertrophic scars.

- Surgical excision
- Radiation therapy (controversial due to carcinogenic effects)
- Pressure dressings
- Silicon gel sheeting
- Laser surgery (pulsed dye laser or a pulsed CO_2 laser)
- Corticosteroids (intralesional triamcinalone injections)
- Intralesional 5-fluorouracil
- Cryosurgery (less desirable in dark-skinned people due to permanent hypopigmentation)
- Interferon therapy (intralesional injections are initially painful, then well tolerated, and very effective)

Miscellaneous therapies include-topical retinoic acid; antihistamines to stabilize mast cells, thereby reducing histamine release; intralesional verapamil; and numerous others.

17. Describe the first-line approach to treating keloids and hypertrophic scars of the face.

Intralesional corticosteroids are limited to between 2.5 and 20 mg/ml due to increased risk of atrophy and telangiectasia formation. Injections are administered at intervals of 4 to 6 weeks for several months or until the scar is flattened.

18. How are earlobe keloids generally treated?

Keloids of the earlobe are generally excised. Daily application of pressure earrings is essential to maintain cosmetic improvement. Deposteroid injection into the developing scar is said to inhibit keloid formation.

19. Describe the most appropriate method to repair a wound on the face.

Because the face is a non-pressure-bearing area, a wound closure strip may be used if the wound edges can be exactly approximated. If exact apposition is not possible, nonabsorbable fine suture should be used and then removed in 3–5 days due to the vascular nature of the face.

20. Describe the clinical considerations for lidocaine use in wound closure.

Lidocaine is most commonly used in concentrations of 0.5% or 1.0%. Lidocaine's advantages include: rapid onset of action, 2- to 3-hour duration of activity, and minimal risk of allergic reaction. Epinephrine can be added in concentrations of 1:100,000 or 1:200,000. Maximum safe doses for lidocaine are 3–4 mg/kg without epinephrine, and 7 mg/kg with epinephrine.

CONTROVERSIES

21. What is the role of nutrition, vitamins, and trace elements in wound healing?

Proper nutrition is essential to prevent the development of pressure ulcers and to support adequate and timely wound healing. Additionally, research and clinical observation suggest nutrients play a major role in wound healing. For information on how the nutrients vitamin A, vitamin C, zinc, calories, protein, and fluids are used in wound healing and recommendations regarding use of supplements, see references 2, 3, and 5.

BIBLIOGRAPHY

1. Adzick SN: Wound healing. In Sabiston DC, Lyerly KH (eds): Textbook of Surgery. Philadelphia, PA, W.B. Saunders Company, 1997, pp 207–220.
2. Andrews M, Gallagher-Allred C: The role of zinc in wound healing. Adv Wnd Care 12:137–138, 1999.
3. Ayello EA, Thomas DR, Litchford MA: Nutritional aspects of wound healing. Home Hlthcare Nurs 17:719–29; quiz 730, 1999.
4. Braddock M, Campbell CJ, Zuder D: Current therapies for wound healing: Electrical stimulation, biological therapeutics, and the potential for gene therapy. Int J Derm 38:808–817, 1999.
5. Carlson GL: The influence of nutrition and sepsis upon wound healing. J Wnd Care 8:471–474, 1999.
6. Cohen KI, Diegelmann RS, Yager DR, et al: Wound Care and wound healing. In Schwartz SI, Shires TG, Spencer FC, et al (eds): Principles of Surgery. New York, McGraw-Hill, 1999, pp 263–295.
7. Karukonda SR, Flynn TC, Boh EE, et al: The effects of drugs on wound healing—Part 1. Int J Derm 39:250–257, 2000. The effects of drugs on wound healing—Part II. Specific classes of drugs and their effect on healing wounds. Int J Derm 39:321–333, 2000.
8. Kramer SA: Effect of povidone-iodine on wound healing: A review. J Vasc Nurs 17:17–23, 1999.
9. Kudravi SA, Reed MJ: Aging, cancer, and wound healing. In Vivo 14:83–92, 2000.
10. Kunimoto BT: Growth factors in wound healing: The next great innovation? Ostomy Wnd Mgt 45:56–64; quiz 65–66, 1999.
11. Lawrence TW: Wound healing biology and its application to wound management. In O'Leary PJ, Capote RL (eds): The Physiologic Basis of Surgery. Baltimore, MD, Williams & Wilkins, 1996, pp 118–135.
12. Osmon DR: Antimicrobial prophylaxis in adults. Mayo Clin Proc 75:98–109, 2000.
13. Russell L: Understanding physiology of wound healing and how dressings help. Br J Nurs 9:10–12, 14, 16 passim, 2000.
14. Ruszczak Z, Schwartz RA: Modern aspects of wound healing: An update. Derm Surg 26:219–229, 2000.
15. Samuels P, Tan AK: Fetal scarless wound healing. J Otolaryng 28:296–302, 1999.
16. Urioste SS, Arndt KA, Dover JS: Keloids and hypertrophic scars: Review and treatment strategies. Semin Cut Med Surg 18:159–171, 2000.

83. TRACHEOTOMY

Sheri A. Poznanovic, M.D., and Bruce W. Jafek, M.D., FACS, FRSM

1. What are the indications for a tracheotomy?

The most critical indication for a tracheotomy is **airway obstruction.** Causes of airway obstruction include large tumors, ingestion of corrosive substances, smoke inhalation, congenital anomalies, severe maxillofacial trauma, and inflammatory swelling of the neck. A tracheotomy is also indicated if a patient is in need of long-term **ventilatory support.** Tracheotomies facilitate suctioning of excessive **airway secretions** and contribute to the **prevention of aspiration.**

2. How does a tracheotomy differ from a tracheostomy?

A tracheotomy is a temporary alternative airway, while a tracheostomy is a permanent or semipermanent tracheocutaneous fistula. In practice, the two terms are often used interchangeably.

3. How is an elective tracheotomy performed?

The first incision is made horizontally, midway between the sternal notch and cricoid cartilage, usually approximately two fingerbreadths above the sternal notch. This incision is continued down through the skin, subcutaneous tissue, and platysma. At this point, the surgeon separates the sternohyoid and sternothyroid muscle pairs ("strap muscles") with a midline vertical dissection. These muscles are pulled to either side with retractors, thus revealing the isthmus of the thyroid gland. The isthmus is transected vertically, and each side is suture-ligated; alternatively, the isthmus may be retracted superiorly, being careful to avoid the thyroid ima vein. A cricoid hook, placed between the cricoid cartilage and the first tracheal ring, is used to pull the trachea superiorly while the tracheal incision is placed.

4. Who standardized this tracheotomy technique?

Chevalier Jackson in 1909. It reduced operative mortality from 25% to 2%.

5. What is the best method of entering the trachea?

Some surgeons feel that an inferior-based flap, also known as the **Björk flap,** is the safest entry. With this method, the anterior portion of either the second or third tracheal ring is sutured to the inferior skin margin. This method protects against accidental decannulation and makes reinsertion of the tube easy if accidental displacement does occur. The Björk flap poses the threat of a subsequent tracheocutaneous fistula, and therefore it should not be used in cases of temporary tracheotomy or in children.

Other surgeons prefer to enter the trachea with a vertical incision; still others prefer to remove a square centimeter section of one tracheal ring.

6. If you feel that you have created an enterocutaneous fistula with the introduction of the tracheotomy, are prophylactic antibiotics indicated?

A tracheotomy is a clean-contaminated wound. Experience has shown that the tracheotomy is always colonized with bacteria. The use of prophylactic antibiotics will only result in colonization with resistant organisms.

7. How is a tracheotomy performed in a child?

The pediatric tracheotomy is performed in a similar fashion to the adult procedure. However, the trachea is almost always entered with a simple vertical incision into the second and third tracheal rings.

8. What are stay (guide) sutures?

Stay sutures are advised in pediatric tracheotomies. A suture is placed on either side of the vertical tracheal incision. These sutures help to guide the replacement of the tube into the trachea if it is accidentally displaced.

9. Where should an elective tracheotomy be performed?

The surgeon is often most comfortable in the setting of the operating room, where all of the instrumentation, proper lighting, and familiar nursing staff are available. The surgeon must consider the patient's status, keeping in mind the potential hazards of transport. In some cases, tracheotomies should be performed in the ICU, if the room can safely and efficiently accommodate the procedure.

10. What is the significance of tube cuff pressure?

Cuff pressures should not exceed **25 mmHg,** or the approximate capillary perfusion pressure. If the cuff pressure exceeds the perfusion pressure, mucosal ischemia, followed by tracheal stenosis, may result.

11. How do you determine the proper tracheotomy tube size?

The outer diameter of the tracheotomy tube should be approximately two-thirds the diameter of the trachea at the insertion site. Although a smaller caliber tube may decrease the risk of tracheal stenosis, it may increase the risk of mucosal ischemia, as high cuff pressures are necessary to keep the tube aligned. In addition, a small tube may cause difficulties with tracheal care, airway suctioning, ventilation, and fiberoptic bronchoscopy. In contrast, tubes that are too large prevent adequate cuff inflation, which may lead to mucosal abrasion by the rigid tube. An insufficient seal poses an aspiration risk.

12. What are the complication and mortality rates with tracheotomy?

The complication rate is 15%, with the most common complication being hemorrhage, followed by tube obstruction and tube displacement. The incidence of complications in pediatric tracheotomy is generally higher than in adults. The incidence of complications in emergency tracheotomies is 2 to 5 times that found in elective procedures. The mortality rate of tracheotomy is less than 2%. The mortality rate in children is higher, and has been reported as being as high as 25% when used chronically.

13. What are the *intraoperative* complications of a tracheotomy?

Violation of the cupula of the lung may result in **pneumothorax, subcutaneous emphysema,** or **pneumomediastinum.** All of these may result from excessive dissection of tissue planes, blockage of the cannula, or assisted ventilation with excessive pressure causing dissection of air along the pretracheal fascia.

A **tracheoesophageal fistula** may result if the posterior membranous tracheal wall is lacerated. The surgeon can prevent this complication by opening the trachea against a protective cannula, such as an endotracheal tube. If detected at the time of surgery, a posterior tracheal laceration must be immediately repaired to avoid mediastinitis or pneumothorax. Postoperatively, the diagnosis should be suspected clinically by coughing during eating, recurrent aspiration, and pneumonia.

The **recurrent laryngeal nerve,** running in the tracheoesophageal groove, may be severed. Use careful midline dissections to avoid this.

Great vessels of the neck also necessitate the need for careful dissection. Reports of intraoperative **hemorrhage** range from 1–37%. Even **minor bleeding** may become critical if it obscures the identification of the trachea. Frequent sites of minor bleeding are the anterior jugular veins, the thyroid isthmus, and vascular variants such as the thyroid ima artery. Minor bleeding can usually be controlled by packing the incision lightly with Surgicel around the cuffed tracheotomy tube.

14. What are the *early postoperative* complications of a tracheotomy?

Mucous plugging is the most common complication in the early postoperative period. For this reason, meticulous tracheotomy care must begin immediately after surgery. Frequent sterile saline washes followed by suctioning often prevent most plugging problems. Humidification may also be of value.

Tube displacement may be a problem, especially in the pediatric population. The child's undeveloped soft neck tissue is at special risk in the presence of the soft pliable pediatric tube. Stay sutures can assist with reinsertion of a displaced tracheotomy tube in a child.

Respiratory arrest may result in patients who receive a tracheotomy after they have labored with partial airway obstruction for some time. Prior to the procedure, hypoxia maintains their drive to breathe. A tracheotomy may suddenly eliminate this hypoxic drive, thus leading to the arrest.

A patient presenting with frothy sputum immediately following tracheotomy may be suffering from **postobstructive pulmonary edema.** This phenomenon may also occur immediately postoperatively in patients who have labored with airway obstruction for a significant time. Prior to the procedure, these patients exhibit extremely negative intrathoracic pressures during inspiration and extremely positive pressures during expiration. The introduction of the tracheotomy causes a sudden loss of these aberrant pressures, subsequently leading to an increase in venous return and thus a hydrostatic pressure gradient across the alveolar membrane.

Severe wound infection, including mediastinitis, clavicular osteomyelitis, and necrotizing fasciitis, following tracheotomy is rare. Transient tracheitis and stomal cellulitis may occur and are associated with mucosal injury. Pulmonary complications, such as pneumonia or lung abscess, may arise due to aspiration of infected secretions. The causative organisms in most infections are *Staphylococcus aureus, Pseudomonas,* and other mixed flora.

15. And the *late postoperative* complications of tracheotomy?

Tracheal stenosis is the most common late complication and may occur at the level of the stoma, cuff, or tube tip. Patients at increased risk for tracheal stenosis include children and patients tracheotomized for closed head trauma.

Bleeding at the tracheotomy site within the first 48 hours probably originates from the incision. Patients who bleed 48 hours after surgery, especially if bright red is seen (a "sentinel bleed" from the vasa vasorum of the innominate artery, which usually precedes arterial rupture by several hours) should be evaluated for a **tracheal-innominate fistula.** This serious complication commonly occurs because the tracheotomy has been improperly placed below the third tracheal ring. At this level, the tracheotomy tip may erode the tracheal wall. Erosions from a high cuff pressure, tube torsion, and infection can also lead to fistula formation. Sixty percent of tracheal-innominate fistulas occur within 2 weeks of the tracheotomy. This complication carries an 80–90% mortality rate.

Tracheal granulation and persistent **tracheocutaneous fistula** can cause continual tracheal secretions, with skin irritation, disturbed phonation, and frequent infections.

16. How is a tracheal-innominate fistula treated?

Attempt to control the hemorrhage by overinflating the tracheotomy tube cuff or inserting an endotracheal tube below the level of the bleeding, to control the airway. Also, compress the innominate artery by compressing anteriorly against the sternum with a finger inserted through the tracheotomy wound anterior to the trachea. Definitive treatment involves dividing and suture-ligating the two ends of the innominate artery.

17. When should a fenestrated tracheotomy tube be used?

Fenestrated tracheotomy tubes promote spontaneous speech in patients who are being weaned from mechanical ventilation or are spontaneously breathing. These tubes have multiple small holes, or fenestrations, on their greater curvature. When the inner cannula is removed, patients can occlude the stomal port and speak through their native airway. In patients who are not at risk for aspiration, the cuff may be deflated to improve natural laryngeal airflow.

18. What is the role of one-way tracheotomy valves?

One-way valves, such as the Passy-Muir valve, are placed on the stomal port of a fenestrated tube and are used to promote speech. These one-way valves allow the passage of air through the tracheotomy tube during inspiration, but close during expiration. They guide expiratory airflow through the fenestration and natural upper airway, thus promoting speech.

19. You have concerns about a patient's tracheotomy. What are five important points in evaluating the tracheotomy?

1. *What is the tracheotomy brand?* Brands vary in size, pliability, shape, and material. Residents become familiar with the specific properties and limitations of each brand. Knowing this information can help the resident give you better suggestions about the care of the specific tracheotomy.

2. *Does the tracheotomy have an inner cannula?* Plugging can easily be managed if the cannula is properly cleaned. If no cannula is present, however, and the tracheotomy is plugged, the resident may need to evaluate the situation personally.

3. *Is the tracheotomy tube fenestrated?* A fenestrated tracheotomy has a hole in the tube, allowing potential communication between the upper and lower airway.

4. *Does the tracheotomy have a cuff?* Cuff status is important when evaluating leaks and aspiration risks.

5. *What is the tube size?* Narrow tubes may be troublesome when cleaning, as they tend to plug easily. The tube diameter must also be considered when evaluating airway pressures.

20. What is a tracheal button?

Tracheal buttons are used to assist in weaning from the tracheotomy tube. This plastic tube maintains the stomal patency, as its distal end opens into the anterior tracheal wall.

21. Which type of nutrition is used in a patient who has received a tracheotomy in the ICU?

The addition of a tracheotomy in a critically ill patient opens the option for oral nutrition, which is unavailable to the translaryngeally intubated patient. A tracheotomy may, however, interfere with swallowing function, and tube feedings may predispose to aspiration. A recent study investigating the relationship between tracheotomy and aspiration found that pre-tracheotomy aspiration status in 20 patients did not differ from post-tracheotomy status.

With appropriate precautions, tube feeding can enhance alimentary nutrition and present several advantages over parental nutrition. Oral feeding is less expensive than parental nutrition. It also ameliorates the risk of central line sepsis. Tube feedings promote the intestinal mucosal barrier, protecting the patient against endogenous sepsis. Enteral feeding in the presence of a tracheotomy may be associated with several complications, however, including aspiration pneumonia, mucosal ulceration, tracheoesophageal fistula, and purulent sinusitis.

22. A patient is believed to need a tracheotomy after evaluation for obstructive sleep apnea. What type of tracheotomy is recommended?

Once a patient is thoroughly evaluated with an extensive polysomnograph, and it is believed that the occlusive problem could benefit from a tracheotomy, management is often with a fenestrated tube. During the waking hours, the tube is plugged, allowing for a functioning voice. At night, the patient unplugs the tube to facilitate respiration. Since this is a "permanent tracheostomy," the Björk flap is usually used (see Question 5).

23. What is a percutaneous dilatational tracheotomy (PDT)?

PDT is a modified Seldinger technique for placing a standard or modified tracheostomy tube. A needle and guidewire are placed percutaneously through the subcricoid membrane or below the first or second tracheal ring. Serial dilators are introduced through the tract into the trachea over the guidewire. A tracheotomy tube loaded onto a final dilator is then placed through the dilated tissue structures.

This technique has become increasing popular in critically ill patients in the ICU requiring long-term ventilation. Note that PDT has never been found to be safer or more effective than standard elective tracheotomy. Proponents of this technique prefer its use over surgical tracheotomy because of shorter operative time, ability to perform the technique at the bedside, lower expense, ease with which the technique can be taught, and lack of need to transport the patient to the operating room.

24. What are the complications associated with PDT?

The main, immediate complications include misplacement of the dilator tracheotomy tube in a paratracheal position within the soft tissues of the neck or laryngeal structures, hemorrhage, subcutaneous emphysema, and damage to the posterior tracheal wall. Long-term complications parallel those of standard tracheotomy. Patients with suboptimal anatomy are found to have a significantly increased complication rate.

Theoretically, the dilation process causes a symmetric dilatation of a hole in the anterior tracheal wall, increasing the chance for tearing of tracheal cartilage and eventual development of tracheal stenosis. When performing PDT in the intubated patient, the endotracheal tube must be withdrawn to near the level of the vocal cords to allow space for the needle and dilators. During this procedure, it is possible for the endotracheal tube to become displaced and cause an acute, life-threatening loss of airway. **Bronchoscopic monitoring** of the technique can add significantly to its safety and decrease the incidence of complications.

25. When should a cricothyrotomy be used?

There are three situations in which a cricothyrotomy is recommended:
- In **emergency situations,** it is often the preferable method to secure the airway. The cricothyroid membrane is usually easily palpable at the skin surface, and very little dissection is necessary to access this portion of the airway.
- It may also be used for **palliative treatment.** For example, a terminally ill patient may require respiratory hygiene.
- It is indicated in the presence of **anatomic variations** that prevent the standard tracheotomy. These situations are rare.

26. When is the cricothyrotomy not recommended?

There are three situations in which the cricothyrotomy is not indicated:
- Pediatric patients
- Presence of laryngeal infection or inflammation
- Endotracheal tube already in place for > 1 week.

27. How is a cricothyrotomy performed?

The right-handed surgeon stands on the patient's right side. The thyroid cartilage should be secured with the right hand, while the left index finger locates the cricothyroid membrane 2–3cm below the thyroid notch. This membrane is located 1.5–2 cm below the vocal cords, averaging 10mm in height. With the scalpel in the right hand, a quick stab is placed through the overlying skin and directly through the cricothyroid membrane. When the knife blade has pierced the membrane, the knife handle is inserted into the subglottic space and twisted vertically, thus enlarging the access for tube placement.

28. Should a transcricothyroid puncture with a 14-gauge catheter (mini-tracheotomy) be used to help ventilate a patient for a short period of time?

The difficulty posed by this technique is the inability of an adult to respire through such a catheter. To compensate for this, a method to supply oxygen under pressure (via an anesthesia machine or pressurized tank or wall circuit) is needed. Some means of intermittently inflating the lungs and controlling peak pressures is also desirable. The risk of pneumothorax is present if oxygen is delivered under high pressure. Overinflation of the lungs with resulting pneumothorax can occur if there is obstruction at the level of the glottis. In this scenario, a second catheter may have to be placed through the cricothyroid membrane to allow a route for oxygen escape.

CONTROVERSIES

29. Should a cricothyrotomy be used as a definitive long-term airway?
Some surgeons have reported favorable results, but most surgeons reserve the cricothyrotomy for emergency situations, converting the access to a standard tracheotomy if a surgical airway is to be needed for > 3–5 days. Most feel that this conversion decreases the risk of **subglottic stenosis.**

30. Is a postoperative chest radiograph needed after tracheotomy?
Recent literature suggests that after a routine, uncomplicated tracheotomy, chest radiography is a low-yield procedure that incurs unnecessary expense. In the past, post-tracheotomy chest radiography was considered essential to detect serious complications such as pneumothorax and pneumomediastinum as well as confirm correct tube placement. The reported incidence of post-tracheotomy pneumothorax ranges from 0% to 17%. Several authors suggest the following indications for post-tracheotomy radiography: pediatric patient, emergent procedure, displaced tube, clinical indications for pneumothorax, and a difficult procedure.

31. Which is the preferred bedside procedure: open surgical tracheotomy or percutaneous dilatational tracheotomy?
According to PDT advocates, the advantages to this technique include a smaller incision, less dissection and tissue trauma, fewer infections, fewer cosmetic deformities, and a faster procedure. PDT, however, is known to have a higher incidence of minor perioperative complications. Use of an open surgical technique avoids the expense of the higher-costing PDT kit and the need for bronchoscopy. PDT is not recommended in obese patients, patients with calcified tracheal rings, nonintubated patients, or patients with head and neck cancer. PDT is also contraindicated in patients with enlarged thyroid glands, a nonpalpable circled cartilage, and previous neck surgery.

Any user of the PDT technique should be knowledgeable in the open procedure, since conversion to an open tracheotomy may be necessary in difficult cases. Open surgical tracheotomy can be safely performed at the bedside, provided lighting, suction, and an experienced assistant are available. This may be preferable to transporting a critical patient, or one requiring a number of monitoring devices, to and from the operating room via an elevator.

BIBLIOGRAPHY

1. Dulguerov P, Gysin C, Pemeger TV, et al: Percutaneous or surgical tracheostomy: A meta-analysis. Crit Care Med 8: 1617–1625, 1999.
2. Esses BA, Jafek BW: Cricothyroidotomy: A decade of experience in Denver. Ann ORL 96:519, 1987.
3. Godwin HC: Special critical care considerations in tracheostomy management. Clin Chest Med 12:573–583, 1991.
4. Goldenberg D, Gov EG, Golz A, et al: Tracheotomy complications: A retrospective study of 1130 cases. Otolaryngol Head Neck Surg 123: 495–500, 2000.
5. Heffner JE: Tracheotomy. In Parsons PE, Wiener-Kronish JP (eds): Critical Care Secrets, 2nd ed. Philadelphia, Hanley & Belfus, 1998, pp 62–67.
6. Johnson JT, Rood SR, Stool SE, et al: Tracheotomy: A Self-Instructional Package from the Committee on Continuing Education in Otolaryngology. Washington, DC, American Academy of Otolaryngology–Head and Neck Surgery Foundation, 1988.
7. Leder SB, Ross DA: Investigation of the causal relationship between tracheotomy and aspiration in the acute care setting. Laryngoscope 110: 641–644, 2000.
8. Smith DK, Grillone GA, Fuleihan N: Use of postoperative chest x-ray after elective adult tracheotomy. Otolaryngol Head Neck Surg 120: 848–851, 1999.
9. Weissler MC: Tracheotomy and intubation. In Bailey BJ (ed): Head and Neck Surgery–Otolaryngology, 2nd ed. Philadelphia, J.B. Lippincott, 1998, pp 803–818.

84. AIRWAY CONTROL AND MECHANICAL VENTILATION

Michael F. Spafford, M.D., Catherine P. Winslow, M.D., and Joel H. Witter, M.D.

1. What are some indications for intubation and assistance with ventilation?

Strive to avoid respiratory emergencies by *timely intervention*. Upper airway obstruction, refractory hypoxia, and inadequate ventilation are the most general indications for airway control and ventilatory assistance. A patient with progressive upper airway compromise for any reason should be intubated (externally [tracheotomy] or internally) to provide an unobstructed airway. The hypoxic patient, who is unable to maintain a PaO_2 >50 mmHg despite noninvasive measures, should receive a secure airway and assistance with breathing. Proper management of hypercapnea (defined as $PaCO_2$ > 45 mmHg) requires a history of the rate of change. Chronic $PaCO_2$ elevation is often well-compensated and well-tolerated, and should not be normalized. Acute elevation produces acidemia and symptoms that require airway control and assisted ventilation.

2. What does a patient's response to oxygen therapy tell you about the etiology of hypoxia?

Hypoxia is defined as PaO_2 < 60 mmHg. Ventilation-perfusion mismatch (e.g., pneumonia, COPD, emphysema, asthma, interstitial lung disease), intrapulmonary or intracardiac right to left shunting (atalectasis, pulmonary edema, pneumonia, pulmonary embolism, vascular anomalies), and alveolar hypoventilation (sedation, weakness, high altitude, inadequate inspired oxygen) are the significant causes of hypoxia. An increase in inspired oxygen improves the oxygen saturation of arterial blood in almost all situations; the exception is a right-to-left shunt > 30%.

3. What are the permanent neurologic sequelae of hypercapnea?

Hypercapnea is defined as a $PaCO_2$ of > 45mmHg. Unlike hypoxia, hypercapnea produces neurologic changes that are completely reversible. Patients with COPD may tolerate elevations of $PaCO_2$ as high as 100 mmHg. Therefore, hypercarbia is a relative indication for initiating or increasing ventilatory support.

4. What is the target PaO_2 when providing oxygenation to a patient with chronic hypoxia and hypercapnea?

Because of compensation for chronically elevated $PaCO_2$, these patients often have a respiratory drive that is not mediated by hypercapnea, but by hypoxia. Therefore, overly enthusiastic oxygenation can lead to respiratory depression, acute hypercapnea, and CNS depression. The target PaO_2 should be approximately 50–60 mmHg or higher, if tolerated.

5. What are CPAP and biPAP? How can they be useful in preventing intubation?

Continuous positive airway pressure supplied by face mask (CPAP) increases oxygenation by opening previously collapsed groups of alveoli, thus decreasing intrapulmonary shunting. BiPAP provides both inspiratory and expiratory positive airway pressure (PAP). The inspiratory PAP given is a function of PCO_2, and the expiratory PAP is a function of PO_2. A standard starting parameter for biPAP is 8/4, which provides 8 cm O_2 during inspiration and 4 cm O_2 on expiration. These methods may decrease the need for intubation in certain groups of patients, such as those with COPD and chronic hypercapnea.

6. What are the types of ventilator modes? How do you decide which is appropriate for a given patient?

Pressure-cycled: These ventilator settings deliver a pre-set pressure. The tidal volume is variable. (Tidal volume and inspiratory time are related to compliance.)

- *Pressure-support ventilation* (*PSV*): This setting delivers breath to pre-set pressure, regardless of volume, and is generally supplied for 90% of the duration of the breath. Tidal volume and flow rate are not set by the ventilator. This mode is good for difficult-to-wean patients because the work of breathing is decreased. However, the pressure must be adjusted to ensure an adequate tidal volume.
- *Pressure-control ventilation* (*PCV*): This setting is similar to PSV, but delivers pressure throughout the entire breath. It is often used with inverse-ratio ventilation (IRV). IRV prolongs ventilatory time and minimizes alveolar collapse, but patients are at an increased risk for barotrauma. *Volume-cycled:* These ventilator settings deliver a pre-set volume. The pressure is variable.

Synchronized intermittent mechanical ventilation (SIMV): The machine delivers breaths at a pre-set tidal volume and rate per minute, regardless of patient effort. Nonetheless, the breaths can be synchronized with patient effort. The patient must generate his or her own tidal volume for additional breaths. This setting is good for weaning, but requires more respiratory effort than assisted-controlled ventilation.

Assisted-controlled ventilation (AC): Each patient-initiated breath is "assisted" by the ventilator to the set tidal volume. In addition, the ventilator initiates "backup" or "control" breaths if the patient is breathing more slowly than the set rate. This setting is good for "resting" patients as it minimizes the work of breathing, but it is difficult to wean patients in this mode, and hyperventilation is possible.

7. What are the starting parameters for the volume-controlled ventilator?

Tidal volume	10–12 ml/kg (in general, about 700–900 ml for an adult)
Rate	10–15 breaths/min, dependent on mode
O2 concentration (FiO2)	Start at 100% and wean rapidly if able
PEEP	0–5 cm H2O
Minute volume	8–10 liters/min.

8. What type of monitoring is appropriate for patients on mechanical ventilation?

Check arterial blood gas (ABG) at regular intervals (every 15–30 minutes) and make ventilator adjustments until desired blood gas levels are reached and the patient is stable. Then check the ABG every morning while the patient is on the ventilator or if the clinical condition changes. Monitor airway pressures to prevent barotrauma. Monitor continuous pulse oximetry, and closely follow vital signs. Intake and output are monitored to prevent pulmonary edema. Obtain a chest x-ray immediately after intubation and at least once a week thereafter. Remember that changes such as tachycardia, hypotension, and agitation may be the result of improper ventilator settings.

9. What is the significance of an elevated plateau pressure?

The peak pressure is that pressure required to deliver a pre-set tidal volume. The portion of that pressure required to overcome the elastic recoil forces of the lungs and chest wall is called the plateau pressure. It is measured by occluding the expiratory port of the ventilator circuit at the completion of a full inspiration. A sudden elevation in peak pressure alone usually signifies a problem with the circuit or airway (kinking or biting the tube, mucus plugging, bronchospasm). An elevation in the plateau pressure signals a lung or chest wall problem (tension pneumothorax, atelectasis, pulmonary edema).

10. A postoperative head and neck cancer patient with a history of COPD requires a period of intubation and ventilatory support. Shortly after you order initial ventilator settings, you are called to the ICU emergently. Your patient is acutely hypotensive, has new onset atrial fibrillation, and, although making obvious respiratory effort, is not triggering the ventilator to deliver an assisted breath. What is the most likely problem?

This patient has been over-ventilated. He is experiencing dynamic hyperinflation with auto-

PEEP. Because of his obstructive pulmonary disease, he requires a longer time to exhale than allowed by the ventilator. Therefore, he has positive end-expiratory airway pressure at the time of the next mechanically supplied breath. This causes progressive pulmonary hyperinflation, increased intrathoracic pressure, decreased central venous return, decreased cardiac output, and hypotension. In addition, excessive ventilation of patients with chronic hypercarbia may cause alkalemia and cardiac arhythmias. Finally, auto-PEEP increases work of breathing. A mechanical ventilator must detect a negative inspiratory pressure of (-)1–2 cm H_2O to deliver an assisted breath. This patient must generate an additional inspiratory effort equal to the auto-PEEP before triggering the ventilator. One corrective measure is to supply external PEEP to a level just below the auto-PEEP.

11. As you finish stabilizing the first patient, the nurse across the hall calls out to you. One of your previously stable intubated and ventilated patients has become acutely hypoxic. Increasing the percentage of inspired oxygen does not help. Lung sounds are absent on the left. She is nonetheless hemodynamically stable. What is the differential diagnosis and most likely problem?

Clinical evaluation, including vital signs and physical exam, are mandatory. ABGs should be obtained, as well as a chest x-ray and EKG if clinically indicated. The differential diagnosis includes reasons for right to left shunt, such as pneumothorax, pulmonary embolism, mucous plug with massive atelectasis, and pulmonary edema. Reasons for ventilation-perfusion mismatch are also included, such as pneumonia, asthma and interstitial lung disease, as are reasons for insufficient inspired oxygen, such as disruption of the ventilator circuit. The FiO_2 should be increased, and consideration should be given to increasing PEEP. Hypoxia refractory to oxygen therapy indicates shunting of pulmonary blood flow, narrowing the differential. In the absence of hemodynamic instability, mucus plugging of the left mainstem bronchus and massive atelectasis is the most likely diagnosis.

12. What is PEEP? What are the hazards of PEEP?

PEEP is positive end-expiratory pressure. It can help prevent atelectasis by redistributing alveolar H_2O into the perivascular space. It can also be used to treat hypoxia by recruiting more lung units and decreasing intrapulmonary shunting. However, it does not decrease extravascular pulmonary H_2O; it can decrease cardiac output; and it can cause barotrauma.

13. How do you wean a patient from the ventilator?

There are several commonly used methods:

The patient may be weaned on IMV by simply decreasing the rate of intervals (once the patient is stable on an $FiO2$ of 40% and a PEEP of 5) and monitoring the patient's tolerance. If the patient does well on a rate of 2, parameters and an ABG are evaluated.

A T-piece can deliver oxygen with the patient still intubated but receiving no additional mechanical support, if the patient's tolerance is questionable.

A pressure support wean is advocated for the difficult-to-wean patient. The pressure support is decreased at regular intervals, while the patient's tolerance is closely followed. The patient may be weaned for several hour intervals throughout the day, and "rested" at a higher pressure support (or AC) at night. If the patient is stable on a pressure support of < 5 mmHg, he or she is probably ready to extubate.

14. What parameters predict a successful wean?

Some commonly used weaning parameters are as follows:

Tidal volume	> 5 ml/kg
Respiratory rate	< 20 breaths/min
Negative inspiratory pressure	< −30 cm H_2O
Vital capacity	> 10 ml/kg
Minute volume	< 12 liters/min
FiO_2	< 40%

A ratio of respiratory frequency/tidal volume of < 100 is an excellent predictor of a successful wean. The patient should be awake and cooperative at the time of extubation.

15. What is barotrauma? Who is at risk?

Barotrauma results from overdistension and rupture of the airways and alveoli under positive pressure. Many complications, such as subcutaneous emphysema, pneumothorax, and systemic air emboli, can ensue. If peak airway pressure is < 50 cm H_2O, the risk of barotrauma is negligible. The risk of barotrauma increases rapidly after this point, with an incidence approaching 50% at pressures > 70 mm H_2O.

16. What is the ventilated patient's risk of infection?

The risk for nosocomial pneumonia may approach 5% per day in mechanically ventilated patients, although the risk appears to fall with long-term ventilation. Nosocomial sinusitis is present by CT scan in 70% of patients who require both nasotracheal and nasogastric intubation for 1 week. If both tubes are placed orally, the risk is 34%.

17. Describe the pathophysiology of injury from long-term intubation.

Capillary perfusion pressure is the most important factor in intubation injury. If the pressure of the endotracheal tube is greater than mucosal capillary pressure, ischemia occurs, followed by epithelial injury. The mucociliary flow is interrupted, causing stasis of secretions and infection. Next, the underlying perichondrium, which supplies blood flow to cartilage and a surface for epithelial regeneration, may be injured. After loss of perichondrium and epithelium, the injured area heals by secondary intention. The deposition of new collagen may continue for months after removal of the endotracheal tube. With maturation of the wound, firm scar tissue left in the airway contracts with time, causing such lesions as subglottic and posterior glottic stenosis.

18. How can laryngeal injury from intubation and mechanical ventilation be minimized?

The smallest tube that allows adequate ventilation should be chosen. In children, uncuffed endotracheal tubes that allow a leak with 20 cm H_2O ventilation pressure should be used. In adults, low-pressure high-volume cuffs, containing only the minimum volume needed to occlude the airway, should be used.

In addition, tube motion can cause mucosal trauma. This can be minimized by adequate stabilization of the tube. Some have argued that a nasotracheal tube is better stabilized by the tissues of the nasopharynx and nose than an orotracheal tube. The ventilator tubing should be suspended to protect the patient from the shearing motion of the mechanical ventilator. Excessive patient movement and coughing can be minimized by adequate sedation and proper suctioning technique.

Infection may also complicate the pathophysiology, and antibiotics may be indicated. Gastroesophageal reflux aggravates the local intubation injury and may be exacerbated by the presence of a nasogastric tube. Finally, and most importantly, limiting the duration of intubation is the most important way to minimize laryngeal injury.

19. What parts of the larynx are most at risk in long-term intubation?

Endotracheal tubes lie in and exert pressure on the posterior larynx. Most damage occurs at three sites:

• The medial surfaces of the arytenoid cartilages, cricoarytenoid joints, and vocal processes
• The posterior glottis and interarytenoid region
• The inner surface of the cricoid cartilage in the subglottis.

20. What is the narrowest part of the airway?

In children, the narrowest part of the airway is the subglottis at the level of the cricoid. In adults, it is the glottis at the level of the true vocal cords.

21. Discuss the common injuries from long-term endotracheal intubation.

An **intubation granuloma** is a rounded, pedunculated mass arising from the vocal process and medial surface of the arytenoid, causing symptoms that range from dysphonia to airway obstruction.

An **interarytenoid adhesion** is a transverse fibrous bridge that tethers the vocal cords together, leaving a small posterior and larger anterior airway with partial obstruction.

Posterior glottic stenosis represents transverse scar tissue between the arytenoids at the glottic level, which may extend downward into the subglottic region.

Subglottic stenosis is a narrowing of the area below the vocal cords and above the inferior margin of the cricoid cartilage sufficient to cause respiratory compromise. Complete obstruction can occur at any of these levels.

Ductal retention cysts result from irritation and obstruction of mucous glands in the subglottic region. These can become quite large and obstructive up to months after extubation.

Vocal cord paralysis, most often unilateral, is thought to result from endotracheal tube compression of the recurrent laryngeal nerve between the arytenoid and laryngeal cartilages.

Dislocation of the arytenoid cartilage, most commonly on the left (most intubations are right-handed), may present as hoarseness and odynophagia after extubation.

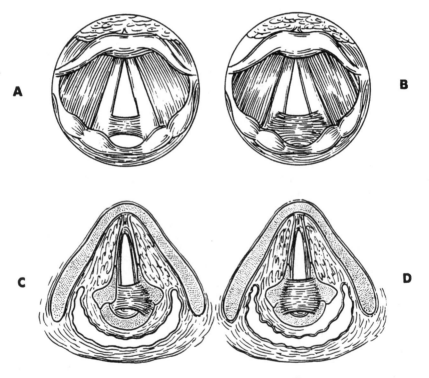

Posterior glottic stenosis. *A,* Interarytenoid adhesion with mucosally lined tract posteriorly. *B,* Posterior commissure and interarytenoid scar without mucosally lined tract posteriorly. *C,* Posterior commissure scar extending into right cricoarytenoid joint. *D,* posterior commissure scar extending into both cricoarytenoid joints (From Cummings CW, et al (eds): Otolaryngology—Head and Neck Surgery, 3rd ed. St. Louis, Mosby-Year Book, 1998, with permission.)

22. How is endotracheal tube size chosen?

The smallest tube that provides adequate ventilation should be chosen. In adults, the upper size limit is generally 7–8 mm inside diameter in males and 6–7 mm in females. For neonates, 2.5- to 3.0-mm tubes are generally chosen, and 3.0- to 3.5-mm tubes are used for ages 3–9 months.

For children 1 year of age or more, the formula [age in years + 16]/4 predicts the correct size tube in over 95% of children. In emergencies, or when history is lacking, a tube is chosen that is approximately the width of the fifth (pinkie) fingernail, a method that predicts the correct tube size in 91% of children.

CONTROVERSIES

23. How long can an adult be safely endotracheally intubated?
There is no definite safe time limit for endotracheal intubation. One study reported severe injury after 17 hours of intubation in adults. Several studies have shown that 7–10 days of intubation is acceptable, after which the incidence of laryngotracheal complications increases. Other authorities advocate intubation for no longer than 5–7 days without endoscopic evaluation of the airway.

24. How long can a child be safely endotracheally intubated?
This decision is also controversial, and the duration varies with the age of the patient. Most authorities agree that neonates with properly sized, uncuffed endotracheal tubes and skilled neonatal intensive care can be intubated for extensive periods (weeks to months) with a low incidence of complications. It is thought that the laryngeal cartilages in infants may mold and yield to pressure more than those of older children and adults. However, duration of intubation remains the chief risk factor for long-term complications.

EVOLUTIONARY REGRESSION?

Liquid ventilation, an idea currently being trialed in the pediatric population, is increasingly being discussed as a possible future trend in ventilation. A review of the available literature indicates that this treatment provides effective gas exchange and has a number of potential advantages. These include lower airway pressures, decreased alveolar surface tension, alveolar recruitment, and removal of pulmonary exudate. While not yet widely accepted, use of liquid ventilation may expand in the future. If it is, those caring for patients treated in this way will require knowledge of the mechanics and physiological changes involved, as well as the potential hazards of this modality.

BIBLIOGRAPHY

1. Anonymous: Part 6: Advanced cardiovascular life support. Section 3: Adjuncts for oxygenation, ventilation, and airway control. Resuscitation 46:115–125, 2000.
2. Benjamin BR: Prolonged intubation injuries of the larynx: Endoscopic diagnosis, classification, and treatment. Ann Otol Rhinol Laryngol Suppl 160:1–15, 1993.
3. Bhuta T, Henderson-Smart DJ: Elective high frequency jet ventilation versus conventional ventilation for respiratory distress syndrome in preterm infants. Coch Database Syst Revs [computer file]. (2):CD000328, 2000.
4. Blackwood B: The art and science of predicting patient readiness for weaning from mechanical ventilation. Int J Nurs Stud 37:145–151, 2000.
5. Bresnahan M: Liquid ventilation: A future modality? Austral Crit Care 12:104–8, 1999.
6. Cotton RT, Zalzal GH: Glottic and subglottic stenosis. In Cummings CW, et al (eds): Pediatric Otolaryngology–Head and Neck Surgery, 3rd ed. St. Louis, Mosby-Year Book, 1998, pp 303–324.

7. Cross AM: Review of the role of non-invasive ventilation in the emergency department. Emerg Med J 17:79–85, 2000.
8. Einarsson O, Rochester CL, Rosenbaum S: Airway management in respiratory emergencies. Clin Chest Med 15:13–34, 1994.
9. Ely EW: The utility of weaning protocols to expedite liberation from mechanical ventilation. Resp Care Clin NA 6:303–319, 2000.
10. Houston P: An approach to ventilation in acute respiratory distress syndrome. Can J Surg 43:263–268, 2000.
11. Krishnan JA, Brower RG: High-frequency ventilation for acute lung injury and ARDS. Chest 118:795–807, 2000.
12. Leatherman JW, Ingram RH: Respiratory failure. In Dale DC, Federman DD (eds): Scientific American Medicine, Section 14, Chapter VIII, p1. New York, WebMD Corp (www.webmd.com), 2000.
13. Mutlu GM, Factor P: Complications of mechanical ventilation. Resp Care Clin North Am 6:213–52, 2000.
14. Plant PK, Elliott MW: Noninvasive positive pressure ventilation. J Roy Coll Phys London 33:521–525, 1999.
15. Polkey MI, Lyall RA, Davidson AC, et al: Ethical and clinical issues in the use of home noninvasive mechanical ventilation for the palliation of breathlessness in motor neurone disease. Thorax 54:367–371, 1999.
16. Sinha SK, Donn SM: Weaning from assisted ventilation: Art or science? Arch Dis Childhood Fetal Neonatal Edition 83:F64–70, 2000.
17. Spence K, Barr P: Nasal versus oral intubation for mechanical ventilation of newborn infants. Coch Database Syst Revs [computer file]. (2):CD000948, 2000.
18. Tobin MJ: 1999 Donald F Egan Scientific Lecture. Weaning from mechanical ventilation: What have we learned? Resp Care 45:417–431, 2000.
19. Tobin A, Kelly W: Prone ventilation—it's time [see comments]. Anaesth Int Care 27:194–201, 1999.
20. Weissler MC: Tracheotomy and intubation. In Bailey BJ (ed): Head and Neck Surgery–Otolaryngology. Philadelphia, J.B. Lippincott, 1998.

85. CARDIOPULMONARY RESUSCITATION AND ADVANCED CARDIAC LIFE SUPPORT

Mark Edward Miller, M.S. III

1. What are the common causes of cardiac arrest?
In infants and children, most cardiac arrests are preceded by respiratory compromise and hypoxia. For adults, the etiology is usually myocardial ischemia, which results in decreased contractility and electrical instability.

2. What are the ABCD's of treating a patient in cardiac arrest?
When you are first on the scene of an unconscious patient, assess responsiveness, call for assistance, and do the **primary survey:**
A—Open the **airway,** either with a head-tilt chin-lift maneuver or, if cervical spine injury is suspected, with a jaw thrust.
B—Assess **breathing.** If the patient is apneic, ventilate with an oropharyngeal airway and bag-mask apparatus.
C—Assess **circulation** and begin chest compressions if carotid artery pulse (or brachial pulse in infants) is absent. The pulse check is no longer required to avoid false-negative results; instead, assess for signs of circulation (normal breathing, coughing, or movement).
D—**Defibrillate** appropriate patients as soon as possible. If a defibrillator is available immediately, "D" takes priority over "ABC."

3. What is the secondary survey?
Once the primary survey is completed, ABCD stands for:
A—**Airway** assessment and management with endotracheal intubation.
B—**Breathing** assessment via verification of endotracheal tube placement.
C—**Circulation.** Continue CPR and establish IV access.
D—**Differential diagnosis.** Assess patient history and clinical presentation to identify possible causes of the arrest and reversibility of the patient's condition.

4. How does CPR differ for infants, children, and adults?

AGE	BREATHS/ MINUTE	CHEST COMPRESSIONS/ MINUTE	COMPRESSION DEPTH	HAND PLACEMENT
Infants < 1 yr	20	> 100	0.5–1 in	2 fingers. 1 finger-width below horizontal nipple line
Children 1–8 yrs	20	100	1–1.5 in	Heel of 1 hand. Lower half of sternum 2 finger-breadths above xiphoid
Children > 8 yrs, adults	> 8–12	80–100	1.5–2 in	Same as for children, but with 2 hands with interlocking fingers

5. List the potential complications of CPR.
Survivors must be assessed for possible complications and treated promptly.
• Skin injury: chest burns, abrasions, contusions
• Intrathoracic trauma: rib or sternal fractures, barotrauma, pulmonary embolus, pneumothorax, hemothorax
• Cardiac trauma: tamponade, contusion, pericarditis
• Airway injury: oral trauma, tracheal trauma, aspiration
• Abdominal injury: gastric perforation, splenic or hepatic laceration

6. Why does vasopressin require less frequent administration than epinephrine?

Vasopressin is an adrenergic agent that possesses the equivalent positive effects of epinephrine and may be used as an alternative for treatment of shock-refractory cardiac arrest with ventricular fibrillation (VF) or ventricular tachycardia (VT). Vasopressin (also known as antidiuretic hormone) requires less frequent administration than epinephrine because it has a longer half-life of 10–20 minutes (compared with the 3–5 minute half-life of epinephrine). Current research does not support a second dose of vasopressin and therefore epinephrine should be used for further therapy if there is no response to vasopressin.

7. What is adequate CPR?

The presence of:
- Palpable femoral and carotid pulses with compressions
- Chest movement, no air leak, and bilateral breath sounds with bag-mask or endotracheal tube ventilation
- End-tidal CO_2 >10 mmHg. This has been correlated with cardiac output, perfusion pressure, and successful outcome in experimental animal models.

8. Who should be defibrillated?

Only patients with VF or pulseless VT should be defibrillated. Patients with stable VT should be monitored and treated pharmacologically. Patients with VT and a pulse who have hypotension, chest pain, dyspnea, or other signs or symptoms of hypoperfusion should be treated emergently with synchronized cardioversion.

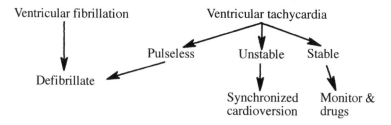

9. What is the procedure for emergent defibrillation?

Note: all defibrillation situations are emergent!

1. Confirm dysrhythmia and pulselessness.
2. Charge machine to 200 joules.
3. While charging the defibrillator, apply conductive gel pads to chest at right sternal border and cardiac apex.
4. When the defibrillator is charged, apply paddles firmly to sternum and apex over the gel pads.
5. State firmly, "All clear," and look around to confirm team members are not touching the patient or bed.
6. Press both paddle discharge buttons simultaneously.
7. Recharge to 200–300 J and assess rhythm and pulse. If unchanged, defibrillate immediately.
8. Recharge to 360 J and assess again. If unchanged, defibrillate immediately.
9. If the rhythm at any point converts to a viable rhythm, assess pulse and blood pressure and do *not* defibrillate.

10. What are common errors in defibrillation?

- Waiting too long to charge the defibrillator. It takes up to 11 sec to charge the machine. If the charge is not needed, i.e., the patient's rhythm changes, the paddles can be returned to the defibrillator holders or turned off.
- Improper paddle placement.

- Insufficient paddle pressure on the chest. Less than 25 pounds of pressure per paddle results in patient burns and electrical arcing when discharged.
- Not doing verbal and visual "all clear."
- Having the synchronized button on for defibrillation, which results in the machine not discharging on command.

11. How does synchronized cardioversion differ from defibrillation?
Synchronized cardioversion is a timed discharge of electricity that occurs at the peak of the R wave in the ventricular complex, thus preventing the dangerous R-on-T phenomenon which can precipitate lethal ventricular dysrhythmia. In defibrillation, the discharge occurs as soon as the discharge buttons are depressed, and thus it is not timed with the cardiac cycle.

Synchronized cardioversion is reserved for patients with unstable tachycardia with a pulse, while defibrillation is used for patients with ventricular dysrhythmias without a pulse. Common rhythms responsive to synchronized cardioversion include unstable VT, paroxysmal supraventricular tachycardia, supraventricular tachycardia with aberrancy, atrial flutter, and uncontrolled atrial fibrillation.

12. Describe the procedure of synchronized cardioversion.
1. Energy levels for supraventricular dysrhythmias begin at 50 J, with doubling of the energy level on successive attempts. For VT, start with 100 J, then 200, 300, and 360 if rhythm is refractory to lower levels.
2. The patient may be conscious with unstable tachycardias. If so, consider IV sedation or anesthesia support if immediately available.
3. The defibrillator/cardioverter monitor leads must be attached to the patient and display a rhythm with prominent R waves of greater amplitude than T waves.
4. The "synch" button must be on. Assess proper function by visualizing the heavy green line "synch" markers superimposed on every R wave marching across the monitor.
5. After "all clear," keep the discharge buttons depressed until the discharge is appreciated. It may take a few seconds, unlike the immediate discharge of defibrillation.
6. The "synch" mode must be reset after each discharge. Most machines default to the unsynchronized defibrillation mode after each discharge.

13. What signs indicate that the need for tracheal intubation is imminent in patients with an asthmatic crisis?
Findings of obtundation
Profuse diaphoresis
Poor muscle tone
Findings of severe agitation, confusion, and fighting against the oxygen mask
Clearly rising PCO_2

14. What are the common signs and symptoms of transient ischemic attack (TIA) and stroke?
Unilateral paralysis   Unilateral numbness
Language disturbance   Monocular blindness
Vertigo   Ataxia

15. When is transcutaneous pacing used in treating cardiac arrest?
Hemodynamically unstable bradycardia ($<$ 50 bpm)
Mobitz type II second-degree AV block
Third-degree heart block
Bilateral bundle branch block (BBB)
Left anterior fascicular block
Newly acquired or age-indeterminate left BBB

Right or left BBB and first-degree AV block

Initial treatment with atropine is indicated only when serious signs and symptoms are related to the bradycardia. Evidence does not support routine use of transcutaneous pacing for asystole.

16. What is pulseless electrical activity (PEA)?

PEA is the absence of pulse and blood pressure in a patient with a viable electrical rhythm. It was formerly known as **electromechanical dissociation.** It is a very disconcerting scenario with a very high mortality (90–100%) unless its etiology can be quickly ascertained and corrected. The differential diagnosis includes:

Cardiac tamponade	Hypoxia	Hyper-/hypokalemia
Massive pulmonary embolism	Hypovolemia	Tension pneumothorax
Acidosis	Hypothermia	Massive acute myocardial infarction

Drug overdose (tricyclic antidepressants, beta-blockers, calcium channel blockers)

17. What are the requirements for confirmation of tracheal tube placement

Primary confirmation: Once a tracheal tube is placed, it is first verified by physical examination techniques. With the first breath delivered by the bag-valve unit:

1. Listen over the stomach and observe the chest wall for movement. If you hear gurgling, you have intubated the esophagus.

2. Reattempt intubation after reoxygenating the victim (15–30 sec with 100% oxygen).

3. If the chest wall rises and no stomach gurgling is heard, listen to the lung fields in the left and right anterior and left and right midaxillary regions. Then listen over the stomach again. Stop ventilating if you are unsure.

4. Use the laryngoscope to observe the tube passing through the vocal cords if you are still unsure.

5. If the placement is correct, reconfirm the tube mark at the front teeth.

6. Secure the tube with a commercial device.

7. Once secured, insert a bite block, oropharyngeal airway, or both, to prevent the patient from occluding the airway.

Secondary confirmation: A new recommendation from Guidelines 2000 (see references) is secondary confirmation by nonphysical examination techniques such as esophageal detector devices, qualitative end-tidal CO_2 indicators, and quantitative end-tidal CO_2 capnographic and capnometric devices. These devices are classified as IIa for patients not in full cardiac arrest, but in cardiac arrest and low pulmonary flow they are rated IIb because they may falsely indicate esophageal intubation.

18. What are automated external defibrillators (AEDs)? How effective are they?

In most settings where AEDs have been introduced, there has been a significant increase in survival of out-of-hospital cardiac arrests. They are now part of BLS training. However, no benefit was shown in some systems where EMS response time is already rapid or when there were long arrest-to-shock times. Also, the other steps in the chain of survival (i.e., activating EMS and performing CPR) must be intact before implementation of a public access defibrillation program is successful. Randomized controlled trials are necessary to determine the full effectiveness of and best locations for AEDs.

19. What are the timeframes for and contraindications of fibrinolytics in treatment of stroke and acute MI?

Stroke: IV tissue plasminogen activator (tPA) is recommended, if it can be administered within 3 hours of the onset of stroke symptoms, and the patient does not have contraindications to fibrinolytic therapy. Contraindications include evidence of intracranial hemorrhage, suspicion of subarachnoid hemorrhage, previous stroke, serious head trauma, recent intracranial or intraspinal surgery, uncontrolled hypertension at time of treatment, seizure at stroke onset, active internal bleeding, current use of anticoagulants, and platelet count $<100,000/\mu l$.

Acute MI: Patients with ischemic pain and ST-segment elevation that present within 12 hours of pain onset receive the greatest benefit. However, fibrinolytic therapy is associated with an increased risk of hemorrhagic stroke. Risk factors for causing stroke include age > 65 years, weight < 70 kg, and initial hypertension. Contraindications include pain that is persistently present for >24 hrs, systolic BP >175 mmHg or diastolic BP >110 mmHg. Third-generation fibrinolytics have been developed that have longer plasma half-lives and show greater vessel patency at 90 minutes, but 30-day mortality rates are no different than those seen with tPA.

20. What resuscitation medications can be given down the endotracheal tube?

Think of the mnemonic **NAVEL**. Note that doses are generally 2–2.5 times those given by the IV route for adults. Be sure to dilute endotracheal drugs in 10 ml of normal saline.

Naloxone
Atropine
Valium
Epinephrine
Lidocaine

21. What is the preferred drug for the initial treatment of hemodynamically stable, wide-complex tachycardia?

Amiodarone and procainamide are now recommended ahead of lidocaine and adenosine for the initial treatment of hemodynamically stable, wide-complex tachycardia.

22. How long must a patient be resuscitated in refractory cardiac arrest?

- Asystole most often represents a confirmation of death. If pacing, medications, and intubation do not serve to restore the patient to a viable rhythm, termination of efforts should be considered.
- If a patient is responding to interventions, the resuscitation should continue.
- The probability of defibrillating a patient back to a viable rhythm decreases from 2–10% with each passing minute.
- Certain special circumstances, such as hypothermia and cold-water drowning, require prolonged resuscitation and special procedures, even in a seemingly refractory patient.

23. What is the initial management of unstable angina and non-Q-wave MI presenting with ST-segment depression?

These patients are treated with both heparin and aspirin. If they meet high-risk criteria (ST depression ≥ 1 mm, persistent symptoms, diffuse ECG abnormalities, depressed LV function, CHF, positive troponin or CK-MB) then glycoprotein IIb/IIIa inhibitors should be added. Patients without contraindications should receive beta-blockers. Recurrent angina may be treated with nitrates and then calcium channel blockers. Fibrinolytic therapy does *not* provide benefit for patients with ST-segment depression.

24. What is the success rate of CPR?

The likelihood of survival decreases with each minute of cardiac arrest. The longest period of time the brain can endure without blood flow at normal temperatures and with complete recovery is 4 to 5 minutes. Even the best CPR yields a cardiac output only 30% of normal. Basic CPR alone merely slows the decline of decreasing survivability. If a patient in VF or VT can be defibrillated immediately, as might occur in an ICU or cath lab, survival can be 70–80% or more. Generally, patients < 70 years old have a 16.2% survival until discharge, while those > 70 years old have a 12.4% chance, according to one large study. If cardiac arrest occurs during an acute illness in the hospital, survival to discharge declines to 10–17%. For aged patients with chronic illness, in-hospital cardiac arrest survival rates are 0–5%. Finally, of all survivors, half sustain permanent neurologic injury.

25. What about postresuscitation management?

The most important goal in the 30 minutes following successful resuscitation is to optimize oxygenation and perfusion to limit brain injury. Specific actions include:

- Perform ABGs, chest x-ray, EKG, and cardiac enzymes
- Support blood pressure to a normal or slightly elevated level with fluids or vasopressors
- Elevate the head of the bed to promote cerebral venous drainage
- Treat dysrhythmias
- Prevent/treat fever
- Diagnose the precipitating cause of the arrest and any complications of CPR.

CONTROVERSIES

26. Does high-dose epinephrine have a role?

Yes: In 1992, the American Heart Association adopted for ACLS an alternative to the 1 mg IV every 5 minutes dosage in certain algorithms, and instead offered moderate or high-dose epinephrine (0.1 mg/kg IV every 3–5 minutes) as Class IIb choices. Increased survival has been demonstrated in children. Physiologically, epinephrine increases systemic vascular resistance, perfusion pressure, coronary and cerebral blood flow, and electrical activity in the myocardium.

No: Although there is an increased rate of return of spontaneous circulation, initial high-dose epinephrine has never statistically been shown to improve survival until hospital discharge in adults. Retrospective studies suggest *worse* hemodynamic and neurological outcomes and toxic hyperadrenergic states in the postresuscitation period.

27. Do alternative CPR techniques have any role?

Several new techniques—such as interposed abdominal compression (IAC) CPR, active compression/decompression (ACD) CPR, and the CPR vest—have shown improved blood pressure in small studies with improved survival at 24 hours. These three techniques have received class IIb approval as alternatives for in-hospital resuscitation by adequately trained personnel. There are also many different automated/mechanical devices available, but most have limited use due to size, weight, cost, risk of sternal fractures, and instability on the chest. Studies with these devices have not demonstrated an improvement in survival, but they may be used in special circumstances when manual compressions are difficult, such as prolonged transport. Simultaneous ventilation-compression is inferior to standard CPR and not available for clinical use.

EXPECTATIONS FOR CPR. WHO LIVES?

Nationally accepted resuscitation courses offer few guidelines for terminating unsuccessful cardiopulmonary resuscitation (CPR). Data collected from 305 physicians and nurses in 1988/1989 and 401 physicians, nurses, and laypersons in 1998/1999 assessed their attitudes and expectations about adult and pediatric CPR. Respondents felt pediatric CPR efforts should continue longer than adult CPR efforts. Respondents in 1998/1999 felt CPR efforts did not need to continue as long as the 1988/1989 respondents believed they should. Laypersons thought that 52% of adult CPRs and 63% of pediatric CPRs were successful. Although lower than laypersons' expectations, healthcare professionals' expectations of CPR success were also unrealistic: physicians believed 24% of adult and 41% of pediatric CPRs were successful, and nurses believed 30% of adult and 45% of pediatric CPRs were successful. Healthcare professionals also indicated that they had a clearer idea of when to terminate adult CPR than pediatric CPR.

~Roberts, Am J Emerg Med 18:465, 2000

———————

BIBLIOGRAPHY

1. Anonymous: Part 1: Introduction to the International Guidelines 2000 for CPR and ECC: A consensus on science. Circulation 102(8 Suppl):I1–11, 2000.
2. Anonymous: Guidelines 2000 for Cardiopulmonary Resuscitation and Emergency Cardiovascular Care. Part 2: Ethical aspects of CPR and ECC. Circulation 102(8 Suppl):I12–21, 2000.
3. Chamnanvanakij S, Perlman JM: Outcome following cardiopulmonary resuscitation in the neonate requiring ventilatory assistance. Resuscitation 45:173–180, 2000.
4. Cummins RO, et al (eds): Guidelines 2000 for Cardiopulmonary Resuscitation and Emergency Cardiovascular Care: An international consensus on science. Circulation 102(8 supp): I1–I358, 2000.
5. Cummins RO, Hazinski MF: Guidelines based on fear of type II (false-negative) errors: Why we dropped the pulse check for lay rescuers. Circulation 102(8 supp): I377–I379, 2000.
6. Cummins RO, Hazinski MF: The most important changes in the international ECC and CPR guidelines 2000. Circulation 102(8 supp): I371–I376, 2000.
7. Donnelly P, Assar D, Lester C: A comparison of manikin CPR performance by lay persons trained in three variations of basic life support guidelines. Resuscitation 45:195–199, 2000.
8. Newman DH, Greenwald I, Callaway CW: Cardiac arrest and the role of thrombolytic agents. Ann Emerg Med 35(5): 472–480, 2000.
9. Roberts D, Hirschman D, Scheltema K: Adult and pediatric CPR: Attitudes and expectations of health professionals and laypersons. Am J Emerg Med 18:465–468, 2000.
10. Safar P: Advanced cerebral resuscitation: The cutting edge of ACLS aiming at maximal functional recovery. In Schwartz GR (ed): Principles and Practice of Emergency Medicine, 4th ed. Baltimore, Williams and Wilkins, 1999.
11. Stiell IG, et al: Improved out-of-hospital cardiac arrest survival through the inexpensive optimization of an existing defibrillation program: OPALS study phase II. JAMA 281(13): 1175–1181.
12. Thel MC, O'Connor CM: Cardiopulmonary resuscitation: Historical perspective to recent investigations. Am Heart J 137(1): 39–48, 1999.
13. Verstraete M: Third-generation thrombolytic drugs. Am J Med 109(1): 52–58, 2000.
14. Wik L: Automatic and manual mechanical external chest compressions devices for cardiopulmonary resuscitation. Resuscitation 47: 7–25, 2000.

86. SHOCK

Gregory J. Martin, M.D. and Matthew L. Robertson, M.D.

1. Define shock.

Shock is an acute, generalized, inadequate perfusion of tissues that ultimately leads to malfunction of the total body cellular metabolism. This metabolic dysfunction causes irreversible cell, tissue, and organ damage and can lead to death unless it is promptly and aggressively treated. Note that shock is *not* defined or diagnosed by blood pressure parameters.

2. What are the four categories of shock?

Hypovolemic shock, the most common, is caused by a decrease in circulating intravascular volume. Hemorrhagic shock is the most common subtype of hypovolemic shock.

Septic shock develops as a result of the systemic effects of infection. Such infections are usually bacterial or fungal.

Cardiogenic shock is caused by reduced cardiac output, leading to inadequate tissue perfusion.

Neurogenic shock is commonly seen in trauma and describes hypotension secondary to CNS injury and subsequent loss of autonomic vasomotor control.

3. List some of the causes of hypovolemic shock.

Hemorrhage, protracted diarrhea or vomiting, burns, trauma, pancreatitis, nephrotic syndrome, and malnutrition. In burns and trauma, fluid is lost to injured tissues. In nephrotic syndrome and malnutrition, there is a decrease of intravascular oncotic pressure with a relative loss of intravascular volume.

4. How does the body respond to hypovolemic shock?

A decrease of intravascular volume results in decreased venous return and a corresponding decrease in cardiac output. This total-body hypoperfusion results in a reflex neurohumoral response in an attempt to adapt to volume losses. Baroreceptors in the carotid and aorta respond to decreased cardiac output and systemic arterial pressure by increasing sympathetic tone. In addition to increasing heart rate and contractility, catecholamines cause vasoconstriction. The pituitary releases antidiuretic hormone, and the kidney, in response to inadequate perfusion, activates the renin-angiotensin axis. All of this is aimed at increasing intravascular volume and systemic arterial pressure. If the cause of hypovolemic shock is hemorrhagic, there will be a decrease in hemoglobin and oxygen-carrying capacity, an increase in anaerobic activity and lactic acid, and a decrease in pH.

5. How is hypovolemic shock diagnosed?

Diagnosis of shock should be obtained by a global assessment of tissue perfusion. The first signs of hypovolemic shock include tachycardia and orthostatic hypotension. As volume losses continue, altered mental status, cutaneous vasoconstriction, supine hypotension, and oliguria ensue. Depending on the degree of hypovolemic shock, the patient may complain of feeling cold or thirsty.

6. Based on this information, what simple steps should be taken to help confirm hypovolemic shock?

1. *Collect serial vital signs.* Is the patient tachycardic with a weak, thready pulse? Does the patient exhibit orthostatic or supine hypotension?

2. *Look at and feel the skin.* Is it cold, clammy, and pale? Are subcutaneous veins visible? Is capillary refill delayed?

3. *Monitor urine output by inserting a Foley catheter.* Normal urine output and urine osmolality is > 0.5 ml/kg/hr and 500–850 mosm/kg, respectively.

4. *Look for alterations in mental status.* Is the patient restless, confused, agitated, obtunded, or even comatose?

7. Summarize the different degrees of severity of hypovolemic shock.

Clinical Classification of Hypovolemic Shock

SEVERITY OF HYPOVOLEMIA	DEFICIT OF BLOOD VOLUME	PATHOPHYSIOLOGY	MANIFESTATIONS
Mild	$< 20\%$	Decreased perfusion of nonvital tissues (skin, fat, skeletal muscle) Compensatory adrenergic vasoconstriction	Pale, cool, clammy skin Postural changes in BP and pulse Patient complains of feeling cold Delayed capillary refill Concentrated urine
Moderate	20–40%	Decreased perfusion of vital tissues (kidney, gastrointestinal)	Decreased urine output, oliguria Patient complains of thirst Occasionally, low BP and pulse while supine
Severe	$> 40\%$	Decreased perfusion of brain and heart	Restless, agitated, confused, obtunded, or "drunk" Low BP Tachypnea Cardiac arrest

BP = blood pressure
Adapted from Holcroft JW, Wisner DH, Ways LW: *Current Surgical Diagnosis and Treatment.* Norwalk, CT, Appleton & Lange, 1994, p 187, with permission.

8. In general, how should you go about treating hypovolemic shock?
Remember the **ABCs** of basic life support—Airway, Breathing, Circulation. With hypovolemic shock, the clinician should remember **ABCIC**—Airway, Breathing, Circulation, and Intravenous Crystalloid.

9. Summarize the steps taken in ABCIC.
A Establish an airway and maintain its patency.
B Ensure adequate ventilation via supplemental oxygen or bag-valve mask if necessary.
C Control external hemorrhage by direct pressure.
IC Establish two large-gauge intravenous catheters for sufficient fluid resuscitation. Use crystalloid solution that approximates the sodium concentration of plasma (e.g., lactated Ringer's) for initial resuscitation. At the same time, draw blood for type and cross-match.

10. How much crystalloid should be used?
The severity of shock determines the rate and amount of fluid given. In general, 2 L of crystalloid should be rapidly infused, followed by clinical reassessment. Since crystalloid solutions redistribute into the extravascular space, they must be infused in a 3:1 ratio based on suspected blood losses. For example, a 70-kg man with a 20% blood loss (1000 ml) requires 3000 ml of initial crystalloid resuscitation.

11. Should blood or blood products be used to correct hypovolemic shock?
Usually no, unless hypovolemic shock is complicated by coagulopathy or persistent hemorrhage. Even during hemorrhage, blood should be withheld until bleeding is controlled to mini-

562   Shock

mize the loss of transfused blood cells. However, patients who remain unstable after the initial
crystalloid infusion present an exception.

12. How much blood should be given to hemorrhagic shock victims?
In young patients with normal cardiovascular function, the hematocrit should be raised into
the mid 20s. In older patients, the hematocrit should be brought into the low to mid 30s, depending on their state of health.

13. What is septic shock?
Septic shock develops as a result of the systemic effects of **infection.** It is the second most
common type of shock in surgical patients, with overall mortality exceeding 30%.

14. What are the two stages of septic shock?
Early or "warm," and late or "cold."

15. Describe the clinical features of the two stages of septic shock.
Patients in **early or "warm" septic shock** are hypotensive but normovolemic. They have a
normal pulse pressure, stroke volume, and normal to high cardiac output. Since patients are va-
sodilated with low systemic vascular resistance, their skin is warm, flushed, and dry. Marked
tachycardia and tachypnea is often present. Oxygen delivery is good, but oxygen consumption is
reduced. Arterial blood gases indicate a moderate respiratory alkalosis with a comparatively mild
change in bicarbonate.
Late or "cold" septic shock results from impaired organ function, namely renal and pulmonary systems. Intravascular volume is depleted secondary to increased capillary permeability
and cellular dysfunction. The cardiac index (a measure of cardiac output relative to body surface
area) falls below normal. Bicarbonate levels decrease, lactate levels increase, and pH decreases.
Vasoconstriction occurs in response to depleted intravascular volume and the skin becomes cold,
clammy, and cyanotic. The patient frequently becomes lethargic and confused. Death often ensues.

16. What are the primary pathogens responsible for septic shock?
Gram-negative organisms from the genitourinary system are the most common etiologic
agents of septic shock. These include, but are not limited to, *Pseudomonas aeruginosa, Klebsiella,
Serratia,* and *Bacteroides.* Endotoxin is responsible for inducing an inflammatory cascade with
tumor necrosis factor (TNF) and interleukin-1 (IL-1) as critical mediators. These agents result in
the ultimate cellular and chemical dysfunction observed in septic shock.

17. How do you treat a patient who has septic shock?
Early recognition and treatment of infection *before* the onset of shock is crucial. However,
once septic shock presents clinically, the mainstay of treatment is **control of infection.** This is accomplished by early identification of the source accompanied by surgical debridement or
drainage. Appropriate and specific antibiotic therapy is initiated. Adjunctive measures may include fluid replacement, vasopressors, inotropes, and blood products if necessary. Treating septic shock is a complex process, and patients often die despite the best medical management.

18. Define cardiogenic shock.
Cardiogenic shock is hypoperfusion of critical organs due to pump failure. More specifically,
cardiogenic shock occurs when cardiac output declines to a point where cardiac index is < 1.8
(normal is 2.8–4.2).

**19. Describe the pathophysiology of cardiogenic shock. How does it differ from congestive
heart failure and other kinds of shock?**
In congestive heart failure, there is normal to increased systemic arterial pressure. Cardiogenic shock results in hypotension, but unlike hypovolemic shock, patients can be normovolemic.

As the cardiac index falls, the body attempts to compensate by reflexively increasing sympathetic tone, thus increasing systemic vascular resistance and decreasing organ perfusion. In essence, this only aggravates the problem by increasing the demand on an already failing heart. Vasodilation in patients with neurogenic and early septic shock produces warm extremities. In cardiogenic shock, systemic vascular resistance is increased, producing cool extremities. Hypovolemic shock is much more common than cardiogenic shock in surgical patients, and the former is not the result of an acute, major insult to cardiac function.

20. What are the etiologies of cardiogenic shock?
Acute myocardial infarction is most common cause of cardiogenic shock. Other etiologies include valvular heart disease, arrythmia, cardiomyopathy, and cardiac contusion.

21. What is the main goal in the treatment of cardiogenic shock?
To improve cardiac function without significantly increasing the metabolic demands of the heart. This includes vigilant volume management, inotropes, vasodilators, and possibly mechanical support.

22. Describe some of the defining characteristics of neurogenic shock.
Neurogenic shock is defined as hypotension secondary loss of autonomic vasomotor control. This type of shock most commonly results from trauma. Cardiac output and oxygen delivery are normal or possibly elevated. Acid-base status, renal function indices, and hemoglobin levels are usually unaffected.

23. How does the prognosis differ for the various categories of shock?
Prognosis varies depending on the type of shock, its duration, the patient's age, and other associated injuries. For example, 80% of young healthy patients survive **hypovolemic shock** in the absence of other life-threatening injuries. However, **cardiogenic** and **septic shock** have mortality rates exceeding 70% when associated with multiple organ system failure. Prognosis for **neurogenic shock** depends on the severity of the trauma.

24. Outline the common signs and symptoms that distinguish the four categories of shock.

A Comparison of the Common Clinical Manifestations in the Different Categories of Shock

	HYPOVOLEMIC	SEPTIC	CARDIOGENIC	NEUROGENIC
Vascular resistance	↑	↓ (early) ↑ (late)	↑	↓
Heart rate	↑	↑	↑	↓
Respiratory rate	↑			Variable
Skin changes	Cold, clammy	Warm, flushed (early) Cold, clammy (late)	Cold, clammy	Warm
Neck veins	Flat	Flat (late)	Distended	Flat
Acid-base	Metabolic acidosis	Respiratory alkalosis (early) Metabolic acidosis (late)	Metabolic acidosis	Normal
Cardiac index	↓	Normal to ↑ (early) ↓ (late)	↓	Variable

25. A 60-year-old woman underwent endoscopic and open surgery for chronic sinusitis. There was no evidence of infection at the time of surgical debridement. Postoperatively she was placed on cephalexin and prednisone, and packing was removed on postop day 5. Three weeks later, the patient returned with a sudden onset of sore throat, fever, vomiting, and

abdominal rash. She experienced a syncopal episode in the ED. After hospital admission for possible sepsis, CT scan revealed clouding of the sinuses. Sinus cultures grew *Staphylococcus aureus*. What is the diagnosis?

Toxic shock syndrome. Toxic shock has been reported in several cases of nasal or sinus surgery. The normal nose is often colonized with *S. aureus*. With surgery, the bacteria have access to traumatized mucosa. Bacterial growth is then supported by postoperative packing, which establishes a closed environment in which toxins may accumulate.

Toxic shock is a potentially life-threatening syndrome caused by the toxins of *S. aureus*. Fatality rates as high as 10% have been reported. Toxic shock syndrome has four major disease characteristics:

- Fever $> 38.9°C$ (102°F)
- Diffuse macular rash
- Skin desquamation of the palms and soles occurring 1–2 weeks after the onset of illness
- Hypotension.

CONTROVERSIES

26. Which fluids should be administered when resuscitating a shock victim?

While fluid resuscitation remains the mainstay of treatment for hypovolemic shock, some disagree about what type of solution should be administered. For example, some still consider albumin-containing solutions to be good volume-expanders for hypovolemic shock. However, recent studies suggest that albumin solutions only transiently increase intravascular volume and are not justified in the treatment of hypovolemic shock. Crystalloids are balanced salt solutions and are the preferred treatment to raise intravascular volume in hypovolemic shock. The one colloid exception is red cells, which are large enough to remain in the intravascular space. In addition, red cells increase the amount of hemoglobin available. Artificial blood and plasma substitutes are also on the horizon as alternatives.

27. Name some controversial drugs which can be used in shock management.

Drugs available for the treatment of shock include inotropes, vasodilators, antibiotics, diuretics, and chronotropic agents. Each drug class provides both potential benefits and detrimental side effects. For example, inotropes such as dopamine and dobutamine can improve cardiac output in cardiogenic shock. However, they also place mechanical strain on the heart, increase vasoconstriction, and can increase heart rate sharply. Therefore, inotropes should be used cautiously and only in closely monitored ICU patients. Norepinepherine, an inotrope and vasoconstrictor, can be used in the late stages of septic shock to raise blood pressure and systemic vascular resistance. However, the increase in vascular resistance can also result in necrosis of the ears and fingertips.

TOXIC SHOCK SYNDROME WITH NECROTIZING FASCIITIS

Streptococcal toxic shock syndrome (strep TSS) with associated necrotizing fasciitis is a rapidly progressive process that kills 30–60% of patients in 72–96 hours. Violaceous bullae, hypotension, fever, and evidence of organ failure are late clinical manifestations. The challenge to clinicians is to make an early diagnosis and to intervene with aggressive fluid replacement, emergent surgical debridement, and general supportive measures. Superantigens such as pyrogenic exotoxin A interact with monocytes and T lymphocytes in unique ways, resulting in T-cell proliferation and watershed production of monokines (e.g., tumor necrosis factor-α, interleukin 1, interleukin 6), and lymphokines (e.g., TNF-β, interleukin 2, and gamma-interferon). Penicillin, though efficacious in mild *Streptococcus pyogenes* infection, is less effective in severe infections because of its short post-antibiotic effect, inoculum effect, and reduced activity against stationary-phase organisms. Emerging treatments for strep TSS include clindamycin and intravenous gamma-globulin.

~Stevens, Ann Rev Med 51:271, 2000

BIBLIOGRAPHY

1. Dabrowski GP, Steinberg SM, Ferrara JJ, et al: A critical assessment of endpoints of shock resuscitation. Surg Clin North Am 80:825–844, 2000.
2. Edwards S: Hypovolaemia: Pathophysiology and management options. Nurs Crit Care 3:73–82, 1998.
3. Hajjeh RA, Reingold A, Weil A, et al: Toxic shock syndrome in the United States: Surveillance update, 1979–1996. Emerg Inf Dis 5:807–810, 1999.
4. Harken AH: Shock. In Harken AH (ed): Surgical Secrets, 4th ed. Philadelphia, Hanley & Belfus, 2000.
5. Holliday MA: Extracellular fluid and its proteins: Dehydration, shock, and recovery. Pediatr Nephrol 13:989–995, 1999.
6. Holm C: Resuscitation in shock associated with burns. Tradition or evidence-based medicine? Resuscitation 44:157–164, 2000.
7. Ince C, Sinaasappel M: Microcirculatory oxygenation and shunting in sepsis and shock. Crit Care Med 27:1369–1377, 1999.
8. McGee S, Abernethy WB, Simel DL: Is this patient hypovolemic? JAMA 281:1022–9, 1999.
9. Merli GJ, Weitz HH: Medical Management of the Surgical Patient. Philadelphia, W. B. Saunders, 1998.
10. Mikhail J: Resuscitation endpoints in trauma. AACN Clin Iss 10:10–21, 1999.
11. Rozenfeld V, Cheng JW: The role of vasopressin in the treatment of vasodilation in shock states. Ann Pharm 34:250–4, 2000.
12. Scalea HS: Resuscitation in the new millennium. Surg Clin North Am 79:1259–67, 1999.
13. Singhi S: Management of shock. Indian Peds 36:265–88, 1999.
14. Stevens DL: Streptococcal toxic shock syndrome associated with necrotizing fasciitis. Ann Rev Med 51:271–88, 2000.
15. Wheeler DS, Kiefer ML, Poss WB: Pediatric emergency preparedness in the office. Am Fam Phys 61:3333–42, 2000.

87. FEVER IN THE CRITICAL CARE PATIENT

John W. Hollingsworth II, M.D. and Joseph A. Govert, M.D.

1. Why are we concerned with fever?

Fever is a common complaint of patients who are seeking medical care. The causes of fever are extensive and can range from a simple problem requiring reassurance to a problem necessitating ICU admission. Fever occurs in 29–36% of medical inpatients. Medical inpatients in whom fever develops have a 13% mortality rate, while those who remain afebrile have a 3% mortality rate.

2. How is fever defined?

Fever is a symptom. A "set-point" increase in the hypothalamic thermoregulatory center causes an elevation of the body temperature above the normal circadian variation. Elevated temperature accompanies many illnesses and is a valuable marker of disease activity. Normal body temperature is 37°C (98.6°F) and has a normal circadian variation of 0.5–1.0°C, with the peak in the late afternoon. Quantitatively, the *Society of Critical Care Medicine* defines fever in the ICU as a temperature > 38.3°C (≥101°F). In humans, fever rarely exceeds 41.1°C.

3. How does hyperthermia differ from fever?

Fever must be distinguished from hyperthermia, which is an elevation in temperature that is not associated with a change in the hypothalamic thermoregulatory set-point. Hyperthermia usually refers to a special group of critical illnesses characterized by excessive heat production, decrease in heat dissipation, and loss of thermoregulation. In contrast, most fevers are due to inflammatory processes, in which the rise in body temperature is caused by circulating pyrogens. Hyperthermia has a higher risk of mortality and must be treated more aggressively. Regardless of the cause, temperature > 41.1°C can result in serious organ dysfunction and injury, especially to the liver, kidneys, and brain.

4. What causes hyperthermia?

There are many etiologies of hyperthermia. It could be due to an **increased heat production,** as seen in exercise-induced hyperthermia, thyrotoxicosis, malignant hyperthermia, pheochromocytoma, and neuroleptic malignant syndrome. It may also be due to a **decreased heat loss,** as seen with heat stroke, drug-induced fever, autonomic dysfunction, dehydration, occlusive dressing, and excessive clothing. **Hypothalamic disorders,** such as infections (granulomatous disease), tumors, trauma, vascular accidents, and drug-induced disorders (i.e., phenothiazine toxicity), may also result in hyperthermia.

5. What are the differences between exogenous and endogenous pyrogens?

Pyrogens are substances that cause fever. **Exogenous pyrogens** are microbes, microbial products, or toxins. Gram-negative bacteria have lipopolysaccharide endotoxins in their outer membrane, while gram-positive bacteria have lipoteichoic acid, peptidoglycans, various exotoxins, and enterotoxins which induce fever. Exogenous pyrogens cause fever by inducing the release of endogenous pyrogens.

Endogenous pyrogens include interleukin-1, TNF-α, interleukin-6, and interferon-α (i.e., cytokines). They are produced by many cells and typically act locally, initiating autocrine and paracrine effects, but also bind in the preoptic region of the anterior hypothalmus.

5. How does your body control thermoregulation and cause fever?

Endogenous pyrogens (EP) are produced, released into the circulation, reach the anterior hypothalamus via the arterial system, and penetrate the blood-brain barrier in the region of the organum vasculosum laminae terminalis. This penetration stimulates the release of arachidonic acid from the endothelial lining of this specialized cluster of neurons. The arachidonic acid is rapidly metabolized into prostaglandin E2. Prostaglandin modulates the hypothalamic thermoregulatory centers by increasing cAMP levels, which subsequently increase the normal thermic set-point. Mediated by sympathetic efferents, this alteration induces peripheral vasoconstriction, shivering, and behavioral changes such as posturing and seeking warm environments. This process continues until the warmer blood reaches the hypothalamus and matches the new set-point, or until the concentration of EP falls or EP-induced prostaglandin synthesis is blocked by antipyretics.

7. Is fever protective?

Despite extensive study into the pathophysiology of fever, it remains unclear whether fever is a defense mechanism that enhances survival or a harmful response that accompanies injury or stress. The beneficial role of fever during infection has not been established, but is strongly speculated. There are three basic protective mechanisms of fever: (1) The growth and virulence of several bacteria species are impaired by increases in temperature (e.g., pneumococcus), while other organisms cannot survive with fever (e.g., gonococcus); (2) fever causes increased phagocytic and bactericidal polymorphonuclear leukocyte activity and increased cytotoxic lymphocytic activity; (3) because of the inhibition of RNA, DNA, and protein synthesis, fever has adverse effects on many types of tumor cells.

Limited human clinical studies support the benefit of fever. A small retrospective study of patients with gram-negative bacteremia reported a positive correlation between maximum temperature on the day of bacteremia and survival. Furthermore, in patients with subacute bacterial peritonitis, it has been reported that a temperature > 38°C increased survival.

8. How does fever affect normal physiology?

Fever increases metabolism. Each 1°C increase results in a 10–13% increase in oxygen consumption. Increased metabolic demands may place a burden on the cardiovascular system by increasing cardiac output, even precipitating **cardiac failure** or **ischemia.** Increased metabolic demands and increased muscle catabolism can lead to a **negative nitrogen balance** and **loss of body weight. Caloric requirements** are increased in a febrile patient. There is a 10–15% increase in **insensible water loss** for each 1°C elevation (8% per °F). This loss often requires an additional 500 ml or more of salt-free water per day in febrile patients. Fever decreases **mental acuity,** leading to delirium and stupor. Some febrile children may develop generalized **seizures.**

9. When do you treat a fever?

Treatment should be reserved for patients with discomfort or patients at high risk of complications. High-risk patients include children at risk of febrile seizures, pregnant women, patients with cardiac or pulmonary insufficiency, and patients with impaired cerebral function. Although they can improve patient comfort, antipyretics are often used without a therapeutic rationale. Hyperpyrexia (fever ≥ 41°C) is clearly an exception, as both antipyretics and physical cooling are necessary.

10. What do you use to treat a fever?

Antipyretics include nonsteroidal anti-inflammatory drugs (NSAIDs), acetaminophen, and glucocorticoids. There are also some endogenous antipyretics, including arginine vasopressin, adrenocorticotropin, α-melanocyte-stimulating hormone, and cortisol-releasing hormone. **NSAIDs** are antipyretic, analgesic, and anti-inflammatory. They act both centrally and peripherally by inhibiting cyclooxygenase (prostaglandin synthetase). Side effects include GI irritation, reversible inhibition of platelet aggregation, transaminase elevations, and potential renal toxicity. **Aspirin** causes irreversible inhibition of platelet aggregation and should be avoided in children because of the risk of Reye's syndrome. **Acetaminophen** acts centrally as an antipyretic and is also an analgesic. It is potentially hepatotoxic and should be used carefully in patients with hepatic insufficiency. **Glucocorticoids** are potent antipyretics with potent immunosuppressive and antiphagocytic effects. This limits their use to febrile states in which inflammation is the major pathogenic factor (e.g., bacterial meningitis, pericarditis, vasculitis).

11. How do you treat hyperthermia?

Once again, fever must be distinguished from hyperthermia. If the patient has hyperthermia, defined as an increase in core temperature without an increase in the hypothalamic set-point, treatment is definitely indicated. Heat stroke and malignant hyperthermia are medical emergencies. Treatment with conventional antipyretics (aspirin, NSAIDs, steroids) is *not* effective, and hyperthermia must be treated by other means. Hypothermic (cooling) blankets, though requiring careful monitoring, may be helpful. However, they should be discontinued when the temperature drops below 39°C. Ice baths are reserved for extreme cases of hyperthermia.

12. How do you begin an evaluation of fever in the ICU?

The evaluation of the febrile ICU patient requires a **meticulous** and **thoughtful** approach to ensure that the cause of the fever is identified accurately and treated appropriately. The causes of fever can be broadly divided into two categories, **infectious** and **noninfectious**. Elicit a thorough history, and perform a complete physical exam. Direct your initial investigation toward identifying an infectious etiology. Blood cultures should be preformed in all ICU patients with new fever. Other laboratory studies may include; a complete blood count with differential, sputum Gram stain and culture, urinalysis, blood chemistries, and stool studies. Pertinent radiologic studies may include chest x-ray, CT, or ultrasound. *A haphazard approach to the febrile patient in the ICU is very inefficient and expensive.* Diagnostic modalities should be chosen according to each individual patient. If no source of infection can be found, consider noninfectious causes.

13. Why draw two sets of blood cultures?

Primarily two reasons: to assist in interpretation of a possibly contaminated culture, and to increase the sensitivity of the test. Blood cultures are affected by many factors, including: type of infection, skin preparation, timing of draw, procurement techniques, volume of blood obtained, and number of cultures. The optimal time to obtain blood cultures is when the magnitude of microorganisms is the greatest in the bloodstream. This has been shown in experimental animals to occur 1–2 hours *before* the onset of fever or chills. Therefore, cultures should be drawn as soon as symptoms occur.

Sensitivity of a single blood cuture is 80–92%, while sensitivity of two sets of cultures is 89–99% (Mylotte, 2000). The incidence of blood culture contamination is 2% in a single study. Use clinical judgement in evaluating positive blood cultures. Multiple positive cultures usually represent pathogens. Organisms such as *Escherichia coli, Streptococcus, Staphylococcus aureus,* and *Candida* usually represent pathogens, while organisms such as diptheriods and *Bacillus* species more frequently represent contamination.

14. What are common noninfectious etiologies of fever in the ICU?

Some common causes of noninfectious fever are neoplasias, CNS disease, myocardial infarction, drug reactions, procedures, drug withdrawal, transfusions, pancreatitis, aspiration pneumonitis, DVT, subarachnoid, and gastrointestinal hemorrhage.

15. Which drugs can cause fever?

Drug fever, largely a diagnosis of exclusion, is relatively uncommon. Drugs have been documented to be the cause of 2–6% of fevers on internal medicine services. Drug fever is most likely an immunologic phenomenon in which the formation of immune complexes stimulates the release of endogenous pyrogen. Antibiotics, particularly b-lactams, are the class of drugs most commonly associated with fever. α-Methyldopa, quinidine, procainamide, and diphenylhydantoin can cause fever.

16. Can procedures cause fever in the absence of infection?

Yes. Repeated intramuscular injections can cause fever. This is especially important to remember in the ICU setting, where patients undergo many different procedures. Bronchoscopy causes fever in the absence of infection in up to 10% of patients undergoing bronchoalveolar lavage.

17. What is the most common etiology of fever in the ICU?

Infection is the most common cause of fever. There are several major sources of nosocomial infections, including pneumonia, bacteremia, and catheter-related infection. Other sources include *Clostridium difficile* colitis, abdominal sepsis, and wound infections.

In the 1980s, urinary tract infections accounted for 25–50% of all ICU infections. Currently it is thought that the majority of these cases represent asymptomatic bacturia or colonization, which is common with indwelling urinary catheters. Criteria have not been developed to differentiate urinary colonization from infection. Clearly, patients with recent urinary tract manipulation/surgery, nephrolithiasis, or urinary tract obstruction should be treated in the presence of bacteruria.

Sinusitis occurs in the critically ill patient and is usually associated with nasal intubation or nasogastric tubes. Although not all agree that sinusitis causes fever or systemic signs of infection, it is best treated by removal of nasal tubes, drainage of sinuses, and usually broad-spectrum antibiotics.

Many factors influence the risk of nosocomial infection in ICU patients, including underlying diseases, severity of illness, type of ICU, duration of ICU stay, and use of invasive devices and procedures.

18. On postop day 3 after a modified radical neck dissection, a 62-year-old man has a temperature of 38.8°C. He appears diaphoretic and pale, but is alert. A nasogastric tube, endotracheal tube, indwelling urinary catheter, and a central venous catheter are in place. There is mild erythema at the site of the central catheter, but no drainage. The neck incisions have mild serosanguineous drainage without swelling, warmth, or tenderness. Chest exam reveals diffuse crackles and decreased breath sounds over the right lower lobe. Over the past 24 hours, the patient has required increased ventilator support and has had increased endotracheal secretions. What is the cause of this patient's fever?

Ventilator-associated pneumonia (VAP) is the most likely diagnosis. This diagnosis refers to a bacterial pneumonia developing in patients with acute respiratory failure who have received mechanical ventilation for at least 48 hours. The diagnosis is strongly suggested by fever, changes on physical exam and chest radiographs, leukocytosis, purulent tracheobronchial secretions, and positive tracheal aspirate on Gram stain and culture. VAP has been reported in approximately 25% of ventilated patients and has a high mortality.

Definitive diagnosis of VAP is difficult. Invasive tests, such as bronchoscopy with bronchoalveolar lavage or protected specimen brush, are often used to define VAP. The impact of bronchoscopy on patient outcomes remains controversial. The most important factor affecting outcome is early initiation of appropriate antibiotic coverage. Definitive identification of pathogens does allow narrowing of antibiotic coverage and may result in cost savings as well as reduced selection of resistant organisms.

19. Do intravascular lines cause fever?

Intravascular devices are well-documented causes of sepsis, and therefore attention should be focused on the presence of phlebitis and infection of IV lines. Risk factors for such infections include the degree of sterile technique when the IV was inserted, endothelial damage produced during insertion of large-bore needles, length of time the line is left in place, frequent manipulation of catheter, use of thrombogenic catheter material, and use of occlusive transparent plastic dressing. Nosocomial septicemia in patients with intravascular devices is usually caused by *S. aureus,* coagulase-negative *Staphylococcus,* aerobic gram-negative bacilli, or enterococci. Diagnosis generally is based on clinical suspicion and blood cultures.

20. What is a fever of unknown origin (FUO)?

FUO is defined as a documented fever > 38.3°C (101°F) that lasts 3 weeks and defies diagnosis after 1 week of intensive medical investigation. Recently, however, this definition has been challenged with the advent of nosocomial FUO and AIDS FUO.

21. List the most common etiologies of FUO.

Infectious (39%)	**Neoplastic** (17%)	**Miscellaneous** (16%)	**Collagen/vascular** (18%)
Endocarditis	Lymphoma/leukemia	Pulmonary embolus	Systemic lupus
Abdominal abscess	Carcinoma	Sarcoidosis	erythematous
Hepatobiliary	Miscellaneous	Hypersensitivity	Rheumatoid arthritis
Mycobacterial			Miscellaneous
Brucellosis			
Bone/joint			
Meningitis, bacterial			
Viral disease			
Miscellaneous			

22. What are the most common causes of postoperative fever? When would you expect each to occur?

To remember the traditional most common causes of postoperative fever, think of the 5 W's:

Wind—*pulmonary atelectasis/pneumonia.* This condition is thought (by some) to cause fever within the first 48 hours postoperatively. Important exceptions include soft tissue infection, leakage of bowel anastomosis, and aspiration pneumonia.

Water—*urinary tract infections.* UTIs are highly suspected on postop days 2–3.

Wound—*an incision infection,* commonly occurring around postop days 3–5. Inspect and palpate the wound edges for evidence of inflammation or drainage. Culture any drainage. Treatment includes facilitating drainage, surgical debridement, and antibiotics.

Walk—*deep venous thrombosis (DVT) or intravascular lines.* Fever associated with infection of intravascular devices should be suspected around postop days 3–4. Inspect for thrombophlebitis and suppurative phlebitis. *S. aureus* or *Staphylococcus epidermidis* are the most common pathogens. Fever secondary to DVT or pulmonary embolism should be considered around postop days 7–10, but can occur anytime.

Wonder drugs—*drug-induced fever.* These can cause fever at any time and are usually a diagnosis of exclusion.

CONTROVERSY

23. Can atelectasis cause postoperative fever?

Many surgical textbooks state that atelectasis is the usual cause of postoperative fever in the first 48 hours, but a number of physicians challenge this theory. It may be assumed that, because pulmonary atelectasis is common postoperatively, it is the cause of fever, but there is no data to support this assumption. In fact, there is evidence that fever occurring in patients with atelectasis indicates concurrent pulmonary infection.

Two groups of investigators induced atelectasis in animals, and neither group was able to demonstrate the occurrence of fever with atelectasis unless there was coexisting pulmonary infection. Two more recent prospective clinical studies have also weakened the link between atelectasis and postop fever. The first study included 100 patients scheduled for elective abdominal surgery: 31% developed atelectasis, and 18% developed fever. Of those who had a fever, 4 patients had atelectasis and 14 did not. There was no significant association between atelectasis and fever.

Another, more recent study looked at 100 postop cardiac surgery patients. In this group, the daily incidence of atelectasis increased from 43 to 69 to 79%. However, the incidence of fever (> 38°C) fell from 37 to 21 to 17%. When fever was defined as temperature $\geq$ 38.5°C, the daily incidence fell from 14 to 3 to 1%. Using chi-squared analysis, no association could be found between fever and atelectasis.

Furthermore, fever does not occur in experimental animals when atelectasis is induced by ligation of a mainstem bronchus. We conclude that atelectasis probably does *not* cause fever in the absence of pulmonary infection.

BIBLIOGRAPHY

1. Arnow P: Fever of unknown origin. Lancet 350: 575–580, 1997.
2. Durack DT: Fever of unknown origin—reexamined and redefined. Curr Clin Topics Infect Dis 11:35–51, 1991.
3. Engoren M: Lack of association between atelectasis and fever. Chest 107:81–84, 1995.
4. Gerberding, J., National Nosocomial Infections Surveillance (NNIS) System Report, Data Summary from January 1990-May 1999. AJIC 1999; 27:520–32.
5. Marik P: Fever in the ICU. Chest, 117:855–864, 2000.
6. Meduri GU: Diagnosis and differential diagnosis of ventilator associated pneumonia. Clin Chest Med 16:61–93, 1995.
7. Mylotte JM: Blood Cultures: Clinical aspects and controversies. Eur J Clin Microbiol Infect Dis 19:157–163, 2000.
8. O'Grady N: Practice guidelines for evaluating new fever in critically ill adult patients. Clin Infect Dis 26: 1042–59, 1998.
9. Perez-Aispuro I, et al: A reconsideration of postoperative fever due to pulmonary atelectasis. Gac Med Mex 127:27–30, 1991.
10. Wallace W: New epidemiology for postoperative nosocomial infections. Am Surg 66:874–878, 2000.

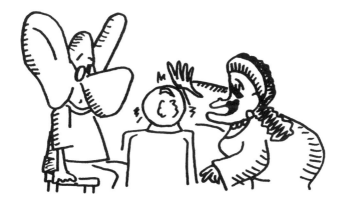

"Roy was horrified to learn that in a previous life he had been an EAR & NOSE specialist."

Jim Gough

88. TELEMEDICINE IN OTOLARYNGOLOGY

Arlen D. Meyers, M.D., MBA and Bruce W. Jafek, M.D., FACS, FRSM

1. Define telemedicine.

Telemedicine is the use of advanced telecommunications technologies to exchange health information and provide healthcare services across geographic, time, social, and cultural barriers. Telemedicine presents unique opportunities for both patients and clinicians when it is implemented in direct response to clear clinical needs.

2. What is the difference between telemedicine and eHealth?

e-Health refers to the use of the Internet for the transmission of medical information.

3. What kind of telemedicine technologies are there?

Several. They include telephone, radio, picture phones, audio-graphics, fax, computer images, broadcast video, compressed video, full-motion video, and virtual reality.

4. Describe the application of telemedicine in otolaryngology.

Telemedicine technology can be used to inform, diagnose, and treat patients at a distance.

5. What is the difference between store-and-forward and real-time technology?

Store-and-forward means that data is transmitted to a web site and then retrieved and analyzed at the viewer's convenience. For example, an image of an abnormal larynx would be sent by a referring provider to a consultant's web site. The consultant would then review the image and clinical data within a reasonable time and then email an opinion back to the inquiring provider.

Real-time transmission means that the referring provider, the patient, and the consultant transmit information at the same time. For example, using the Web or videoconferencing, practitioners would exchange information. A telephone conversation is another example of a real-time transmission.

6. Why don't more people use telemedicine?

Three basic reasons. First, practitioners are reluctant to learn and use a *new technology* unless there is a clear value to its adoption. Second, practitioners need *access to hardware and software* to conduct telemedicine consultations. Finally, there are significant legal, regulatory, ethical, and socioeconomic *barriers* to full implementation of telemedicine in medicine.

7. What kind of barriers prevent implementation of telemedicine?

Take licensure, for example. Since each state decides who can be licensed to practice in the state, there are significant variations in the ability of licensed physicians to practice telemedicine between the states. If , for example, you are licensed to practice medicine in Colorado, you may not be able to "see" patients using telemedicine in Kansas unless you are licensed to do so in Kansas. These barriers are not unique to the United States.

8. Are there risks involved?

Excessive reliance upon this technology to the detriment of traditional clinician-patient relationships and complacency regarding the risks and responsibilities—many of which are as yet unknown—of distant medical intervention, consultation, and diagnosis represent significant risk.

9. What should I do if I want to start practicing telemedicine?

Contact your hospital Audiovisual or Information Systems department to find out what kind of communications capability they have. Once you get the system up and running, put together a plan to implement it.

10. What should the plan include?

First, consider the *financial issues* and make a budget. The rules concerning reimbursement for telemedicine are changing rapidly and will vary depending on your circumstances. Second, do a needs assessment, in which you will select the right technology and decide who will manage and run the system. Third, decide about daily operational issues, and write a policy and procedures manual. Finally, determine when an evaluation to improve the system would be appropriate.

11. Where can I learn to do these things?

There are several telemedicine courses offered nationally and locally. A good place to start is the American Telemedicine Association at http://www.ata.org and the Association of Tele-health Service Providers at http://www.atsp.org. Two telemedicine journals are *Telemedicine Journal* and *Telemedicine & Telecare*.

CONTROVERSY

12. Is telemedicine cost-effective?

Establishing systems for patient care using telecommunications technologies is feasible, but there is little firm evidence yet of clinical benefits. The initial studies were generally inadequately designed or conducted, and it is difficult to perform a traditional meta-analysis. These studies provided variable and inconclusive results for other outcomes such as psychological measures, and no analyzable data about the real cost-effectiveness of telemedicine systems. Furthermore, there are a number of disturbing features common to these studies, including the omission of the number of consultations or patients, almost nonexistent longitudinal data collection, and lack of uniformity in cost analyses. Therefore, it is premature for any statements to be made, either positive or negative, regarding the cost-effectiveness of telemedicine in general. There is a need for further research and randomized trials of telemedicine applications. Policy makers should be cautious about recommending increased use and investment in these new technologies until these trials are completed.

BIBLIOGRAPHY

1. Aires LM, Finley JP: Telemedicine activity at a Canadian university medical school and its teaching hospitals. J Telemed Telecare 6:31–5, 2000.
2. Currell, R, Urquhart, C, Wainwright, et al: Telemedicine versus face to face patient care: Effects on professional practice and health care outcomes. Cochrane Effective Practice and Organization of Care Group—Database of Systematic Reviews. (2): CD002098, 2000.
3. Fujimoto M, Miyazaki K, von Tunzelmann N; Complex systems in technology and policy: Telemedicine and telecare in Japan. J Telemed Telecare 6:187–92, 2000.
4. Mair FS, Haycox A, May C, et al: A review of telemedicine cost-effectiveness studies. J Telemed Telecare 6 Suppl 1:S38–40, 2000.
5. Mitchell J: Increasing the cost-effectiveness of telemedicine by embracing e-health. J Telemed Telecare 6 Suppl 1:S16–9, 2000.
6. Reid J: A Telemedicine Primer: Understanding the Issues. Billings, Montana, Innovative Medical Communications, 1996.
7. Rissam HS, Kishore S, Trehan N: Telemedicine: Applications, barriers and medico-legal aspects. J Assoc Phys India 47:811–817, 1999.
8. Stanberry B: Telemedicine: Barriers and opportunities in the 21st century. J Int Med 247:615–628, 2000.
9. Tachakra S, Dawood M: Telemedicine—the technology and its applications. Emerg Nurse 7:6–8, 2000.
10. Wright D, Chestnutt L: Telemedicine in the twenty-first century: Report of a workshop. J Telemed Telecare 6:120–123, 2000.
11. Yellowlees PM: Intelligent health systems and third millennium medicine in Australia [editorial]. Telemed J 6:197–200, 2000.
12. Zollo S, Kienzle M, Loeffelholz P, et al: Telemedicine to Iowa's correctional facilities: Initial clinical experience and assessment of program costs. Telemed J 5:291–301, 1999.

XII. Conclusion

89. MINUTIAE IN OTOLARYNGOLOGY
(Things You Really Shouldn't Be Expected to Know, But That Will Really Impress the Attending on Rounds or in Conferences)

Bruce W. Jafek, M.D., FACS, FRSM

1. How did otolaryngology originate?

The specialty of otolaryngology is a product of the 20th-century amalgamation of two specialties having quite different origins, otology and laryngology. Otologists ("aurists") trace their origins to the mid-19th century efforts of Toynbee, Wilde, von Tröltsch, and Politzer. Laryngology had a more specific birthdate, September 1854, when Manuel Garcia first visualized his own larynx with a mirror (although he was not the first to visualize the living human larynx; see Question 6). Türck and Czermak popularized the new discipline of laryngology. As laryngologists herniated upward into the airway via the larynx, and otologists probed deeper into the ear via the eustachian tube, the two disciplines met a unifying organ, the nose, and the specialty of otorhinolaryngology, shortened by some to otolaryngology, was born.

2. Where was the first chair of otology located?

The first chair of otology was created at the University at Vienna, and the first otology clinic was also founded there in 1873. Billroth, the great general surgeon, supported the creation of the chair noting, "It is desirable to give this small and yet not unimportant subject a place in the curriculum of the universities." Billroth characterized otology as a "difficult and thankless" discipline. Josef Gruber and Adam Politzer were codirectors.

3. Where was the first chair of laryngology located?

Vienna, also.

4. Was the first laryngology clinic in Vienna, too?

No. In 1863, Morell Mackenzie, the great English laryngologist, opened The Metropolitan Free Dispensary for Diseases of the Throat and Loss of Voice in London, beating the Viennese in this area. But Morell wasn't always so highly regarded. More about that later.

5. Why do otolaryngologists wear head mirrors?

John Avery, a British surgeon, was one of the first to use a head mirror to reflect light into a patient's mouth to visualize the tongue, larynx, etc., freeing the hands for holding retractors or to manipulate mirrors. A candle was his light source.

6. So who was the first to observe the human larynx?

In Frankfurt in 1807, **Philip Bozzini** used an exotic, double-barreled instrument called a "lichleiter," illuminated by a wax candle, to inspect a variety of canals, including the pharynx. It is doubtful, however, that he ever actually saw the larynx. **Benjamin Babington,** a physician at

Guy's Hospital in London, described his "glottiscope" to the London Hunterian Society in 1829. A colleague at Guy's, **Thomas Hodgkin,** characterized Babington's invention as a "laryngoscope," but it is questionable whether Babington actually ever viewed the glottis with his complex spatula/mirror invention. (Babington also described hereditary hemorrhagic telangiectasia 30+ years before Randu or Osler, but that is a secret for another book.)

John Avery, a London surgeon, mounted a curved mirror on his head and used a candle as his light source in approximately 1848. He *probably* saw larynges with his cumbersome laryngoscope, but didn't receive credit for this.

Manuel Patricio Garcia, a Spanish Professor of Singing, had dreamed of seeing "a healthy glottis exposed in the very act of singing." His dream was achieved as he coordinated a series of mirrors to see his *own* larynx, a process characterized as "autolaryngoscopy." This was done in late 1854 to early 1855 and presented to the Royal Society of Medicine in 1855. Garcia is generally credited with being the first to visualize the human larynx, although it is probably more correct to say that he was the first to *popularize* the procedure, an example of an early marketing success, and is regarded as the "father of laryngology." Actually, **Ludwig Türck** and **Johann Czermak,** Viennese physicians, really popularized laryngoscopy.

7. What was the early understanding of the function of the ear?
Pliny located the seat of the memory to the ear, while Noury felt that the seat of Nemesis, the goddess of retribution, was behind the right ear.

8. If in Morocco on March 25th, what ritual might you witness?
Moroccans have traditionally collected rainwater on March 25th. Moroccan history recounts that this ritual was performed yearly to ward off all diseases of the ear and nose.

9. What happened on July 18, 1856?
Trick question. Nothing of significance in the field of otolaryngology that I know of. Otolaryngology attendings and residents are occasionally guilty of a trick question, as are members of other disciplines.

10. Who did the first tracheotomy?
Galen credited **Asclepiades of Bithynia** (2nd century AD) with the origin of this operation. The term *trachea* was not introduced until the 16th century. At this time, a tracheotomy was performed only in the direst of emergencies. Nearly another century passed before it came into common acceptance.

11. When was the myringotomy introduced?
The myringotomy was probably first naturally introduced when the first caveperson (or cave child) suffered acute otitis media, as their tympanic membrane may have perforated spontaneously. But **Thomas Willis** (better known for his description of the arteries of the base of the brain, the circle of Willis, and cofounder of the Royal Society of England), Antonio Valsalva (also better known for his description of the maneuver to inflate the middle ear via the eustachian tube, originally used to try to rid the middle ear of pus), and William Cheselden all perforated the tympanic membrane of dogs to see if their hearing diminished. Sir Astley Paston Cooper, however, popularized the procedure in London in the early 1800s as "an operation for the removal of a particular species of deafness." He even described the special trochar and cannula that he used.

12. Who described the eustachian tube?
(Hint: It was not Gabriele Falloppio. That was a different tube.) Another Italian, **Bartolomeo Eustachio,** one of the great pioneers of otology, was one of the foremost anatomists of his era (the 1500s), possibly greater than Falloppio. Personal physician to the Pope, Eustachio made his greatest contribution in providing a precise description of the tubular structure that bears his name. He also recognized the functional nature of the tube. Incidentally, Eustachio also discovered the stapes in the course of his anatomic investigations.

13. For whom is the organ of Corti named?

Getting a little easier. **Marquis Alfonso Corti** (1822–1888) was a well-known Italian histologist whose microscopic observations of this organ made a major contribution to Helmholtz's "resonance" theory—i.e., that vibration of the basilar membrane is a factor in hearing.

14. What otolaryngologic disease contributed to George Washington's death?

The answer remains a matter of debate and might be quinsy (peritonsillar abscess or peritonsillitis), bacteremia, or the inappropriate attempts of an early surgeon. However, it is known that Washington had a severe sore throat with fever and was treated by blood-letting, a form of therapy to release the "evil humors" (early barber-surgeons marked their offices with a red and white-striped pole, representing the soiled bandages from blood-letting). Shortly thereafter, he died, possibly of any of the above. Otolaryngologists like to tell stories of surgical misadventures by members of other disciplines.

15. Which American presidents had cancer?

Two had cancer of the head and neck region: Ulysses S. Grant (cancer of the tongue base) and Grover Cleveland (maxilla, or hard palate). Ronald Reagan had colon cancer. Some also think Franklin D. Roosevelt may have had a melanoma above his eyebrow (which may have metastasized intracranially and bled, leading to his "stroke"), but that was never verified.

16. Tell me more about Grant's cancer.

In early 1884, 7 years after the completion of his Presidency, Grant noted the onset of a sore throat, especially when eating peaches, "of which he was fond." Then 62 years old and a stubborn man, Grant delayed seeking medical advice. However, at the insistence of his wife, he was examined by a physician named Da Costa. Grant was spending the summer with his family in Long Beach, New Jersey, and was advised to see his personal physician, Dr. Fordyce Barker, on his return to New York. As Dr. Barker was vacationing in Europe at the time, Grant received no additional evaluation until 12 weeks later, in October. When Barker examined the ex-president, he referred him immediately to Dr. John H. Douglas. Dr. Douglas was a leading "throat specialist" of the day. On October 22, 1884, Douglas described a lesion of the right tonsil with a small neck node (today classified as a T1N1M0, Stage 3 tumor) of "epithelial" origin. To Grant, Douglas characterized the tumor as "serious . . . sometimes capable of being cured."

Grant was both a heavy smoker, preferring cigars, and a heavy drinker, predisposing him to squamous cell carcinoma of the oral cavity. This tonsillar lesion was initially treated with a combination of cessation of smoking, topical iodoform, salt-water gargles, dilute carbolic acid gargle, and 4% topical cocaine solution applied topically for pain relief. These measures did not slow the tumor growth and by December, it had spread extensively to involve the tongue base and palate.

A biopsy was obtained in February 1885, suggesting a tumor that would today be diagnosed as squamous cell carcinoma. The pathologic examination was done with a new instrument, a microscope, regarded as a toy at the time. Radical excision, involving a resection of the lateral tongue, lateral palate, and involved upper cervical nodes, was considered via a lateral mandibulotomy, but "in the best interests of the distinguished patient, the surgeons did not feel inclined to recommend the procedure." It was felt that the surgery "did not offer a guarantee of complete tumor removal" (but what cancer operation does?) and that there was a "risk to life by the severe shock to a constitution already much enfeebled." Clearly, the surgeons of the time "blinked," but in their defense, it must be remembered that general anesthesia was only 41 years old and modern techniques of sterility, blood transfusion, and antibiotics were unknown. The patient likely would have died of the surgery, and the surgeons probably made a wise choice.

As Grant's tumor advanced, he developed apprehensions that he might choke to death in his sleep and slept sitting up (and as little as possible to avoid choking). He undertook the completion of writing his memoirs, both to justify his decisions as well as to try to recoup some of his financial losses. During the latter part of his illness, he was unable to speak and his gasping, breathing, and gurgling could be heard for some distance.

On June 16, 1885, Grant was moved to Mount McGregor, New York, a small village outside of Saratoga known for its fresh mountain air. He died there 5 weeks later, completing his memoirs 3 days before his death.

17. How about Grover Cleveland?

Grover Cleveland, the only President of the United States who served two different disconnected terms, was a large bull of a man. Shortly after his second inauguration, in 1893, he was found to have a sore area of ulceration in the roof of his mouth. Biopsies were nondiagnostic (the science of pathology was yet in its infancy!), but a friend of the President and an eminent surgeon, Dr. Joseph Bryant, concluded, "Were it in my mouth, I would have it removed at once." This was not simply accomplished, as 1893 was a year of economic crisis and Cleveland was regarded as the leader to give the country stability and leadership during this crisis. His medical condition was therefore concealed, lest it should cause panic.

On the evening of June 30, 1893, Cleveland boarded a yacht, the Oneida, heading out of New York's East River into Buzzard's Bay. On board were Drs. W.W. Keen (Professor of Neurosurgery at Jefferson Medical College and an eminent neurosurgeon), Ferdinand Hasbrouck (a dentist and anesthesiologist of note), Edward Janeway (a prominent New York physician), Robert O'Reilly, and J.F. Erdman. All were sworn to secrecy.

On July 1, 1893, an intraoral partial maxillectomy was performed in the yacht's saloon, which had been converted into an operating room. Bone was removed from the bicuspid region on the left side as far back as the palatine bone, carefully avoiding external incisions. The tumor was gelatinous in nature, suggesting a sarcoma. The procedure took 1.5 hours, with blood loss of 168 cc. The Oneida returned to port on July 5, and the public was told that the President had caught a cold, suffered a toothache, and had required an extraction. He was subsequently fitted with a maxillary obturator made of vulcanized rubber. Cleveland served out his entire term and died, apparently tumor-free, in 1908 of unrelated causes.

The operation was not concealed for long. Rumors and leaks continued to surface until 1917, when Keen released the story to the *Saturday Evening Post*. Mystery, however, continued to surround the diagnosis. Dr. William M. Welch, of Johns Hopkins, was said to have confirmed the initial diagnosis of sarcoma. By 1917, Keen felt that the diagnosis was carcinoma. Others subsequently questioned the diagnosis of malignancy, in view of the President's "cure," and raised the possibility of ameloblastoma, a benign salivary mixed tumor, and even necrotizing sialometaplasia or a syphilitic gumma. The specimen remained in the Mutter Museum of the College of Physicians of Philadelphia until 1980, when a definitive examination revealed verrucous carcinoma, partially accounting for the good prognosis.

18. Had Grant and Cleveland lived today, how might they have fared?

Renehan offers a comprehensive discussion of how Grant's and Cleveland's tumors might have been handled today. Cleveland's might have been handled with the laser, and certainly the prosthetic rehabilitation would have been superior. But the result—apparent cure and no evidence of disease at death—could not have been improved upon. Grant, on the other hand, would have been the beneficiary of a number of major advances in the field and could have expected a greater than 50% 5-year survival rate for his T1N1M0, Stage 3 tonsillar fossa tumor.

19. What famous German leader died of laryngeal cancer?

Crown Prince Frederick ascended the German throne as Frederick III but lived only 99 days in this position, dying on June 15, 1888. Many feel that his young successor, Wilhelm I, was heavily influenced by the militant Chancellor Bismark, contributing to Germany's provocation of World War I. The management of this famous patient has been repeatedly analyzed, and is briefly recounted here.

Frederick had an English wife who encouraged his evaluation by the most noted laryngologist of the time, **Morell Mackenzie** of England. Mackenzie apparently simply missed the diagnosis, thinking that he might be observing a syphilitic gumma. A biopsy was initially misread by the best-known pathologist of the time, Virchow (although it must be admitted that pathology and pathologic diagnosis was in its infancy), and treatment was delayed. By the time the proper diagnosis was made, laryngectomy was impossible (although laryngectomy was also in its infancy, having first been performed by Billroth 5 years previously), and only a palliative tracheotomy was performed. It should also be admitted that few surgeons even considered a laryngectomy. Who would want to be remembered as the surgeon whose royal patient died under the knife? Mackenzie was subsequently criticized and censured by the Royal Society of Surgeons and the British Medical Association and forced to resign from the Royal College of Physicians.

Robert J. Ruben, Chair of Otolaryngology at Albert Einstein College of Medicine of Yeshiva University, offers another spin: "If you read Virchow's pathology report, there is a credible hypothesis that the reason why Mackenzie did not say what the Crown Prince had is because he did not want to embarrass his patron and good friend, Queen Victoria, by saying that one of his relatives had picked up 'the Spanish disease.'" Harrison disputes this position, pointing out that the this "rumour . . . was based on the unsubstantiated allegation that the Crown Prince had contracted syphilis in Suez, on or about 16 November 1887, from a beautiful woman named Dolores Cada." He concluded that this rumor was "a personal act of revenge" by "a vindictive French journalist, Jean de Bonnefon," as "a personal act of revenge for the recovery of Alsace-Lorraine by Germany after the Franco-Prussian War."

The autopsy, by Virchow, showed cancerous destruction of the larynx with metastatic lymph nodes. But speculation continues to this day.

20. What otolaryngologists received a Nobel Prize?

Gyorgy von Békésy, a Hungarian, won the Nobel Prize in 1947 for developing the semiautomatic audiometer. This advancement produced threshold measurements, which were valuable in the differentiation of conductive and sensorineural hearing loss. Another winner was **Robert Barany,** who was awarded the 1914 Nobel Prize for his work on the physiology and pathology of the vestibular apparatus. He was a prisoner of war in Russia (WWI) and was in a prisoner of war camp in Turkestan when he learned of the award and was released to receive it. (Alertly contributed by Nasir Ahmad, MD, FRCS(C), FACS, who hereby corrects my error in the first edition of ENT Secrets.) Ruben (see Question 19) points out that Barany was an enlisted man at the time of his capture because, being Jewish, he was not allowed to be an officer, and certainly was not considered a gentleman. After the Swedish ambassador got him out of the Russian Prisoner of War Camp, and he was received in Stockholm, he never returned to Vienna.

21. Is all of this historical stuff really important?

Walter Howarth, a rhinologist, observed, "We are so much preoccupied nowadays with the problems of the present and the future that our debt to the past is sometimes apt to be overlooked. We are, in fact, inclined to take our present state of knowledge for granted, and when we think of the generations which have preceded our own, we are apt to do so with a sense of superiority and of pity for their mistakes, rather than with a sense of humanity and of admiration for their achievement."

22. Who are some of the 20th century gurus of otolaryngology?

This is a toughie, because many friends will be overlooked (my apologies to them, and my assurances that they will be in the third edition!). **Carl Olaf Nylén** developed the operating microscope, and **Jack Urban** perfected the binocular operating microscope and its many attachments, allowing microscopic surgery to evolve. **Sourdille** and **Lempert** (about whom a whole book could be written or, more appropriately, a soap opera) pioneered surgery for otosclerosis, but **Sam Rosen** and **John Shea** simplified it to surgery of the stapes. **Howard House** and **Harold Schuknecht** developed the stapes prosthesis. **Zöllner** and **Wullstein** developed tympanoplasty, now facilitated with a variety of prostheses, via several (e.g., trans-canal, canal-up, canal-down) approaches. **Bill House** reported a number of procedures around the skull base, founding neurootology. **Blair Simmons** did much of the early American work on the cochlear implant, along with Bill House. Otitis media was relieved by **Beverly Armstrong**'s collar button tube, although the indications for placement remain subject to debate (and if you ask who "she" is, you probably don't know that *he* published his results in 1954, either).

Mosher and **Cottle** are two of the best-known older rhinologists, while the development of the Hopkins rod endoscope has allowed the development of transnasal functional endoscopic surgery by **Messerklinger, Stammberger, Wigand,** and **Kennedy. Jacques Joseph** is the best-known early plastic surgeon of the nose, with subsequent contributions by **Goldman, Anderson,** and **Tardy. McCullough** and Tardy have popularized facial plastic surgery within the field of otolaryngology. A number of otolaryngologists contributed to the evolution of the modern endoscope, especially the development of distal, fiberoptic lighting and fiberscopes.

The treatment of head and neck cancer recognizes **John Conley, John Loré, John Kirchner,** and **Joseph Ogura** as four of its guiding lights, while **Paul Ward** trained a number of the leading educators of the field, building on the tradition founded by **John Lindsey** and **Cesar Fernandez,** of the University of Chicago. **Blom** and **Singer** pioneered the tracheoesophageal puncture and valved prosthesis for surgical voice rehabilitation after laryngectomy. **George Reed** was deeply committed to education within our field, assisted by (at the time) several young academicians, including **Brian McCabe, Jim Donaldson,** and **Bobby Alford. Jim Snow** was instrumental in establishing the discipline at the NIH and assisted in the establishment of the National Institute of Deafness and Communicative Disorders and served as its Director.

Iapologize again to many friends, colleagues, and mentors who have contributed mightily to the development of the field of otolaryngology and whose names I have omitted. Next edition . . .

23. Who is Bruce W. Jafek, and what did he do?

Bruce W. Jafek wrote this chapter and others, and helped to edit this book. And that's the last question and final answer for which we'll hold you responsible. Thanks for reading *ENT Secrets, 2nd edition,* and thanks for your curiosity about the interesting and challenging field of otolaryngology!

P.S.—Bruce Murrow, MD, PhD, has assumed Anne Stark's coediting responsibilities. Anne Stark, the former coeditor, is now a scientist at the Nucleus Corporation in Denver, Colorado.

ROLE OF THE EDUCATOR

The need for continuing, solid teaching is obvious. Effective teaching is the essence. Are we teaching with such effectiveness that young men and women change and discipline their lives, or are we giving them a kind of theoretical/theological Twinkie—filled with froth and empty calories?

~Paraphrased from a talk by Jeffrey R. Holland

BIBLIOGRAPHY

1. Brooks JJ, Enterline HT, Aponte GE: The final diagnosis of President Cleveland's lesion. Trans Stud Coll Physician Phila 2(1), 1980.
2. Keen WW: The surgical operations on President Cleveland in 1893. Saturday Evening Post (Sept 22):24–25, 1917.
3. Renehan A: The oral tumours of two American presidents: What if they were alive today? J RSoc Med 88:377–383, 1995.
4. Weir N: Otolaryngology: An Illustrated History. London, Butterworths, 1990.
5. Harrison D: Felix Semon 1849–1921. A Victorian Laryngologist. London, Royal Society of Medicine Press, Ltd., 2000.
6. Catlin G: Shut Your Mouth and Save Your Life, 6th ed. London, Trübner, 1875.
7. Politzer A: History of Otology. Volume 1. Phoenix, Columella Press, 1981.

INDEX

Page numbers in **boldface type** indicate complete chapters.